PEDIATRIC REHABILITATION

SECOND EDITION

This volume is one of the series,
Rehabilitation Medicine Library,
edited by John V. Basmajian.

New books and new editions published, in press or in preparation for this series:

BASMAJIAN (ROGOFF): Manipulation, Traction and Massage, third edition*

BLOCH AND BASBAUM: Management of Spinal Cord Injuries

BRANDSTATER AND BASMAJIAN: Stroke Rehabilitation

EHRLICH: Rehabilitation Management of Rheumatic Conditions, second edition

FISHER AND HELM: Comprehensive Rehabilitation of Burns

GRANGER AND GRESHAM: Functional Assessment in Rehabilitation Medicine

HAAS AND AXEN: Pulmonary Therapy and Rehabilitation: Principles and Practice, second edition

JOHNSON: Practical Electromyography, third edition*

LEHMANN: Therapeutic Heat and Cold, fourth edition

REDFORD: Orthotics Etcetera, third edition*

* *Originally published as part of the Physical Medicine Library, edited by Sidney Licht.*

PEDIATRIC REHABILITATION

SECOND EDITION

Edited by

Gabriella E. Molnar, M.D.

Director
Department of Pediatric Rehabilitation
Children's Hospital Medical Center of Northern California
Oakland, California

Medical Director
Pediatric Unit
Golden State Rehabilitation Hospital
San Ramon, California

Clinical Professor
Department of Rehabilitation Medicine
University of California
Davis, California

Clinical Professor
Department of Pediatrics
University of California
San Francisco, California

WILLIAMS & WILKINS
BALTIMORE · HONG KONG · LONDON · MUNICH
PHILADELPHIA · SYDNEY · TOKYO

Editor: John P. Butler
Managing Editor: Linda Napora
Copy Editor: Shelley Potler
Designer: Bert Smith
Illustration Planner: Wayne Hubbel
Production Coordinator: Charles E. Zeller

Copyright © 1992
Williams & Wilkins
428 East Preston Street
Baltimore, Maryland 21202, USA

Accurate indications, adverse reactions, and dosage schedules for drugs are provided in this book, but it is possible that they may change. The reader is urged to review the package information data of the manufacturers of the medications mentioned.

Printed in the United States of America

First Edition 1985

Library of Congress Cataloging-in-Publication Data

Pediatric rehabilitation / edited by Gabriella E. Molnar.—2nd ed.
    p.   cm.—(Rehabilitation medicine library)
    Includes bibliographical references.
    Includes index.
    ISBN 0-683-06118-6
    1. Physically handicapped children—Rehabilitation.   I. Molnar, Gabriella E.,
1926- . II. Series.
    [DNLM: 1. Rehabilitation—in infancy & childhood.   WS 368 P371]
RJ138.P38   1992
617'.03—dc20
DNLM/DLC
for Library of Congress   91-7275
                                              CIP

92 93 94 95
2 3 4 5 6 7 8 9 10

Series Editor's Foreword

In my Foreword to the first edition, I described this book as "... a gem in its field. It is truly unique, threatening to drive ambitious future authors of books on children's rehabilitation to despair for years to come. True, no book can live forever, but this one will serve its time with great vigor."

My predictions proved prophetic. Indeed, the book continues to stand in splendid uniqueness with no other that even approaches it in quality. But time has passed and a great deal of equally splendid new knowledge has appeared in the literature.

Conscientious and perceptive as always, Dr. Molnar has not only swept clean the gathering cobwebs but she has completely rebuilt the structure with all-new materials and creative insights.

The birth of the first edition of this special volume in the Rehabilitation Medicine Library was the cause for great pleasure and congratulation. It became a "best-seller." Now matured, it has become a vigorous and exciting second edition of which I am very proud. Editor Gabriella Molnar has, with her outstanding team of authors, produced a living classic. It has become equally lively, friendly, and eminently useful to all disciplines with an interest in the health and the disabilities of children.

JOHN V. BASMAJIAN, M.D.

Preface

Pediatric rehabilitation integrates the principles of rehabilitation medicine with those of child development. This book illustrates a consolidation of those two viewpoints into one comprehensive volume.

In this second edition, we have retained the organizational structure of the initial publication. Section I addresses the adaptation of diagnostic and treatment methods to the changing needs and abilities of children. Section II is a discussion of specific disabilities. Each chapter has been revised to include clinical and technological advances that have taken place since the inception of the first edition. The updated bibliography will serve as an extended guide for further reading. The chapter on pediatric rehabilitation nursing is an entirely new contribution. We hope that practitioners, residents, and students of medicine and allied rehabilitation professions will find this volume helpful in their work with childhood disabilities.

I would like to express my gratitude to all of the contributors for their commitment to this project and for their outstanding work in condensing large amounts of information into well-focused chapters.

This book is dedicated to the children and families whose confidence and trust enables us to provide care and guidance in preparation for adulthood.

GABRIELLA E. MOLNAR, M.D.

Contributors

Michael A. Alexander, M.D.
Chief of Rehabilitation, Alfred I. duPont Institute, Wilmington, Delaware

Angeles Badell, M.D.
Chief, Division of Rehabilitation Medicine, Long Island Jewish Medical Center and Schneider Children's Hospital, New York, New York; Associate Professor of Rehabilitation Medicine, Albert Einstein College of Medicine, Bronx, New York

Helga Binder, M.D.
Associate Physiatrist, Children's National Medical Center; Associate Professor, Department of Pediatrics, George Washington University Medical School, Washington, D.C.

James Boyd, M.D.
Department of Pediatric Rehabilitation, Children's Hospital, Oakland, California; Assistant Clinical Professor, University of California, Davis Medical Center, Sacramento, California

Yasoma Challenor, M.D.
Clinical Professor, Physical Medicine and Rehabilitation, Columbia University College of Physicians and Surgeons, New York, New York; Director, Department of Rehabilitation Medicine, Blythedale Children's Hospital, Valhalla, New York

Susan Pasternack Chinitz, Psy.D.
Director, Early Childhood Center; Assistant Clinical Professor of Pediatrics, Albert Einstein College of Medicine, Bronx, New York

Jessie K.M. Easton, M.D., M.P.H.
Clinical Associate Professor of Pediatrics, University of South Dakota School of Medicine, Sioux Falls, South Dakota

Gloria D. Eng, M.D.
Chairman, Department of Physical Medicine and Rehabilitation, Children's National Medical Center; Professor of Medicine and Pediatrics, George Washington University Medical Center, Washington, D.C.

Carol Z. Feder, Ph.D.
Director, Pediatric Psychology Service, The Rusk Institute of Rehabilitation Medicine, NYU Medical Center, New York, New York

Shirley P. Hoeman, Ph.D., M.P.H., R.N., C.N.A.A., C.R.N.N.
Administrative Director, Center for Human Development, Morristown Memorial Hospital, Morristown New Jersey; President, Health Systems Consultations, Long Valley, New Jersey

Ruth K. Kaminer, M.D.
Associate Director for Medical Services, Children's Evaluation and Rehabilitation Center, Rose F. Kennedy Center; Associate Professor, Pediatrics, Albert Einstein College of Medicine, Bronx, New York

Wilma C. Kellerman, M.D.
Director, Inpatient Rehabilitation Unit, Sacred Heart Hospital and Rehabilitation Center, Norristown, Pennsylvania; Clinical Assistant Professor, Department of Rehabilitation Medicine, University of Pennsylvania, Philadelphia, Pennsylvania

Barbara M. Koch, M.D.
Attending Physiatrist, Children's Hospital; Associate Professor, George Washington University School of Medicine, Washington, D.C.

Dennis J. Matthews, M.D.
Medical Director and Chairman, The Children's Hospital and Rehabilitation Center, Denver, Colorado

Gabriella E. Molnar, M.D.
Director, Department of Pediatric Rehabilitation, Children's Hospital Medical Center, Oakland, California; Medical Director, Pediatric Unit, Golden State Rehabilitation Hospital, Clinical Professor, Department of Rehabilitation Medicine, University of California, Davis, California; Clinical Professor, Department of Pediatrics, University of California, San Francisco, California

Maureen R. Nelson, M.D.
Assistant Professor, Baylor College of Medicine, Departments of Physical Medicine and Rehabilitation, Department of Pediatrics, Chief of Rehabilitation, Texas Children's Hospital, Houston, Texas

Jane C.S. Perrin, M.D.
Medical Director, Rehabilitation Service, William Beaumont Hospital, Royal Oak, Michigan; Clinical Associate Professor, Pediatrics; Associate Professor, Physical Medicine and Rehabilitation, Wayne State University School of Medicine, Detroit, Michigan

Phoebe Saturen, M.D.
Professor, Clinical Rehabilitation Medicine, New York Medical College, Valhalla, New York

Anjali Shah
Director, Rehabilitation Engineering, Alfred I. duPont Institute, Wilmington, Delaware

Lydia H. Soifer, Ph.D., C.C.C.
Director, Total Learning Center in Westchester, Inc., Harrison, New York

Patricia J. Taggert, M.B.A., P.T.
Manager, Pediatric Rehabilitation, Children's Hospital Medical Center of Northern California, Oakland, California

Contents

Section I. Principles of Diagnosis and Treatment

Section II. Rehabilitation of Childhood Disabilities

Principles of Diagnosis and Treatment

1

History and Examination

GABRIELLA E. MOLNAR AND WILMA C. KELLERMAN

The concept of disability as a functional impairment is essential to the understanding of rehabilitation. This viewpoint requires an assessment of dysfunction resulting in, but distinguished from, organic pathology (49). While diagnosis elucidates the nature of the underlying disease, the evaluation process entails a further step to determine functional status. At the conclusion of this inquiry, the traditional intent to assign a diagnostic label is broadened into an inventory of functional assets upon which the intervention phase of rehabilitation is based (49).

In the assessment of handicapped children, the principal elements of pediatric history-taking and examination are retained (7, 38, 60, 72) with an orientation toward the neuromuscular and other functional consequences created by the presenting disease or injury. A framework for the interpretation of findings is provided by the behavioral and developmental achievements expected of children at different ages (7, 34, 35, 41).

Continuing re-evaluation is necessary as the child grows. Progress needs to be appraised to take advantage of newly acquired abilities. Dysfunction is assessed to correct existing deficits and to avert the occurrence of preventable secondary complications.

The diagnostic evaluation in pediatric rehabilitation explores the functioning of the family unit, the style of parenting, child-rearing practices, and the dynamics to cope with having a handicapped child. It is essential that the child be viewed as a part of a family, which has a strong formative influence on preparing that child for the future role of adulthood (51, 58, 79, 87). Information should be gathered about school achievements and social opportunities, for these experiences contribute to ultimate functioning in society (56, 57).

History

This chapter only intends to highlight the essential components of a systematic anamnesis in pediatric rehabilitation. Details pertaining to specific disabilities are discussed in respective chapters of this volume.

2

Clinical history is a fundamental tool of medical diagnosis. For the infant or young patient, information is obtained from the parents or caretakers. Most school-aged children are able to participate in the diagnostic interview when asked in concrete terms. Preadolescents and adolescents can provide a description of their abilities and limitations.

Privacy and adequate time are necessary to establish good communication with the family and the child. It has been shown that the physician's skill of history-taking and attitude about the child's handicap contribute to developing a supportive relationship with the family and to the family's ability to participate in the proposed program (65, 85, 90).

The pediatric physiatrist's history-taking has two phases: a medical diagnostic inquiry and a functional inventory. Historical information-gathering for the purpose of diagnosis follows the customary principles of directed inquiry regardless of whether the cause of disability is in question or, as is often the case, already established. The functional inventory focuses on current accomplishments and includes information about all aspects of development and daily life. There should be an equal emphasis on noting the child's abilities, limitations, and compensatory functional solutions.

PRENATAL AND PERINATAL HISTORY

Because a number of childhood disabilities are caused by abnormalities of pregnancy and labor, a history of gestation and delivery should be obtained (83). Prenatal and intranatal complications arouse the suspicion of central nervous system damage and the possibility of cerebral palsy. Maternal disease, acute illness during gestation, a history of drug use or treatment may account for fetal malformations (20, 44). Congenital anomalies following gestational rubella, thalidomide syndrome, fetal alcohol syndrome (43), and sacral agenesis with myelodysplasia in maternal diabetes (63) are some well-known examples. Decreased fetal movements may be reported in diseases with severe congenital weakness, such as spinal muscular atrophy, high level of myelodysplasia, or arthrogryposis.

History of the newborn period should be explored (13, 31, 38, 48). Complications of the neonatal course manifested by cardiorespiratory distress, feeding difficulties, lethargy or irritability, seizures, and abnormal neurologic signs suggest central nervous system dysfunction of prenatal or perinatal origin and the possibility of cerebral palsy. Primary muscle weakness due to congenital myopathy or spinal muscular atrophy may present with predominant respiratory and feeding difficulties (27). Birth weight, together with the length of gestation is basic information for identifying small-for-gestational age infants (31). Apgar scores give an indication of the infant's condition at birth.

Prematurity, especially very low birth weight, is the most frequent cause of diplegic cerebral palsy, whereas large birth weight predisposes to traumatic labor and potential injury to the brain, spinal cord, or brachial plexus

(31). A description of deformities or malformations as they appeared at birth or a photograph of the infant provides comparison with findings on later examination.

DEVELOPMENTAL HISTORY

A fundamental requirement in the assessment of handicapped children is a thorough developmental history, which should encompass all areas of function and behavior discussed in Chapter 2. Accomplishment of major landmarks in gross motor function, fine motor and adaptive skills, language, and personal social behavior should clarify whether the disability is confined primarily to the neuromuscular system or involves deficits in other areas as well. Coexistent multiple dysfunction will influence the rehabilitation plans, intervention methods, and ultimate expectations. An essential question is to distinguish slow pace of development from regression of function (30, 54, 83). However, one must realize that slow deterioration in a progressive neurologic disease may be masked for a while by the relatively fast early maturational process.

The logical culmination of developmental history is a comprehensive survey of the child's current accomplishments. An account should be obtained from the parents and, whenever possible, from the child. The assessment should include all aspects of daily life. Physical and educational achievements are as relevant as gaining insight to the child's functioning and behavior at home, school, and in social contacts.

GENERAL HEALTH

In the customary review of systems and past illnesses (7, 38, 60, 72), one should keep in mind those problems that are likely to accompany certain disabilities. Seizures, feeding difficulties, and pulmonary and urinary system complications are some examples.

The incidence and risk of seizure disorder is increased in static and progressive diseases of the central nervous system (66). Clinical manifestations, changes in the type of seizures or their frequency, anticonvulsant medications, and possible side effects should be recorded.

The examiner should review the history of feeding in suspected or known physical handicaps, which may be accompanied by oral motor incoordination or by facial and bulbar weakness and often herald dysarthric speech problems at a later age (66, 83). Difficulties with introducing pureed and, particularly, solid foods are early signs of pseudobulbar palsy associated with bilateral spasticity or dyskinesia in cerebral palsy. In bulbar weakness, such as presented by spinal muscular atrophy or some types of congenital myopathy, taking liquids may be more difficult.

Nutrition, an often neglected aspect of history should be reviewed (5, 7, 18, 22, 23). Children with feeding difficulties or behavior problems may consume inadequate calories and essential nutrients or their dietary intake may be lower than required for the high energy expenditure during physical activities (37). Conversely, caloric intake may be excessive for the activity level of the child and account for the obesity that occurs most often in wheelchair-bound youngsters with spina bifida or muscular dystrophy (85). Dietary habits are fundamental information when regulation of neurogenic bowel incontinence is planned. Family eating patterns should be taken into consideration. Caloric requirements must be calculated according to age-appropriate standards with allowance for growth (Table 1.1). (5, 7, 18, 22, 23). Injuries, such as burns, fractures, and spinal cord or head trauma, are followed by a catabolic state (18, 23). Monitoring weight as well as nutritional and fluid intake is essential (3, 12, 18), particularly during the early phase of inpatient rehabilitation for major injuries while supplementary and oral feedings are adjusted.

A history of respiratory complications should be explored in a number of disabilities (39). Intercostal muscle paralysis caused by high thoracic paraplegia, spinal muscular atrophy, and muscle diseases are some examples where inefficient pulmonary ventilation and handling of secretion predispose to recurrent bouts of infection. A similar situation may be created by incoordination of the respiratory musculature associated with severe neuromuscular dysfunction of cerebral palsy. Coexistent feeding difficulties with minor aspirations or restrictive pulmonary disease due to spinal deformity often aggravate these problems. Ankylosing spondylitis and severe systemic onset of juvenile rheumatoid arthritis result in restricted mobility of the spine and thoracic cage. Exercise dyspnea may suggest a pulmonary compromise. However, an excessive increase in respiratory rate on exertion may merely reflect a low state of conditioning and/or high energy cost of activities in the presence of any physical deficit. Nightmares, insomnia, and night sweating are complaints associated with hypercapnia and may be reported by patients in advanced stage of muscular dystrophy or atrophy. Cardiac decompensation, especially right-sided failure is a potential complication of pulmonary dysfunction in any of the aforementioned instances. In the absence of heart failure, myopathic conduction defects and arrhythmias are generally symptom free.

In view of the high incidence of visual and hearing deficits among physically handicapped children, inquiry about these aspects of function should not be neglected (53, 55, 66, 67). History of prenatal infections, asphyxic or infectious encephalopathy, metabolic diseases, meningitis, hydrocephalus, head injury, or antibiotic treatment warrants exploration of the status of vision and hearing.

The category of general information includes immunizations, allergies, and medications taken regularly or occasionally. Diagnostic tests, injuries related or unrelated to the disability, surgical procedures, medical treatment, and hospitalizations should be recorded.

Handicapped children are prone to have a variety of illnesses as do other youngsters. However, one should keep in mind that, in some instances, acute symptoms may be directly related to complications associated with a specific disability. In children with myelodysplasia or diplegic cerebral palsy caused by prematurity, vomiting, headache, irritability, or lethargy may be prodromal signs of intercurrent illness or could indicate decompensating hydrocephalus and shunt malfunction. Recurrent headaches may be a manifestation of autonomic dysreflexia precipitated by bladder or bowel distension in spinal cord injury. After all other causes of fever have been excluded, hyperthermia due to sudorimotor paralysis should be entertained in high thoracic paraplegia. Central hyperpyrexia may occur in severe head injury. In the presence of neurogenic bladder, urinary tract infection always should be considered as the cause of a febrile episode. A history of the pattern and amount of voiding and fluid intake, keeping in mind pediatric norms (8, 36, 47), is essential in neurogenic bladder dysfunction (Table 1.1). Systematic daily recording of this information is a guide for bladder training.

Table 1.1.
Selected Physiologic Guidelines in Childhood[a]

Calorie and Fluid Requirements (3, 7, 12, 18, 22, 23, 37, 60)			
Age	Cal/kg	Protein gm/kg	Water ml/kg
Infancy	120	2.2	120–150
1 yr	110	2.0–2.2	120–135
2–3 yr	100	1.8–2.0	100–125
4–6 yr	85–90	1.5–1.6	90–110
7–10 yr	80–85	1.5	75–100
11–14 yr	60–70	1.2	50–70
15–18 yr	50–60	0.8–1.0	40–60

Blood Pressure and Heart Rate (68, 72)			
	Systolic	Diastolic	Heart Rate/min
Age	In Seated Position		At Rest
Infancy	80	55	125
1 yr	90	55	120
2–5 yr	90–94	55	100–110
6–9 yr	95–98	55–60	90–100
10–13 yr	98–109	60–65	85–90
14–18 yr	110–115	63–68	70–80

Vital Capacity (39)			
Newborn	5 years	10 years	15 years
100 cc	1300 cc	2300 cc	4000 cc

Urinary Output (7, 60):		2 ml/kg/hr	Infants and young children
Bladder Capacity (8, 36, 47):	Newborn:	16–25 ml	
	1–14 years:	(age in years + 2) × 30 = ml	

[a]Numbers in parentheses refer to references.

SCHOOL, BEHAVIOR, AND PSYCHOSOCIAL HISTORY

Knowledge of the child's scholastic achievements and identification of problem areas are essential since proper educational planning is a prerequisite of vocational preparation. Parental consent should be secured to obtain school reports, especially when the child's performance or the appropriateness of educational placement is questionable (7).

A number of physical handicaps of childhood are associated with intellectual deficit or learning disability (66). A suitable educational program for these children has to match their intellectual abilities with environmental adaptations for physical dysfunction. Educational reintegration presents a special set of problems in a child with acquired central nervous system dysfunction. This is particularly true after head injury if memory and attention deficits, impaired judgment, and personality changes persist. The physician must be familiar with educational facilities in the community and establish a collaborative relationship with the school system.

The examiner should inquire about the child's behavior in terms of characteristics expected of different age groups and of those reflecting individual personality. Sleeping and eating habits, activity level, temperament (19), drive and motivation, compliance or discipline problems, special interests, and dislikes are revealing information about behavior and adjustment. A valuable insight into the child's life experience and the family's child-rearing style can be obtained by asking a description of a typical daily schedule including regular and occasional activities on a weekday and weekend. Time spent in school, in therapy, or homework, or at play should be noted together with the nature of leisure and other activities the child does with family members, friends, or alone (56). This appraisal may point out the need for behavioral and psychosocial intervention or it may reveal areas of strength to be further developed.

FAMILY HISTORY

Information on this aspect of history is often incomplete until repeated exploration brings to light additional data. Pictures of relatives or a family album can be helpful to demonstrate abnormal facial or other dysmorphic features (44). Consanguinity increases the risk of genetic diseases. Family pedigree with an affected member of either sex in each generation is characteristic of autosomal recessive conditions. However, some autosomal dominant diseases have a wide spectrum of clinical manifestations. A mild form of the disease may be overlooked until evident signs in a proband lead to more thorough investigation of other family members (83). Congenital myotonic dystrophy and fascioscapulohumeral dystrophy are some examples that may present such history. Affected males with familial history on the maternal side are the hallmark of an X-linked disease. A more complex situation is encountered in multifactorial inheritance, such as represented by spina bifida (7).

Referral to genetic counseling is mandatory whenever a familial disease is suspected or known to exist. Pregnant mothers of affected children should be informed about prenatal diagnosis if a test for detection in the fetus is available (7).

Examination

This discussion presents only the general principles of examination and is intended as a complement to subsequent chapters that provide a description of diagnostic evaluation in specific disabilities.

The pediatric rehabilitation examination entails an assessment of pathologic signs to provide or confirm a diagnosis. A problem-oriented interpretation of findings will identify the nature and extent of dysfunction and differentiate primary disabilities due to the underlying pathology from secondary preventable or correctable complications. A concurrent assessment of residual and potential abilities completes the examination. Throughout each phase of examination, the physician must be sensitive to the developmental stage of the child (34, 35, 41).

CONSIDERATIONS FOR AGE

Infants and Young Children

Cooperation is essential for a thorough examination, especially for performing a reliable and informative functional assessment. To achieve this, the examiner must create a relaxed atmosphere and devote sufficient time for establishing a relationship of trust. An assortment of toys, games, and books should be available to put the child at ease. A warm, cheerful room and an examiner who is not wearing a white coat creates a nonthreatening environment. Friendly advances while the history is obtained allay the child's fear in preparation for the actual examination. The customary structured systematic examination used in older children and adults is replaced by a flexible approach. The basic plan is to proceed from observation to interactive play; actual physical handling and manipulation are the final step. The examiner should be prepared to improvise if a complete examination is to be obtained.

Observation is the first and, sometimes, the most informative part of the examination. It begins when the child is brought in or walks into the office and continues during the history-taking. Infants and children under 2 yr of age who are often afraid of strangers are held in the parent's lap. A child who can sit and walk may be seated at a low table to play. A great deal of information can be obtained about the neuromuscular system, alertness, behavior, affect, and parent-child interaction by observing the child in spontaneous activities and at play (16). Developmental testing can be incorporated in this phase of the examination by presenting selected toys and objects.

For the second part of the examination, the child is gradually undressed, but remains in the parent's lap or comforting vicinity. The examiner should approach the child in a friendly manner, talking quietly, and offer a toy to initiate interactive play. Gentle touch, tickling, or funny sounds may break the ice with an anxious child. Vision, hearing, cranial nerves, reaching, and fine manipulatory skills are assessed at this time, together with inspection and palpation of body parts.

Handling and manipulation is the last stage of examination with anxiety-provoking or painful tests deferred to the end. Fears allayed by the preceding experience, the child is placed on the table or floor to examine gross motor function noting abnormal movements and postures that suggest weakness, incoordination, or other characteristics of a movement disorder. With a very anxious infant or child, this aspect of the examination may be conducted through the parent. Testing of tone, range of motion, and positional manipulation to elicit primitive reflexes require "laying on of hands" and should be done after evaluation of active mobility. Examination of sensation, fundi, ears, oral function, and other tests that need instrumentation are reserved for the conclusion of the evaluation.

Preschool Child

The format of examination resembles that described for infants. Observation and play remain the principal methods of evaluation and testing. The growing child's expanding functional repertoire should be reflected by the scope of examination. Developmental testing is broadened by assessment of skills in self-care and other activities of daily living. By 4 to 5 yr of age, the examination becomes more structured. Formal testing of motor function and strength may be applied with variable success and reliability. Explaining what will be done and sometimes demonstrating on the examiner or parent assures the child's cooperation.

School Age to Adolescence

The customary methods of systematic medical examination are applicable to this age group (17, 38). However, children with a cognitive deficit may have to be approached according to their mental age rather than chronological years. A screening test of the three major areas of scholastic skills—reading, writing, and arithmetic—is part of a comprehensive assessment at this age, although it is not a substitute for formal psychologic and psychoeducational evaluation.

PHYSICAL EXAMINATION

Growth Assessment

The examination of pediatric patients includes measurement of height and weight to compare the child's physical development with standards for that age, as discussed in Chapter 2. Head circumference is measured in all children under 3 yr of age and continued thereafter when deviations are present. Serial monitoring is mandatory in youngsters who have or are at risk for hydrocephalus. Extremity length and girth discrepancy should be recorded in localized growth disturbances associated with neurogenic weakness, epiphyseal fractures, or arthritis. A child with unexplained hemihypertrophy needs investigation for renal tumor (11).

Inspection

The examiner should observe the child's general appearance. Unusual facial features, such as epicanthal folds, anomalies of the external ear, fingers, and toes, or other dysmorphic signs suggest prenatal, possibly teratogenic or genetic etiology. Often a thorough inspection will detect associated anomalies that may identify a specific syndrome. Asymmetry of the face, palpebral fissure, and pupils indicate facial palsy or Horner syndrome (83). Weak or involuntary movements of the extraocular muscles, face, and tongue reflect cranial nerve damage, myopathy, or other neurologic disease. Craniofacial asymmetry and vertical strabismus generally accompany congenital torticollis.

The skin is inspected for teleangiectasia, nevi, cafe-au-lait spots, and lesions located over the spine as signs associated with progressive diseases of the central nervous system or spinal cord malformation (30, 54, 83). Skin rash may be a manifestation of collagen disease or some infectious arthritides (7, 60, 72). A thorough observation of the skin should be done on every examination of children with sensory deficit. Callus formation on the medial or lateral border of the foot is a good indication of abnormal weight-bearing. Hyperkeratosis over the knees and dorsum of the feet is a telltale sign that crawling is the preferred mode of locomotion in an older child. Multiple scars, bruises, and abrasions in various stages of healing arouse the suspicion of child abuse.

Development of the skeletal musculature should be observed noting the presence, localization, and distribution of atrophy or anomalies, such as absent pectoralis muscle. Congenital club feet or multiple joint deformities may be manifestations of intrauterine weakness or muscle disease of prenatal onset, for example, arthrogryposis, spina bifida, or myotonic dystrophy (15, 31, 69). Multiple joint contractures may accompany genetic anomalies but their association with fusiform, dimpled joints, and sloping shoulders is typical of arthrogryposis. Position of the lower extremities indicates the distribution of weakness affecting specific muscles in a newborn with spina bifida. Generalized muscle hypertrophy may be present in the rare myotonia congenita (83). A convincing sign of effective crutch walking and independent wheelchair function is hypertrophy of the shoulder girdle and upper extremities.

Palpation

In infants and young children, the fontanelles and cranial sutures should be felt for patency, size, and tension preferably in sitting position; however, a bulging fontanelle in a vigorously crying infant does not necessarily signify hydrocephalus with increased intracranial pressure. Shunt reservoir should be located and checked for ease of emptying and rapidity of refill.

The skin is palpated for texture, excess or lack of perspiration when sudorimotor paralysis is suspected. Lesions of subcutaneous or underlying structures may be detectable, for example, by palpation of hard calcific deposits in dermatomyositis, by feeling the soft mass of a lipomeningocele, or neurofibromatous nodules along the course of peripheral nerves. In arthritis, each joint should be palpated for the cardinal signs of inflammation, warmth to touch, synovial thickening and intra-articular effusion.

Muscles with lower motor neuron paralysis have reduced bulk and tone and may feel fibrotic when paralysis is long-standing. The psuedohypertrophic muscle of Duchenne dystrophy has a characteristic rubbery, doughy consistency. A fibrotic nodule usually can be palpated in the sternocleidomastoid with torticollis due to birth injury and, in the quadriceps, with knee extension contracture following repeated intramuscular injections in infants. Localized pain and swelling accompany acute injuries to soft tissue and bone. When tenderness affects many muscle groups and is associated with weakness, fatigue, or skin rash, myositis due to parasitosis, viral infection, or collagen disease are differential diagnostic possibilities.

Examination of Organ Systems

The primary health care of handicapped children remains the responsibility of pediatricians. Nevertheless, the physiatrist should perform a selective general physical examination. The focus is on health problems for which there is an enhanced risk in certain handicaps and which may necessitate a modification of rehabilitation plans.

In disabilities that cause ineffective ventilation, especially when complicated by threat of minor aspirations, auscultation of the lungs should be part of the examination. In myopathies and collagen diseases with the possibility of associated heart disease, cardiac auscultation and pulse rate recording should be performed. Blood pressure should be measured in all children with neurogenic bladder, spinal cord injury, residual poliomyelitis, and Guillain-Barré syndrome (68). Abdominal and rectal examinations to explore bladder distension, rectal fullness, and anal sphincter tone should be done in children with neurogenic bowel and bladder dysfunction. Table 1.1 shows selected physiologic parameters at different ages in childhood.

EXAMINATION OF MOTOR FUNCTION

Neuromuscular System

Testing of reflexes, tone, active motion, coordination, and strength constitute the principal aspects of assessing neuromuscular function. Beyond 4 to 5 yr of age, the conduct of examination and the interpretation of findings are not different from the standard neurologic evaluation.

In infancy, reflex examination is extended to include those responses that are related to immaturity of the central nervous system or, conversely, signal the process of maturation. The development of infantile reflex behavior and its implications are discussed in Chapter 2.

Muscle tone in newborns and young infants shows a great deal of variation depending on their state of activity, alertness, and comfort (4, 13, 28, 31). Examination of tone should not be attempted when the infant is anxious, resistant, or crying. Repeated testing may be needed for reliable assessment. Flexor tone predominates in the first few months of life (2). Damage to the corticospinal system and basal ganglia results in hypertonicity. Hypotonic extremities or muscles feel limp and offer no resistance to passive manipulation (27). An infant with generalized hypotonicity is floppy and, in severe cases, may feel like a "rag doll" on handling. Hypotonia is the manifestation of anterior horn cell disease, myopathy (15, 27, 83) neuropathy (29), and cerebellar dysfunction. In infancy, it may be a transient stage following perinatal cerebral anoxia or it may precede the appearance of spasticity or dyskinesia of cerebral palsy (27). Tone abnormalities in infancy and childhood are manifested by characteristic postures that are described in Chapters 14 and 18. In spasticity, distribution of hypertonia and the resulting postures are influenced by body position in space and in relation to gravity. Therefore, examination should be performed in supine, prone, and vertical positions. Resistance to passive motion should be tested by both fast and slow stretch to differentiate spasticity (91) from rigidity.

Children under 4 to 5 yr of age will rarely cooperate adequately for formal testing of active movements and strength. Knowledge of infantile reflexes, normal motor development, and kinesiology (2, 4, 6, 40, 41, 46, 62) will help to detect weakness caused by muscle disease or lesions of the upper or lower motor neuron. During infancy, developmental reflex responses can be used to examine the function of certain muscle groups (45). The Moro and palmar grasp reflexes, for example, require shoulder abduction and finger flexion, respectively. Asymmetrical responses in a newborn may signify weakness in these muscles and the presence of Erb or Klumpke paralysis. Unilateral absence of protective arm extension after 6 months of age suggests weakness of the extremity, possibly a hemiparesis. When a myopathy with proximal involvement is suspected, scapular winging due to serratus anterior weakness can be demonstrated in the prone position as the infant elevates the trunk on the arms and in a young child by the wheelbarrow maneuver (83).

Young children will move in any way they can and show great inventiveness in developing their own functional solutions. Observation of compensatory methods gives a clue about localization and extent of muscle weakness; an example is the combat crawl seen in paralysis of both lower limbs. Infants and children are also quick to learn vicarious movement substitutions in case of isolated muscle weakenss. For example, a child with paralyzed deltoid may fling the arm forward by momentum or substitute the long head of the biceps for shoulder flexion. Abnormal attitudes or deformities of the joints accompany paralytic muscle imbalance and identify segmental or peripheral distribution of weakness in lesions of the lower motor neuron.

When using indirect functional and observational methods to detect muscle weakness, one must know what is expected of children at different ages. For example, walking on tiptoes, squatting, and rising to stand without using the arms for help, and sitting up from supine without first rolling to prone are accomplished around 3 yr of age (34). Failure to perform these tasks in a mature pattern prior to that age should not be interpreted as weakness of the plantar flexors, hip and knee extensors, or abdominals, respectively. Similarly, testing for Trendelenberg sign of grading the strength of triceps surae by rising on the toes a designated number of times is not applicable until after 4 yr when children acquire adequate balance for standing on one leg (34).

The standard technique of manual muscle testing (21, 24, 46, 61) is appropriate from school age unless the child has a severe behavior problem or mental retardation. The scoring system of zero to normal or zero to five grades is used as in adults. The limitations of manual muscle testing in upper motor neuron lesions should be recognized. Since children are very adept in using substitution movements, the examiner must pay particular attention to precise technical conduct of testing in order to avoid spurious results. Above fair grade, which stipulates complete range of active motion against gravity, experience is needed to appreciate what is good or normal strength at a given age. There is an inherent subjectivity in judging the strength of children, because of growth and the wide range of normal variations (59).

Quantitative measurements are recommended when precise information is essential. Comparing identical muscles on two sides of the body by manual testing is usually adequate to demonstrate even mild neurologic weakness. However, disuse atrophy in strong muscles, like the quadriceps, tends to escape detection by this method. Quantitative strength determination comparing the two legs is advisable, especially in knee injuries of adolescent athletes. Before training for competition is resumed, the quadriceps of the affected leg should be nearly as strong as that on the normal side.

Impaired coordination is a common sign of central movement disorders. Apraxia may produce a motor ineptitude (66). Sensory deficits caused by parietal lobe damage or proprioceptive loss can also interfere with coordinated movements. Cerebellar dysfunction, basal ganglion disease, dyskinetic movement disorders, and spastic incoordination are distinguishable by the nature of the characteristic movement abnormalities (52). In infancy, delayed motor development is a general manifestation of coordination deficits. Detection of incoordinated movements is based mostly on observing gross and fine motor activities in children under 2 to 3 yr of age. Thereafter, the examination becomes more directed and should reflect developmental considerations in respect to age appropriateness of a task and quality of performance. For example, most children are able to walk a straight line unsteadily by placing one foot in front of the other around 3 yr of age (34); however, the comparative facility of tandem walking by 5 yr illustrates the significance of age in continuing refinement of motor control (35). The physician may be called upon to evaluate the appropriateness of coordination in children without an overt movement disorder (86). Among other subtle symptoms, clumsiness of handwriting and drawing, difficulties with physical education, and sports are frequent complaints. These children may have a motor incompetency of an apraxic nature, which, in some cases, is associated with learning and behavioral dysfunction (66). A number of tests have been described for examining motor proficiency as a function of age in normal children (10, 14). Tasks such as imitation of gestures (9), hopping (25), hand tapping (26), and pegboard performance (33, 89) yield information about maturation and deviant motor behavior (86).

Musculoskeletal System

In addition to muscle testing, examination of the musculoskeletal system (70, 84) entails inspection and palpation of bones and soft tissues, assessment of stance and gait (42, 50, 81), and measurement of active and passive range of motion (21, 84). As in previous parts of this chapter, only developmental variations are emphasized.

Variations in muscle tone, joint mobility, and bone configuration produce differences in range of motion during early development (78, 84). In the first 3 months of life, elbow extension may lack as much as 25° due to predominant flexor tone. Hip extension is incomplete at birth with an average of 30° limitation that decreases to less than 10° by 3 to 6 months (32, 78). External rotation of the hips exceeds internal rotation at birth and in early infancy (32, 78, 88). A gradual increase of internal rotation coincides with the resolution of the initial hip flexion attitude. A difference in hip abduction range with asymmetry of gluteal and upper thigh skin creases arouses the suspicion of congenital hip dysplasia (84, 92). In contrast to the predominant flexor tone of full-term neonates, joint hyperextensibility and hypotonia allow increased passive motion in preterm infants (2, 28, 31, 74). The scarf sign is a good illustration of excessive joint mobility of prematures. Holding the infant's hand, the examiner draws the arm across the chest, like a scarf, toward the contralateral shoulder. The elbow will cross the midline in premature infants (28). On straight leg raising, the popliteal angle is 180° in the preterm baby (2, 74). In the mature newborn, it is decreased to about 90° as a result of predominant flexor tone and retroversion of the proximal tibia. Anatomic preparations showed that both the tibia and the femur change in configuration from birth to adulthood. The angle of femoral inclination is 160° and anteversion of the femoral neck may be up to 60° in the newborn (78, 84) compared to the adult measurements of 125° and 10° to 20°, respectively (78). Retroversion of the proximal tibia that contributes to the flexed knee position in young infants, disappears by 10 yr of age (78). The physiologic varus configuration of the tibia is responsible for the bowlegged appearance until the age of 2 to 3 yr (78, 84).

A systematic review of the examination of the spine and extremities and analysis of normal and pathologic gait is beyond the scope of this discussion (1, 42, 50, 64, 76, 77, 80–82, 84). Table 2.3 shows the most significant developmental changes of posture and gait in childhood (81, 84). Variations in stance and gait that are characteristic of normal maturation should not be mistaken for pathology in growing children (77, 80, 81, 84).

Sensory Examination

A complete examination of peripheral sensory modalities, including proprioception, is feasible only in older children (17). In early infancy, crying and squirming to move away from pinprick demonstrates that pain sensation is perceived (16). A sleepy infant may be slow to respond, necessitating repeated application of stimuli. Withdrawal to touch or pinprick representing isolated distal spinal cord reflex activity may be confused with volitional response and misinterpreted as a sign of preserved sensation in spinal cord dysfunction at the thoracic level. Contrasting the infant's reaction to noxious stimuli on the arms and face helps distinguish the area of sensory deficit. Older infants will signal perception of touch and vibration by turning or moving away from the stimulus. The presence of superficial reflexes indicates that both afferent and efferent components of the reflex arc are intact. The neurosegmental levels for abdominal reflexes are T8 to T12; for the cremasteric reflex, L1 to L2; and for the anocutaneous reflex, S4 to S5. Their absence generally coincides with sensory deficit of the respective dermatomes in spina bifida. In young children who cannot be tested, ataxia and incoordination suggest the possibility of proprioceptive loss; objective evaluation of position sense can usually be performed by school age.

Cortical sensory function may be impaired when the parietal lobe is damaged (17, 66). Poor spontaneous function and visual monitoring while the extremity is used are suspicious signs. In general, objective examination can be conducted after 5 to 6 yr of age in the same manner as in adults to assess stereognosis and two-point discrimination and to detect topagnosia on single or double sensory stimulation (17, 66). At this age, testing for graphesthesia may be attempted by drawing a circle or cross on the palms; around

8 yr, the traditional number identification method provides a more accurate examination (17). Cutaneous sensation, proprioception, and adequate intellectual ability are prerequisites of testing cortical sensory function.

Examination of the special senses must be adapted to the child's ability to cooperate. Vision is tested by using a bright light or moving an attractive object across the infant's visual field. An infant is expected to follow to midline by 1 month and through 180° by 3 months. The STYCAR test (73, 75) and the illiterate E chart may be used for screening preschool children at risk for visual deficits. Unilateral loss or impairment of vision and visual field deficits, such as hemianopsia, are more likely to escape detection at an early age than are bilateral deficits. A child having strabismus or suspicion of diminished vision should be referred for an ophthalmologic evaluation as soon as these signs are discovered (53). Central dysfunction of visual attentiveness, discrimination, and information processing (51) may be misinterpreted as diminished vision and require both ophthalmologic and neuropsychologic investigation.

Screening of auditory function is a routine procedure in the neonatal nursery, pediatric office, and school (55, 67). Response to speech, tuning fork, or cricket toy is a gross screening method of hearing that should be included in the examination of handicapped infants and young children. Absent, lost, or delayed speech, articulation deficit, inattentiveness to sound, a history of otologic complaints, or failure to pass the screening test are some indications to refer a child for complete evaluation of auditory function (51, 55, 66, 67).

Functional Evaluation

The pediatric rehabilitation examination would be meaningless if the physiatrist did not construct from it a coherent picture of the child's functional accomplishments. This evaluation both complements and integrates the variety of information derived from all phases of the examination.

A convenient approach for functionally oriented assessment of infants and preschool children is offered by the developmental diagnostic evaluation (34, 35). Language, fine motor and adaptive skills, gross motor abilities, and personal-social behavior are the four major areas of function in the organizational framework of developmental testing. The same functional considerations are applicable to the evaluation of older children and adolescents. However, the examination will encompass a broader range of developmental expectations and abilities required for functioning in school and society. Skills in activities of daily living and gross motor function must be appraised in this context. In addition to speech, testing of language function entails other forms of communication, reading, writing, and spelling (7, 66). Drawing, design construction, arithmetic problems, and response about handling hypothetical situations of daily life provide a brief preliminary screening of mental abilities and learning (7, 66).

The essential feature of functional examination in children is to assess both physical and developmental disabilities. Comprehensive evaluation is based on the contributions of the multidisciplinary team.

Informing Interview

Informing the family about the findings of the examination and their implications is a responsibility for which the physician must be adequately prepared (85, 90). This role calls for a complex process of communication that must convey factual information in an attitude of caring (56, 87). Informing the parents about a newly established diagnosis should be regarded as a crisis intervention (71, 85). A diagnostic label is insufficient without explanation of its meaning. The parents need to know an estimate of prognosis in terms of medical implications and functional outlook. However, the uncertainties of early prognostication have to be pointed out, particularly in central nervous system dysfunction with the possibility of multiple handicaps. The parents should be advised about management of all aspects of function projected over the years. The importance of avoiding focus only on the physical disability and considering the child's developmental and social needs should be emphasized. Effective counseling and communication skills (65, 85, 90) are essential to establish a partnership between the physician and the parents for the success of the rehabilitation process.

REFERENCES

1. Alexander JE: The limping child. *Curr Probl Diagn Radiol* 16:229–270, 1987.
2. Amiel-Tison C, Grenier A: *Neurologic Assessment during the First Year of Life.* New York, Oxford University Press, 1986.
3. Arnold WC, Kallen RJ (eds): Fluid and electrolyte therapy. *Pediatr Clin North Am* 37:2, 1990.
4. Baird HW, Gordon EC: *Neurologic Evaluation of Infants and Children.* Clinics in Developmental Medicine no. 84/85. Philadelphia, JB Lippincott, 1983.
5. Barness LA: Nutrition and Nutritional Disorders. In Behrman RE, Vaughan VC (eds): *Nelson's Textbook of Pediatrics,* ed. 13. Philadelphia, WB Saunders, 1987.
6. Basmajian JV, De Luca CJ: *Muscles Alive,* ed. 5. Baltimore, Williams & Wilkins, 1985.
7. Behrman RE, Vaughan VC (eds): *Nelson's Textbook of Pediatrics,* ed. 13. Philadelphia, WB Saunders, 1987.
8. Berger RM, Maizels M, Morgan GC, Conway JJ, Firlit CF: Bladder capacity. *J Urol* 129:347–349. 1983.
9. Berges J, Lezine I: *The Imitation of Gestures.* Clinics in Developmental Medicine no. 18. London, W Heinemann Medical Books Publ, 1965.
10. Bialer I, Doll L, Winsber BG: A modified Lincoln-Oseretsky motor development scale. Provisional standardization. *Percept Motor Skills* 38:599–614, 1974.
11. Bishop M, Betts J, Chatten J: Partial nephrectomy for Wilms tumor in a child with hemihypertrophy. *Med Pediatr Oncol* 13:37–39, 1985.
12. Boineau FG, Lewy JW: Estimation of parenteral fluid requirements. *Pediatr Clin North Am* 37:257–266, 1990.
13. Brazelton TB: *Neonatal Behavioral Assessment Scale.* Clinics in Developmental Medicine no. 88. Philadelphia, JB Lippincott, 1984.

14. Broadhead GD, Bruininks RH: Factor structure consistency of the Bruininks-Oseretsky test—short form. *Rehab Lit* 44:13–18, 1983.
15. Brooke M (ed): *A Clinician's View of Neuromuscular Diseases,* ed 2. Baltimore, Williams & Wilkins, 1986.
16. Brown SB: Neurologic examination during the first 2 years of life. In Swaiman KF, Wright FS (eds): *The Practice of Pediatric Neurology.* St. Louis, CV Mosby Co, 1982.
17. Brown SB: Neurologic examination of the older child. In Swaiman KF, Wright FS (eds): *The Practice of Pediatric Neurology.* St. Louis, CV Mosby Co, 1982.
18. Bursztein S, Elwyn DH, Askanazi J, Kinney JM: *Energy Metabolism, Indirect Calorimetry and Nutrition.* Baltimore, Williams & Wilkins, 1989.
19. Carey WB: Clinical appraisal of temperament. In Lewis M, Taft LT (eds): *Developmental Disabilities, Theory, Assessment and Intervention.* New York, SP Medical and Scientific Books, 1982.
20. Chasnoff IJ: Drug use in pregnancy: parameters of risk. *Pediatr Clin North Am* 35:1403–1412, 1988.
21. Cole TM, Barry DT, Tobis JS: Measurement of musculoskeletal function. In Kottke FJ, Lehman JF (eds): *Krusen's Handbook of Physical Medicine and Rehabilitation,* ed. 4. Philadelphia, WB Saunders, 1990.
22. Committee on Dietary Allowances, Food and Nutrition Board, National Research Council: Recommended Dietary Allowances, ed. 9. Washington DC, National Academy of Sciences, 1980.
23. Committee on Nutrition American Academy of Pediatrics: *Pediatric Nutrition Handbook,* 1985.
24. Daniels L, Worthingham C: *Muscle Testing Techniques of Manual Examination,* ed. 5. Philadelphia, WB Saunders, 1986.
25. Denckla MB: Development of coordination in normal children. *Dev Med Child Neurol* 16:729–741, 1974.
26. Denckla MB: Development of speed in repetition and successive finger movements in normal children. *Dev Med Child Neurol* 15:635–645, 1973.
27. Dubowitz V: *The Floppy Infant.* Clinics in Developmental Medicine no. 76. Philadelphia, JB Lippincott Co, 1980.
28. Dubowitz V, Dubowitz L: *The Neurological Assessment of the Preterm and Fullterm Infant.* Clinics in Developmental Medicine no. 79. London, W. Heinemann Medical Books, 1981.
29. Dyck PJ (ed): *Peripheral Neuropathy,* ed. 2. Philadelphia, WB Saunders, 1984.
30. Fenichel GM: *Clinical Pediatric Neurology. A Signs and Symptoms Approach.* Philadelphia, WB Saunders, 1988.
31. Fenichel GM: *Neonatal Neurology.* New York, Churchill Livingstone, 1980.
32. Forero N, Okamura LA, Larson MA: Normal ranges of hip motion in neonates. *J Pediatr Orthop* 9:391–395, 1989.
33. Gardner RA: Purdue Pegboard. Normative Data (Revised) Examiner Manual for the Purdue Pegboard Test. Chicago, Science Research Associates, 1978.
34. Gesell AL, Halverson HM, Thompson H, Ilg FL, Castner BM, Ames LB: *The First Five Years of Life.* New York, Harper and Row, 1946.
35. Gesell AL, Ilg FL: *The Child from Five to Ten.* New York, Harper and Row, 1946.
36. Gierup J: Micturition studies in infants and children. *Scand J Urol Nephrol* 4:191–207, 1970.
37. Gines DJ: *Nutrition Management in Rehabilitation.* Frederick, MD, Aspen Publishers, 1990.
38. Green M: *Pediatric Diagnosis: Interpretation of Symptoms and Signs in Different Age Periods,* ed. 4. Philadelphia, WB Saunders, 1985.
39. Hansen TH, Tooley WH: Lung function in infancy and childhood. In Rudolph AM, Hoffman JIE (eds): *Pediatrics,* ed. 18. Los Altos, CA, Appleton and Lange, 1987.

40. Hollinshead WH, Jenkins DB: *Functional Anatomy of the Limbs and Back,* ed. 5. Philadelphia, WB Saunders, 1981.
41. Illingworth RS: *Development of the Infant and Young Child: Normal and Abnormal.* New York, Churchill Livingstone, 1987.
42. Inman VT, Ralston JH, Todd F: *Human Walking.* Baltimore, Williams & Wilkins, 1981.
43. Jones KL: Fetal alcohol syndrome. *Pediatr Rev* 8:122–125, 1986.
44. Jones KL: *Smith's Recognizable Patterns of Human Malformations,* ed. 2. Philadelphia, WB Saunders, 1988.
45. Johnson EW: Examination for muscle weakness in infants and small children. *JAMA* 168:1306–1313, 1958.
46. Kendall FP, McCreary EK: *Muscles, Testing and Function,* ed. 3. Baltimore, Williams & Wilkins, 1983.
47. Koff SA: Estimating bladder capacity in children. *Urology* XXI: 248, 1983.
48. Korobkin R, Guilleminault C: *Progress in Perinatal Neurology.* Baltimore, Williams & Wilkins, 1981.
49. Kottke FJ, Lehman JF (eds): *Krusen's Handbook of Physical Medicine and Rehabilitation,* ed. 4. Philadelphia, WB Saunders, 1990.
50. Lehman JF, DeLateur BJ: Gait analysis, diagnosis and management. In Kottke JF, Lehman JF (eds): *Krusen's Handbook of Physical Medicine and Rehabilitation,* ed. 4. Philadelphia, WB Saunders, 1990.
51. Lewis M, Taft LT (eds): *Developmental Disabilities. Theory, Assessment and Intervention.* New York, SP Medical and Scientific Books, 1982.
52. Lockman LA: Movement disorders. In Swaiman KF, Wright FS (eds). *The Practice of Pediatric Neurology.* St. Louis, CV Mosby, 1982.
53. Martin LJ: Pediatric ophthalmology. In Behrman RE, Vaughan VC (eds): *Nelson's Textbook of Pediatrics,* ed. 12. Philadelphia, WB Saunders, 1983.
54. Menkes JH: *Textbook of Child Neurology,* ed. 4. Philadelphia, Lea & Febiger, 1990.
55. Milstein JM: Abnormalities of hearing. In Swaiman KF, Wright FS (eds): *The Practice of Pediatric Neurology,* ed. 2. St. Louis, CV Mosby Co, 1982.
56. Molnar GE: A developmental perspective for the rehabilitation of children with physical disabilities. *Pediatr Ann* 17:766–776, 1988.
57. Molnar GE: Intervention for physically handicapped children. In Lewis M., Taft LT (eds): *Developmental Disabilities. Theory, Assessment and Intervention.* New York, SP Medical and Scientific Books, 1982.
58. Molnar GE: The influence of psychosocial factors on personality development and emotional health in children with cerebral palsy and spina bifida. In Heller BW, Flohr LM, Zegans LS (eds): *Psychosocial Intervention with Physically Disabled Persons.* New Brunswick, Rutgers University Press, 1989.
59. Molnar GE, Alexander J, Gutfeld N: Reliability of quantitative strength measurements in children. *Arch Phys Med Rehabil* 60:218–221, 1979.
60. Oski FA, De Angelis CD, Feigin RD, Warshaw JB (eds): *Principles and Practice of Pediatrics.* Philadelphia, JB Lippincott, 1990.
61. Pact V, Sirotkin-Roses M, Beatus J: *The Muscle Testing Handbook.* Boston, Little, Brown & Co, 1984.
62. Paine RS, Brazelton TB, Donovan DE, Drorbaugh JE, Hubbel JP, Sears EM: Evolution of postural reflexes in normal infants and in the presence of chronic brain syndromes. *Neurology* 14:1036–1048, 1964.
63. Perrot LJ, Williamson S, Jimenez JF: The caudal regression syndrome in infants of diabetic mothers. *Ann Clin Labor Sci* 17:211–220, 1987.
64. Phillips WA: The child with a limp. *Orthop Clin North Am* 18:489–501, 1987.
65. Quill TE: Recognizing and adjusting barriers in doctor-patient communication. *Ann Intern Med* 111:51–57, 1989.

66. Rapin I: *Children with Brain Dysfunction. Neurology, Cognition, Language and Behavior.* International Review of Child Neurology Series. New York, Raven Press, 1982.
67. Rapin I: Children with Hearing Impairment. In Swaiman KF, Wright FS (eds): *The Practice of Pediatric Neurology,* ed. 2. St. Louis, CV Mosby Co, 1982.
68. Report of the Second Task Force on Blood Pressure Control in Children. *Pediatrics* 79:1–25, 1987.
69. Rodriquez JL, Garcia-Alix A, Palacios J, Paniaguara R: Changes in the long bones due to fetal immobility caused by neuromuscular disease: a radiographic and histologic study. J Bone Joint Surg 70-A:1052–1060, 1988.
70. Rosse C, Clawson DK (eds): *The Musculoskeletal System in Health and Disease.* Hagerstown, MD, Harper and Row, 1980.
71. Rubin AL, Rubin RL: The effects of physician counseling technique on parent reaction to mental retardation diagnosis. *Child Psychiatry Hum Dev* 10:213–221, 1980.
72. Rudolph AM, Hoffman JIE: *Pediatrics,* ed. 18. Los Altos, CA, Appleton and Lange, 1987.
73. Savitz R, Valadian I, Reed R: Vision Screening of the Pre-School Child. Children's Bureau Publication no. 414.
74. Sher PK: Neurologic examination of the premature infant. In Swaiman KF, Wright FS (eds): *The Practice of Pediatric Neurology.* St. Louis, CV Mosby Co, 1982.
75. Sheridan MD: Manual For The STYCAR Vision Tests, ed. 3. Windsor, NFER, 1976.
76. Singer JI: The cause of gait disturbance in 425 pediatric patients. *Pediatr Emerg Care* 1:7–10, 1985.
77. Staheli LT: In-toeing and out-toeing in children. *J Fam Pract* 16:1005–1011, 1983.
78. Steindler A: *Kinesiology of the Human Body.* Springfield, CC Thomas, 1955.
79. Strax TE: Psychological problems of disabled adolescents and young adults. *Pediatr Ann* 17:756–761, 1988.
80. Sutherland DM: *Gait Disorders in Childhood and Adolescence.* Baltimore, Williams & Wilkins, 1984.
81. Sutherland DM, Olshen R, Cooper L, Woo-Sam J: The development of mature gait. *J Bone Joint Surg* 62A336–353, 1980.
82. Sutherland DM, Olshen R, Cooper L, Wyatt M, Leach J, Mubarak S, Schultz P: The pathomechanics of gait in Duchenne muscular dystrophy. *Dev Med Child Neurol* 23:3–22, 1981.
83. Swaiman KF, Wright FS (eds): *The Practice of Pediatric Neurology,* ed. 2. St. Louis, CV Mosby Co, 1982.
84. Tachdjian MO: *Pediatric Orthopedics,* ed. 2. Philadelphia, WB Saunders, 1990.
85. Taft LT, Matthew SW, Molnar GE: Pediatric management of the physically handicapped child. In Barness LA (ed): *Advances in Pediatrics.* Chicago, Year Book Medical Publishers Inc, 1980.
86. Touwen BCL: *Examination of the Child With Minor Neurologic Dysfunction,* ed. 2. Clinics in Developmental Medicine no. 71. Philadelphia, JB Lippincott, 1980.
87. Wallender JL, et al: Disability parameters, chronic strain and adaptation of physically handicapped children and their mothers. *J Pediatr Psychol* 14:23–42, 1988.
88. Waugh KG, Minkel JL, Parker R, Coon VA: Measurement of selected hip, knee and ankle joint motion in newborns. *Phys Ther* 63:1616–1621, 1983.
89. Wilson BC, Iacovillo JM, Wilson JJ, Risucci D: Purdue pegboard performance in normal preschool children. *J Clin Neuropsych* 4:125–130, 1982.
90. Wolraich ML: Communication between physicians and parents of handicapped children. *Except Child* 48:316–327, 1982.
91. Young RR, Delwaide PJ: Spasticity. Parts I and II. *N Engl J Med* 304:28, 96, 1981.
92. Yousafzadeh DK, Ramilo JL: Normal hip in children: correlation of ultrasound with anatomic and cryomyotome myotonic sections. *Radiology* 165:644–655, 1987.

2

Growth and Development

GABRIELLA E. MOLNAR AND
RUTH K. KAMINER

The essential distinguishing features of pediatrics are: (*a*) the patient is growing and developing; and (*b*) the professional relationship is among physician, child, and parent. The work of childhood is growing up to be a well-functioning adult. The impact of illness or disability and of treatment must be viewed against the yardstick of this outcome. When a handicap occurs early in the life of a child, it may interfere with more areas of function, whereas if it is acquired later, the child tends to have greater difficulty in accepting a change in his or her own status.

In planning the goals of intervention, the physician must consider both immediate results and the long-term effect on overall growth and development. It is the physician's responsibility to ensure that short-term goals for attaining specific skills do not conflict with the long-term aim of achieving maximal emotional maturity and self-reliance. Because of the nature of the professional relationship when the patient is a child, the physician needs skills in working with both parents and child, an awareness of how the usual parenting practices may be affected by having a child at risk or with proven handicap, and how this may influence the child's development (33).

Growth

Growth is an increase in physical measurements. Its rate is variable; the two most rapid phases occur during infancy and from prepubescence through adolescence (4). Various body parts grow at selective rates and with relative predominance during certain periods: the head in infancy; the trunk in infancy and adolescence; and the extremities from 1 year to puberty (32). Changing body proportions result in a shift of the center of gravity from the xiphoid process in the newborn to the sacral promontory by late childhood (45). Individual differences in growth are considerable, depending on genetic, environmental, and other factors. The range of expected variations for different ages is a bell-shaped normal distribution curve.

The rate of growth is a far more sensitive indicator of health or disease

Table 2.1
Growth from Birth to Maturity[a]

Height		Weight		Head Circumference	
Birth	50 cm	Birth (full-term)	3400 gm	Birth	35 cm
12 months	75 cm	5 months	Double	4 months	6-cm increment
4 years	100 cm	12 months	Triple	12 months	6-cm increment
Early school age	5 cm annually	Until adolescent growth spurt	2 kg annually	Until maturity	10-cm increment
Prepubescence/ adolescence	5–8 cm annually				

[a]Average values compiled from various sources (4, 32, 51).

than absolute size at a given age. Growth trends should be monitored by serial longitudinal measurements as they tend to be consistent in individual children. Values outside ± 2 SD range or significant persistent shift in relative growth trends warrants investigation. Growth charts on which serial measurement can be plotted are useful tools in clinical practice (4).

Table 2.1 is a brief guide to growth in the most important physical measurements. Most noteworthy is the marked growth velocity in the first year. The average newborn is 3.4 kg at birth, doubles his or her weight by 5 months, and triples it by 1 yr. Birth length, which averages 50 cm, will increase by 50% in 1 year and head circumference, which averages 35 cm at birth, increases by 12 cm, representing more than one half of the total anticipated growth until maturity.

Height

Adult height can be estimated by doubling body length at 2 yr. Accurate prediction is made by skeletal age from the Bayley-Pinneau tables that are based on the Greulich-Pyle standards (24). Appearance of the ossification centers and epiphyseal closure are indicators of bone age and of the remaining anticipated growth. Girls show maximal growth velocity prior to menarche and, in most cases, growth ceases 2 yr thereafter. Boys achieve maximal growth velocity in late puberty, which is identifiable by the appearance of facial hair on the cheeks and chin (17).

Generalized growth retardation accompanies certain types of endocrine dysfunction or systemic skeletal diseases (51, 57). Children with cerebral palsy, as a group, were found to have a shift to the left in height and weight measurements (60). Epiphyseal trauma sustained before maturity leads to localized disturbance in growth (43, 49, 57). Neurologic lesions may be associated with selective atrophy of the affected extremities. Shortening of a limb is generally more significant in lower motor neuron lesions, such as neonatal brachial plexus palsy (15) or myelodysplasia, than in spastic paralysis; for example, congenital or early acquired hemiparetic cerebral palsy (25).

Familiarity with prediction of growth trends is relevant to selecting the method and timing of treatment for leg length discrepancy and scoliosis where progression is expected to occur during the rapid adolescent spinal growth (1, 31, 48, 57). Anticipated growth is considered in orthotic and prosthetic prescriptions for children.

Weight

Newborns below 2500 gm at birth are considered low birth weight infants, which includes those who are small for gestational age if they are born at term and premature infants if they are delivered less than 37 weeks from the first day of the last menstrual period (4). The distinction between these two groups has prognostic importance, but may be difficult to make since menstrual histories can be unreliable. Serial sonographic evaluations of the size of the fetus and newborn assessment of gestational age by physical and neurologic examination, most often using the Dubowitz scale (14), improve the accuracy of determining gestational age. Because of neurological immaturity and more frequent complications leading to anoxic and hemorrhagic brain damage, premature infants are at a greater risk for cerebral palsy than those who are small for gestational age. The latter group, on the other hand, has an increased incidence of congenital anomalies (11).

Head Circumference

The considerable increase in normal head size during infancy is related to rapid brain growth. Head circumference is measured over the most prominent area of the occiput and supraorbital ridges. Estimates by observation are misleading; since normal values are in a narrow range, only actual measurements are reliable.

Head circumference measurements are routinely obtained on children up to age 3 yr and plotted on growth charts, of which the Nellhaus graph is the most commonly used (42). A child whose head is growing at the expected rate does not give cause for concern, even if the size is in the 2nd or 98th percentile. However, a head circumference outside 2 SD from the mean or "crossing percentiles," due to deceleration or acceleration of head growth, requires further investigation. For children over 3 yr of age, head circumference measurements are obtained when the child is suspected of having central nervous system pathology.

A very small head circumference or marked deceleration in growth usually reflects defective brain development. Values of 3 SD below the mean are generally associated with intellectual deficit. Since the fontanelles are open until 12 to 18 months and calvarial sutures do not unite firmly until about puberty, intracranial pathology can lead to excessive head growth. An enlarged head or gradual relative increase in head size results most often from elevated intracranial pressure due to a space-occupying lesion or to hydrocephalus, which is frequently associated with myelodysplasia (56). Cerebral palsy may also be associated with alteration in head size; enlargement, due to hydrocephalus, particularly after intracranial hemorrhage in premature infants, or microcephaly, as a result of cerebral atrophy in severe anoxic encephalopathy (56, 63).

DEVELOPMENT

Development is the acquisition and refinement of skills (30). Increasing complexity of behavior is related to maturation of the central nervous system and to experience, with adequacy in both areas needed for optimal functioning. Superiority in either sphere may compensate for deficits in the other, as when a well-endowed infant succeeds despite a minimally adequate environment. Conversely, the follow-up of premature and at-risk infants indicates that socioeconomic and educational status of the family is positively correlated with better outcome (18).

Attainment of new developmental skills follows a generally applicable sequence and timetable with a range of normal individual variations (27). The sequence in which skills are acquired tends to be more constant than the rate of their acquisition. Progress in various areas of development may proceed at different rates even in normal children. Motor skills are attained in a cephalocaudad progression; first, head control, followed by voluntary reaching and grasping, sitting, and, finally, walking. Behavior patterns evolve from generalized movements and responses to more discrete, refined, and complex actions (12, 26, 35).

Normal development may appear to be a static body of knowledge since the biological aspects of development have not changed from the time descriptions became available. However, changes occurring in the physical and social environment affect children's development pre- and postnatally and make different demands on their ability to adapt. As societal values change, they are reflected in the expectations parents and other adults have of children's performance on various tasks. These issues have direct relevance for children with disabilities, since even motor impairments do not affect only a child's motor functioning, but also the child's self-image and total adaptation to societal demands.

New challenges to the successful development of children have resulted both from the scientific advances that make survival of more fragile infants, such as prematures, possible and from the social problems that result in the birth of greater numbers of fragile or compromised infants, such as those who have been exposed to drugs or infected with AIDS. Providing appropriate environments for the development of these vulnerable infants has acted as a stimulus to new research in the area of infant development and to an exploration of ways to enhance it.

Neonatal intensive care has led to societal expectations that even very small and premature newborns will survive and have successful outcomes. Neonates weighing 2500 gm or less, 6.8% of all U.S. births, are defined as low birth weight, but their progress is seldom reported in the literature since they are expected to do well. Published follow-up studies focus on the very low birth weight (VLBW) group weighing 1500 gm or less who constitute 1.2% of U.S. births and have a 10–20% rate of neurologic and developmental handicap (4). Even those who are free of major handicap are at greater risk for academic and emotional problems. Learning to be the parent of a small premature infant, who, even if not critically ill, may be unable to suck, is hypotonic, or not clearly awake or asleep poses unique challenges. Support and guidance to families in adapting their parenting to their child's needs is the first step in the rehabilitation program for the child.

A purely descriptive study of development offers only a survey of the surface phenomena. Theoretical formulation concerning the neurological foundations of behavior, the development of cognition, and of personality connect these phenomena into a coherent picture (40).

DEVELOPMENTAL DIAGNOSIS

Gesell and associates (21–23) viewed development as a process in which differentiation of structure is reflected by specialization of function. They provided a methodical inventory of developmental milestones in terms of typical behavior patterns in four distinct areas of function.

1. *Gross motor behavior*—Preambulatory skill, walking, and other advanced physical activities;
2. *Fine motor-adaptive behavior*—Prehension, manpulatory skills, and utilization of the sensorimotor system in encounters of daily life;
3. *Language behavior*—Vocalization, comprehension, and expression in oral and other modes of communication;
4. *Personal-social behavior*—Acquisition of the standards of society and culture in which the child lives.

The developmental examination compares a child's function with expected standards for that age (30). This evaluation is complementary to the classical neurological examination designed to elicit abnormal findings, with emphasis on signs that localize the nervous system lesion. All tasks on developmental tests are expected of normal children. The observed behavior patterns are indices of maturity and integrity of the nervous system (30). Developmental assessment entails observation of selected behavioral and performance items in each area. It is important to ascertain from the parent what the child is able to do at home and whether the sample of observed behavior is representative of the child's usual function. Besides determining which tasks a child can perform, the examiner must also note the quality of the performance and the child's style of coping with difficult tasks. Developmental assessment is best performed before the child is undressed or manipulated in any way. Careful observation of a child performing developmental tasks often provides the most revealing information concerning neurological function, such as muscle strength and coordination.

The Denver II, a revision of the Denver Developmental Screening Test (DDST) (19), is a commonly used tool that has been well validated and should be used as part of standard well child care, not only when a disability is suspected. It is based on the Gesell Standards as well as on several other scales for assessing young children's development from which items were selected for their consistency, reliability, and ease of administration. The Denver II is organized in the four areas of behavior described by Gesell and is designed to be used by trained paraprofessionals to categorize the children as passing the screening test, failing, or being questionable. The Denver II, like other developmental screening tests, is intended to select children who fall below age expectancy and will need more comprehensive evaluation, as well as those who are questionable and will require rescreening. The Early Language Milestone Scale is another useful screening tool developed to assess the language skills of infants and children up to age 3 yr (13). Such tests should not be used for diagnostic labeling of the child nor do they eliminate the need to listen to parental concerns and observe child behavior at all medical encounters. When the results on the original DDST were compared to standardized psychological testing, 81% of children were correctly identified, with most of the errors being due to overreferral of normal children (36).

The pattern of functional deviations detected on developmental assessment provides a guide for further diagnostic inquiry. Isolated or predominant delay of gross and fine motor milestones arouses the suspicion of neuromuscular dysfunction. Intellectual deficit is usually manifested by slowness in all areas, with gross motor development and personal social skills being areas of relative strength. It is noteworthy that motor development is the area most easily scored and the least valuable for overall assessment of a child's cognitive ability (27). Parents attach great significance to the onset of independent walking as a measure of developmental intactness, but studies have shown that most children who begin walking after 17 months have normal intelligence (41). While the incidence of delayed gross motor development is increased in mental deficiency, a majority of retarded children who do not also have a neuromotor disability begin walking before 17 months of age (29).

Delayed or defective language skills may indicate hearing loss, a specific language or affective disorder (3, 47, 64), or may be the first indication that the child is mentally retarded. Parental observations of delayed speech and language skills are usually correct, and require further evaluation of the reason for the delay, which may or may not be due to an isolated problem in the speech and language area. Formal audiometric testing is mandatory in any child with delayed language acquisition. Language development may be the most useful indicator of cognitive ability in physically handicapped children, whose adaptive and personal social skills are impeded by their motor deficits. However, it is essential to rule out a hearing deficit before assessing language comprehension skills, particularly in view of the fact that many of the risk factors for hearing loss and for cerebral palsy are the same. One must also recognize a possible impairment of peripheral speech mechanism that can interfere with verbal communication, such as is seen in cerebral palsy with bilateral spasticity or dyskinesia.

INFANTILE REFLEX DEVELOPMENT

Motor behavior in neonates and young infants reflects the immaturity of the central nervous system and is influenced by primitive reflexes (10, 44, 58). Maturation is signaled by a gradual suppression of infantile reflexes as volitional control is acquired (5, 10, 37, 56). Concurrent with this process, more sophisticated postural responses emerge that remain operative throughout life to provide a background supportive mechanism for coordinated motor performance (5, 10, 27). Both processes of infantile reflex development progress simultaneously and follow a fairly well-defined timetable that has a chronological association with the attainment of motor milestones. Twitchell (61, 62) has described the relationship between grasp reflexes and various stages in the development of prehension. The observation of Milani-Comparetti and Gidoni (38, 39) suggested a similar relationship between gross motor milestones and the two processes of infantile reflex behavior.

Table 2.2 provides a description of selected infantile reflexes with particular emphasis on those that are relevant to motor behavior and to detection of a neuromuscular deficit. Reflexes that are part of the standard neurologic examination at all ages, such as pupillary and other ocular reflexes or superficial and deep tendon reflexes, are not included. Their significance and any age-related differences are mentioned in Chapter 1.

Persistence of primitive reflex activity beyond the expected age can be interpreted as a sign of delayed maturation of the central nervous system and may be the earliest indication of a neuromuscular dysfunction, for example, of a static encephalopathy in cerebral palsy or some progressive neurologic disease (5, 10, 37, 44). On the other hand, absent reflex responses should arouse the suspicion of weakness (28) related to muscle disease or to interruption of the peripheral reflex arc, for example, spinal muscular atrophy, myelodysplasia, or neuropathy of traumatic or hereditary etiology.

COGNITIVE DEVELOPMENT

Piaget is a psychologist who studied the question of how a child comes to know what he or she knows and the process by which he or she acquires the ability to reason logically (46). His view is that infants formulate "schemas," which are a combination of a sensory and motor experience, and then repeat

Table 2.2
Infantile Reflex Development[a]

Reflex	Stimulus	Response	Suppression	Clinical Significance
		PRIMITIVE REFLEXES; Present at Birth, Suppressed with Maturation		
Asymmetric tonic neck	Head turning or tilting to the side	Extension of the extremities on the chin side, flexion on the occiput side	Suppressed by 6–7 months	Obligatory abnormal at any age Persistent suspicious of CNS pathology
Symmetric tonic neck	Neck flexion Neck extension	Arm flexion, leg extension Arm extension, leg flexion	Suppressed by 6–7 months	Obligatory abnormal at any age Persistent suspicious of CNS pathology
Moro	Sudden neck extension	Arm extension abduction followed by flexion-adduction	Suppressed 4–6 months	Abnormal if persists
Tonic labyrinthine	Head position in space, strongest at 45° angle to horizonal Supine Prone	Predominant extensor tone Predominant flexor tone	Suppressed 4–6 months	Abnormal at any age if hyperactive or if persistent
Positive supporting	Tactile contact and weight-bearing on the sole	Leg extension for supporting partial body weight	Suppressed by 3–7 months and replaced by volitional standing	Abnormal at any age if obligatory or hyperactive; suggests spasticity of the legs
Rooting	Stroking the corner of mouth, upper or lower lip	Moving the tongue, mouth, and head toward the site of stimulus	Suppressed by 4 months	Searching for nipple Diminished in CNS depression; obligatory persistence may be immature CNS development
Palmar grasp	Pressure or touch on the palm, stretch of finger flexors	Flexion of fingers	Suppressed by 5–6 months	Diminished in CNS depression; absent in lower motor neuron paralysis; persistence suggests spasticity, i.e., cerebral palsy

Reflex/Response	Stimulus	Response	Timing	Significance
Plantar grasp	Pressure on sole just distal to metatarsal heads	Flexion of toes	Suppressed by 12–18 months	Absent in lower motor neuron paralysis; persists and hyperactive in spasticity, i.e., cerebral palsy
Automatic neonatal walking	Contact of sole in vertical position tilting the body forward and from side to side	Automatic alternating steps	Suppressed by 3–4 months	Variable activity in normal infants; absent in lower motor neuron paralysis of the legs
Placing	Tactile contact on dorsum of foot or hand	Flexion to place the leg or arm over the obstacle	Suppressed before end of first year	Absent in lower motor neuron paralysis or extensor spasticity of the legs
PHYSIOLOGIC POSTURAL RESPONSES: Emerge with Maturation, Present throughout Life, Modulated by Volition				
Head righting	Visual and vestibular	Align face vertical mouth horizontal Prone Supine	Emerge at 2 months 3–4 months	Delayed or absent in CNS immaturity or damage or motor unit disease
Body, head righting	Tactile proprioceptive vestibular	Align body parts	Emerge from 4–6 months	Delayed or absent in CNS immaturity or damage or motor neuron disease
Protective extension or propping	Displacement of center of gravity outside of supporting surface	Extension-abduction of the extremity toward the side of displacement to prevent falling	Emerge between 5 and 12 months	Delayed or absent in CNS immaturity or damage, or motor unit disease
Equilibrium or tilting	Displacement of center of gravity	Adjustment of tone and trunk posture to maintain balance	Emerge between 6 and 14 months	Delayed or absent in CNS immaturity or damage, or motor unit disease

[a]Compiled from various sources (5–7, 10, 14, 27, 38, 39, 44, 58, 61, 62).

and modify them to conform to new situations. They progress through stages of cognitive functioning that can be recognized by the children's method of solving problems. The stages are seen as consecutive, each based on the previous one, and resulting from an active process on the child's part. Each stage is a plateau and its attainment permits the child to reason in a qualitatively more complex manner (46).

The sensorimotor stage, from birth to 2 yr, spans the transition from immature reflex and sensorimotor responses to purposeful activity. Cognitive ability at this stage is practical and action oriented. During the preoperational stage that follows and lasts from 2–7 yr, the ability to use symbols is consolidated and manifested by the expanded use of language and the capacity to deal with objects and events not present in the immediate situation. The age of 7–11 yr is the time when basic logical thinking emerges and is called the stage of concrete operational thought. The stage of formal operational thought is reached after 11 yr of age and is characterized by the ability to use abstract reasoning and to entertain hypothetical ideas (46).

PERSONALITY DEVELOPMENT

Many prevailing theories on emotional development of children originate from Freud's system of psychology, which he developed to describe and explain the phenomena observed in adult patients undergoing psychoanalysis. His psychoanalytic theories were applied to children (20) and modified by Mahler (34) and Erikson (16), using direct observations. Mahler focuses on the child's process of separation and individuation from the mother, which occurs at 5 months to 2 yr (34). During this time, the child develops the concept of himself or herself as a person apart from the mother, to whom the mother is available as a source of nurturing and assistance, initially by her physical presence, and eventually, through an internalized image that gives the child comfort in times of stress.

Erikson's formulation (16) accepts the concept of innate aggressive and sexual drives and attempts to integrate social and cultural factors into the theory. Each stage of development is seen as a crisis, whose resolution is the task of the child during that particular period. The issue in the first year of life is basic trust vs. mistrust. If the infant's needs are satisfied, he or she is able to develop the expectation that these will continue to be met and, thus, the child can acquire a sense of trust. Long hospitalizations required by some premature infants may interfere with the development of this relationship. For those babies who are difficult to feed and handle, professional help is needed to enable the mother to satisfy her infant's wants. The crisis of the second year of life is autonomy vs. shame and doubt. The process of separation and individuation studied by Mahler is acknowledged by Erickson, but his main focus is on the child's achievement of control over locomotion and sphincters. Success in this stage means that the child derives a sense of autonomy in controlling his or her own body while conforming to some parental expectations. The issue of autonomy is a critical one for disabled individuals throughout their lives and requires professional sensitivity at all times. Otherwise, even well-intentioned therapeutic interventions may inadvertently encourage a child to assume a passive role by rewarding compliance and discouraging independent action. The stage of initiative vs. guilt, from 3–5 yr, is when children become aware of their own sex and prefer the parent of the opposite sex. At the resolution of this crisis, they come to identify with the parent of the same sex. Industry vs. inferiority are the issues from 5 yr to puberty. In all cultures this is the stage at which children receive systematic instruction in the skills of their society. The arena of much of the child's activity shifts from the home to the school as children seek their place among their age peers. For children with limitations in their ability to learn or to compete successfully in recreational activities such as sports, this period brings special challenges. The adolescent faces the crisis of identity vs. identity diffusion. Young people are "concerned with what they appear in the eyes of others as compared with what they feel they are, and with the question of how to connect the roles and skills cultivated earlier with the occupational prototypes of the day" (16). This is an age at which disabled youngsters benefit from expert counseling to assist them in forming an identity that recognizes their strengths and capabilities as well as acknowledging their disabilities.

Another theoretical framework for studying personality development is the learning theory that deals with how behaviors change as a result of experience. This approach is characterized by the premise that behavior is learned and by the assumption that learning occurs through the association of events. It focuses on what the person does, rather than on inferences about the individual's attributes or motives; this approach stresses empirical investigation. Learning is viewed as characterized by pairing of external stimuli with autonomic or instrumental events, with feedback from the reinforcing consequences that perpetuate the behavior. It is assumed that environmental factors external to the child are primarily responsible for the child's social behavior patterns. While the learning theories generally do not offer a comprehensive view of development, Bandura (2) and others attempted to construct a theory of child development within the orientation of this school of thought. They proposed a social learning theory, which deals with the development of social behavior. This viewpoint acknowledges a central "cognitive" mechanism that codes and organizes inputs and formulates the hypotheses that lead to rules of behavior. They see the human learner as an individual who actively processes information and then uses the restructured information to guide future behavior. Perception and interpretation of stimuli generate learned rules and patterns of behavior and influence the individual's responses. Learning theory has been criticized for its inadequacy in explaining emotional development, particularly in light of recent observations about the ability of infants to express emotions. Additionally, learning theory does not account for the accumulating evidence about biological preparedness of infants for interacting with the social and physical world, nor for their ability to elicit behaviors from caretakers, rather than just respond to their actions.

However, this theoretical position leads to a useful therapeutic approach, the behavior therapy techniques. Since all behavior is seen as learned, abnormal behavior is felt to be continuous with normal behavior, only an exaggeration of it. Behavior therapy relies on an analysis of behavior to explain observable actions in terms of functional relationships and then attempts to modify these behaviors by methods developed in the laboratory. In practice, the use of these methods does not require a belief in the underlying theories. The social learning view is that behavioral change following therapy or experience is partly due to the individual's increased expectation of "personal efficacy," which is the sense of mastery resulting from successful performance. Social learning leads to the development of a set of expectations for a given situation.

Just as an individual can learn to anticipate mastery of a situation, the opposite may also occur. "Learned helplessness," is a behavior pattern described in individuals who perceive situational outcomes as independent from their behavior (50). This concept is very relevant to working with disabled children, for whom it is essential to know that they are not helpless and can anticipate a predictable impact on their environment. Behavior intervention techniques have proven useful in altering maladaptive behaviors and interactions of children and are especially applicable in working with those who are retarded.

DEVELOPMENTAL MILESTONES

The most significant milestones in the four descriptive areas of development and the simultaneous cognitive and emotional stages are shown in Table 2.3. Descriptions of children's behavior at key ages are given below.

Newborn

Flexor tone predominates in the full-term newborn who usually lies with extremities semiflexed, head to one side and hands fisted. He can suck, swallow, sneeze, and cough. Behavior is largely based on reflex responses according to the patterns described previously. However, recent studies have shown that neonates have greater capacity than previously assumed. Using the neonatal behavior assessment scale devised by Brazelton (6–8), newborns can be shown to quiet and turn their heads to a rattle or voice and to follow a brightly colored object. They are also capable of habituation, which consists of the ability to give successively decreasing responses to repeated stimuli. All responses are highly dependent on the state of alertness of the infant. The neonates' cuddliness is such a striking characteristic that it is included in the Brazelton scale (6).

Table 2.3.
Milestones in Child Development[a]

Age	Gross Motor	Fine Motor Adaptive	Personal/Social	Speech and language	Cognitive	Emotional
Newborn	Flexor tone predominates In prone, turns head to side Automatic reflex walking Rounded spine when held sitting	Hands fisted Grasp reflex State dependent ability to fix and follow object	Habituation and some control of state	Cry State dependent quieting and head turning to rattle or voice	*Sensorimotor period* 0–24 months Reflex stage	*Basic trust vs. basic mistrust*—first year Normal symbiotic phase—does not differentiate between self and mother
4 months	Head midline Head held when pulled to sit In prone, lifts head to 90° and lifts chest slightly Turns to supine	Hands mostly open Midline hand play Crude palmar grasp	Recognizes bottle	Turns to voice and bell consistently Laughs, squeals Responsive vocalization Blows bubbles, "raspberries"	"Circular reaction" the interesting result of an action motivates its repetition	"Lap baby," developing a sense of basic trust
7 months	Maintains sitting, may lean on arms Rolls to prone Bears all weight; bounces when held erect Cervical lordosis	Intermediate grasp Transfers cube from hand to hand Bangs objects	Differentiates between familiar person and stranger Holds bottle Looks for dropped object "Talks" to his mirror image	Uses single and double consonant-vowel combinations		At 5 months began to differentiate between mother and self, i.e., beginning of separation individuation Has a sense of belonging to a central person
10 months	Creeps on all fours Pivots in sitting Stand momentarily Cruises	Pincer grasp, mature thumb to index grasp Bangs 2 cubes held in hands	Plays peek-a-boo Finger feeds Chews with rotary movement	Shouts for attention Imitates speech sounds Waves "bye-bye"	Can retrieve an object hidden in his view	Practicing phase of separation—individuation, practices initiating separations

Table 2.3.
Milestones in Child Development—*Continued*

Age	Gross Motor	Fine Motor Adaptive	Personal/Social	Speech and language	Cognitive	Emotional
10 months	Slight bow leg Increased lumbar lordosis; acute lumbo-sacral angulation			Uses "mama" and "dada" with meaning Inhibits behavior to "no"		"Love affair with the world"
14 months	Walks alone, arms in high guard or midguard Wide base, excessive knee and hip flexion Foot contact on entire sole Slight valgus knees and feet Pelvic tilt and rotation	Piles two cubes Scribbles spontaneously Holds crayon full length in palm Casts objects	Uses spoon with overpronation and spilling Removes a garment	Uses single words Understands simple commands	Differentiates available behavior patterns for new ends, e.g., pulls rug on which is a toy	Rapproachement phase of separation— individuation; ambivalent behavior to mother *Stage of autonomy vs. shame and doubt (1–3 yr)* Issue of holding on and letting go Pleasure in controlling muscles and sphincters
18 months	Arms at low guard Mature supporting base and heel strike Seats self in chair Walks backwards	Emerging hand dominance Crude release Holds crayon butt end in palm Dumps raisin from bottle spontaneously	Imitates housework Carries, hugs doll Drinks from cup neatly	Points to named body part Identifies one picture Says "no" Jargons	Capable of "insight", i.e., solving a problem by mental combinations, not physical groping	
2 yr	Begins running Walks up and down stairs alone Jumps on both feet in place	Hand dominance is usual Builds eight-cube tower	Pulls on garment Uses spoon well Opens door turning knob	Two-word phrases are common Uses verbs Refers to self by name	*Preoperational period (2–7 yr)* —able to evoke an object or event not present	

Age	Gross motor	Fine motor/adaptive	Personal-social	Language	Cognitive	Psychosexual/Psychosocial
		Aligns cubes horizontally Imitates vertical line Places pencil shaft between thumb and fingers Draws with arm and wrist action	Feeds doll with bottle or spoon Toilet training usually begun	Uses 'me', 'mine' Follows simple directions	—object permanence established —comprehends symbols	
3 yr	Runs well Pedals tricycle Broad jumps Walks up stairs alternating feet	Imitates three-cube bridge Copies circle Uses overhand throw with anteroposterior arm and trunk motion Catches with extended arms hugging against body	Most children toilet trained day and night Pours from pitcher Unbuttons; washes and dries hands and face Parallel play Can take turns Can be reasoned with	Three-word sentences are usual Uses future tense Asks 'what', 'who', 'where' Follows prepositional commands, i.e., 'put it under' Gives full name May stutter in eagerness Identifies self as boy or girl Recognizes three colors	Preoperational period continues Child is capable of: —deferred imitation —symbolic play —drawing of graphic images —mental images —verbal evocation of events	*Stage of initiative vs. guilt* (3–5 yr) Deals with issue of genital sexuality
4 yr	Walks down stairs alternating feet Hops on one foot Plantar arches developing Sits up from supine position without rotating	Handles a pencil by finger and wrist action, like adults Copies a cross Draws a frog-like person with head and extremities Throws underhand Cuts with scissors	Cooperative play-sharing and interacting Imaginative make-believe play Dresses and undresses with supervision distinguishing front and back of clothing and buttoning Does simple errands outside of home	Gives connected account of recent experiences Questions 'why', 'how', 'when' Uses past tense, adjectives, adverbs Knows opposite analogies Repeats four digits		

Table 2.3.
Milestones in Child Development—*Continued*

Age	Gross Motor	Fine Motor Adaptive	Personal/Social	Speech and language	Cognitive	Emotional
5 yr	Skips; tiptoes Balances 10 sec on each foot	Hand dominance is expected Draws man with head, body, and extremities Throws with diagonal arm and body rotation Catches with hands	Creative play Competitive team play Uses fork for stabbing food Brushes teeth Is self-sufficient in toileting Dresses without supervision except tying shoelaces	Fluent speech Misarticulations of some sounds may persist Gives name, address, age Defines concrete nouns by composition, classification, or use Follows three-part commands Has number concepts to 10		*Stage of industry vs. inferiority* (5 yr to adolescence) Adjusts himself to the inorganic laws of the tool world
6 yr	Rides bicycle Roller skates	Prints alphabet; letter reversals still acceptable Mature catch and throw of ball	Teacher is an important authority to child Uses fork appropriately Uses knife for spreading Ties shoelaces Plays table games	Shows mastery of grammar Uses proper articulation		Stage of industry vs. inferiority continues
7 yr	Continuing refinement of skills		Eats with fork and knife Combs hair Is responsible for grooming		*Period of concrete operational thought* (7 yr to adolescence) Child is capable of logical thinking	

[a]Compiled from various sources (3, 4, 6, 9, 21–23, 27, 30, 32, 52–54, 57).

During the first 4 months of life, the infant is a "lap baby," his or her behavior is largely controlled by reflexes, depending on the mother (or primary caretaker) for satisfaction of all needs. However, even at this age, the infant is not totally passive and possesses individual temperamental characteristics capable of eliciting specific responses from caretakers (6, 30). Thomas and Chess (59) have followed the temperamental characteristics, which they refer to as the "how" of behavior, rather than the "what" or "why," of a group of children from infancy to adulthood. They found significant correlations between certain infant temperamental characteristics and subsequent behavior problems. Their work emphasizes the infant's contribution to the parent-child interaction. They urge professionals providing guidance to parents to obtain information on the child's temperament prior to offering advice.

Piaget and Inhelder (46) call this age the reflex stage of the sensorimotor period. Erikson (16) and Mahler (34) view this as the normal symbiotic phase when the infant does not differentiate between self and mother, a position that has recently been questioned by Stern (53). As his or her needs are satisfied, the infant begins to acquire a sense of basic trust.

Four Months

By 4 months, the baby has coordinated his or her vision and prehension. The infant has attained head control, predominantly midline head position, and a crude palmar grasp. The baby's hands can meet in the midline, permitting hand play and he or she can turn from prone to supine (21, 27, 30, 32). Many of the primitive reflexes are beginning to be suppressed while the postural responses may not be present yet (38, 39). The baby not only smiles spontaneously, but laughs, makes vowel sounds, blows "raspberries," and turns to voice consistently, without the previous dependence on state. He engages in "conversations" with caretakers wherein the infant pauses when the adult imitates the baby's vocalizations and then proceeds to repeat the sound. Stern's videotaped observations of these mother-child communications demonstrate that the infant controls the interactions (53). The child determines the duration of the episodes of mutual gaze and alternating vocalization between self and mother by looking away from her when tired and then looking back in response to her efforts to engage him or her.

At this stage, Piaget and Inhelder (46) note that the interesting result of an action motivates its repetition. An example of this "circular reaction" is grasping a mobile repeatedly to make it move. At this point, the infant is assumed to make no distinction between the action performed and the results obtained. On an emotional level, the increasing skills and comprehension will shortly lead to an end of the symbiotic phase (34).

Seven Months

The 7-month-old infant can maintain sitting, transfer a cube from hand to hand, and has begun to differentiate strangers from familiar people. The child can now roll from supine to prone and reach with one hand in the prone position. When erect, the baby can bear all his or her weight and bounces when held. Cervical lordosis becomes evident. The baby uses single and some double consonant-vowel combinations. The infant holds his or her own bottle and if an object is dropped, looks for it. The circular reactions are expanded as the infant uses learned ways to achieve different ends (46).

The process of separation and individuation began at 5 months as the baby differentiated between mother and self (34). Behavior indicative of this process is preferential smiling at the mother and reaching for her face and mouth. The infant develops a sense of belonging to a central person, and by 7 or 8 months, behavior toward strangers differs from that with familiar people. This behavior, which has been termed "stranger anxiety," is manifested by crying in some infants whereas others only look wary and more sober when handled by strangers.

Ten Months

Independent mobility by means of creeping, a refined pincer grasp (30), and the concept of permanence of objects (46) are the major achievements of the 10-month-old. The 10-month-old child sits securely and can pivot in this position; can creep on all fours; can stand momentarily and cruises, i.e., walks around furniture holding on. The baby has slightly bowed legs, increased lumbar lordosis, and acute lumbosacral angulation. He or she picks up small objects neatly with a mature thumb to index finger pincer grasp and can bang two cubes held in his or her hands. Manipulative skills enable the child to finger feed himself or herself and the child is able to chew food with a rotatory jaw movement. The baby understands the meaning of gestures and uses such gestures as waving bye-bye. On hearing "no," the child inhibits behavior, and uses "mama" and "dada" with meaning.

The baby now demonstrates more complex acts of practical intelligence (46). He or she sets out to obtain a given result independent of the means to be employed; the coordination of means and ends is invented differently for each situation. If an object is covered in the infant's view, he or she may pull off the covering or move the hand of an adult in the direction of the hidden item. The game of "peek-a-boo," a favorite at this age, provides an opportunity to deal with the disappearance and reappearance of a face, a subject of cognitive and emotional interest to the infant.

The newly mobile infant is in the practicing phase of separation and individuation (34). The child cheerfully experiments with separations and reunions that he or she initiates; the 10-month-old has been described as having a "love affair with the world."

Fourteen Months

The term toddler aptly describes the ambulation of the 14-month-old (52). Besides toddling, the 14-month-old is also saying a few words, using two objects in relation to each other, and behaving ambivalently toward the mother.

The toddler walks on a wide base with arms in high or midguard (9, 39). In the swing phase of gait, the child shows excessive hip and knee flexion and foot contact takes place on the entire sole in early stance phase. Pelvic tilt and rotation are emerging gait determinants. Posture is characterized by valgus attitude of the knees and feet (32, 57). At this stage, the crayon is still held full length in the palm. Casting objects is a characteristic pattern. Daily living skills have advanced so that the child removes a garment and uses a spoon with overpronation and spilling. Communication proceeds to the use of single words and comprehension of simple commands (21, 30, 32).

In this state of the sensorimotor period, the child develops the "behavior pattern of the support," such as reaching a toy by pulling its string. The ability to combine two objects in relation to each other is seen in piling two cubes, scribbling on paper with a crayon, and attempts at using a spoon (21, 30, 32).

Ambivalent behaviors are characteristic of this age; the child clings to the mother and pushes her away and struggles with holding on and letting go in terms of sphincter control. In this rapprochement phase of separation and individuation, the child is aware of separateness from the mother. Pleasure in physical autonomy and in the ability to speak are mitigated by the sense of vulnerability that separateness engenders. Erikson (16) views this as the beginning of the stage of autonomy vs. shame and doubt, when the child has a "violent wish to have a choice, to appropriate demandingly, and to eliminate stubbornly." The child takes pleasure in controlling his or her musculature and sphincters.

Eighteen Months

While all skills are improved and consolidated as the child reaches 18 months, the most important change occurs in the area of cognition, as the child becomes capable of "insight."

Walking is accomplished on a mature supporting base within the lateral dimensions of the body; the arms are at low guard and stance phase begins with heel strike (9, 53, 54). The child can also walk backwards and seat himself or herself in a small chair. Crude release of objects is seen and a crayon is held butt end in palm; some children show hand dominance. Children are expected to drink from a cup neatly. Speech and language development includes the ability to say "no," identify a picture, point to a body part, and use jargon, which is complex babbling with the inflection of a sentence (21, 30, 32).

The last stage of the sensorimotor period is now reached and the child becomes capable of finding new means of doing something, not by trial and error, but by mental combinations that lead to sudden comprehension or "insight" (46). When the child is presented with a small transparent bottle containing a raisin and finds that it cannot be pulled out with the finger, the child is able to get it out by inverting the bottle without requiring a demonstration. Beginning comprehension of symbols is manifested by treating a doll like a baby and by identifying a picture of an object. The child continues to deal with the issue of autonomy and rapprochement with the mother (34). Imitation of observed activities, such as housework, is usual.

Cognitive ability in the sensorimotor stage is practical and action oriented (46). A physical handicap that impedes the infant's access to active exploration and experimentation may potentially interfere with cognitive development at this stage. This consideration provides one rationale for early intervention programs that can provide the child with alternative experiences for learning about the environment. The nature of learning in this stage dictates that therapeutic intervention should be presented to infants and young children by means of a variety of activities and by offering opportunities of guided experimentation. Individuals with profound or low-level severe mental retardation usually function in the sensorimotor stage their entire lives.

Two Years

Although progress in speaking is the most obvious accomplishment of the 2-yr-old, the ability to understand and use symbols is the invisible prerequisite for this skill.

The 2-yr-old child is beginning to run, can go up and down stairs alone, and jump in place. Hand dominance is usually established and a pencil is held in a mature grasp with the shaft between thumb and fingers. Drawing is performed with arm and wrist action and advances from scribbling to imitation of a vertical line. In using blocks, the child can build an eight-cube tower or align them horizontally (21).

The improved understanding and coordination is evidenced in the daily activities of pulling on a garment, efficient self-feeding with a spoon, and the ability to open a door by turning the knob. Toilet training is usually begun at this age, although there is considerable cultural variation in the age at which infants are trained (21).

A sense of individual identity and autonomy is achieved. The child knows he or she is a separate person capable of any independent actions and is fond of asserting this fact. The child uses "me," "mine," refers to himself or herself by name, follows directions, and usually converses in two-word phrases.

In cognitive terms, the 2-yr-old has entered the preoperational stage that lasts until age 7 yr (46) and is described further in the section on the 3-yr-old.

Three Years

A 3-yr-old child has the necessary skills in all areas that enable him or her to leave mother willingly for hours at a time and function with a small group of peers under adult supervision. Motor skills are being refined; the child runs well, alternates feet walking up stairs, can jump down one step, broad jump, and pedal a tricycle. The 3-yr-old is becoming more adept at handling a ball and throws overhand with anteroposterior arm and trunk motion and catches with extended arms, hugging the ball against the body (21).

Self-care and interpersonal skills are at a level permitting longer periods of time without direct adult attention. The child is toilet trained, eats alone with a spoon, washes and dries his or her hands and face, unbuttons and removes clothes. The 3-yr-old likes to play near other children and can take turns, but periods of interaction around a given toy or game are brief. The ability to pretend in games is a newfound skill (21).

The achievement of the Piagetian preoperational stage enables the child to evoke concepts, objects, and events that are not present since he or she can now represent them by a symbol, such as a word or a picture (46). The behaviors that illustrate this ability, listed in order of increasing complexity consist of deferred imitation, i.e., imitation that occurs after the disappearance of the model; symbolic play in which the child pretends, by using toys or actions to perform familiar activities or to enact events; drawings; and verbal evocation of events not occurring at the time. The ability to use symbols, including words, enables a child to deal with ideas, feelings, and events outside the immediate time and place in which the 3-yr old finds himself or herself.

However, thinking in the preoperational stage remains concrete, egocentric, bound by the surrounding field of perception. The ability to classify objects by similarity, difference, and use indicates development of elementary concrete concept formation. Maturation of perceptual motor organization is manifested by the ability to draw and construct increasingly complex designs and structures. Imaginative play activities, characteristic of this stage, are an integral part of learning and serve to organize the variety of daily experiences. In the preoperational stage, playing remains the primary mode of delivering treatment, although verbal communication on a concrete level has an increasing role as an instructional medium.

Speech now usually consists of three-word sentences and can be about an object that is not present. The newly acquired ability to use the future as well as the present tense reflects the child's grasp of the concept of time other than "now." A child can give his or her first and last name; sex; ask "what," "who," and "where" questions; understand propositions such as "under" and "behind"; and recognize some colors by name. As the child puts more complex ideas into words, some dysfluencies may be transiently present (21) and parents should be encouraged to ignore them.

Children with cerebral dysfunction may show a discrepancy of maturation in different areas. Unless there is a central communication disorder, language development tends to be an area of relative strength in comparison with sensorimotor integration. This discrepancy between language and perceptual function should be considered both in assessment and in treatment. Good verbal and social skills on the part of a child do not obviate the necessity for evaluating visual perceptual and graphomotor abilities, which are also necessary for preacademic performance. Moderately retarded trainable persons function on a cognitive level consistent with this stage of development even as adults.

Erikson's stage of initiative vs. guilt is a time when children become aware of genital sexuality, show a preference for the parent of the opposite sex, and competitiveness with the parent of the same sex (16). The child's urge is for attack and conquest, but it is balanced against the inability to compete successfully with an adult. Resolution of this crisis is considered a necessary step in the development of moral responsibility.

Four Years

The major progress observed at age 4 yr consists of improved peer group interaction and greater complexity in language use.

All motor skills are being refined. The child can now walk down stairs alternating feet, hop on one foot, and sit up from supine without rotating. He handles a pencil by finger and wrist action, like an adult, copies a cross and begins to draw a human figure, which often resembles a frog since it has a face with extremities protruding from it, but no body. The 4-yr-old also cuts with scissors and throws underhand. The child dresses with some supervision and can button (21).

Parallel play is largely replaced by cooperative interaction and simple individual pretending turns into complex joint games of make believe. The child can follow longer stories and is able to relate recent experiences in a connected sequential manner using the past tense. Sentences now include adjectives and adverbs. "Why" is a favorite question used both to keep the adult talking as well as to get information about causality. Opposite analogies such as "mother is a woman, father is a man" are understood. Increased flexibility in the use of language is also manifested by playing with language, i.e., silly rhyming, using profanity for its effect, and whispering (21).

Five Years

At 5 yr the child enters the stage of industry vs. inferiority where he or she adjusts to the "inorganic laws of the tool world" (16). Acquisition of skills and interaction with peers become the focus of the child's energies.

Skipping is a new achievement and a favorite means of locomotion. Five-yr-olds can also tiptoe, walk on their heels, and perform a running broad jump. Excessive pelvic tilt and knock knees are decreasing. Adeptness in ball play and improved social skills now permit competitive team play. A child of this age throws with diagonal arm and body rotation, catches with the hands, and kicks a ball well. Self-care skills require almost no adult intervention, only cutting meat, tying shoelaces, and help with combing hair. Clearcut hand dominance is expected (22).

Since, at this age, more than before, many of the expected behaviors are learned skills, it is crucial to assess them in terms of parental expectations and the child's educational experience. A 5-yr-old can copy a triangle and his or her drawing of a person includes a body as well as the head and extremities. Speech is fluent with only rare misarticulations and concrete nouns can be defined by their composition, classification, and use. The child is able to follow commands consisting of three different parts, i.e., "take the pencil from the box, the paper from the shelf, and sit down at the table." The child knows factual information, such as counting 10 objects, first and last name, address, and age (22).

The stage of industry that continues until adolescence is viewed as a time when the child sublimates sexual wishes and learns to win recognition by producing things and through acceptance by peers (16).

Six Years

In our culture, 6-yr-olds are expected to begin learning to read. Children's abilities increase gradually from age 5–6 yrs, but educational demands increase abruptly. Although kindergarten programs still include large amounts of play time, a first grader is expected to spend most of the full day at school working on academic tasks while sitting quietly at a desk (22).

Motor skills now include riding a bicycle without training wheels, roller skating, and mature catching and throwing of a ball. Self-care skills include using a fork appropriately, using a knife for spreading, and tying shoelaces. Although children must be able to identify letters before they can begin reading, in writing letters, some reversals are still acceptable. Reading requires mastery of two kinds of skills, decoding the written words and understanding the content of a passage, either of which may present problems to children with central nervous system dysfunction. Children begin to play table games with rules, such as dominoes, cards, and board games. They show practical mastery of the rules of grammar and speak with proper articulation. The authority of teachers tends to be highly respected by children at this age (22).

Seven Years

The 7-yr-old enters the stage of concrete operational thought during which basic logical thinking and reasoning emerge (46).

Perceptual motor efficiency, mastery of language, and the ability to concentrate and attend to an imposed task make the child ready for academic learning. The ability to analyze, associate, and retrace thoughts applied to concrete material enables children to acquire scholastic skills at this age. Interest in motor activities expands to a variety of sports. The earlier egocentric viewpoint of the world is replaced by appreciation of the needs and wishes of others. Seven-yr-old children play and work cooperatively. Good table manners and responsibility for grooming are accomplished (22).

Individuation and separation are enhanced by the establishment of relationships outside the home and by a broadening knowledge of the world at large (34).

From this stage on, training and instructions in the traditional verbal conceptual mode are appropriate, taking into consideration the differnces in emotional maturity at various ages. Youngsters with central nervous system dysfunction may have attentional disorders and deficits in perceptual organization, sequencing, and conceptualization. These problems can lead to difficulties in scholastic learning, in acquisition of skills of daily life, or in training for such activities. Individuals in the mildly retarded range of intellectual functioning develop to the stage of concrete operational thought. They are able to achieve academic skills up to fourth to sixth grade level but remain limited in judgment and abstract thinking.

Preadolescence and Adolescence

The 10th to 11th years herald the beginning of the stage of formal operational thought (46). Cognitive function is characterized by the ability to think abstractly, to plan based on hypothetical ideas, to solve mental problems, to have insight into motives and a sense of morality and social judgment. Social and cultural factors play a significant role in shaping various aspects of cognitive development. Increasing poise, expanding interests, and the importance of friendship are typical of the preteen years (23).

Adolescence is an age of profound physical, physiologic, and emotional changes. Accelerated growth rate is accompanied by a similar increase in strength and endurance (32). Interest in the opposite sex and in conforming to the rules of peer groups influence social behavior at this age. With the eventual resolution of the identity crisis, the adolescent is ready to cross the threshold to young adulthood (16).

The cognitive stage of formal operational thought is achieved only by persons of normal intelligence. Disabled children are often hindered in achieving separation, in controlling their environment, and in developing self-sufficiency. A perpetuation of dependency and unresolved identity crisis may interfere with the developmental thrust toward a mature personality. The sudden changes in body dimensions, which call for considerable readaptation in motor performance and the tendency to develop progressive deformities during the accelerated phase of growth may lead to regression or loss of marginal physical achievements in more severely handicapped adolescents.

Conclusion

The influence of growth and its possible deviations are important considerations in the management of children with physical disability. Developmental assessment that translates behavior into age values (30) requires an adjustment for motor dysfunction and for cognitive or other associated disabilities when such deficits are present. A well-planned treatment program must be based on guidelines derived from the principles of growth and development.

REFERENCES

1. Anderson, M, Green WT, Messner MB: Growth and prediction of growth in the lower extremities. *J Bone Joint Surg* 45A:1, 1963.
2. Bandura A: *Social Learning Theory.* New Jersey, Prentice Hall, 1977.
3. Bax M, Hart H, Jenkins S: Assessment of speech and language in the young child. *Pediatrics* 66:350–354, 1988.
4. Behrman RE, Vaughan VC (eds): *Nelson's Textbook of Pediatrics.* Philadelphia, Saunders, 1987.
5. Bobath K: *A Neurophysiologic Basis for the Treatment of Cerebral Palsy.* Clinics in Developmental Medicine no 75. Philadelphia, JB Lippincott, 1980.
6. Brazelton TB: *Neonatal Behavioral Assessment Scale.* Clinics in Developmental Medicine no. 88. Philadelphia, JB Lippincott, 1984.
7. Brazelton TB: Behavioral competence of the newborn infant. In Avery GB (ed): *Neonatology: Pathophysiology and Management of the Newborn.* Philadelphia, JB Lippincott, 1987.
8. Brazelton TB, Cramer BG: *The Earliest Relationship.* New York, Addison Wesley, 1990.
9. Burnett CN, Johnson EW: Development of gait in childhood. *Dev Med Child Neurol* 13:196–206, 207–215, 1971.
10. Capute AJ, Accardo PJ, Vining EPG, Rubenstein JE, Harryman S: *Primitive Reflex Profile.* Baltimore, University Park Press, 1977.
11. Cassady G, Strange M: The small-for-gestational-age (SGA) infant. In Avery GB (ed): *Neonatology: Pathophysiology and Management of the Newborn.* Philadelphia, JB Lippincott, 1987.
12. Connolly KJ, Prechtl HFR (eds): *Maturation and Development: Biological and Psychological Perspectives.* Clinics in Developmental Medicine no 77,78. Philadelphia, JB Lippincott, 1981.
13. Coplan J: *Early Language Milestone Scale.* Tulsa OK, Modern Education Corp, 1983.
14. Dubowitz V, Dubowitz L: *The Neurologic Assessment of the Preterm and Fullterm Infant.* Clinics in Developmental Medicine no 79. London, W. Heinemann Medical Books, 1981.
15. Eng GD, Koch B, Smokvina MD: Brachial plexus palsy in neonates and children. *Arch Phys Med Rehabil* 59:458–464, 1980.
16. Erikson EH: *Childhood and Society.* New York, WW Norton, 1963.
17. Finkelstein JW: The endocrinology of adolescence. *Pediatr Clin North Am* 27:53–70, 1980.
18. Fitzhardinge PM: Follow-up studies of the high-risk newborn. In Avery (ed) *Neonatology: Pathophysiology and Management of the Newborn.* Philadelphia, JB Lippincott, 1981.
19. Frankenburg WK, Dodds J, Archer P, Bresnick B, Maschka P, Edelman N, Shapiro H: *Denver II Technical Manual.* Denver, Denver Developmental Materials, Inc., 1990.
20. Freud A: *Normality and Pathology in Childhood: Assessment of Development.* New York, International Universities Press, 1965.
21. Gesell A, Halverson HM, Ilg Fl, Thompson H, Castner BM, Ames LB, Amatruda CS: *The First Five Years of Life.* New York, Harper & Row, 1940.
22. Gesell A, Ilg Fl: *The Child From Five to Ten.* New York, Harper & Row, 1946.
23. Gesell A, Ilg FL, Ames LB: *Youth, the Years From Ten to Fifteen.* New York, Harper & Row, 1956.
24. Greulich SS, Pyle SI: *Radiographic Atlas of Skeletal Development of the Hand and Wrist.* ed 2. Stanford, Stanford University Press, 1959.

25. Holt KS: Growth disturbances. *Hemiplegic Cerebral Palsy in Children and Adults.* Clinics in Developmental Medicine no 4. London, National Spastics Society, 1961.
26. Holt KS (ed): *Movement and Child Development.* Clinics in Developmental Medicine no 55. Philadelphia, JB Lippincott Co, 1975.
27. Illingworth RS: *The Development of the Infant and Young Child: Normal and Abnormal.* Edinburgh, New York, Churchill Livingstone, 1987.
28. Johnson EW: Examination for muscle weakness in infants and small children. *JAMA* 168:1306–1313, 1958.
29. Kaminer RK, Jedrysek E: Age of walking and mental retardation. *Am J Public Health* 73:1094–1096, 1983.
30. Knobloch H, Stevens F, Malone AF: *Manual of Developmental Diagnosis: The Administration and Interpretation of the Revised Gesell and Amatruda Developmental and Neurological Examination.* Hagerstonwn, MD, Harper & Row, 1980.
31. Lovell WW, Winter RB (eds): *Pediatric Orthopedics,* ed. 2. Philadelphia, JB Lippincott Co, 1986.
32. Lowrey GH: *Growth and Development of Children.* Chicago, Year Book Medical Publishers, 1986.
33. Mac Keith RC: The feelings and behavior of parents of handicapped children. *Dev Med Child Neurol* 15:524–527, 1973.
34. Mahler, ML: Thoughts about development and individuation. *Psychoanal Study Child* 18:307–326, 1963.
35. McGraw MB: *Neuromuscular Maturation of Human Infants.* New York, Hafner Press, 1963.
36. Meier J: Screening and assessment of young children at developmental risk. The President's Committee on Mental Retardation. Department of Health Education and Welfare Publication no. 73–90, 1973.
37. Menkes JH: *Textbook of Child Neurology,* ed. 4. Philadelphia, Lea & Febiger, 1990.
38. Milani-Comparetti A, Gidoni EA: Pattern analysis of motor development and its disorders. *Dev Med Child Neurol* 9:625–630, 1967.
39. Milani-Comparetti A, Gidoni EA; Routine developmental examination in normal and retarded children. *Dev Med Child Neurol* 9:631–638, 1967.
40. Mussen PH, Conger JJ, Kagan J: *Child Development and Personality,* ed. 5. New York, Harper & Row Publishers, 1979.
41. Neligan G, Prudham D: Potential value of four early developmental milestones in screening children for increased risk of later retardation. *Dev Med Child Neurol* 11:423–431, 1969.
42. Nellhaus G: Head circumference from birth to eighteen years. Practical composite international and interracial graphs. *Pediatrics* 41:106–114, 1968.
43. Ogden JA: Injury to the growth mechanism of the immature skeleton. Skeletal Radiol 6:237, 1981.
44. Paine SR, Brazelton TB, Donovan DE, Drorbaugh JE, Hubbell JP, Sears EM: Evolution of postural reflexes in normal infants and the presence of chronic brain syndromes. *Neurology* 14:1036–1048, 1964.
45. Palmer CD: Study of the center of gravity in the human body. *Child Dev* 15:99, 1944.
46. Piaget J, Inhelder B: *The Psychology of the Child.* New York, Basic Books, 1969.
47. Rapin I: *Children with Brain Dysfunction Neurology, Cognition, Language and Behavior.* International Review of Child Neurology Series. New York, Raven Press, 1982.
48. Risser JC: Scoliosis: Past and present. *J Bone Joint Surg* 46A:167–199, 1964.
49. Salter RB, Harris WT: Injuries involving the epiphyseal plate. *J Bone Joint Surg* 45A:587–622, 1963.
50. Seligman MEP: *Helplessness.* San Francisco, WH Freeman, 1975.
51. Smith DW: Growth and its disorders: Basics and standards, approach and classification, growth deficiency disorders, growth excess disorders, obesity. *Major Probl Pediatr* 15:1–155, 1977.

52. Statham L, Murray MP: Early walking pattern of normal children. *Clin Orthop* 79:8–24, 1971.
53. Stern DS: *The Interpersonal World of the Infant.* New York, Basic Books, 1985.
54. Sutherland DH, Olshen R, Cooper L. Woo-Sam J: The development of mature gait. *J Bone Joint Surg* 62A:336–353, 1980.
55. Sutherland DM: *Gait Disorders in Childhood and Adolescence.* Baltimore, Williams & Wilkins, 1984.
56. Swaiman KF, Wright FS (eds): *The Practice of Pediatric Neurology,* ed. 2. St. Louis, CV Mosby Co, 1982.
57. Tachdjian MO: *Pediatric Orthopedics,* ed. 2. Philadelphia, WB Saunders, 1990.
58. Taft LT, Cohen HJ: Neonatal and infant reflexology. In Hellmuth J (ed): *Exceptional Infant.* Seattle, Special Child Publications, 1967, vol 1, pp 81–120.
59. Thomas A, Chess S: Temperament and follow-up to adulthood. In Porter R, Collins GM (eds): *Temperamental Differences in Infants and Young Children.* London, Pitman, 1982.
60. Tobis JS, Saturen P, Larios G, Posniak AO: Study of growth pattern in cerebral palsy. *Arch Phys Med Rehabil* 42:475–480, 1961.
61. Twitchell TE: Attitudinal reflexes. *Phys Ther* 45:411–418, 1965.
62. Twitchell TE: Normal motor development. *Phys Ther* 45:419–423, 1965.
63. Volpe JJ, Hill A: Neurologic disorders. In Avery GB (ed): *Neonatology: Pathophysiology and Management of the Newborn.* Philadelphia, JB Lippincott, 1987.
64. Yule W, Rutter M (eds): *Language Development and Disorders.* Clinics in Developmental Medicine no. 101/102. Philadelphia, JB Lippincott Co, 1987.

3

Psychological Assessment

SUSAN PASTERNACK CHINITZ AND
CAROL Z. FEDER

Psychological evaluation contributes to the understanding and management of the handicapped child. It provides an assessment of overall development and its rate relative to other children. It describes the child's learning style, possible impediments to learning, and the extent to which the child has built upon previous learning experiences. The evaluation culminates in a proposal of the type of educational program most likely to meet the child's needs. It describes behavioral and cognitive strengths and weaknesses that can be addressed at home and in school to foster the child's overall development.

Conditions that alter the child's physical integrity or central nervous system functioning can manifest in a wide variety of learning and/or behavioral problems. Psychological consultation is appropriate whenever there is a question regarding development, intellectual and learning capabilities, or behavioral management. Referral is particularly helpful as part of a multidisciplinary evaluation when initial diagnosis is being established and interventions are planned for a young child, when an appropriate educational program must be designed for a school-aged child, and for periodic assessment of developmental progress throughout childhood and adolescence to determine if needs have changed.

Components of a Psychological Evaluation

An adequate assessment results in description of the child's cognitive abilities as elicited by samples of both verbal and nonverbal competencies and problem-solving strategies. The availability and quality of expressive and receptive language are investigated, as are perceptual and information processing skills. Social-adaptive functioning, including academic accomplishments, behavior, and emotional characteristics are described.

48

A complete psychological assessment is culled from different sources of information. Ideally, the psychologist assesses the child after medical evaluation is completed so that appropriate assessment procedures can be determined. Since there is no one standard procedure for the psychological assessment of all children, medical information should communicate the cause of the child's exceptionality and describe probable areas of deficit or diminished skill in sensory or motor areas. Specific medical or etiologic events, interventions such as shunts, the presence of seizures, or the administration of medications that could affect behavior is important information for the psychologist.

PARENT INTERVIEW

The evaluation includes a parent interview from which the psychologist seeks to estimate the child's rate of development prior to the time of the evaluation. It is important to determine the child's attainment of developmental milestones, as well as the parents' perception of the child's current level of functioning. Parents re-create for the psychologist a picture of how the child participates in everyday life including usual activities, opportunities for and style of socialization with family members and peers, and perceived strengths and weaknesses. It is through this contact that the psychologist has the opportunity to explore the emotional climate of the home and to understand and integrate relevant family circumstances in the child's overall assessment.

BEHAVIORAL OBSERVATION

In the context of an evaluation, the child exhibits many behaviors that are observed and evaluated for purposes of diagnosis and intervention. The examiner notes the behavior of the child to determine how this may have influenced performance on formal evaluation, as well as functioning outside of the testing situation. Though sometimes the child's behavior is transient or situational, usually these observations reflect characteristic behavioral patterns that are prognostic for future course and adjustment. In making such determinations, norms of child behavior are considered. Some behaviors are expected at one age but not at another, while others are atypical or abnormal at any age. Behavioral observations of significance include the child's social relatedness and interpersonal skills. Mobility and general coordination are noted. Working methods are observed, including attention span and problem-solving techniques. Aspects of mood and temperament, such as level of perseverance and frustration tolerance are noted. An incorrect or specific pattern of response may reveal a deficit that has previously gone undetected, such as impaired vision or hearing. Good ability to grasp novel tasks may suggest that limited levels of attainment are on the basis of environmental deprivation or lack of educational experience, in contrast to a child who shows generalized deficits in comprehension.

PSYCHOLOGICAL TESTING

Psychological tests are tools for eliciting specific behaviors or attributes in a standard way and under uniform conditions. Results of testing are expressed in quantitative terms that tell something about the child's performance in a comparative way. Standard scores represent a child's standing in a given group based on the mean and standard deviation for that group. Percentile scores tell what proportion of a comparison group scores below the child in question. Age or grade equivalents are frequently employed. Since the child's position relative to his or her group has to be considered, all standardized tests provide information on the typical performance of that group. Test "norms" should refer to a clearly defined population as obtained from a representative sample. The populaton should be the group to whom users of the test would ordinarily compare the tested child. This might include a stratified national sample of 12-month-olds or 4th graders in urban school districts, for example.

Additional criteria for selecting assessment instruments and interpreting results include test reliability and validity. Reliability refers to the consistency of test results from one administration to another. Reliability coefficients represent the extent to which an obtained score represents a true measurement of the characteristic versus measurement error. Validity refers to the extent to which the test actually measures what it has been designed to measure. This is usually determined by the degree of correlation of test scores with external or other criteria regarded as evidence of the trait to be measured by the test.

For some physically handicapped children, testing can be accomplished through traditional means and by instruments designed for nonhandicapped children. In other cases, alternate instruments and/or adaptations of existing scales have to be employed so that physical limitations are taken into consideration. Otherwise, test results would lead to inaccurate conclusions. Children with severe or multiple handicaps may be impeded in testing by limited motor abilities, dysarthria, and a tendency toward easy fatigability. The nature and severity of the child's handicaps must dictate test selection and procedures for administration. Item content, mode of response, and the nature of test materials must be considered in planning the testing procedures. Although the large majority of children are testable by some procedure, standard administration of traditional test batteries is sometimes precluded for children with significant handicaps as scores in such cases would largely reflect the extent of the impairment and thus fail to represent existing abilities accurately.

Deviation from standardized procedures, however, requires modification in the interpretation of test results as standardized scoring is unwarranted in these situations. To communicate results, one may qualitatively describe the child's strengths and weaknesses by means of a clinical analysis of the tasks accomplished. Alternatively, the examiner might rely on test norms to provide age-level equivalencies for individual test items or subtests that were possible to adminster.

Infant Testing

Historically, referrals for psychological testing of infants were made primarily when a physician encountered a young child who showed delays in one or more areas of development and was concerned about the possibility of mental retardation. The advent of Public Law 99–457, the Education of the Handicapped Amendments of 1986, has resulted in considerably more widespread attention to, development of, and application of assessment methodologies in order to identify and to provide early intervention for those infants and toddlers the legislation is intended to serve (69). Part H of the law encourages the development of statewide comprehensive services for handicapped infants and toddlers and their families. For infants from birth to 2 years old the definition of handicapped includes those children with established delays as measured by appropriate diagnostic instruments, children with existing conditions that almost invariably lead to delay or disability (e.g., cerebral palsy, myelomeningocele, and Down's syndrome) and, at the state's discretion, extends to children who are "at risk" due to medical/biologic factors, such as prematurity and/or adverse environmental factors.

Evaluation of infants' cognitive-developmental functioning is one component of a multidisciplinary evaluation needed for purposes of diagnostic formulation and assessment of the child's strengths and weakness for purposes of individual program planning. Diagnostic assessment typically relies on norm-referenced instruments that convey the child's standing relative to a normative peer group, while program planning relies on criterion-referenced inventories that assess the child's level of achievement, independent of a comparison group, to assist in targeting the next developmental achievement in a sequence toward which activities may be planned. Most of the instruments discussed in this section are norm-referenced scales administered by psychologists to determine if an infant is developing slowly or otherwise differently than other infants the same age and, if so, the extent of the delay (Table 3.1). Criterion-referenced tests are typically used by infant educators within the context of an early intervention program to plan curriculum for individual infants. These instruments are numerous and will not be covered in this chapter.

GESELL DEVELOPMENTAL SCHEDULES

The Gesell Developmental Schedules (34) are the oldest of the infant tests and provided the groundwork for much subsequent work in this area. The scales were developed in the 1920s when Gesell and his colleagues began a

Table 3.1.
Infant Scales

Test	Age Range	Scope and Value	Limitations
Gesell Developmental Schedules	4 weeks to 6 years	The forerunner in the systematic observation of infant development; a useful standardized procedure for evaluating and observing behavior in four major areas of functioning; provides a developmental quotient in each area	Representativeness of standardization sample is limited; use of ratio-derived developmental quotient hampers interpretation and comparability from one age to another
Bayley Scales of Infant Development	Birth to 30 months	Provides separate mental and motor scales; excellent psychometric properties including broad standardization sample and use of standard scores; Infant Behavior Record permits assessment of qualitative aspects of child's social-emotional behaviors and goal-orientation in addition to developmental status	Like most infant tests, scales are most useful for providing an indication of current developmental levels; heavily weighted with motor-based items, which limits predictive validity especially for physically handicapped children
Griffiths Mental Developmental Scale	Birth to 2 years; 2–8 years	Divided into subtests tapping different areas of function; useful in formulating a profile of child's developmental strengths and weaknesses	Averages scores on all subtests to produce a General Quotient where locomotor skills are given equal weight; normed on British, not American sample; uses ratio quotients
Infant Mullen Scales of Early Learning	Birth to 3 years	Examines intradomain functions of receptive and expressive abilities in all areas assessed; designed to translate into intervention strategies; good psychometric properties	Relatively new instrument; little clinical or research background available as yet
Fagen Test of Infant Intelligence	6–12 months	Uses a visual information processing paradigm to assess cognitive skills free from reliance on motor or verbal output	Applicable only for children in a restricted age range at present

longitudinal study of the course of infant development using an empirical observational approach. Gesell believed that development followed predictable patterns that invariably emerged as the child grew and matured; he hoped to use these derived schedules to detect delayed or atypically developing infants for whom special services were needed. Rather than focusing solely on mental ability, Gesell intended to measure the child's developmental status in a more global way. The resulting scale assesses the infant's behavior in five areas: gross motor, fine motor, adaptive, language, and personal-social abilities. Testing is conducted by observing the infant's response to standard stimulus items and is supplemented by information provided by parents. Items are grouped by age levels that are organized by 4-week intervals during the first year and 6-month intervals thereafter. A Development Quotient is calculated by dividing the child's developmental age by his or her chronological age in each of the five areas. Although Gesell disavowed claims that developmental quotients were synonymous with IQs, results have often been erroneously interpreted this way.

Gesell's foremost contribution was in the organization of age-related schedules of observable infant behaviors and the design of tasks through which developing competencies could be elicited. Items from the schedules have been incorporated, to a large extent, in subsequent infant tests. Although the standardization base has been expanded over the years, its representativeness is still limited. The use of a ratio-derived developmental quotient hampers interpretation and comparability from one age to another.

GRIFFITHS MENTAL DEVELOPMENT SCALES

The Griffiths (36) was developed in England and actually consists of two scales, one for children from birth to 2 years and an upward extension for children from 2 to 8 years of age. The infant scale is composed of five subscales for the measurement of abilities in locomotion, personal-social skills, hearing/speech, eye-hand coordination, and performance. The test yields a subquotient for each of the five major areas, as well as an overall Mental Age and General Quotient, which is an average of the subscale scores.

Subtest scores permit the creation of a developmental profile that contributes to a more accurate differential diagnosis than is possible with infant tests that yield only a global summary score. The span of items from birth to 8 years permits ongoing comparison on the same scale for purposes of follow-up. This continuous age span also allows for testing of delayed or handicapped children in the 2- to 3-year range who may be at the ceiling of other infant tests but unable to succeed on enough items in traditional preschool tests to assess their skills adequately. Drawbacks of the Griffiths include its reliance on ratio scores (mental age divided by chronological age) and its non-American standardization sample.

THE BAYLEY SCALES OF INFANT DEVELOPMENT

The Bayley Scales of Infant Development (4) consists of three instruments, each tapping different domains that Bayley considered relevant to the comprehensive assessment of the infant. The Mental Scale is designed to assess processes of learning, problem-solving, and the development of expressive and receptive language. Item content is varied, beginning with those designed to assess the young infant's responsiveness to sensory-perceptual events, proceeding through sensorimotor stages of object exploration and the development of object constancy, and culminating in more conceptual tasks that begin to approximate beginning items on preschool tests. The Motor Scale is designed to provide an evaluation of fine and gross motor development. The child's performance on the Mental and Motor Scales is expressed in standard scores. Age equivalents can be calculated if needed. The Infant Behavior Record provides a description of the infant's behavior as observed during administration of the Mental and Motor Scales and includes ratings of the infant's social orientation, goal directedness, attention span, adaptability, and general emotional tone.

The Bayley is the best developed infant test from a psychometric perspective. Its standardization sample is considerably more extensive than that of the previously described instruments and was more carefully constructed to represent an even distribution of the U.S. population across variables such as geographic region, urban and rural settings, ethnicity, and socioeconomic status. The provision of standard scores is more psychometrically sound than ratio scores and permits comparability of scores from one age to another. Finally, by including the Infant Behavior Record, the Bayley is the only scale that formally assesses qualitative behavioral features of sociability, motivation, and endurance, all of which are highly relevant in the evaluation of at-risk or disabled babies beyond quantitative assessment of developmental level.

INFANT MULLEN SCALES OF EARLY LEARNING (MSEL)

The Infant MSEL (70) is a recent downward extension of Mullen's original assessment instrument for toddlers and preschoolers. The full instrument is now applicable to children from birth to 3½ years. Its most unique contribution is that it goes beyond the measurement of separate domains to an examination of intradomain functions of receptive and expressive abilities. The resulting scales include Visual Receptive Organization (visual-spatial facility, visual discrimination, and visual memory), Visual Expressive Organization (eye-hand coordination and fine motor skills), Language Receptive Organization and Language Expressive Organization, and a scale to assess the Gross Motor Base for learning in other areas. The MSEL has strong psychometric underpinnings, including national norms stratified to represent geographic, ethnic, and socioeconomic variables, and the use of standard scores to assess infants' developmental strengths and weaknesses. It was designed to translate into strategies for effective intervention for youngsters with delayed and/or uneven skill development.

INTERPRETATION OF INFANT TESTS

Results of infant tests are best interpreted as a measure of an infant's current developmental status relative to a normative peer group (Table 3.1). An early impetus in the development of infant scales was the desire to find reliable means for the early appraisal of intelligence. However, research on the prediction of later intelligence from these assessments has been disappointing. Repeated studies have found low correlations between abilities measured on infant tests and later childhood IQs (64, 84). The reliability of the tests seems to be well documented and indicates that this is not the reason for the lack of predictive power (17). The explanation seems to lie in the fact that modalities of learning and overtly observable behaviors during infancy vary considerably from those available in later stages of childhood. Observable development during the first 18 months is characterized by advances in sensorimotor competencies noted as the infant solves practical, concrete problems through his or her interactions with objects. Infant tests have traditionally tapped the emergence of these nonsymbolic, motor function-dependent skills, whereas ability tests for older children have more verbal and symbolic content reflecting the increasing role of verbal conceptual skills in intellectual functioning. This accounts for the slightly better predictive value of infant test scores beginning at about 18 to 24 months when language and symbolic functions typically emerge.

Despite the fact that infant tests are not highly predictive for the typical child, they are sensitive indicators of early developmental problems that may have continuing effects later in the child's life if markedly delayed development is noted. Several studies have shown that while test-retest correlations for samples of children scoring in the normal range are low, the correlations are substantially higher for children who score significantly below average in infancy (25, 54, 86). Thus, whereas the course of cognitive development in normal children shows considerable variability and later outcome cannot be reliably predicted from tests in infancy, a finding of subnormal development may be an important indicator of significant deficits in cognitive development that will affect later functioning. Finding of depressed performance on an infant test should be followed by a plan for intervention and follow-up testing. It is essential that infant test results be considered provisional and followed by periodic re-evaluation for further diagnostic and prognostic clarification.

TESTING PHYSICALLY HANDICAPPED INFANTS

Further caution is warranted in the cognitive assessment of the physically handicapped infant. Because infant tests rely heavily on motor responses to assess the child's interest and learning, it is difficult to draw inferences about the child's current or future intellectual abilities in the presence of known physical limitations. Kearsley (49), Zelazo (93), and Fagen and Singer (30) discuss theoretical and methodological shortcomings of procedures often used to assess the cognitive status of physically disabled infants. They question the adherence to a sensorimotor theory of cognitive development with its assumptions that infants' motor interaction with the object world provides the necessary substrate for mental development and that sensorimotor dysfunction is indicative of a more generalized deficit inclusive of intellectual functions. Studies which established that one third of a large sample of children with cerebral palsy identified in infancy displayed normal intelligence as adults (18) and the follow-up of children with severe physical malformations associated with thalidomide are used to support their contention that motor and cognitive development, although mutually facilitating, may proceed independently of one another.

Recent developments in infant research have greatly expanded knowledge of how infants learn and what infant responses provide us with windows into their mental processes. It is now known that infants have the ability to attend to and discriminate perceptual events and to establish memory stores for such events almost from the time of birth, long before they could demonstrate this through motor or language modalities. Fantz (31) identified infants' looking at patterns as a correlate of visual preference and introduced the paired-comparison technique as a way to assess visual interest and attention. Discovery of infants' tendency to habituate or respond progressively less to a stimulus over time (presumably due to its loss of novelty) has resulted in additional paradigms to assess mental processes. To see if an infant can discriminate two objects, one presents the first, repeatedly, for a "familiarization" period. A second stimulus is then substituted for the expected presentation of the first. If the infant notices, he or she will dishabituate or look at it a lot, as initially done for the first presentation. If the infant cannot tell the difference, habituation will continue, she or he will look as little at the new stimulus as at the initial one after seeing it repeatedly. Finally, if an infant shows preferential looking at a novel stimulus that has been paired with a previously seen object, this indicates that the infant can recognize or remember the initial stimulus as familiar. By controlling the manner in which novel and previously exposed stimuli vary, investigators have explored the development of the infant's ability to discriminate and remember patterns as well as more abstract classes of information and temporal sequences of events.

These paradigms have been applied to the field of infant assessment in an attempt to develop methodologies appropriate for use with physically compromised children. As an alternative to conventional infant tests, Kearsley (49) and Zelazo (93) propose a perceptual-cognitive information-processing approach that assesses the child's reactivity to sequential visual and auditory events using the habituation/dishabituation paradigm and, based on the infant's demonstrable interest in the "moderately discrepant" event. The procedure involves the presentation of a standard sequence of events over a specified number of trials, the introduction of a moderately discrepant variation of the event, which is repeated for a fixed number of presentations, and the subsequent reintroduction of the original standard. This paradigm remains constant for each of five events, two visual and three auditory. These engaging dynamic visual and auditory events function as perceptual-cognitive "puzzles" for the infant to solve. The standard trials provide the infant with an opportunity to attend, to process, and to assimilate a complex event. Transformation trials offer discrepancies that require rapid adaptation, while return trials allow the infant to demonstrate the capacity to retain a memory for the standard event and recognize its return. Testing takes place in a darkened room equipped to resemble a puppet theater, with the child facing a stage. Windows in the curtain of the stage allow observers to record targeted behaviors such as visual fixation, smiling, vocalizing, and pointing, as indices of attention and learning. In addition to these behavioral measures, an electrocardiogram recording is taken to reflect changes in heart rate as a measure of attention. The stimulus event is also recorded, and all parameters are integrated on a polygraph recorder. Age-related changes in behavioral clusters noted at different points in the events have been established and serve as normative guides. In contrast to traditional methods of assessment, the perceptual-cognitive approach taps the child's ability to process information actively, rather than providing a static assessment of stored knowledge. Not yet available as a clinical tool, it has been used in longitudinal research and shows promise as a measure of cognition in studies of concurrent and predictive validity.

The Fagen Test of Infant Intelligence (29) is currently being used in a variety of research and clinical settings (Table 3.1). It is based on visual preference and habituation paradigms and was designed to be used as a screening device to differentiate normal from potentially cognitively delayed infants within groups of infants suspected to be at risk for later intellectual deficit due to various prenatal or postnatal conditions. The basic component of the test is a visual novelty problem in which pictures are presented in a box-like stage for viewing by the infant. For each novelty problem, the infant is first exposed to a stimulus (usually a picture of the face of a man, woman, or infant) until he or she has looked at it for a standard period of time. A tester, sitting behind the apparatus, out of the infant's view, observes the infant's visual fixations through a peephole and records the length of time of the fixations by pressing a timing key on a computer. When the standard study time has been reached, the tester withdraws the picture from the infant's view and immediately pairs it with a novel picture. The two are presented to the infant simultaneously for a specified test time. Still observing the infant's looking behavior through the back of the stage, the tester is able to determine if the infant is looking at either of the two stimuli by observing the corneal reflection of the stimuli over the pupils of the infant's eyes and records the amount of viewing time devoted to each picture on the computer. The computer computes a "novelty score," which consists of the amount of fixation during the test phase devoted to the novel picture divided by the total fixation time to both the novel and familiar picture. Novelty problems were carefully constructed to tap emerging cognitive abilities at different ages within the first year. The Fagen test does not yield a numerical score. Rather, it determines the degree of correspondence between an infant's preference for novelty compared with other children of the same age. Those whose novelty preferences are comparable are likely to have normal intelligence, whereas failure to demonstrate age-appropriate novelty preference is presumed to be associated with later mental retardation. These children are designated "at risk." The Fagen test, like the perceptual-cognitive approach, provides an opportunity to observe the child's capacity to process and assimilate information free from the constraints of speech or gross motor performance. It has been found to be particularly useful in the clinical assessment of infants with severe motor handicaps, such as cerebral palsy (24).

Predictive validity using various types of information processing tests is higher in a number of studies than has traditionally been found for conventional infant tests (75, 79, 80). It is contended that information-processing assessment techniques tap skills that are more closely related to those behaviors deemed components of intelligent behavior in older children. Intelligence tests given to children of preschool or school age call upon abilities to encode and retain new information, categorize stimuli, and retrieve useful information for problem-solving. Whereas conventional infant tests tap primarily sensorimotor skills, it is hypothesized that methodological advances in the study of infants' perception and recognition memory have made it possible to elicit conceptually similar capacities for encoding, retaining, categorizing, and retrieving information at this age.

Assessment of Cognitive Functioning in Preschool and School-aged Children

Most referrals for psychological evaluation of preschool or school-aged children center around the need to assess the child's intellectual or cognitive abilities and to plan an appropriate educational program (Table 3.2). Intelligence tests, the most widely used instruments in the psychological evaluation of children, grew out of attempts to develop procedures that would enable educators to predict the likelihood of students' success in a traditional academic program and to detect, early on, those students who might have difficulty and require special services. The strength of intelligence tests still lies in their correlation with school performance. Total scores, historically called IQs but also referred to as the "Full Scale Score," "Test Com-

Table 3.2.
Cognitive Assessment Instruments for Preschool and School-aged Children

Test	Age Range	Scope and Value	Limitations
Stanford-Binet Intelligence Scale: Fourth Edition	2 years to adult	Assesses functioning in four areas of cognitive ability; yields standard scores for each area in addition to a global score; guidelines for testing children with certain handicapping conditions are provided	Examiner's choice of subtests can influence results; tasks too difficult for significantly developmentally delayed preschoolers
Wechsler Preschool and Primary Scale of Intelligence: Revised	3–7 years	Both instruments yield a Verbal Score, a Performance Score, and a Full Scale Score; assess a broad variety of skills and permit delineation of child's strengths and weaknesses; widely used instruments with broad clinical and research base	Both require intact sensory and motor skills, particularly for performance items; not appropriate for children with severe developmental delays
Wechsler Intelligence Scale for Children: Revised	6–16 years		
McCarthy Scales of Children's Abilities	2½–8½ years	Yields standard scores in five areas of ability, in addition to a General Cognitive Index; motor abilities are scored separately; items are appealing to preschool-aged children; Kaufman and Kaufman (47) provide guidelines for testing handicapped children	Lengthy administration; not appropriate for young children with severe developmental delays
Kaufman Assessment Battery for Children	2½–12½ years	Measures mental processes independent of the content or acquired knowledge component of most existing scales; particularly useful for children from disadvantaged backgrounds; yields Mental Processing Composite and separate Achievement score; has a nonverbal scale for use with non-English-speaking children or children with language problems	Subtests assigned to "Successive" or "Simultaneous"; processing subtests do not always tap these processes exclusively; over-reliance on this distinction can be misleading

posite Score," or "General Cognitive Index," are most appropriately interpreted as a measure of behavior that reflects the probability of standard academic achievement.

In addition to information provided by the overall score, it is equally important to know whether the child's abilities are evenly developed or whether there are patterns of strengths and weaknesses that are relevant to learning and general adaptation. A global summary score does not provide meaningful information about the child who shows highly developed abilities in some areas and specific or circumscribed deficits in others. Although the forerunner of all intelligence tests, the Stanford-Binet, was rooted in Binet's theory of intelligence as a unitary power, most tests currently in use employ a multifactorial model which posits that there are various types of intellectual abilities that can manifest as relative strengths or weaknesses within any individual profile and contribute to the child's success or difficulty in school.

STANFORD-BINET INTELLIGENCE SCALE

The Stanford-Binet Intelligence Scale is the oldest of the individually administered intelligence scales. Although it has undergone several revisions since its introduction in this country in 1916, only the most recent revision has resulted in major changes in its theoretical underpinnings and test construction.

The original scale was developed to measure global intellectual abilities, conceived by Binet to consist of the powers of judgment, reasoning, and abstraction. Many different types of test items were developed to measure these abilities and items were arranged by age levels beginning with those appropriate for a 2-year-old child. A mental age was calculated by determining how far up the increasingly difficult scale the child progressed. It was later reasoned that this mental age could be divided by the child's chronological age to produce a ratio called an intelligence quotient or "IQ" (mental age divided by chronological age, multiplied by 100). The average score was assumed to be 100, as this represented an exact equivalence between mental age and chronological age. Scores below 100 indicated less than average rates of development, while scores above 100 indicated accelerated rates of mental development. Subsequent revisions of the scales were aimed at changing the problematic ratio scoring to the more psychometrically sophisticated use of standard deviation scores and at updating norms to keep up with changing demographics and learning patterns of children (83). However, the basic format of the test remained unchanged. Earlier versions of the Stanford-Binet test were widley used and well established as reliable instruments for the assessment of overall cognitive abilities, with particular applicablity for very young children and for older children with moderate to severe retardation. Problems were posed by the strong verbal emphasis of the scale, which penalized children with limited English proficiency and underestimated the cognitive abilities of children with specific language impairments. In addition, the division of items into age levels rather than skill areas and the provision of one global score made it less than optimal for assessing children's varying abilities in different areas.

The 1986 revision, resulting in the Stanford-Binet Fourth Edition (85), was aimed at providing a more detailed diagnostic assessment of the child's functioning across a number of different areas and to help differentiate between children who have more global versus more circumscribed learning problems. The age-scale format used in previous editions has been replaced by 15 subtests. Each comprises a series of similar items designed to measure a specific cognitive skill. Four broad areas measured by these tests include Verbal Reasoning, Abstract/Visual Reasoning, Quantitative Reasoning, and Short-Term Memory. The Composite Score that appraises general reasoning ability is retained by the 4th Edition, but is supplemented by Standard Age Scores for each of the four subscales and for each of the individual tests comprising the subscales, providing a richer data base for understanding the child's learning patterns. Certain tests lend themselves to nonverbal administration for children with limited proficiency in English and/or with language impairments. In addition, the Examiner's Handbook (20) provides guidelines for meeting the specific testing needs of children with hearing, visual, or motor handicaps.

WECHSLER SCALES OF INTELLIGENCE

The Wechsler series includes two tests for children, the Wechsler Preschool and Primary Scale of Intelligence—Revised (89) for children from 3 to 7 years of age and the Wechsler Intelligence Scale for Children—Revised (88) for children from 6 to 16 years of age. The organization of both scales is the same. Reflecting Wechsler's theory that intelligence is multidimensional, subtests were developed that measure a variety of abilities thought to reflect different aspects of intelligence. Twelve subtests on each test are grouped into two broad subscales measuring Verbal and Performance abilities. The verbal tests are similar in that each consists of a group of questions asked orally by the examiner and answered orally by the child. Receptive and expressive language processes are tapped, as are verbal reasoning and verbal concept formation. Performance tests assess the child's ability to solve novel problems with visually based concrete materials that require visual-perceptual organization, facility for spatial relationships, and visual-motor coordination. Although verbal skills are required to understand performance test directions and may be used by the child to mediate or guide a response, the child's mode of expressing the solution is free of verbal demands. The WPPSI-R and WISC-R both provide a Verbal Score, a Performance Score, and a Full Scale Score, which is a composite or summary score.

The Wechsler scales have been studied extensively and have been found to be highly reliable and valid. They were the first to be organized by subtests reflecting different skills and abiliites and, therefore, have been found to be very useful in identifying children's individual strengths and weaknesses. Most subsequent tests have adapted this general format. Revisions of the original Wechsler scales have kept their standardization samples up to date and reflective of the diversity in regional, ethnic, and socioeconomic backgrounds of American children based on census data. These revisions also have permitted modernization of out-dated content. The Wechsler scales call for the manipulation of small materials; standard presentation would penalize children with motor handicaps, especially on performance tests, many of which are timed. In addition, because standard scores have not been derived for extremely variant performance, the Wechsler scales are not very useful for children with severe levels of mental retardation.

MCCARTHY SCALES OF CHILDREN'S ABILITIES

The McCarthy Scales of Children's Abilities (65) were designed to assess the cognitive abilities of children from 2½ to 8½ years of age. Eighteen subtests are grouped into five scales. The Verbal Scale assesses verbal expression and verbal concept development. The Perceptual-Performance Scale assesses nonverbal reasoning and problem-solving through the manipulation of concrete materials. The Quantitative Scale measures the child's facility with numbers and quantitative concepts. The General Cognitive Index is a composite of the child's performance on the Verbal, Perceptual-Performance, and Quantitative Scales and reflects the child's cognitive level in relation to other children of the same age. In addition, there is a Memory Scale, which assesses visual and auditory short-term memory, and a Motor Scale, which assesses gross and fine motor coordination. The psychometric properties of the McCarthy Scales are good and the items and materials are appealing to young children. Kaufman and Kaufman (47) provide guidelines for retesting children with handicapping conditions using the McCarthy Scales.

KAUFMAN ASSESSMENT BATTERY FOR CHILDREN (K-ABC)

The Kaufman Assessment Battery for Children (48), developed for the cognitive and psychoeducational evaluation of children from 2½ to 12½ years of age, has significantly different conceptual underpinnings than other psychological tests for children. The K-ABC is based on a neuropsychological model of information processing. It was designed to measure mental processes separate from the content or acquired knowledge component of existing scales in an effort to separate active problem-solving abilities from those that are highly influenced by exposure to formal or informal cultural or educational experiences. Acquired knowledge is not dismissed as irrelevant in the comprehensive evaluation of the child, but tasks that require the retrieval and/or application of factual knowledge are placed on a separate scale of the K-ABC, the Achievement Scale, to be used in comparison to the Mental Processing Composite. The Mental Processing Composite reflects the child's performance on subscales designed to capture two primary modes of information processing. In one mode, called Simultaneous Processing, information is taken in a holistic manner in order to solve a problem. Such tasks, frequently visuospatial in nature, require the ability to perceive a gestalt. In the other mode, termed Successive Processing, stimuli are arranged or processed sequentially and information is meaningful only in serial or temporal relationship to other information. Each of the Simultaneous and Successive Scales is comprised of several subtests designed to assess these respective competencies. The Achievement Subtest consists of measures of expressive vocabulary, general information, and early reading skills.

A major objective in designing the Mental Processing subtests was to minimize the role of receptive or expressive language in order to be able to assess the cognitive abilities of children with significant language impairments and/or children from different language backgrounds who are not English proficient. In fact, it is possible to derive a nonverbal score based only on those subtests that are fully free of language demands. The distinction between problem-solving and acquired information is highlighted in order to assess fairly the cognitive abilities of children from socioeconomically disadvantaged backgrounds whose environments do not foster the development of verbal and preacademic readiness skills. The excellent standardization of the K-ABC includes the provision of supplementary sociocultural norms that reflect an individual child's standing relative to children from similar backgrounds. For all children, the K-ABC was meant to offer strategies for educational remediation based on assessment of the indiviudal child's processing strengths and weaknesses. For example, a different reading program may be indicated depending upon whether the child uses successive or simultaneous modes more efficiently.

ALTERNATIVE INSTRUMENTS FOR ASSESSMENT OF COGNITIVE ABILITIES

Most of the widely used intelligence tests depend to some degree on language and include tasks that are presented, and responded to, verbally. This is because the bulk of our learning and thinking is mediated by language. For the nonhandicapped child and in relation to traditional academic skills, aptitude for learning can be tested more effectively by tasks that involve language than by those that do not. However, for some groups of handicapped children, such as those with hearing deficits, central language impairments, or the severe articulatory disorders that are part of the motor deficit of cerebral palsy, an alternative form of assessment is needed (Table 3.3). Tests which are nonverbal in nature or do not make demands on expressive language have been developed for this purpose. These alternative instruments

Table 3.3.
Alternative Tests of Intelligence

Test	Age Range	Scope and Value	Limitations
Peabody Picture Vocabulary Test: Revised	2–18 years	Effective test of receptive language; particularly useful for testing children with severe speech and/or motor impairments	Measures only one area of intellectual functioning (hearing vocabulary); can be misleading to generalize from this to other areas of intellectual or language ability
Columbia Mental Maturity Scale	3–10 years	Tests perceptual discrimination and concept formation; designed for use with children with cerebral palsy; calls for no expressive language and a minimum of motor response	Limited range of abilities is sampled
Leiter International Performance Scale	2–18 years	Designed for use with deaf children and is useful in the assessment of speech and motor handicapped children; measures nonverbal intelligence; test administration allows for observation of learning ability	Limited range of abilities is sampled
Raven's Progressive Matrices	6 years to adult	Measures nonverbal intelligence and concept formation using visual analogy type of tasks	Subject to distortion by the visual perceptual difficulties that commonly prevail among handicapped children
Pictorial Tests of Intelligence	3–8 years	Consists of five subtests designed to measure intellectual ability of multiply handicapped children with motor and/or speech defects	Requires receptive language abilities
Hiskey-Nebraska Test of Learning Aptitudes	4–12 years	Designed for deaf children; standardized on deaf and hearing children	Does not evaluate language skills

are particularly useful in testing physically handicapped children who are limited in modalities of motor expression. Unlike tests that call for the manipulation of concrete materials to solve a problem, presentation of alternative tests requires only minimum motor responses, such as pointing to the correct answer from an array of choices. Where even such a response is not possible, the examiner may point to the available choices successively, eliciting whatever "yes" or "no" response the child is capable of making. The validity of these tests as measures of general intelligence is based on reasonably good correlations with the Stanford-Binet and Wechsler scales. Their most important limitation is that they measure a restricted range of cognitive functioning. Caution must be used in generalizing findings from a relatively small behavioral sample to more global intellectual abilities.

Among the various types of tasks represented on children's ability tests, vocabulary tests typically show the strongest correlation with overall intellectual ability and school success. This has led to the development of picture vocabulary tests designed to provide an abbreviated or alternative tool for the estimation of general intelligence. The Peabody Picture Vocabulary Test—Revised (PPVT-R) (26) is the most well-known instrument in this category. The PPVT-R provides an estimate of the child's verbal intelligence by measuring receptive vocabulary. Presented with a series of plates, each containing four pictures, the child listens to a word and is asked to identify the picture that best illustrates it. The PPVT-R is normed for children aged 2 years and older. Results are expressed in standard scores, percentiles, and age equivalents. The Pictorial Test of Intelligence (33) is designed to measure the intellectual ability of multiply handicapped children with motor and/or speech impairments who are 3 to 8 years of age. Like the Peabody Picture Vocabulary Test, it requires and makes use of receptive language abilities.

The Columbia Mental Maturity Scale (12) was designed to measure the intelligence of children with cerebral palsy. For each item, the child is asked to look at several pictures on a card and select the one that is different from or unrelated to the others. In order to do this, the child must formulate a mental rule for organizing the pictures so as to exclude just one. At the early levels, correct response calls for relatively simple perceptually based discriminations involving color, size, and shape. As the test progresses, correct response is more demanding of categorical thinking and abstract reasoning abilities. No formal language processes are required.

The Raven's Progressive Matrices (73) require the child to select the one of the several visual stimuli that correctly completes a drawing or a series of drawings. It employs a visual analogy type of task and tests visual reasoning in addition to concepts involving number, shape, spatial orientation, and seriation. The number of corerct responses is translated into a percentile score in accordance with the child's age. The Raven's is used primarily for school-aged children.

The Leiter International Performance Scale (59) was originally designed for use with deaf children. In this test, which uses matching and association tasks, the child is asked to slide pictures mounted on blocks into stalls on a response frame that displays corresponding pictures or concepts. Instructions are given nonverbally by demonstration and repeated trials are allowed until the child has grasped the nature of the task. The scale covers skills ranging from simple matching to the comprehension of more complex relationships involving space, category, and analogy. There are four items on each successive age level beginning at 2 years of age. Credit is assigned from a basal age at which all subtests are passed and testing is discontinued once a ceiling has been reached. Results are expressed in terms of a mental age and IQ. The Hiskey-Nebraska Test of Learning Aptitude (41) was also designed for deaf children and has been standardized on both deaf and hearing populations. It is applicable for children from 4 to 12 years of age. The test comprises multiple subtests that primarily tap visual memory, visual sequencing, and visual reasoning abilities. No language skills are evaluated.

The instruments so far described provide alternatives to standard assessment for most handicapped children, but require a minimal ability to comprehend at least preschool-level symbols. The Haeussermann Evaluation (38) provides a set of procedures for determining the level of comprehension of those preschool-aged children most severely involved either physically or intellectually. The Haeussermann approach consists of items that can be responded to with the minimum of a consistent "yes" or "no" response. It also establishes means of simplifying demands or retreating to more basic levels for the less capable child. The competencies measured include a gross evaluation of sensory intactness, recognition of objects, perception of color, form and amount, language comprehension, and concept formation. Materials are modified to the abilites of the child but, for the most part, consist of concrete life-sized objects and large clear pictures. The presentation of items is arranged so that there is always a choice of at least two alternative responses, which the child can designate by any means at his or her disposal. The physical arrangement of response choices and the child's position are designed to yield optimal performance and to preclude errors of interpretation. Results are not expressed in a total score, but age equivalents are provided for the different competencies the child is judged to have mastered.

Assessment of Perceptual and Perceptual-Motor Abilities

Visual perception and perceptual-motor functions, the integration of visual and motor channels for the execution of a complex and coordinated act, are two modes of information processing that are basic to school-related learning, particularly in the early grades. Many instruments have thus been developed to assess these abilities (Table 3.4). One of the most widely used tests in this area is the Bender Gestalt (8), which is used to evaluate visual-motor maturity in children and to detect delays or impairments in visual

Table 3.4.
Perceptual Evaluations

Test	Age Range	Scope and Value	Limitations
Bender Visual Motor Gestalt Test	5 years to adult	Assesses visual-motor functioning in relation to maturation; nonthreatening, easy to administer, well researched	Open to overinterpretation; requires functional graphomotor skills to provide useful information
Beery and Buktenica Developmental Test of Visual-Motor Integration	2–16 years	Assesses visual-motor performance; is useful in the evaluation of younger children compared to the Bender Gestalt	Unlike the Bender Gestalt does not allow for observation of child's ability to organize work
Wepman Auditory Discrimination Test	5–8 years	Examines ability to detect likeness and difference in pairs of words presented aurally	Requires mastery of basic language concepts to follow through on test instructions

perceptual skills and/or eye-hand coordination. The test consists of nine geometric designs, each printed on a 3 × 5-inch card. The cards are presented to the child serially and he or she is asked to copy them on an unlined 8 × 11-inch piece of paper. Test performance is evaluated in terms of the adequacy of the reproduction. Scoring is usually based on a system developed by Koppitz (56) in which rotation of designs, distortion of forms, failure to integrate components of the designs, and/or perseveration in the execution of designs are counted as errors. Norms are provided for children from 5 to 11 years of age. The test has good concurrent validity with other tests of perceptual-motor ability but only marginal ability to predict academic success, although it is helpful in discerning the sometimes severe processing problems of children with central nervous system involvement.

The Beery-Buktenica Developmental Test of Visual-Motor Integration (5) is similar to the Bender Gestalt in that the child is required to copy geometric shapes. However, the shapes are more varied in level of difficulty and, therefore, are suitable for children from ages 2 to almost 16. The manual presents scoring criteria to determine whether the child's reproduction of the model form passes or fails. The total score is expressed as an age equivalent. Techniques for determining specific areas of difficulty in the visual-motor spectrum are provided in the manual.

In addition to visual perceptual problems, children with neurologic and developmental disabilities sometimes exhibit difficulties in auditory, kinesthetic, or tactile functioning and/or in the integration of these functions. A variety of instruments are available to test for these disabilities. The Wepman Test for Auditory Discrimination (90) assesses the child's ability to distinguish between similar sounding words presented orally. The Visual Aural Digit Span Test (VADS) (57) assesses visual and auditory memory using oral and motor response modalities, thus enabling analysis of cross-modal information processing. Various neuropsychological tests assess functioning within discrete sensory-perceptual modalities, including visual, aural, and tactile processing, as well as cross-modal integration of information received through, or expressed via, different sensorimotor channels (76).

Academic Achievement Tests

Achievement tests are designed to evaluate the child's performance in school subject areas such as reading and mathematics. Scores on achievement tests are typically given in terms of school grade equivalents which provide an estimate of the child's level of academic skill, as well as standard scores which are based on age norms (Table 3.5). Achievement tests vary greatly in characteristics that can be critical in the examination of children with handicapping conditions. Many are group-administered paper and pencil tests that penalize handicapped children for their slower pace, poorer attention, or difficulty keeping track of their place on a page. In such instances, results may give a distorted picture of the actual mastery of content being tested. In the context of a psychological evaluation, instruments of choice are those that are designed for individual administration and, thus, permit observation of task approach in addition to quantitative results.

The Wide Range Achievement Test—Revised (WRAT-R) (45) is a frequently used individually administered test of achievement in reading, spelling, and arithmetic from kindergarten age. The reading score is based on letter matching and letter identification at the lowest level and word recognition and decoding thereafter. The spelling test calls upon the child to write a series of words dictated by the examiner. At the lowest level, visual-motor copying is assessed as the child is asked to reproduce geometric forms from a model. The arithmetic test involves counting, identifying numbers, and solving simple addition and subtraction problems orally at the younger level, and solving written computation problems of increasing complexity at the more advanced levels. The value of the WRAT-R lies in its ability to provide a quick estimate of the child's academic proficiency and progress from one evaluation to another. A limitation is that the reading test measures only word recognition and not reading fluency or comprehension, which are salient to a child's success with academic material. These are explored in more depth on other reading tests. The Gray Oral Reading Paragraphs (35) and Spache Diagnostic Reading Scales (81) are diagnostic tests

Table 3.5.
Academic Achievement Tests

Test	Age Range	Scope and Value	Limitations
Wide Range Achievement Test: Revised	K to 12th grade	Used to assess quickly level of academic skills and improvement from one evaluation to the next	Reading subtest does not tap comprehension
Peabody Individual Achievement Test	K to high school	Provides an overview of achievement in mathematics, reading, spelling, and general information; requirement for only a pointing response and use of large clear response choices make it useful in the evaluation of handicapped children	Considered by authors to be a screening instrument; manual suggests use of alternative instruments when more intensive study is required
Gray Oral Reading Paragraphs Spache Diagnostic Reading Scales	K to high school	Give important information on level of accomplishment and types of error in decoding and comprehension; helpful in planning intervention	Independent reading tests that may prove difficult for children with severe perceptual problems

designed to analyze the child's strengths and weaknesses in skills inherent to the reading process and to suggest the causes of reading difficulties.

The Peabody Individual Achievement Test (27) is another test that samples several academic areas including mathematics, reading recognition, reading comprehension, spelling, and general information. Several of the subtests use a multiple choice format in which the child can point to the correct response from a choice of four. Thus, execution of a complex motor or verbal response is minimized, making the PIAT particularly adaptable for the assessment of children with various disabilities.

Assessment of Adaptive Abilities

Comprehensive assessment of a handicapped child should include a description of his or her social and adaptive abilities for the conduct of everyday activities. To understand fully the range of abilities and disabilities, the clinician must know the child's means and level of achievement in locomotor, communication, and self-care areas, such as feeding, dressing, and toileting. The child's mode of interaction with those around him or her, both family members and peers, and his or her ability to assume increasing levels of responsibility should be determined (Table 3.6).

The ages at which children usually achieve such competencies have been documented and scales have been developed to permit assessment of social-

Table 3.6.
Social/Adaptive Scales

Test	Age Range	Scope and Value	Limitations
Vineland Adaptive Behavior Scale	Infant to adult	Questionnaire-type instrument for the measurement of general social competence; yields Adaptive Behavior Composite in addition to separate scores in communication, socialization, daily living skills, and motor skills; updated standardization includes supplementary norms for handicapped populations	Data are obtained through interview with an informant who may not be able to provide reliable information in all areas investigated
AAMD Adaptive Behavior Scale	3 years to adult	In addition to items that assess the child's status in activities of daily living, the scale also provides items that give full evaluation of deviant or maladaptive behaviors; provides a public school version of the questionnaire, which was originally developed for an institutionalized population	Several of the items may be upsetting to parents; information is probably best obtained from those involved in intervention to assist in program planning
Maxfield-Buchholz Social Maturity Scale for Blind Preschool Children	Preschool	Scale of social development designed specifically for young blind children	Older instrument; items and norms may be dated

adaptive abilities much in the same way as any standardized test of ability is constructed. The most widely used instrument of this type is the Vineland Adaptive Behavior Scales (82), a recent expansion and revision of the original Vineland Social Maturity Scale (23). The revised instrument continues to be applicable from infancy through adult years. Three separate forms, the Survey Forms, the Expanded Form, and the Classroom Edition, are now available for different purposes and for evaluation of the child's performance in the different settings in which he or she participates. The authors of the scale define adaptive behavior as the performance of the daily activities required for personal and social sufficiency. Each version of the scale measures adaptive behavior in four domains: Communication, Daily Living Skills, Socialization, and Motor Skills. Data are obtained by means of a semistructured interview with an informant, usually a parent, who is knowledgeable about the child's functioning in these areas. Standard scores are provided for each of the domains, and an Adaptive Behavior Composite is derived. The 1984 revision provided a greatly expanded item base; it refined or deleted items to reflect societal changes that have occurred since the original scale was developed and significantly improved the scale's psychometric properties, including the standardization sample, which is now substantially larger and more representative of the national population. Supplementary norms are available to permit comparison of a handicapped individual's scores with those of others with similar handicapping conditions. In addition, the Survey Form and the Expanded Form include a Maladaptive Behavior Scale, the administration of which is optional.

The Adaptive Behavior Scales (71), published by the American Association on Mental Deficiency, is another commonly used instrument. One of its two versions is applicable for children aged 3 to 6 years. Similar to the Vineland, it taps several subdomains of social-adaptive functioning and provides norms that permit comparison to children with varying degrees of cognitive ability. The Maxfield-Buchholz Social Maturity Scale for blind preschool children (63) is a scale of social development designed specifically for young, visually impaired children.

The significance of adaptive abilities and their contribution to the child's functional status is emphasized in the definition of mental retardation. Criteria for the diagnosis of mental retardation are met only when a finding of subaverage intellectual skills is matched by a comparable deficit in adaptive functioning.

Emotional Factors and Projective Tests

Psychological evaluation typically includes an assessment of the child's emotional adjustment. In children for whom disruptive emotional problems are present or suspected, it is essential to identify the basis of such difficulties and their impact on the child's overall development and performance. Various techniques are commonly used for this purpose. The first is direct observation of the child's behavior for style of response and interpersonal relatedness. Second is the parent interview wherein family attitudes, demands, and stresses on the child are investigated. Third is the formal evaluation of personality factors through the use of projective techniques (Table 3.7). In projective tests, the child is presented with tasks that afford him or her the opportunity to respond in an individual manner due to the lack of structure inherent in the task. Individual style of response, as well as content and themes elicited, permit inferences that clarify aspects of personality and adjustment.

Because of their broad appeal to children, drawings are probably the most commonly used projective technique in pediatric assessment. Well-known examples are provided by the Draw-a-Person Test (62) and the Kinetic Family Drawing (21). In these procedures, the child's drawings are followed by a request to make up a story about his or her picture or respond to a set of

Table 3.7.
Emotional Assessment Tests

Test	Age Range	Scope and Value	Limitations
Children's Apperception Test	3–10 years	Useful in assessing child's adjustment patterns	Requires good verbal skills for telling a logical story
Rorschach	3 years to adult	Evaluates personality structure including ego strengths, reality testing, and defense mechanisms	Requires good verbal skills expressively and receptively as well as freedom from significant perceptual problems
Figure Drawings	4 years to adult	Reveal self-image and perception of interpersonal relationships in addition to providing an estimate of level of development of intelligence; appealing task for most children	Requires good graphomotor ability in order to interpret for emotional factors

standard questions. Drawings provide insight into the child's body image and its impact on emotional development, as well as his or her perceptions of important interpersonal relationships (55).

The Children's Apperception Test (7) employs a series of pictures of animals or human figures in various situations. The child is asked to provide a story for each illustration. The stories are examined for patterns in the salient characteristics of central figures, the general nature of the situations being faced by figures, and the recurring traits of the people with whom the characters interact.

The Rorschach Test (74) consists of ten ink blot stimuli. Upon presentation, the child is asked what each ink blot might represent. Subsequent to his or her response, an inquiry is made to discover the determinants of the child's response. The child's style of responding, as well as the content of associations, combine to form a global assessment of ego resources, conflicts, fantasies, and preoccupations.

Projective instruments can provide valuable information as part of a comprehensive evaluation. However, many of the more common projective techniques prove to be unsatisfactory with young children, particularly with those who have significant neurologic handicap. The ability to respond to these instruments requires fairly sophisticated drawing or language skills and is impeded by the perceptual-motor distortions that tend to prevail in this group.

Levels of Intellectual Functioning

Individually administered global intelligence tests yield standard scores, sometimes referred to as Test Composite Scores or Full Scale Scores, more popularly known as IQs, are used to designate a child's overall level of intellectual functioning. This is arrived at by comparing an individual child's performance to the performance of hundreds of children in a representative, age-stratified norm group. This system is based on the assumption that intelligence, like many human traits, is normally distributed. On most tests, the mean is 100, which represents average or "normal" intelligence. Classifications of exceptionality, including superior and subaverage intellectual functioning, typically refer to scores that fall two standard deviations above and below the mean, respectively (Fig. 3.1). The statistical properties of

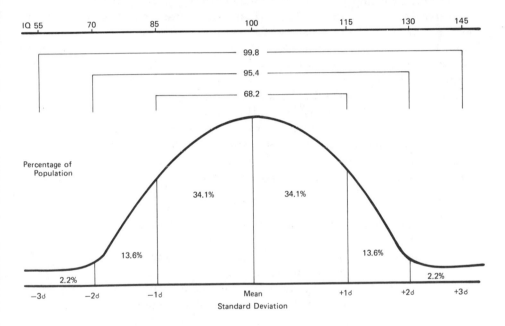

AAMD Classification of Mental Retardation

	Standard Deviation Below the Mean	Measured Intelligence Score	
		Stanford Binet SD = 16	Wechsler SD = 15
Mild	2.01 − 3.00	52 − 67	55 − 69
Moderate	3.01 − 4.00	36 − 51	40 − 54
Severe	4.01 − 5.00	20 − 35	25 − 39
Profound	5.00	20	25

Figure 3.1. Levels of intellectual functioning.

commonly used scales of intelligence vary, so that not all tests have uniform standard deviations. Therefore, classification of intellectual functioning may be represented by slightly different scores depending upon the instrument used. In addition, since all measurement involves some "error," classification of intellectual functioning should take into account the standard error of measurement of the instrument employed. Interpretation of test results should be based on the understanding that a "true" score is likely to fall approximately five points above or below the obtained score.

Overall scores that fall in the range of 90 to 110 are usually designated as normal or average. Scores that range from 80 to 90 and from 110 to 120 are typically considered "low average" and "high average," respectively. A score between 70 and 80 on a standard test of intelligence is usually indicative of functioning within the borderline range of intelligence. Children who score within this range are those who, without being retarded according to formal criteria, are nevertheless well below average with respect to their developmental or intellectual status. As a form of normality, although with problems in conceptual and abstract abilities, these children often travel in the educational mainstream and are sometimes referred to as "slow learners" due to their persistent difficulties in maintaining standard academic progress. In favorable circumstances, with much remedial support, a child so classified may be able to function in a regular class although perhaps not as well as his or her classmates or siblings. In some circumstances, special education will be needed. Prognostically, this intellectual level enables most children to function adequately in social and vocational domains as adults.

MENTAL RETARDATION

The definition of mental retardation includes three components: significantly subaverage general intellectual functioning as determined by an individually administered standardized test of intelligence, concurrent deficits in adaptive behavior, and manifestation during the developmental period, or first 18 years (37). All three criteria must be present in order to diagnose mental retardation formally. In the conduct of a psychological evaluation, a developmental history is obtained to determine when delays were first apparent. Although the definition above refers to subaverage "general" intellectual functioning, most psychologists use this diagnosis to reflect cognitive profiles that are relatively even and show global deficits across all subareas assessed. Assessment of delays in adaptive abilities refers primarily to slower mastery of self-care and personal-social skills in preschool-aged children, but should expand to document failure to achieve academic skills, as well, in school-aged children. The diagnosis of mental retardation is made independent of etiology. There is no need for an identifiable medical entity, nor does a specific medical entity reliably predict the level of intellectual ability. In addition, the diagnosis of mental retardation is one that reflects a child's current functioning and does not necessarily place limits on the child's ultimate outcome, which may vary depending on response to intervention or other individual circumstances.

There are four levels of mental retardation and one of these is usually specified when a diagnosis of mental retardation is made. The classification of *mild* mental retardation encompasses the largest number of children with mental retardation. Developmentally, such children often show delayed language development as toddlers and weakness in the acquisition of preacademic readiness skills in preschool or in the mastery of formal academic skills in the earliest grades. These constitute the common points at which evaluation is usually sought. The "educable" classification commonly used by school systems encompasses approximately the same population as those designated mildly retarded and refers to the fact that children within this range are capable of learning academic skills, albeit at a modified pace and often requiring special education services. Generally, children in this category reach a 3rd to 5th grade level of academic achievement. If associated physical handicaps are mild enough, they may be independent in activities of daily living. For practical purposes, this level of intellectual functioning, especially at the upper range and in the absence of severe social-emotional problems, is generally sufficient for achieving relative independence in adulthood, although support is needed periodically and in relation to certain types of tasks.

Children with moderate mental retardation have a higher incidence of neurological involvement and/or physical stigmata than children with mild mental retardation. This, in conjunction with an even slower rate of attainment of developmental milestones, results in coming to attention often by the time they are toddlers. During school years, children in this category most often attend special classes where they are taught primarily self-care and practical daily living skills; the attainment of only functional academic competencies is expected. Most children are able to acquire language or other communication skills. As adults, many are able to achieve some independence in self-care skills but continue to live with their families or in supervised group homes and, vocationally, function in sheltered workshops or other protected employment.

Children with severe mental retardation often achieve functional language skills but no formal academic skills and special, intensive programming may be required to master independence in activities of daily living. In adulthood, closely supervised and supported care is needed. The profoundly retarded child usually has associated severe motor handicaps, limited language abilities, and limited potential for acquiring self-care skills.

Studies of children with identified involvement of the central nervous system and associated neuromotor handicaps suggest that this population is overrepresented in the lower ranges of intellectual functioning when compared to their nonhandicapped peers. Central nervous system dysfunction is not incompatible with normal intelligence and the degree to which a child will be intellectually impaired cannot be predicted solely on the basis of the physical or motor deficit. However, Hopkins and associates (42), in a study of over 900 children with cerebral palsy during the 1940s through 1950s, found that approximately 50% had intelligence scores within the retarded range. Other investigators have found comparable IQ distributions in the study of children with cerebral palsy (52). Even unilateral cerebral lesions that result in hemiplegia in young children have been found to be associated with significant decreases in intelligence scores (61). Similarly, in an extensive review of the literature, Anderson and Spain (1) discuss evidence for the fact that, among children with spina bifida, particularly those with significant degrees of hydrocephalus, intelligence is skewed, with a peak in the low average to borderline range. Nonetheless, even the presence of hydrocephalus is not incompatible with normal intelligence. Studies have found that some children with hydrocephalus obtain intelligence scores in the average to high average range (21). Central nervous system infection constitutes an important factor in the lower intelligence of children with spina bifida and hydrocephalus (67).

Consistency of Intellectual Classifications

Beginning in the preschool years, when language is well established for most children, there is reasonable correlation between intelligence scores obtained in childhood and those obtained on subsequent testing during the adolescent years. However, IQ, as a measurement of dynamic and multivariate competencies, is never a fixed entity for any child. The literature documents noteworthy inconsistencies in scores, even for nonhandicapped children who test broadly within the normal range of intelligence. This is particularly true for handicapped children whose development takes place under extenuating circumstances and who often show unevenness in the rate of development across different areas.

Klapper and Birch (51) investigated the stability of test-retest scores in a group of young children with cerebral palsy who were re-assessed on follow-up 14 years later. The predictive value of earlier measures was found to vary with the level of intelligence established on the first examination. Initial intelligence scores below 50 or above 90 were excellent predictors of re-test score, whereas initial scores between 75 and 89 were the poorest predictors. Severely impaired children remained as such on follow-up and the children initially identified as normal retained this classification. The most frequent change occurred among children whose initial score placed them within or near the borderline range and occurred mostly in the direction of higher intelligence scores on later testing.

Several influences may account for the finding of higher scores as children grow older. Klapper and Birch suggest that the intellectual functioning of children with cerebral palsy is transiently depressed during their earliest years due to restrictions in sensory and motor experiences. In clinical practice, it is not uncommon to observe improved motor skills and the increased opportunity for varied experiences resulting in advances of cognitive abilities. An intelligence classification can be positively influenced by the provision of an educational program. In recent years, increases in intelligence scores are one of many beneficial effects of early intervention programs for handicapped children. Moreover, positive alterations in medical or behavioral management obtained through medications for seizure control or attention deficits, for example, can make a child more available to learning situations and reflect in improved performance on intelligence testing. Improved performance in later years may also be an artifact of the tests used to assess children's abilities at different ages. Tests for infants, toddlers, and preschool-aged children are often heavily weighted with items that require sensorimotor and perceptual-motor skills, which penalize youngsters with physical and motor handicaps, whereas the increased emphasis on verbal competence inherent to measures of intelligence in later years highlights the relative strength of verbal skills for many of these children. It is also sometimes the case that, in the assessment of a young child with motor dysfunction, too much emphasis is given to speech delays due to dysarthria, with less than adequate attention to other indicators of comprehension, which are detected once alternative means of communication or response modality have been established.

In some cases, children seen in follow-up will score lower on subsequent testing than they did on an earlier evaluation. Rather than reflecting a decline in intellectual ability, this may be explained on the basis of the different cognitive demands of tasks at different age levels. At the preschool level, for example, many test items consist of matching tasks that tap simple perceptual discriminations and focus on the concrete characteristics of objects. This is in contrast to tasks for older children that, increasingly, demand the ability to think categorically, appreciate relationships, and reason inferentially. Often, the verbal fluency and good rote auditory memory characteristic of some children with cerebral deficits lead to the assessment of good mental abilities in the early years but are no longer sufficient to sustain this rating once the child is presented with more complex situations calling for comprehension and the application of past learning. Finally, a downward trend on re-evaluation may reflect the intellectually disadvantageous effects of deteriorating medical conditions such as uncontrolled seizures or progressive neurological disease, or the detrimental effects of an adverse social situation or serious emotional problem.

Specific Learning Problems of Handicapped Children

The determination of overall level of intellectual functioning is just one step in the psychological assessment of the child. A global intelligence score, although it constitutes a starting point in understanding and planning for the child, fails to do justice by itself to the individual variations that can produce a given score or to the individual child's unique learning style. A child may show comparable levels of ability across all areas assessed or marked variation in levels of ability across different types of tasks. Consequently, an assessment of individual strengths and weaknesses and identification of disturbances in underlying psychological processes, which are likely to interfere with learning, are essential components of psychological evaluation. Problems described in the following sections can occur concurrent with mental retardation or may constitute circumscribed deficits.

PERCEPTUAL AND PERCEPTUAL-MOTOR DIFFICULTIES IN CHILDREN WITH CEREBRAL PALSY

Although there are substantial individual differences, studies of children with cerebral palsy have shown that these children, as a group, show evidence of impaired perceptual functioning when compared to their nonhandicapped peers. Most of these difficulties are in the area of visual perception, which is also emphasized here because of the significance of visual-perceptual skills for school-related activities. Children with cerebral palsy have been found to have difficulties in several aspects of visual perception. Often there is greater difficulty in distinguishing figure from background in a visual display, a tendency to be distracted by impinging background stimuli, creating forced responsiveness to irrelevant information and interfering with the perception of more salient features (19). Children with cerebral palsy also exhibit a tendency for dissociation, an inability to relate parts to the total configuration, and difficulty perceiving a figure as an integrated entity. Problems with the spatial organization of size, form, and position are frequently identified in this group, as might be reflected in the child's difficulty with puzzles. Due to motor and visual-perceptual deficits, there are difficulties with visual-motor integration, the ability to execute a motion with the hand as mediated by a visual stimulus. The child with this type of deficit experiences a problem analogous to the one a nonimpaired person would face when trying to reproduce a complex geometric figure while observing the writing hand only through a mirror.

As a result of these difficulties, children with cerebral palsy are likely to obtain higher verbal than performance scores on intelligence tests. Studies of children with spina bifida similarly suggest that visual perception and performance on visual-motor tasks are likely to be impaired in this population (1, 91). Distortions of figure-background relationships are a deterring factor in test items calling for the identification of missing features in a picture. Distortion in spatial comprehension and visual-motor integration show in depressed scores on mazes, block design, puzzle assembly, and graphomotor tasks. Bender designs often show rotations in space, distortion of forms, misshaped angles, and poor integration of parts of figures. Academically, these deficits manifest in difficulties recognizing visual symbols such as letters and numbers, laborious reading, distraction by competing and irrelevant visual stimuli, letter reversals, and poor handwriting.

Studies have shown that under certain conditions, children with visual perceptual problems show improved performance. For example, children seem better able to discriminate figure from background patterns when materials are presented in color, rather than black and white (19). These findings have implications for the adaptation and modification of learning materials to suit the needs of children with such difficulties. The stimulus value of items to which the child's attention should be directed, such as words on a page, might be increased by the use of color, while the stimulus value of background stimuli, like lines or margins, are decreased. Whereas there is evidence for the efficacy of such modification of classroom materials, support for justifying formal programs of perceptual-motor and sensory integration training (3) as remediation for learning disorders remains questionable. Although it is shown that such programs improve performance on the tests with which they are associated, transfer to more remote academic skills, such as reading, is limited (2, 39).

While perceptual and perceptual-motor abilities are important in the development of the mechanics of early reading and writing, such skills become subordinate to verbal competence as the child deals with academic material in the later grades. Thus, many children with good verbal comprehension ultimately learn well despite their visual perceptual or visual-motor deficits. Nonetheless, appraisal of perceptual functioning is an integral part of a psychological evaluation as it does constitute a primary mode of learning and, in some cases, when adequate compensation has not been achieved or problems are severe, perceptual deficits continue to pose a serious learning impediment.

CHARACTERISTICS OF VERBAL BEHAVIOR IN CHILDREN WITH SPINA BIFIDA AND HYDROCEPHALUS

Among children with spina bifida and hydrocephalus, a qualitative style of language is frequently noted, which Diller et al. (22) have described as hyperverbal behavior, referring to the apparent failure to inhibit nonsalient verbal responses in this group of children. Hyperverbal behavior is characterized by superficial verbal fluency, coupled with poor comprehension. Children with this pattern tend to develop early language milestones at the expected times. Further acquisition of vocabulary and syntax seems normal and speech is fluent and well articulated. These children have good auditory memory and learn nursery rhymes and television commercials readily. This fluent verbal behavior is misleading and parents often reinforce it, thinking it is an indication of brightness. Initially, clinicians also tend to interpret this apparent facility with language as a sign of good cognitive function. However, on closer scrutiny, such verbalizations are often tangential and relatively devoid of meaningful content. There is holistic application of previously learned phrases and such children have difficulty staying relevant in conversational exchanges. In contrast to the fluidity of their language productions, these children show deficiencies on verbal tasks that demand reasoning and increasing degrees of abstraction. Recent studies (43) suggest that children with spina bifida and hydrocephalus have more difficulty attending to the relevant aspects of a situation and that this distractibility is responsible, at least in part, for deficits in language functioning.

ATTENTIONAL DIFFICULTIES

Children with central nervous system impairments often show disorders of attention that may influence their performance on formal psychological testing and, more importantly, their functioning at home and in the classroom situation. Such children are noted primarily for their limited attention span and tendency to move quickly from one activity to another. They display marked distractibility and are unable to refrain from reaction to the multiple stimuli occurring in the environment, whether or not they are related to the task at hand. There is an impulsive style of response to the demand characteristics of surroundings and events, as well as to problem-solving in more formal academic situations. Attention deficits often occur in conjunction with motor hyperactivity. In a testing or classroom situation, these children are frequently restless, have difficulty focusing and sustaining concentration, and tend to engage in seemingly purposeless and disruptive motor activity. In some cases, intellectual abilities may be higher than achievement indicates since the quality of behavior makes the child unavailable to learning or prevents him or her from responding completely even when comprehension exists. Klapper and Warner (52) described a related quality of disorganization in problem-solving in these children who, unlike nonimpaired children, are unable to break a task down into its component parts and proceed systematically. Children are also prone to social difficulties because their behavior is offensive or prohibits participation in peer group activities. For children with adequate verbal skills, techniques such as verbal mediation are often used to help think, plan, and monitor their responses in academic and social situations (68).

Perseveration is characterized by persistent repetition or continuation of a response beyond the relevance or adaptiveness of this response and concomitant difficulty shifting from one response to the next. Perseveration may occur on a behavioral or ideational level. A child who tends to perseverate often requires external cues in order to break the pattern.

PSYCHOLOGICAL SEQUELAE OF HEAD INJURY

The psychological sequelae of head injury in children are dependent upon a number of elements, including the type of injury and whether it is local or diffuse, the age of the child, and many other medical and psychosocial factors. Nevertheless, traumatic brain injury during childhood is a potentially devastating event as it impacts on a period of life during which there is normally rapid growth and development in all spheres—physical, linguistic, cognitive, emotional, and social—and will almost inevitably inhibit, delay, or distort these normal developmental processes (58).

Although earlier research suggested that younger children sustain less morbidity or disability following a comparable brain injury than do older children or adults due to the greater presumed plasticity of the young brain (50), this has not been borne out by most of the studies of recent years (58). The plasticity theory suggested that prior to the development of hemispheric specialization, thought to occur around 2 years of age, interhemispheric transfer of function could occur with the undamaged hemisphere taking over for and developing the functional capabilities usually associated with the damaged hemisphere. Specifically, children who sustained an injury to the left hemisphere prior to the age of 2 years were thought to be less likely to suffer permanent language impairment than would older children or adults, as language functions would be taken over by their intact right hemisphere (78). This was believed to be possible, however, only in the case of localized unilateral brain damage (78), which is less likely to be the situation following the type of traumatic head injury typically seen in children, where diffuse brain damage is more likely to result (6, 9). Diffuse generalized damage is more likely to cause impairment of higher cognitive functions than is localized damage (9).

Contrary to the earlier presumed advantage in overcoming injury the young child's brain was thought to have over the older child's or adult's, the infant brain is noted to be more vulnerable to injury due to the fragility of its structures (58, 78). Consistent with this, some studies have found that scores on cognitive testing were lower and later school achievement was more significantly impaired in children who sustained head injury prior to the age of 5 years than in those injured later (15, 28, 78). In fact, as memory impairment is the most common cognitive deficit following brain injury (44, 60, 72) and new learning is affected to a much greater degree than is the retrieval of old, well-ingrained skills and information (15, 77, 78), it follows that children would be at a greater disadvantage than adults following brain injury as the majority of their learning still lies ahead of them.

The long-term cognitive and behavioral sequelae of head injury in children are frequently more impairing to function than are the residual physical sequelae (44). Even children who sustain a mild or minor head injury and manifest no outward physical sequelae can exhibit a variety of problems that can significantly impair their functioning, including decreased attentional and memory capacity; increased irritability, distractibility, and impulsivity; and reduced ability to cope with stress (9).

Effects of childhood brain injury may not be apparent for months or years, until the time when a particular cognitive or behavioral function would be expected to appear in the course of normal growth and development (58). For example, problems with higher order abstract reasoning or impulse control are hard to discern in a 2-year-old who has recently sustained a brain injury, because neither of these functions are usually part of the cognitive or behavioral repertoire of the normal toddler. Thus, deficits in these areas may not become apparent until several years after injury or, frequently, when the child enters school and conceptual abilities and impulse control are expected to be present.

What are the common long-term cognitive, behavioral, and emotional sequelae following moderate to severe head injury in children? Memory deficits, particularly for long-term storage and retrieval of new information, appear to be pervasive and persistent following all classes of head injury (10, 15, 44, 60, 78, 87). Other frequently seen deficits include: shortened attention span; difficulty dividing attention between competing stimuli; impaired concentration; increased distractibility; decreased speed and efficiency of information processing; decreased problem-solving ability, abstract reasoning, social judgment, and tolerance for stimulation; reduced cognitive flexibility; difficulty with integration and generalization of information; problems with initiation and goal setting; problems with organization and self-monitoring; increased anxiety, irritability, aggression, hyperactivity, and impulsivity; decreased frustration tolerance; and increased susceptibility to fatigue and stress, leading to overload and further deterioration in performance (6, 13, 16, 32, 58, 66). In addition, general overall reduction of intelligence scores on tests such as the WISC-R is usual, with scores on visuo-spatial, visual-perceptual, and visual-motor integration tasks showing more severe and sustained impairment than scores on verbal subtests (14, 28, 60, 78), possibly because of the greater reliance on old learning of the latter and the unfamiliarity and speeded performance necessary in the former. However, although functioning on verbal tasks is generally more resistant to the effects of head injury than is performance on visual-motor tasks, many studies have found long-term subtle language deficits in both expressive and receptive domains, as well as in written language (28, 46, 92).

Children with severe head injuries show a high rate of emotional or psychiatric disorders in the years after injury with a relationship seen between the development of these behavioral/psychiatric problems and the child's preaccident behavior, current intellectual level, and the presence of cognitive or psychosocial disturbance within the family system. With the exception of greater prevalence of socially disinhibited behavior, no other specific pattern of psychiatric disorder was found to differentiate head-injured from nonhead-injured children (11). However, lowered self-esteem, sadness, and frank depression are frequently observed as children become aware of many of their deficits and mourn their losses (66). Social isolation can also be an increasing problem, particularly as children get older. Children with brain injuries can often be insensitive to the needs of others, fail to pick up on important social cues, demonstrate behavioral immaturity, and generally act in ways that alienate their peers. In addition, adolescents who are now thrown back into a dependent, often infantile position, vis a vis their parents, during a phase of life when they were beginning to separate and become more independent, frequently are hostile and resentful, only heightening the stress within the family.

The recovery from brain injury in children is long and hard with the majority of gains made in the first 18 months after injury, but subtle and ongoing improvements in function expected at least up to 5 years (6, 53). Psychological evaluation should be repeated at intervals, in order to clarify the evolving process of recovered capacities and sustained deficits.

Scholastic achievement can be profoundly affected following head injury (28). The cognitive sequelae following brain injury in childhood usually require significant modifications both in the child's school setting and in the teaching style used (40). Among the modifications most frequently required are return to a smaller, more structured classroom setting where more individualized instruction is available and stimulation is reduced; the breakdown of tasks into smaller components and a reduction in task demands; teaching through areas of strength and helping to develop compensatory strategies for circumventing areas of weakness; providing external cues or memory aids to facilitate learning; modeling appropriate behaviors and reinforcement; and providing an increased opportunity for repetition and practice on all tasks to facilitate learning and integration of new material as well as relearning of old information (6, 58).

Conclusion of a Psychological Assessment

Psychological assessment should culminate in clear interpretation of data so that test findings are helpful to the family and other clinicians working with the child. Practical recommendations should be made based on the child's diagnosis and observation of individual characteristics in development, learning, and behavior. For an infant or toddler for whom global developmental problems are most likely to be discerned, psychological evaluation may suggest the need for an early intervention program. For preschoolers and school-aged children, the type of educational setting that would be most supportive and specific remedial strategies should be offered. For all children, psychological evaluation should be considered a reflection of the child's current functioning and as a baseline from which interventions are planned, and not as a statement of static abilities used to make long-range predictions. Psychological re-evaluation is usually recommended, particularly for young children and for children with changing pictures, in order to assess changing needs and to provide further diagnostic and prognostic clarification.

REFERENCES

1. Anderson E, Spain B: *The Child with Spina Bifida*. London, Methuen & Co., 1977.
2. Arter J, Jenkins J: Differential diagnosis/prescriptive teaching: A critical appraisal. *Rev Educ Res* 49:517–555, 1979.
3. Ayers J: *Sensory Integration and Learning Disorders*. Los Angeles, Western Psychological Services, 1979.
4. Bayley N: *Bayley Scales of Infant Development*. New York, The Psychological Corporation, 1969.
5. Beery K, Buktenica N: *Development Test of Visual-Motor Integration*. Chicago, Follett, 1967.
6. Begali V: *Head Injury in Children and Adolescents*. Brandon, Clinical Psychology Publishing Co., 1987.
7. Bellak L: *Manual Children's Apperception Test*, ed 4. New York, Grune & Stratton, 1961.
8. Bender L: *The Bender Visual-Motor Gestalt Test*. New York, American Orthopsychiatric Association, 1946.
9. Boll T: Minor head injury in children—out of sight but not out of mind. *J Clin Child Psychol* 12:74–80, 1983.
10. Brooks ND: Cognitive deficits. In Rosenthal M, Griffith E, Bond M, Miller JD (eds): *Rehabilitation of the Adult and Child with Traumatic Brain Injury*. Philadelphia, FA Davis, 1990.
11. Brown G, Chadwick O, Schaffer D, Rutter M, Traub M: A prospective study of children with head injuries: III, Psychiatric Sequelae. *Psychol Med* 11:63–78, 1981.
12. Burgemeister BB, Blum LH, Lorge I: *Manual: Columbia Mental Maturity Scale*, ed 3. New York, The Psychological Corporation, 1972.
13. Burns R, Cook J, Ylvisaker M: Cognitive assessment and intervention. *An Educators Manual*. Southborough, National Head Injury Foundation, 1988.
14. Chadwick O, Rutter M, Brown G, Schaffer D, Traub M: A prospective study of children with head injuries: II, Cognitive Sequelae. *Psychol Med* 11:49–61, 1981.
15. Chadwick O, Rutter M, Thompson J, Schaffer D: Intellectual performance and reading skills after localized head injury in childhood. *J Child Psychol* 22:117–139, 1981.
16. Cohen SB: Educational reintegration and programming for children with head injuries. *J Head Trauma Rehabil* 1:22–29, 1986.
17. Cook MJ, Holder-Brown L, Johnson LJ, Kilgo JL: An examination of the stability of the Bayley Scales of Infant Development with high risk infants. *J Early Intervent* 13:45–49, 1989.
18. Crothers B, Paine R: *The Natural History of Cerebral Palsy*. Cambridge, Harvard University Press, 1957.
19. Cruickshank W, Bice H, Wallen N, Lynch K: *Perception and Cerebral Palsy: Studies in Figure-Background Relationship*, ed 2. Syracuse, Syracuse University Press, 1965.
20. Delaney EA, Hopkins TF: *Examiner's Handbook: An Expanded Guide for Fourth Edition Users*. Chicago, Riverside Publishing Company, 1987.
21. DiLeo J: *Children's Drawings as Diagnostic Aids*. New York, Brunner Mazel, 1973.
22. Diller L, Gordon W, Swinyard C, Kastner S: Psychological and educational studies with spina bifida children. Project No. 5–0412, Washington, D.C., U.S. Department of Health, Education, and Welfare, U.S. Office of Education, 1969.
23. Doll E: *Vineland Social Maturity Scale*. Circle Pines, American Guidance Service, 1965.
24. Drotar D, Mortimer J, Shepherd PA, Fagan JF: Recognition memory as a method of assessing intelligence of an infant with quadriplegia. *Dev Med Child Neurol* 31:391–394, 1989.

25. DuBose R: Predictive value of infant intelligence scales with multiply handicapped children. *Am J Ment Defici* 81:388–390, 1977.
26. Dunn LM, Dunn LM: *Peabody Picture Vocabulary Test—Revised: Manual for Forms L and M*. Circle Pines, American Guidance Service, 1981.
27. Dunn L, Markwardt F: *Manual: Peabody Individual Achievement Test*. Circle Pines, American Guidance Service, 1970.
28. Ewing-Cobbs L, Fletcher J, Levin H: Neuropsychological sequelae following pediatric head injury. In Ylvisaker M (ed): *Head Injury Rehabilitation: Children and Adolescents*. San Diego, College Hill Press, 1985.
29. Fagen JF, Shepherd PA: *The Fagan Test of Infant Intelligence Training Manual*, Vol 4. Cleveland, Infantest Corporation, 1987.
30. Fagen JF, Singer LT: Infant recognition memory as a measure of intelligence. In Lipsitt LP (ed): *Advances in Infancy Research*, Vol 2. Norwood, Ablex, 1983.
31. Fantz RL: A method of studying early visual development. *Percep Motor Skills* 6:13–15, 1956.
32. Fay G, Janesheski J: Neuropsychological assessment of head injured children. *J Head Trauma Rehabil* 1:16–21, 1986.
33. French J: *Manual: Pictorial Test of Intelligence*. Boston, Houghton Mifflin, 1964.
34. Gesell A: *Gesell Development Schedules*. New York, Psychological Corporation, 1940.
35. Gray W: *Standardized Oral Reading Paragraphs*. Indianapolis, Bobbs Merrill, 1967.
36. Griffiths R: *The Abilities of Young Children: A Comprehensive System of Mental Measurement for the First Eight Years of Life*. High Wycombe, The Test Agency, 1970.
37. Grossman H: *Manual on Terminology and Classification in Mental Retardation* (Revised ed). Washington, D.C., American Association on Mental Deficiency, 1977.
38. Haeussermann E: Evaluating the developmental level of preschool children handicapped by cerebral palsy. *J Genet Psychol* 80:3–23, 1952.
39. Hammill D, Bartel N: *Teaching Children with Learning and Behavior Problems*. Boston, Allyn and Bacon, 1975.
40. Heiseken O, Kaste M: Late prognosis of severe brain injury in children. In *Dev Med Child Neurol* 16:11–14, 1974.
41. Hiskey MS: *Manual: Hiskey-Nebraska Test of Learning Aptitude*. Lincoln, University of Nebraska Press, 1966.
42. Hopkins T, Bice H, Colton M: *Evaluation and Education of the Cerebral Palsy Child: New Jersey Study*, ed 2. Washington, D.C., International Council for Exceptional Children, 1955.
43. Horn DG, Lorch EP, Lorch RF, Culatta B: Distractibility and vocabulary deficits in children with spina bifida and hydrocephalus. *Dev Med Child Neurol* 27:713–720, 1985.
44. Jaffee K, Brink J, Hays R, Chorazy A: Specific problems associated with pediatric head injury. In Rosenthal M, Griffith E, Bond M, and Miller J (eds): *Rehabilitation of the Adult and Child with Traumatic Brain Injury*, ed 2. Philadelphia, FA Davis, 1990.
45. Jastak S, Wilkinson GS: *The Wide Range Achievement Test—Revised*. Wilmington, Jastak Associates, 1984.
46. Jordan F, Ozanne A, Murdoch B: Long-term speech and language disorders subsequent to closed head injury in children. *Brain Injury* 2:179–185, 1988.
47. Kaufman A, Kaufman N: *Clinical Evaluation of Young Children with the McCarthy Scales*. New York, Grune & Stratton, 1977.
48. Kaufman A, Kaufman N: *Kaufman Assessment Battery for Children*. Circle Pines, American Guidance Service, 1983.
49. Kearsley R: Cognitive assessment of the handicapped infant: The need for an alternate approach. *Am J Orthopsychiatr* 51:43–54, 1981.
50. Kennard MA: Cortical reorganization of motor function. *Arch Neurol Psychiatr* 48:227–240, 1942.

51. Klapper Z, Birch H: A fourteen year follow-up study of cerebral palsy: Intellectual change and stability. *Am J Orthopsychiatr* 37:540–547, 1967.

52. Klapper Z, Werner H: Developmental deviations in brain injured members of pairs of identical twins. *Quart J Child Behav* 2:288–313, 1950.

53. Klonoff H, Low D, Clark C: Head injuries in children: A prospective five year follow up. *J Neurol Neurosurg Psychiatr* 40:1211–1219, 1977.

54. Knobloch H, Pasamanick B: *Developmental Diagnosis: The Evaluation and Management of Normal and Abnormal Neuropsychological Development in Infancy and Early Childhood*, ed 3. New York, Harper & Row, 1974.

55. Koppitz E: *Psychological Evaluation of Children's Human Figure Drawings*. New York, Grune & Stratton, 1968.

56. Koppitz E: *The Bender Gestalt Test for Young Children*. New York, Grune & Stratton, 1973.

57. Koppitz E: *Visual Aural Digit Span Test*. New York, Grune & Stratton, 1973.

58. Lehr E: *Psychological Management of Traumatic Brain Injuries in Children and Adolescents*. Rockville, Aspen, 1990.

59. Leiter R: *The Leiter International Performance Scale*. Chicago, Stoelting, 1969.

60. Levin H, Eisenberg H: Neuropsychological impairment after closed head injury in children and adolescents. *J Pediat Psychol* 4:389–401, 1979.

61. Levine SC, Huttenlocher P, Banich MT, Duda E: Factors affecting cognitive functioning of hemiplegic children. *Dev Med Child Neurol* 29:27–35, 1987.

62. Machover K: *Personality Projection in the Drawing of the Human Figure: A Method of Personality Investigation*. Springfield, Charles C Thomas, 1949.

63. Maxfield K, Buchholz S: *Manual: Maxfield-Buchholz Scale of Social Maturity for use with Preschool Blind Children*. New York, American Foundation for the Blind, 1957.

64. McCall RB: The development of intellectual functioning in infancy and the prediction of later IQ. In Osofsky J (ed): *Handbook of Infant Development*. New York, John Wiley & Sons, 1979.

65. McCarthy D: *Manual: McCarthy Scales of Children's Abilities*. New York, Psychological Corporation, 1972.

66. McGuire TL, Rosenberg MB: Behavioral and psychosocial sequelae of pediatric head injury. *J Head Trauma Rehabil* 1:1–6, 1986.

67. McLone DG, Czyzrwski D, Raimondi AJ, Sommers RL: CNS infection as a leading factor in the intelligence of children with mylomeningocele. *Pediatrics* 70:338–342, 1982.

68. Meichenbaum DH, Goodman J: Training impulsive children to talk to themselves. *J Abnormal Psychol* 77:115–126, 1971.

69. Meisels SJ, Provence S: *Screening and Assessment: Guidelines for Identifying Young Disabled and Developmentally Vulnerable Children and Their Families*. Washington, D.C., National Center for Clinical Infant Programs, 1989.

70. Mullen EM: *Mullen Scales of Early Learning*. Cranston, T.O.T.A.L. Child, 1989.

71. Nihira K, Foster R, Shellhaas M, Leland N: *AAMD Adaptive Behavior Scales* (revised ed). Washington, D.C., American Association on Mental Deficiency, 1974.

72. Pang D: Pathological correlates of neurobehavioral syndromes following closed head injury. In Ylvisaker M (ed): *Head Injury Rehabilitation in Children and Adolescents*. San Diego, College Hill Press, 1985.

73. Raven J: *Raven's Progressive Matrices*. Dumfries, Scotland, Crichton Royal, 1958.

74. Rorschach H: *Psychodiagnostics*, ed 2. New York, Grune & Stratton, 1942.

75. Rose SA, Wallace IF: Individual differences in infants' information processing: Reliability, stability and prediction. *Child Devel* 59:1177–1197, 1988.

76. Rourke BP, Bakker DJ, Fisk JL, Strang JD: *Child Neuropsychology: An Introduction to Theory, Research and Clinical Practice*. New York, Guilford Press, 1983.

77. Rutter M: Psychological sequelae of brain damage in children. *Am J Psychiatr* 138:1533–1544, 1981.

78. Rutter M, Chadwick O, Schaffer D: Head injury. In Rutter M (ed): *Developmental Neuropsychiatry*. New York, Guilford, 1983.
79. Shepherd PA, Fagen JF: Visual pattern detection and recognition memory in children with profound mental retardation. *Internat Rev Res Ment Retard* 10:31-60, 1981.
80. Sontheimer D: Visual information processing in infancy. *Dev Med Child Neurol* 31:787-796, 1989.
81. Spache GD: *Spache Diagnostic Reading Scales*. Monterey, Test Bureau, 1963.
82. Sparrow SS, Balla DA, Cicchetti DV: *Vineland Adaptive Behavior Scales*. Circle Pines, American Guidance Service, 1984.
83. Terman L, Merrill MA: *Manual: Stanford-Binet Intelligence Scales, Form L-M* (revision 3). Boston, Houghton Mifflin, 1973.
84. Thomas H: Psychological assessment instruments for use with human infants. *Merrill Palmer Quarterly* 16:179-223, 1970.
85. Thorndike RL, Hagen EP, Sattler JM: *The Stanford Binet Intelligence Scale: Fourth Edition: Guide for Administering and Scoring*. Chicago, Riverside, 1986.
86. Vanderveer B, Schweid E: Infant assessment: Stability of mental function in young retarded children. *Am J Ment Defic* 79:1-4, 1974.
87. Vogenthaler DR: An overview of head injury: Its consequences and rehabilitation. *Brain Injury* 1:113-127, 1987.
88. Wechsler D: *Wechsler Intelligence Scale for Children—Revised*. New York, Psychological Corporation, 1974.
89. Wechsler D: *Wechsler Preschool and Primary Scales of Intelligence—Revised*. San Antonio, Psychological Corporation, Harcourt Brace Jovanovich, 1989.
90. Wepman J: *Auditory Discrimination Test*. Chicago, Language Research Associates, 1958.
91. Williamson GG, Szczepanski M (eds): *Children with Spina Bifida: Early Intervention and Preschool Programming*. Baltimore: Brookes, 1987.
92. Ylvisaker M: Language and communication disorders following pediatric head injury. *J Head Trauma Rehabil* 1:48-56, 1986.
93. Zelazo P: Reactivity to perceptual-cognitive events: Application for infant assessment. In Kearsley R, Segal I (eds): *Infants at Risk: Assessment of Cognitive Functioning*. Hillside, Lawrence Erlbaum Associates, 1979

4

Development and Disorders of Communication

LYDIA H. SOIFER

"Conceivably, the only true and unique disorder of man as man is a disorder in his language spoken, written, or perceived."

Travis (119)

Communication

Communication takes many forms, a look, a gesture, or an intonation pattern that contains the real message, the first word, or those rarely occurring well-chosen words that cut right to the heart of the matter. Simple or complex, communication is so characteristic of the human condition that unless the act is interrupted or the skill is impaired, we usually take it for granted.

Essential to the communication process is the setting in which the exchange takes place, the expectations of the speaker and the listener, the knowledge that they share, and the extralinguistic clues, such as gesture and intonation, that are used. There is communication without speech. At times, speech and language are neither necessary nor sufficient for communication and simple gestures may be more efficient.

Our most common communicative experiences are speaking and listening. There are those, however, for whom speaking and/or listening is difficult and, in some cases, impossible.

Language Development

Language is the highest form of communication consisting of production and comprehension. Language production is the process by which speakers encode meaning into messages. Comprehension refers to the processes by which listeners obtain meaning. Speech represents the spoken aspects of the communication act, what is voiced and articulated in the service of oral communication.

88

Traditionally, it was believed that comprehension preceded production in normal language development. A significant body of literature (10, 51, 56, 81) has emerged that counters this view. In fact, comprehension varies as a function of several factors, including context and linguistic complexity. Moreover, regarding language production, imitation had long been considered an important part of learning to speak. Once again, recent research has countered this view (10, 11) and suggests that imitation has less importance in linguistic acquisition than previously thought. In fact, spontaneous production exceeds imitation in many instances.

Bloom and Lahey (12) offer an excellent definition by stating that "language is a code whereby ideas about the world are represented through a conventional system of arbitrary signals for communication." A code is some means of representing one thing with another. A code is generally made up of symbols that represent objects, events, and relationships, but are separate from the meaning they stand for. Symbols can be manual, spoken, or graphic, as in sign, oral, or written language. In conventional spoken and written language, the code symbols are words. Language represents our ideas about the world, our knowledge about objects, events, and relationships. Language is systematic. We come to learn and sometimes need to be taught rules for grammar and spelling. Language is also conventional. Speakers of the same language have a shared knowledge and have made a tacit agreement within the community of users for the rules of the language. Finally, the function of language is to communicate, to give and to receive information, to maintain contact with others, and to help accomplish our goals.

Using the definition of Bloom and Lahey (12) as a basis, it is possible to discuss speech and language as integrated parts of communication. The role of language is to communicate regardless of the code symbol system used. Speech is one manifestation of this function when verbal symbols are used.

LANGUAGE COMPONENTS

Content, form, and use are the three major components of language. For the purpose of this chapter, each component will be dealt with individually, although in actual function they are inseparable.

Content

Content conveys an intended meaning that is presented in the form of words or other symbols used in a given context. Language content or semantics is determined by the ideas a person has to express. It is related to culture, experience, and intellectual level. Therefore, words and sentence structures have different meanings for different users. Word meaning, sentence meaning, and nonliteral meaning are essential components of semantics. Word meaning refers to the number and type of words that one understands and produces. Sentence meaning is involved with the relationship between and among words in a sentence and across sentences as well. Contextual meaning is derived across sentences as we speak or read. The nonliteral aspects of semantic knowledge include idioms ("He hit the roof"), metaphors ("She's as cool as a cucumber"), proverbs ("A bird in hand is worth two in the bush"), and jokes. A mature aspect of semantic development, nonliteral knowledge alerts us that language does not always mean what it says.

The language of children is not the same as adult language. It is not an immature version of adult language because words have different meanings for children as they acquire more mature semantic knowledge. We are familiar with stories of young children in the process of language acquisition who produce "poetic" references in the attempt to communicate their understanding of the world. An example is the 2-yr-old child who comments during a rainstorm, "Mommy, the sky is crying!" Less poetic but similarly strong evidence of the differences in ideas and their reflection in semantics is the language of the 1-yr-old child who refers to all furry, four-legged creatures as "doggy."

Semantics as an emerging function is most closely related to cognitive development. Semantic and cognitive knowledge differ in a subtle but significant way. Cognitive knowledge becomes semantic when it is linked to language (18).

Just as semantics is an indication of ideas about the world, there are developmental similarities in the language content of children and differences from that of adults. Experience and environment account for the individual variations and for those related to cultural background in the vocabulary and concept development of children (13, 84, 107).

Form

Language form can be defined in terms of apparent, observable features of production. The form of an utterance consists of phonetic and grammatical characteristics. For verbalization, form has three components: (a) phonology or sound systems; (b) morphology or meaning in words and inflections; and (c) syntax and grammar, the way in which the units of meaning are combined.

Phonology. The sound system of a language is phonology. In English, there are 44 base sounds or phonemes as well as multiple variations of certain phonemes, particularly vowels. These variations account for regional dialects. The phonemes are patterned into acceptable sequences to form words (Table 4.1).

Traditionally, phonological acquisition was perceived as a unit by unit process of learning each phoneme in a developmental sequence. Recently, we have come to understand that phonological development is not isolated or discrete but integrally related to the language system as a whole. Phonological development progresses with physical maturation, the mastery of

Table 4.1.
Common Phonological Processes

Process	Example	
Syllable structure processes— simplication of words to either consonant-vowel (CV) syllables or CVCV structures	1. reduplication 2. final consonant deletion 3. cluster reduction 4. deletion of unstressed syllables	/dæ dæ/ for daddy /kʌ/ for cup /tɑr/ for star /efɪnt/ for elephant
Substitution processes—one sound is substituted for another depending upon the position in a word	1. fronting 2. stopping 3. gliding	/tʌp/ for cup; /dʌn/ for gun /dʊt/ for juice /wæ bɪt/ for rabbit
Assimilation processes—two phonemes in a word become alike	1. consonant harmony 2. prevocalic voicing	/gɔ gi/ for doggy /dʌb/ for tub

sound features, phonological processes that reflect the linking of sounds to words and meanings, and the growth of semantic and syntactic rule knowledge and ability. Recent theories suggest that there are phonological or natural processes by which children work to master adult level productions. These processes are rule governed and form the basis of the sound sequences that children produce. Table 4.1 identifies common phonological processes in young children. It is now understood that children do not learn separate sounds. Sounds are acquired in relationship to one another and in the framework of the word (36, 54, 55). The phonological system is integral to sound production and later on to spelling and reading. A youngster may be nonverbal but still needs to meet the requirements of a phonological system for understanding. Table 4.2 offers a summary of the sequence of sound acquisition.

Table 4.2.
Phonemic Acquisition—Age at Which 75% of Children Tested Correctly Articulated Consonant Sounds[a]

Age	Sounds
2	m, n, h, p, ŋ (riNG)
2.4	f, j, k, d
2.8	w, b, t
3	g, s
3.4	r, l
3.8	ʃ (shy), tʃ (chin)
4	ð (father), ʒ (measure)
4+	dʒ(jar), θ(thin), v, z

Data from Prather and associates (88).

Morphology and Syntax. The two aspects of language form that create the grammar of a language are morphology and syntax. Bolinger (16, 17) defines a morpheme as the basic unit of language. Through syntax or the way in which words are arranged to form sentences, morphemes are combined, sequenced, and altered in order to code meaning with a particular intention in mind. Morphemes may be unbound (free) or bound. Unbound morphemes can stand alone, such as "argue" or "table." Bound morphemes comprise the affix system of English, including prefixes and suffixes and must be attached to another morpheme. Through the use of bound morphemes, "argue" may become "argument," an example of change in grammatical class, in this instance from verb to noun. Mastery of the morphological system is progressive and explains some of the grammatical errors made by young children. Table 4.3 is a summary of the earliest acquired grammatical morphemes.

Syntax is also complex and intimately related to the systems of semantics and phonology. The rules of syntax dictate how we are able to create a variety of sentence structures and combine words to change meaning.

Observe the following sequence of words:

A tall lady built the tower.

lady the tall a built tower

The first is easier to remember; furthermore, given the second sentence, one might be inclined to rearrange it into an order that gives it meaning. The first is a meaningful sentence that reflects a series of recognition, recall, and comprehension processes. The second is a word string. Knowledge of syntax allows us to vary the way we express the same idea with different emphasis as in the following sentences:

John hit the ball.

The ball was hit by John.

It was John who hit the ball.

In normal development, children are not taught simple declarative sentences, passive constructions, question forms, clausal relations, noun-verb agreement, or any of the transformations necessary to create an infinite number of sentences. They are able to devise these rules by exposure to the language around them. Most children accomplish this in an orderly fashion making predictable errors on the way to mastery. The process begins at birth and continues throughout the early years of life. Table 4.4 shows examples of sentences in early stages of language development.

Use

Language use or pragmatics has been defined both as "the rules governing the use of language in context" (5) and "when to say what, and how to whom"

Table 4.3.
Brown's 14 Grammatical Morphemes[a]

Morpheme	Example
Present progressive (Be + verb(ing))	I am eating
Plural	
(Regular)	Boys
(Irregular)	Men
Preposition	
In	Kermit in there.
On	Doggie on chair.
Past irregular	I went
Possessive	
(Regular)	Tommy's
(Irregular)	Mine
Uncontractible copula	I am a girl
Articles	
(A, some, the)	the car
Past regular	
(-ed)	I kissed it.
Third person singular	
Regular (-s)	He eats the cake.
Third person singular	
Irregular	Daddy has it
Uncontractible auxiliary	I am walking
Contractible copula	I'm a girl.
Contractible auxiliary	I'm going.

[a]Data from Brown (20).

Table 4.4.
Early Sentence Types[a]

Three years
  Possessive: daddy's name
  Negations: I am not here (emerging)
  Interrogative: Is he sleeping? (emerging)
  Wh-Question: What is that? (emerging)
  Contraction: He's watching.
  Imperative: Get out of here!
  Progressive: He is going.
  Do: I did read it.
  Adjective: I have a black dog.
  Pronoun: I was mad.
  And conjunction: Peter is here and you are there.
  Infinitive Complement: I want to play.
Four years
  Conjunction deletion: I see a lipstick and a comb.
  Relative clause: I don't know what he's doing.
  Mastery of negatives and questions.
Five years
  Tag questions: She's here, isn't she?

Data from Menyuk (75).

(52). The pragmatic view focuses on the social dynamics in language use. Emphasis is placed on social interaction and relationships. These are essential as they provide the framework within which content and form relations are understood and produced. Language is a vehicle for socializing and directing the behavior of others (21). Using language in social contexts involves rules for language functions and the choice of linguistic codes for communicating those functions (12). Language functions reflect a communicator's intent. Examples of communicative intentions are greeting, informing, requesting, inquiring, clarifying. To code adequately or to represent an intent, a communicator must be aware of the listener's needs and the context in which they are interacting. When greeting an ambassador, "How do you do?" is appropriate, whereas, "Hi, honey!" is more apt for a 2-yr-old.

Pragmatics is also concerned with conversational competence. Discourse or conversational skills include initiating a topic, coherent organization of utterances, turn-taking, topic maintenance, and appropriate eye-gaze behaviors, to identify but a few (44, 95, 103).

The ability to control form, content, and use in communication is a highly sophisticated skill that has its rudiments in infancy. Dore (33) and Halliday (45) identified several language functions in children. These functions, first observed in infancy, include the instrumental ("I want", "I need"), regulatory ("Do this"), interactional ("Me and you"), and personal ("Here I come") categories. Between the ages of 2 and 5 yr, children expand their uses of language and the number of functions they can control. Categories of language functions used by children 2 to 5 yr (32, 79) and 3 to 7 yr (118) reflect the great variety of uses and functions available to young children. Table 4.5 is a display of these categories.

The mastery of language entails integration and organization of form, content, and use. Progress toward competence includes a knowledge of the cognitive and linguistic rules of form and content as well as the social rules for use in a variety of situations. A disturbance of any of these components may lead to a communicative breakdown. An articulation disorder (disturbance of form), word retrieval difficulties (disturbance of content), or inappropriate responses (disturbance of use) are examples of the possibilities that may result in communicative failure.

CONTRIBUTORY FACTORS IN LANGUAGE DEVELOPMENT

Language learning is based on the acquisition and organization of information derived from experience and interaction with the world. In the normal process of acquiring the rules of language and interpersonal function of communication, we depend on having an array of support systems and functional abilities. Thus, motor, sensory, and cognitive deficits may result in limitations in the information obtained. Central nervous system damage may interfere with processing and organization of information. Affective disorders may curtail interaction with the world. Hearing and the physical

Table 4.5.
Most Frequent Communicative Functions of Children 2 to 7 Years Old

Communicative function of 2-to 5-year-olds[a]

 Moerk[a]
   Imitating
   Asking a question
   Expressing a need
   Answering a question
   Encoding from picture books
   Describing objects or events
   Describing own acts
   Describing plans
   Describing a past experience

 Dore[b]
   Requests information, action, or acknowledgment
   Responds to requests
   Describes
   States facts, rules, attitudes, feelings, and beliefs
   Regulates contact and conversation
   Miscellaneous (complains, jokes, teases)
Communicative functions of 3- to 7-year-olds
 Tough[c]
   Thinking and problem-solving
   Reasoning
   Relating events to one another
   Engage in complex imaginative play
   Control own behavior

[a]Data from Moerk (70).
[b]Data from Dore (33).
[c]Data from Tough (118).

capability to produce speech are necessary for the development of verbal communication.

When any of the essential support systems is impaired, either individually or in combination, language and communication may be impeded or interrupted. It is, however, possible to compensate for deficits and disruptions as attested to by the many physically and intellectually handicapped children and adults who have, through skillful intervention, developed alternative means of communication.

Auditory Function

Hearing is the primary sensory area involved in language acquisition (63, 74). Hearing is a process of energy conversion that transforms sound waves into electrical and chemical impulses. The process is mediated by the three anatomic parts of the ear and by the pathways of the eighth cranial nerve and its supranuclear connections to the auditory centers of the brain. Hearing loss may be either conductive, sensorineural, or mixed. Additionally, auditory dysfunction may exist despite intact peripheral hearing mechanisms. This type of dysfunction is categorized as a central auditory disorder

(110). Central auditory processing defects may have significant impact on the learning disabilities exhibited by some school-aged children. Certain academic problems may have their basis in listening difficulties or inadequate understanding of auditory information. It is common for children with central auditory processing disorder to have deficient comprehension and memory for auditory information (66). A conductive hearing loss or impairment is associated with external or middle ear pathology resulting in decreased hearing sensitivity that usually affects all frequencies of sound. Conductive hearing losses are generally amenable to medical intervention. A sensorineural hearing loss or impairment is associated with pathology of the inner ear, eighth nerve, brain stem, and/or supranuclear auditory structures. This type of hearing loss results in a more selective deviation from normal hearing acuity and may lead to impairment of auditory discrimination as well. Most sensorineural hearing losses are irreversible and not amenable to medical intervention.

Speech Production

Speech is a complex motor act that requires the synchronization of respiration, phonation, and articulation.

Breathing. At rest, breathing is rhythmic with inhalation and exhalation approximately equal in duration. For speech, however, this pattern is altered and exhalation, which provides the air flow for phonation, must be prolonged and sustained. Audible speech production results as the exhaled air flow is modified by movements of the vocal tract.

Phonation. Voice production or phonation is accomplished through coordination of breathing and laryngeal valving to initiate vocal fold vibrations. During regular breathing, the vocal folds are abducted. For sound production they are moved to various degrees of adduction. Aphonia may be related to impaired respiratory control, laryngeal function, or both.

Articulation. Coordinated motion of the muscles of the mandible, lips, tongue, and velum is required when articulating. The same muscles participate in the vegetative functions of sucking, chewing, and swallowing. However, the movements used for articulation are finer, more rapid, and occur in a greater variety of combinations. They must be controlled independently yet be used with considerable temporal overlap.

Traditionally, speech production errors were viewed in terms of omission, substitution, and distortion of sounds. Recent research on the acquisition of phonological rules has described a series of processes operating in the development of mastery, including syllable deletion, assimilation of sounds, and simplification of consonant clusters (53).

Diagnosis and Remediation of Communication Disorders

The collective term of communication disorders includes a diverse group of language and speech deficits caused by a variety of underlying conditions.

This discussion will concentrate on disorders that occur among children with physical handicaps.

ASSESSMENT

Evaluation of speech and language disorders is based on knowledge of normal development. In the physically handicapped child, assessment should take into consideration the neurologic deficit, motor and sensory function, and cognitive development.

Diagnostic procedures are best viewed in the context of process and goal setting for remediation. Language is a complex, interrelated, dynamic system. Attempting to isolate it by individual skill or function sharply narrows the perspective in which language is viewed. Evaluators must be vigilant regarding the interpretation of standardized test results based on norms irrelevant to children whose life experiences are vastly different than the population used for standardization. Formal measures cannot be used reliably and validly for severely or physically handicapped children. The diagnostician must ask three relevant questions prior to an evaluation (77): *Why* are we assessing the child?; *What* are we going to assess?; and *How* are we going to assess the child? Children are assessed to identify potential problems in their development or to define existing problems. Such a definition establishes baseline functioning and permits educators and therapists to measure change within a teaching program. What is assessed is traditionally the language systems of phonology, morphology, syntax and semantics, and the language processes: comprehension, production, pragmatics (communicative functions and conversational competence), and cognition.

Particularly relevant to the needs of the physically handicapped children is the question of "how" we are going to assess language and communication skills. Miller (76) advocates a child-centered approach in which no child is viewed as untestable, an important consideration when dealing with youngsters who have multiple disabilities. Shane (108) suggested a functional communication assessment considering the basic physical requirements, affective needs, significant persons, objects, and events.

The use of standardized tests for all children has come under criticism for the absence of appropriate context (28, 94). Moreover, the vast range of skills and functions interacting in effective language and communication defies containment in one test. Another consideration is the wide range of variables that will affect a "nonstandard" child's performance on standardized testing. These include the testing environment and the tester, as well as attention, memory, motivation and motor, sensory, and perceptual deficits of the child. Standardized testing has limitations in the actual assessment of dynamic language processes and very frequently assesses metalinguistic knowledge (94). Nonetheless, standardized tests are widely used. Table 4.6 lists tests frequently used in language evaluations.

Under these circumstances, developmental scales, nonstandardized tests

Table 4.6.
Frequently Used Standardized Tests for Language Evaluation[a]

	Expressive	Receptive
Form Phonology	Templin-Darley Tests of Articulation (116,117) Assessment Link between Phonology and Articulation (ALPHA) (69) Phonological Process Analysis (122)	Goldman-Fristoe-Woodstock Auditory Discrimination (43) Auditory Discrimination Test (123) Test of Awareness of Language Segments (104)
Morphology	Northwestern Syntax Screening Test (NSST) (68) Grammatic Closure Subtest, Illinois Test of Psycholinguistic Abilities (ITPA) (62)	Northwestern Syntax Screening Test (68) Test of Auditory Comprehension of Language (24)
Syntax	Northwestern Syntax Screening Test (68) Development Sentence Types (67) Patterned Elicitation Syntax Screening Test (130)	Miller-Yoder Test of Grammatical Competence (78) Test of Auditory Comprehension Language (24)
Content Vocabulary	Vocabulary Subtest, Wechsler Intelligence Test for Children-Revised (121) Auditory Association Subtest, Illinois Test of Psycholinguistic Abilities (62) Verbal Expression Subtest, Illinois Test of Psycholoinguistic Abilities (62) The Word Test (60) The Adolescent Word Test (131) Expressive One Word-Picture Vocabulary Test (41) Test of Word Finding (43)	Peabody Picture Vocabulary Test (35) Boehm Basic Concept Inventory (15) Language Processing Test (97) Assessing Semantic Skills through Everyday Themes (ASSET) (4)
Use	Stocker Probe (114) Test of Language Competence (125)	

[a]Numbers in parentheses refer to references.

(often teacher made), and behavioral observation become essential to the diagnostic process. Developmental scales presume that the course of language development is predictable. While this is generally so, the course may be hindered by numerous factors from prematurity to physical handicap. The Early Language Milestone Scale (ELM) (26) covers a variety of communicative behaviors typically occurring in children from birth to 36 months of age. This is a screening device. Thus, a failure in one of the three evaluated areas (auditory-receptive, expressive, visual) indicates the need for further assessment. Other developmental scales for older children include the Environmental Language Inventory (71) and the Preschool Language Scale (132).

Nonstandardized testing is often a combination of tasks derived from standard measures and teacher- or clinician-devised procedures. Such a design is flexible, allowing for consideration of individual needs, physically, neurologically, cognitively, and environmentally. Free speech samples, elicited production, comprehension, and elicited imitation are helpful means for evaluating language behaviors (76).

Behavioral observations can be as simple as observing a child and making notations in regard to performance across time and contexts. The value of behavioral observations in evaluating communicative interaction and play behaviors as part of language acquisition is demonstrated in the recent development of detailed behavioral observation instruments. DuBose (34) developed guidelines for behavioral observations during assessment that included informal assessment of fine and gross motor skills, language, socialization, and self-help skills. More recently, "low structured observation" (25) of caretaker-child interaction by videotape and subsequent review has been included as part of the evaluation procedure for at-risk infants and toddlers. Such a procedure permits the measurement of specific affective and communication interactions as they occur. Weatherby et al. (124) developed a system for analyzing communicative functions in normal children. The children were studied from prelinguistic to multiworded stages of development. Play behavior is recognized as both procursor and partner to language development. Using play with specific materials as a constant, scales have been devised to record interpersonal behaviors and language milestones (25).

In addition to the possibility of a primary language disorder, hearing loss, mental retardation, and experiential deficits must be considered. When a child appears to understand but oral responses are inadequate, the diagnostic possibilities of sensorimotor deficits should be differentiated. When speech production is defective, the processes of respiratory control, laryngeal action, articulation, and their coordination should be investigated.

HEARING IMPAIRMENT

Hearing loss may range from mild to profound and affect a range of frequencies. Table 4.7 shows the classes of hearing loss according to the degree of difficulty in understanding speech.

In order to define a hearing impairment, several factors need to be considered: degree of hearing loss in terms of sensitivity to pure tone; time of onset, whether the loss is congenital or acquired; causative factors, such as injury, infection, structural or neurological deficit, heredity, or other defects; site of dysfunction in the auditory system; and social factors including environment, emotional status, and intelligence. It is difficult to describe the speech and language behaviors of hearing impaired children. Quigley and Kretsch-

Table 4.7.
Classes of Hearing Loss According to Degree of Difficulty in Understanding Speech

dB	Degree of Difficulty in Understanding Speech
<25	No significant difficulty with faint speech
25–40	Slight difficulty only with faint speech
40–55	Mild difficulty with normal speech
55–70	Marked difficulty with loud speech
70–90	Severe handicap—can understand only shouted or amplified speech
90 +	Extreme handicap—usually cannot understand even amplified speech

[a]Data from Silverman (109).

mer (90) consider numerous factors that influence language development in the hearing impaired. These factors include issues of age, degree and slope of hearing loss, amount and type of habilitation, the nature of the language (English or American Sign Language), and communication input (manual or oral).

Northern and Downs (85) recommend that children be fitted with hearing aids as soon as possible after the diagnosis of hearing loss. The determination of which ear to aid is dependent upon several factors including the degree of hearing loss, type of hearing loss, nature of the improvement in the child's social and functional communication ability, and tolerance for amplification. Most crucial of all, however, is the early identification of hearing loss, as the process of language acquisition begins at birth. Approaches to the habilitation of hearing-impaired children have evolved from a greater understanding of language acquisition processes in normal-hearing children. This includes a shift in emphasis to include the social-pragmatic needs of effective communication (64).

The language of hearing-impaired children varies from their peers with normal auditory acuity. The most dramatic finding in the literature that considers language comprehension skills of hearing-impaired children is that a majority do not develop age-appropriate language skills (100). Deficits in sentence structure and vocabulary, distortions in speech production, and pragmatic deficits are consistently observed. Multiple meaning words, verbalization of abstractions, and the complexity of language structure are additional areas of concern in the language of the hearing-impaired child. Studies of hearing-impaired youngsters (91, 98) indicate severe delay rather than deviation in the development of syntactic structures among deaf children.

Although hearing-impaired youngsters may have an adequate store of information and an ability to interact for communication, they often lack the language form to convey content. Sign language is the commonly used substitute language form in these cases. The most widely used system is the American Sign Language (ASL), which will be discussed in conjunction with intervention strategies.

The last decade has brought enormous change to the technology of amplification and use of residual hearing in hearing-impaired children. The use of cochlear implants (46) and artificial hearing devices (86) has opened new vistas for early intervention, improved speech production, and the ultimate quality of written language and reading comprehension.

MENTAL RETARDATION

Many studies have been undertaken in the attempt to understand the differences between the language of retarded and nonretarded children. Most of the studies investigated various aspects of form; phonology (19), morphology (31), and syntax (65, 102). The quantitative results showed some differences but qualitative comparisons suggest strong similarities. The current view is that retarded children acquire language in the same sequence as their nonretarded peers but at a slower rate (129). Basically, cognitive development is seen as a pacer of language acquisition. Thus, the general slowness characteristic of retardation is apparent in language development as well. This is an essential issue from the viewpoint of language training, which can be modeled after the milestones and sequence of linguistic development established for nonretarded children.

There are, however, qualitative differences. Naremore and Dever (83) and Baer (3) reported that the language of older children with retardation is not equivalent to that of younger, nonretarded children with the same mental age. There are differences in linguistic complexity, hesitation phenomenon, and style. Additionally, the mental age concept is an abstraction that cannot account for differences in age and the quality of experience, particularly when comparing normal and deviant populations. Progress in our understanding of the nature of language development to include social and contextual considerations has influenced the way in which language training programs have been conducted (112). Training has been extended to include interpersonal communication needs with consideration of emotional and social development, contextual variables, and the need for generalization (22). Systems to enhance the communication skills of retarded persons include aspects of augmentative communication from manual communication to computer-assisted programs (23).

SPEECH DISORDERS

Speech disorders represent defective development of language form. Language function is a prerequisite of speech acquisition but delayed speech can also hinder language development.

In children with neuromuscular disability, speech disorders may arise as a result of aberrations in respiratory control, phonation, articulation, or any combination of these three processes. Commonly seen breathing problems (82) are rapid respiratory rate, shallow inspiration, difficulty in controlling prolonged exhalation, reverse breathing, involuntary movements, or weakness of the respiratory musculature. Disturbances of phonation may be caused by adductor or abductor spasm of the vocal folds. Poor control and incoordination of the lips, tongue, palate, and mandible lead to disorders of articulation.

A general description of the speech patterns of children with physical disabilities classified on the basis of neurological signs was presented by Berry and Eisenson (6). Spastic speech is characterized by severe articulation problems due to inability to produce graded, synchronous movements of the oropharyngeal structures. The rate of speech production is labored and vocal inflections are lacking. Athetosis is accompanied by a shallow, irregular breathing pattern. Asynchrony of respiration with phonation attempted on inspiration is also common. Phonation and articulation defects range from severe to mild; complete mutism to slight lingual awkwardness representing the two extremes of the spectrum. Attempts to characterize "athetoid speech" defy stereotypes. Continual involuntary shifts in muscle tone and the involvement of muscle sets unrelated to particular movements necessary for speech are common to athetosis. Tongue and jaw movements may be particularly affected. As consonant production is primarily a function of tongue movement, variations in "athetoid speech" may be considerable in individual cases. In ataxia, rhythm is disrupted and articulation may be slurred lapsing into unintelligibility. Table 4.8 summarizes the diagnostic evaluation of speech disorders in children with neuromuscular dysfunction. It is important to realize that the nature and degree of speech production difficulty varies along a continuum (61).

Articulation disorders may accompany neuromuscular disabilities, mental retardation, hearing impairment, or other types of neurologic dysfunction. Those caused by a neurologic deficit affecting the articulatory musculature are called dysarthrias. The mechanism of these disorders may entail weakness of the elevators of the mandible, weakness or incoordination of the muscles of the lips, slow or absent mobility, or involuntary movements of the tongue. Recent research on adult subjects with cerebral palsy and dysarthria (87) showed that abnormalities are similar to those described in children, specifically, inaccurate anterior lingual placement, imprecision of fricative sounds, and inability to produce sounds at the extremes of the vowel quadrant.

Dysarthria must be distinguished from verbal apraxia, a frequently observed speech disorder following brain dysfunction. The mechanism of verbal apraxia is a deficit in the volitional sequencing of movements necessary for speech production. Crystal (27) describes it as "the patient aims to say one sequence of sounds and another comes out." Although some patients may experience both apraxic and dysarthric difficulties, these two conditions may be differentiated on the basis of several features shown in Table 4.9.

Table 4.8.
Evaluating Respiration, Phonation, and Articulation

I. Respiration—breathing patterns
  1. Does the child inhale upon request?
  2. Does the child retain air?
  3. Does the child whisper?
  4. Does the child alternate retention and phonation on a single exhalation (e.g., a-a-a-a-)?
  5. Does the child exhibit reversed breathing or involuntary movement (at rest, during speech)?
  6. Does the rate of inhalation/exhalation exceed 20 bpm?

II. Phonation—laryngeal function
  1. Does the child have adductor spasms resulting in difficulty initiating phonation or an abrupt cessation of phonation?
  2. Does the child have abductor spasms resulting in a breathy voice pattern?
  3. Does the child have pitch, loudness, and quality changes in his or her voice due to changes in tension?
  4. Does the child have increased bodily tension during phonation?

III. Articulation
  1. Does the child have proper oral movements necessary for facilitation of lip closure at rest, during sucking, swallowing, chewing, and speech?
  2. Does the child have any involuntary movements of the lips, tongue, and mandible?
  3. Does the child have any dysarthric pattern in the lips, tongue, and mandible?
    Lips: close on command
               purse and retract
    Tongue: lateralize right/left
               elevate, protrude, point
               dissociate from jaw movement
    Mandible: open mouth, drooling
               hyperextension of mandible
  4. Does the child have the ability to make rapid, alternating movements, i.e., diadochokinesis?

Table 4.9.
Characteristic Features of Dysarthria and Apraxia

	Dysarthria	Apraxia
Vegetative functions	May be impaired	Intact
Error types	Phonetic distortions and omissions	Substitution
Consistency of errors	Errors are consistent in repeated utterances	Variability in error types for repeated utterances; especially for multisyllabic words
Initiation of speech	No difficulty	Frequency: difficulty marked by pauses, fillers, and repetitions

LANGUAGE DISORDERS

Language impairment or disorder is a descriptive term used to identify aberrant comprehension and production. The complexity of language, the extent of its involvement in varying arenas from academic (reading, writing) to social (conversational competence, discourse functions), and the array of theoretical constructs by which it is defined make it difficult to encapsulate a definition of language disorders. The American Speech Language and Hearing Association defines a language disorder as follows:

> "A language disorder is the abnormal acquisition, comprehension or expression of spoken or written language. The disorder may involve all, one or some of the phonologic, morphologic, semantic, syntactic or pragmatic components of the linguistic system. Individuals with language disorders frequently have problems in sentence processing or in abstracting information meaningfully for storage and retrieval from short term and long term memory" (2).

One classification of these disorders is based on using the concepts of form, content, and use to define areas of deficit. There are a number of language disorders which can be considered aberration of form. Omission or misuse of word endings, confusion in word order, telegraphic speech, incomplete sentences, inadequate use of verbs, and other grammatical forms belong to this category. Some examples of language disorders affecting content or meaning are represented by deficits in vocabulary, inability to categorize, or understanding relationships, such as cause and effect or word finding difficulties. Disorders of language use include, among others, inability to provide appropriate and salient information, to use and understand idioms, to be relevant as in the "cocktail party" syndrome of hydrocephalic youngsters (106, 115). As children mature, disorders of use may be demonstrated as ineffective use and mastery of communicative functions and strategies and weaknesses in discourse skills. The concept of communicative functions includes the use of language to solve problems, to reason, to relate a series of events (118). Weakness in communicative strategies, such as taking the perspective of the listener, known as presuppositional ability, are another form of a disorder in the use of language. Inadequate discourse skills are demonstrated in poor conversational ability and in the deficient use of narratives. Narratives are the orderly connection, causally and temporally, of a series of sentences to communicate (59, 113).

Another classification of language disorders is by using the definition of aphasia. Such a classification system may be more appropriate in instances of known nervous system damage. A language disorder associated with cerebral dysfunction, aphasia is characterized by loss or impairment in the use of spoken or written symbols for the formulation, reception, or transmission of ideas (37).

Aram (1) identifies three major groups of language disorders in children: (a) acquired childhood aphasia in which language is lost after a period of normal development; (b) developmental language disorder with known central nervous system impairment, sometimes called developmental or congenital aphasia; and (c) developmental language disorders without consistent or focal neurological findings.

In acquired aphasia, the site and extent of lesion are the most crucial factors in determining language performance. Age, once considered as a primary factor is now seen as less significant (1). Several features are characteristic of acquired aphasia: (a) reduced expressive language, primarily with left hemispheric lesions; (b) comprehension deficits are less frequent than expressive impairment; (c) there is some evidence associating anterior lesions with production deficits and posterior lesions with impaired comprehension; (d) sequelae affecting cognitive and academic performance (47). Head trauma or other neurologic lesions sustained in childhood with or without associated physical handicap may lead to acquired aphasia.

Developmental language disorders with known central nervous system pathology can present diverse symptomatology depending on the site and extent of lesion. As a rule, congenital hemispheric lesions do not present with profound aphasia; however, careful investigation may indicate more subtle deficits. In a recent study demonstrating unilateral lesions on CAT scan, children with congenital right-sided paralysis were found to be inferior to left hemiplegics on performance tasks in speech production, vocabulary, syntactic comprehension, and formulation (92).

Eisenson (37) delineates five differential features in the diagnosis of primary developmental aphasia: (a) perceptual dysfunction; (b) auditory dysfunction; (c) sequencing disturbances; (d) intellectual limitations; and (e) variable language functioning. He warns that these youngsters are frequently misdiagnosed as mentally retarded. *Perceptual dysfunction* is observed in one or more modalities, most outstanding in the auditory area. Perception is essentially an act of categorization in which sensory stimuli are received and, then, responded to by identification, sorting, and attribution of meaning. *Auditory dysfunction* generally exceeds what would be expected as a result of hearing loss. It includes difficulty in sound discrimination and sequencing. Speech is a steady flow of sequenced sounds. Children with this type of auditory dysfunction may be able to hear but not "tune in" and listen to the flow of speech. There is disturbance in *sequencing* auditory and, possibly, visual events. *Intellectual* functioning is inefficient in that performance is depressed beyond the level of measured intellectual ability. Perseveration, low frustration tolerance when confronted with difficult tasks, problems with generalization, and variable performance are observed. *Variability in language* development consists of significant delay in language form, content, and use.

Table 4.10 is a summary of the characteristics of developmental language

Table 4.10.
Patterns of Developmental Language Disability in Children Without Primary
Neuromotor Dysfunction[a]

Deficit Area	Description
Verbal auditory agnosia (word deafness)	Mute and noncomprehending of spoken language; able to process visual (printed) language
Semantics/pragmatics (content) (use)	Fluent and verbal; anomic and often tangential in response; difficulty in comprehending conversation
Phonologic/syntactic (form)	Impaired fluency and expressive ability, comprehension exceeds expression; variable oromotor function
Phonologic programming	Severe expressive disorder; impaired oromotor function; adequate comprehension

[a]Data from Rapin and Allen (93).

disorders without known pathology of the central nervous system as classified by the Child Neurology Society and reported by Rapin and Allen (93).

The diagnosis of developmental aphasia requires a comprehensive assessment and cannot be made in a single observation. Psychological, emotional,
medical, perceptual, and linguistic investigations are part of the multidisciplinary approaches to diagnostic identification. Mental retardation and
hearing loss must be ruled out before making a diagnosis of aphasia. However, it is also important to realize that, in children with brain damage,
including neuromuscular handicap, congenital aphasia may exist concomitant with cognitive and/or hearing deficits. It is essential, although often
difficult, to determine in these cases whether the language disorder is secondary to intellectual or sensory dysfunction. Another important distinction is between primary motor speech disorder and aphasia in children with
cerebral palsy. Severe dysarthria, which completely impedes speech production, is a possibility without primary dysfunction in language conceptualization, formulation, and comprehension. A severe physical handicap can
interfere with accurate assessment of intellectual and linguistic performance. In such cases, even minimal signs of communicative responsiveness
warrant further investigation as developments in nonverbal communication
enable severely physically handicapped children, including those with additional intellectual disability, to accomplish some degree of meaningful
interaction.

Childhood aphasia has serious implications that extend beyond language
function. As so aptly said by Myklebust (81) "to view the spoken word only
in terms of ability to comprehend or to speak no longer suffices as a theoretical framework, nor as a construct for diagnostic or remedial efforts." Childhood aphasia affects all aspects of learning, including social skills and academic performance. The learning disability resulting from brain damage

and/or aphasia is a concern for speech and language pathologists as well as for special educators.

LANGUAGE DISORDERS IN CLOSED HEAD INJURY

One tragic consequence of our ever more fast-paced society is the alarming increase in the incidence of nonpenetrating traumatic head injuries, commonly called closed head injuries. Beyond the potential physical, neuromotor, and sensory insults are the cognitive-communicative disturbances that may affect as many as 75% of closed head injury patients (72). Cognitive-communicative impairments are defined by ASHA as, "those communicative disorders that result from deficits in linguistic and nonlinguistic cognitive processes" (48). The speech-language pathologist is a crucial member of the diagnostic-rehabilitative team with particular respect to cognitive-communicative dysfunctions. In settings such as the Shock Trauma Center of the Maryland Institute for Emergency Medical Services, closed head injury patients are evaluated by a speech-language pathologist within 24 to 48 hours of injury (105).

In patients with closed head injuries, language functioning is now viewed within the context of more global cognitive and communicative impairments (128). This construct of a cognitive-communicative function extends beyond the conceptualizations of cognition and language generally noted in the rehabilitation literature. Attention, memory, learning, perception, organization, and reasoning are among the cognitive processes most commonly considered. Language impairment in head trauma has been traditionally viewed from an aphasia framework. While there is evidence of classically defined aphasia in closed head injury patients (127), it is generally held that, in aphasia, brain damage is more focal rather than the diffuse injury typical of closed head injury.

In a cognitive-communication approach to diagnosis and intervention of closed head injury patients, communicative functions are placed within the context of cognitive deficits. Ylvisaker and Szekeres (128) emphasize cognitive functioning that includes a consideration of a knowledge base and executive functions. "The knowledge base includes an organized system of general information; learned skills or routines; concepts, words, rules, strategies, and procedures; organizational principles and abstracted life scripts." Language and communication as active, rule-governed cognitive and social acts can readily be seen within the context of a "knowledge base." The executive functioning is conceptualized by Ylvisaker and Szekeres as abilities such as goal setting, planning, self-directing and initiating, self-monitoring, self-evaluating, self-correcting, and flexible problem-solving. It is the executive function, Ylvisaker and Szekeres write, "which directs and regulates cognitive activity." The executive function can be viewed as particularly pertinent to the pragmatic aspects of language, especially conversational competence and appropriate social communication behavior. It is also apparent that the concepts of the knowledge base and executive functioning are particularly relevant for children with closed head injury who must resume their formal education.

Relatively few authors have addressed the implications of closed head injury in children and adolescents returning to school (14, 99, 127). The closed head injury student who returns to school may have varying degrees of disruption in functioning physically, communicatively, cognitively, in perceptual-motor skills, behaviorally, and socially (19). For children with closed head injuries who return to school, language problems are identified among the most important deficits that impede academic performance. Language disturbances at phonological and morphological levels are rare in children with closed head injury. Deficits in naming and word retrieval are far more common. However, they are often subtle and not readily identified as impacting on school function (126). Difficulty in language comprehension and expression within the educational setting as the result of disrupted memory, judgment, pragmatic and problem-solving skills are at the forefront of the problems of closed head injury students with readjustment. Table 4.11 lists the emotional and academic characteristics as well as the cognitive-communicative deficits of students with a closed head injury. It is essential to emphasize that closed head injury children and adolescents returning to school are in a vastly different position than their peers or other "handicapped" students. The communication and learning handicaps that

Table 4.11.
Characteristics of Communication Dysfunction in Children with Head Injury

Cognitive Communicative	Academic	Emotional
Word retrieval errors	History of academic success	Sense of being different
Slowness in processing auditory information	Inconsistent performance	Poor judgment
Normal sentence length	Difficulty in organizing, integrating and generalizing information	Loss of emotional control
Inadequate quality of communication, pragmatics	Need for compensatory strategies in learning	Inappropriate behaviors
Ability to provide surface information, but not extended explanation	Ability to rapidly relearn previously learned information	Confusion over discrepancy in ability—some high level abilities intact while lower level skills are disrupted
Reduced verbal reasoning		
Reduced ability to process and represent sematic aspects of language (satire, inferences, sarcasm)		

those students experience are acquired and exist in contrast to premorbid functioning.

REMEDIATION

Speech and language therapy is based on the knowledge of normal sensory, motor, intellectual, and linguistic development. Two basic principles to be applied in all aspects of remediation are sequential learning and the integration of skills. Activities to stimulate speech and language development should begin as soon as there is any indication of developmental delay and/or neuromuscular abnormality.

Language stimulation programs can start in the first year of life to foster skills beginning at the most basic prelinguistic level. The provision of varied visual, auditory, tactile, and motor experiences lays the early foundation for growth in knowledge about the environment and interaction in different contexts. Talking about the surrounding world, naming objects used, activities in progress, relationship in the course of daily management and play offer opportunities for communication and are all predecessors of linguistic training.

Generally, in the child with cerebral palsy, difficulties with sucking, swallowing, and chewing are early indications of impaired oral control and, later, dysarthria. Remediation should begin in infancy concentrating on these oropharyngeal vegetative functions, which are the underlying mechanisms for speech production. Thus, the earliest forms of prespeech training include feeding programs that incorporate techniques to overcome abnormal postures, atypical motor patterns, and reflexes (70, 80). Encouraging vocalization of any kind to heighten awareness of communicative function and improvement of breathing patterns are additional goals. For older children, training in respiratory control is an example of the sequential approach to treatment. Attempting to improve articulation in the presence of uncontrolled exhalation is to ignore the developmental necessities of the prespeech stage.

Inherent in any remedial program is to integrate language skills into a functional, social context. Family, teachers, friends, and other professionals all become remediators so that the child's communicative attempts are used and reinforced in various settings. The sense of social purpose of language must be emphasized in all phases of the child's life while structured training in prelinguistic and linguistic skills takes place. Language therapy follows the sequential nature of development. As an example, recognizing, pointing to, and naming body parts are precursors of talking about their use and other characteristics. Selection of therapeutic goals is based in each case on the level of language comprehension and production in respect to form, content, and use (12).

Historically, the speech-language pathologist did not see physically handicapped children or those at risk for such handicaps until the children were aged 3 yr or older. However, recent advances in identifying and meeting the needs of babies identified as "high risk" has increased awareness of the higher probability of speech and language disorders during toddler (50) and preschool (39) years. Acknowledgment of the increasing number of infants considered to be "at risk" as well as the ultimate benefits of early, comprehensive intervention, prevention, and remediation programs for babies and families is demonstrated in recent legislation, Public Law 99-457 (1986). Knowledge of the benefits of early intervention for at-risk infants and their families has contributed to a change in the role of the speech-language pathologist (38). Speech and language assessment procedures may include patterns of infant vocalization, particularly differentiating cry and noncry vocalizations (89), feeding and related motor patterns (58), the nature of interactions that may affect later communication development (57, 111), gestures as a precursor to verbalization for communication (49), and early comprehension either by vocabulary checklist (96) or by behavior (101).

AUGMENTATIVE COMMUNICATION

General Principles

There are circumstances in which communication by speech or writing may be impossible or inadequate to serve its purpose. Physical limitations, such as cerebral palsy, severe oral motor dysfunction, deafness, intellectual disability, aphasia, or progressive neurological disability may dictate the need for alternative methods of communication.

The study and use of augmentative communication has its genesis in the early communication boards of the 1960s. Since the time those seeds were sown, there has been a virtual explosion in our knowledge and application. Volumes have been written, journals are regularly published, and the early concept of "nonspeech" communication has been supplanted by the more encompassing augmentative communication. The reader is directed to Beukelman and associates (7), Blackstone (8), and Fishman (40) for comprehensive discussions of augmentative communication.

Able-bodied people augment their communication by facial expressions, gestures, and vocal inflections. Similarly, disabled people with speech and language, sensory, cognitive, or physical deficits rely on these standard techniques and also may use an ever-increasing variety of augmentative communication aids and systems. There are several essential considerations to be made when approaching the area of augmentative communication. These include an understanding of communication, the particular needs of the person who will be accessing the augmentative communication device or system, including the reason for that person's need, and the forms of augmentative communication to be developed and used.

Communication, the process of exchanging meaning between individuals, is now understood as the essence of any evaluation or remediation for speech- and language-impaired persons. So too, it is a driving force when augmentative means to disrupted communication are necessary. Thus, augmentative systems should be perceived and developed with the goals of serving the numerous communicative functions: greeting, requesting, giving information, expressing intentions, regulating behavior, problem-solving, describing, learning, and conversing. The concepts of communication need to be considered whether the augmentation is for speaking, writing, or both. When developing, remediating, or re-establishing language skills, knowledge of normal language development and the dynamic nature of language acquisition and/or characteristics of disrupted language functions secondary to brain trauma is imperative. Language learning or relearning must be considered in a purposeful communicative context.

The needs of people who use nonstandard augmentative communication are greatly varied (8). Vanderheiden and Yoder (120) identify four groups of disabling conditions that may lead to varying degrees of reliance on augmented communication. In childhood, they include congenital conditions, such as cerebral palsy, mental retardation and autism, or acquired disabilities, most often head trauma or cervical spinal cord injury. The need may also arise in progressive neurologic diseases, which affect several aspects of speech production, as in muscle diseases or spinal muscular atrophy. In some instances, augmented communication may be used temporarily, for example, in severe facial burns or in patients with tracheostomy. Not only the immediate but also the ongoing needs of these populations will be diverse. Age, environmental demands, and the nature and course of the disability are contributing factors in the development of augmented communication systems. Consider the differing needs of a youngster with cerebral palsy as opposed to those of an adolescent with a cervical spinal cord injury. The child with cerebral palsy will be in the language acquisition process. This child will have an expanding vocabulary, repertoire of sentences, a maturing semantic knowledge, and increasing knowledge and use of language functions and "conversational competencies." Augmentative systems employed according to the child's physical, intellectual, and linguistic status would be part of a naturalistic approach to acquiring normal language skills. For a teenager who premorbidly had normal language and communication skills, but now is physically disabled and has limitations in oral speech production, augmentative communication needs must include other considerations. Educational needs, including writing, must be addressed. Communication contents should span a broad spectrum of subjects, tests, report preparation, all part of the educational curriculum. Social and emotional needs will be different for this teenager than his or her peers and the augmentative communication system would, by necessity, have to include means for the expression of these thoughts and feelings. A child with a progressive neurological disease will experience increasing loss of traditional modes of communication and, as such, become more dependent on typical

Bliss Symbols (CK Bliss (5))

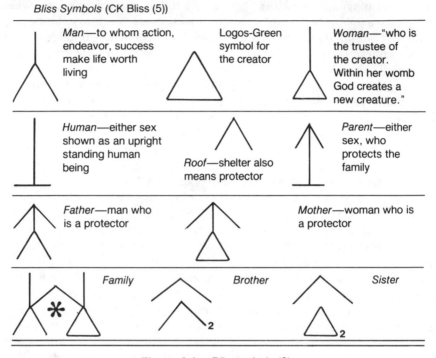

Figure 4.1. Blissymbols (9).

augmentative communication techniques to communicate orally or in writing. These needs will change with the progressive nature of the disease.

There is an ever-increasing variety of augmentative communication aids and systems available to meet the variety of individual needs. They range from basic pointing techniques to an array of available computer systems. Augmentative systems are generally classified into three categories: simple systems, dedicated devices, and multipurpose systems (30). Simple systems may include communication boards that use alphabet, words, pictures, symbols or combinations of them, gestures (pointing, sign, yes/no headshakes), and writing. Dedicated devices reflect the introduction of technology into communication and perform a predesigned limited range of functions. Multipurpose systems are generally computer based. They are created for multiple functions: communication, education, socialization, and are flexible in their ability to adapt to the user's need. Technology has afforded the user of augmentative communication systems a range of opportunities. Simple systems, such as pointing, either by hand, headstick, or light beam may be incorporated with a variety of symbol systems from alphabet to Blissymbols (9) within the context of a computer-based program that can be individualized from a generic type to meet the physical, cognitive, social, emotional, and linguistic needs of the user. Augmentative communication systems can perform a variety of functions: communication, assessment, rehabilitation, and improvement in the quality of life. Blissymbols are a frequently used symbol system that have both ideographic and pictographic components (73). Examples of Blissymbols appear in Figure 4.1.

This chapter was written with the intention of exposing the readers to some ideas that reflect the shift in thinking about the role of speech, language, and communication. Discussion of augmentative communication methods seems an apt terminus to reverse the misconception that communication and language do not exist in the absence of speech.

REFERENCES

1. Aram D: Variation in Child Language Disorders. Paper presented to the 2nd Annual Neuropsychology of Language Conference, New York, December 1981.
2. ASHA Committee on Speech Language and Hearing Services in the Schools. Definitions for communicative disorders and differences. *ASHA* 22:317, 1980.
3. Baer D: Discussion summary-language intervention for the mentally retarded. In Schiefelbusch R, Lloyd L (eds): *Language Perspectives—Acquisition, Retardation and Intervention.* Baltimore, University Park Press, 1974.
4. Barrett M, Zachman L, Huisingh R: Assessing Semantic Skills Through Everyday Themes. Moline, Il, LinguiSystems, 1988.
5. Bates E: Pragmatics and sociolinguistics in child language. In Morehead D, Morehead A (eds): *Normal and Deficient Child Language.* Baltimore, University Park Press, 1976.
6. Berry M, Eisenson J: *Speech Disorders: Principles and Practices of Therapy.* New York, Appleton-Century Crofts, 1956.
7. Beukelman D, Yorkston K, Dowden P: *Communication Augmentation: A Casebook of Clinical Management.* San Diego, College Hall Press, 1985.
8. Blackstone S (ed): *Augmentative Communication: An Introduction.* Rockville, MD, ASHA, 1986.
9. Bliss C: *Semantography-Blissymbols.* Sydney, Australia, Semantography Publications, 1965.
10. Bloom L: Talking, understanding and thinking. In Schiefelbusch R, Lloyd L (eds): *Language Perspective—Acquisitions, Retardation and Intervention.* Baltimore, University Park Press, 1974.
11. Bloom L, Hood L, Lightbown P: Imitation in language development: If, when and why. *Cognitive Psychol* 6:380, 1974.
12. Bloom L, Lahey M: *Language Develpment and Disorders.* New York, John Wiley & Sons, 1978.
13. Bloom L, Lightbown P, Hood L: Structure and variation in child language. Monogr Soc Res Child Dev 40:2, 1975.
14. Blosser J, DePompei R: The head injured student returns to school: Recognizing and treating deficits. *Topics Lang Dis* 9:67, 1989.
15. Boehm A: *Boehm Test of Basic Concepts.* New York, Psychological Corporation, 1970.
16. Bolinger D: *Aspects of Language.* New York, Harcourt-Brace-Jovanovich, 1975.
17. Bolinger D: The atomization of meaning. *Language* 41:555, 1965.
18. Bowerman M: Sematic factors in the acquisition of rules for word use and sentence construction. In Morehead D, Morehead A (eds): *Directions in Normal and Deficient Child Language.* Baltimore, University Park Press, 1976.
19. Bricker W, Bricker D: Assessment and modification of verbal imitation with low-functioning children. *J Speech Hear Res* 15:690, 1972.

20. Brown R: *A First Language.* Cambridge, MA, Harvard University Press, 1973.
21. Brunner J: From communication to language. A psychological perspective. *Cognition* 3:225, 1974–1975.
22. Bryen D, Joyce D: Language intervention with the severely handicapped: A decade of research. *J Spec Ed* 19, 1985.
23. Bull G, Cochran, Snell M: Beyond closed head injuries: computers, language and persons with mental retardation. *Topics Lang Dis* 8:4, 1988.
24. Carrow E: *Test of Auditory Comprehension of Language.* Austin, TX, Urban Research Group, 1973.
25. Coggins T, Olswang L, Guthrie J: Assessing communicative intents in young children: Low structured observation or education tasks? *J Speech Hear Dis* 52:44, 1987.
26. Coplan J: *The Early Language Milestone Scale.* Tulsa, OK, Modern Education Corp., 1983.
27. Crystal D: *Introduction to Language Pathology.* Baltimore, University Park Press, 1980.
28. Darley F: *Evaluation and Appraisal Techniques in Speech and Language Pathology.* Reading, MA, Addison-Wesley Publishing Company, 1979.
29. DePompei R, Blosser J: Strategies for helping head injured children successfully return to school. *Lang Speech Hear Serv Schools* 18:292, 1987.
30. DeRuyter F, Becker M. Augmentative communication: Assessment, system selection and usage. *J Head Trauma Rehab* 3:2, 1988.
31. Dever R: A comparison of the results of a revised version of Berko's test of morphology with the free speech of minimally retarded children. *J Speech Hear Res* 15:169, 1972.
32. Dore J: Requestive systems in nursery school conversations: Analysis of talk in its social context. In Campbell R, Smith P (eds): *Recent Advances in the Psychology of Language: Language Development and Mother-Child Interaction.* New York: Plenum Press, 1975.
33. Dore J: Holophrases, speech acts and language universals. *J Child Lang* 2:21, 1975.
34. Dubose R: Assessment of severely impaired young children. Assessing the handicapped preschooler. *Topics Early Child Sp Ed* 1:2, 1981.
35. Dunn L: *Peabody Picture Vocabulary Test.* Minneapolis, American Guidance Service, 1959.
36. Edwards M, Shriberg L: *Phonology Applications in Communicative Disorder.* San Diego, College Hill Press, 1983.
37. Eisenson J: *Aphasia in Children.* New York, Harper & Row, 1972.
38. Ensher G, Sparks S: Early intervention: Infants, toddlers and families. *Topics Lang Dis* 10:1 (December), 1989.
39. Fein D: The prevalence of speech and hearing impairments, ASHA 25:37, 1983.
40. Fishman I: *Electronic Communication Aids: Selection and Use.* San Diego, College-Hill, 1987.
41. Gardner M. *Expressive One Word Picture Vocabulary Test.* Novato, CA, Academic Therapy Publications, 1983.
42. German D. *Test of Word Finding.* Allen, TX, Developmental Learning Materials, 1986.
43. Goldman R, Fristoe M, Woodcock R: *Goldman-Woodcock Test of Auditory Discrimination.* Circle Pines, MN, American Guidance Service, 1970.
44. Grice H: Logic and conversation. In Cole P, Morgan J (eds): *Studies in Syntax and Semantics, Speech Acts.* Vol 3. New York, Academy Press, 1975.
45. Halliday M: *Learning How to Mean: Explorations in the Development of Language.* New York, Elsevier North Holland, 1975.
46. Hasenstab M: The multichannel cochlear implant in children. *Topics Lang Dis* 9:4, 1989.
47. Hecaen H: Acquired aphasia in children and the ontogenesis of hemispheric functional specialization. *Brain Lang* 3:114, 1976.
48. Herer G: The role of the speech-language pathologist in the habilitation and rehabilitation of cognitively impaired individual. *ASHA* 29:53, 1987.

49. Horstmeier D, MacDonald J: *Environmental Prelanguage Battery.* New York, Psychological Corp, 1978.
50. Hubatch L, Johnson C, Kistler O, Barns W, Moneka W: Early language abilities of high risk infants. *J Speech Hear Dis* 50:195, 1985.
51. Huttenlocher J: The origins of language comprehension. In Sola R (ed): *Theories in Cognitive Psychology: The Loyola Symposium.* New York, Wiley & Sons, 1974.
52. Hymes D: *Language in Culture and Society.* New York, Harper & Row, 1964.
53. Ingram D: *Phonological Disability in Children.* New York, Elsevier North Holland, 1976.
54. Ingram D. Phonological processes in young children. *J Child Lang* 1:97, 1974.
55. Ingram D: *Procedures for the Phonological Analysis of Children's Language.* Baltimore, University Park Press, 1981.
56. Ingram D; The relationship between comprehension and production. In Schiefelbusch R, Lloyd L (eds): *Language Perspectives—Acquisition, Retardation and Intervention.* Baltimore, University Park Press, 1974.
57. Jacobson C, Starnes C, Gassen R: An experimental analysis of the generalization of descriptions and praises for mothers of premature infants. *Human Communication* 12:23, 1988.
58. Jaffe M: Feeding at-risk infants and toddlers. *Topics Lang Dis* 10:13, 1989.
59. Johnston J: Narratives: A new look at communication problems in older language disordered children. *Lang Speech Hear Serv Schools* 13:144, 1982.
60. Jorgenson C, Barrett M, Huisingh R, Zachman L: *The Word Test.* Moline, IL, Lingui-Systems, 1981.
61. Karlin I, Karlin D, Gurren L: *Development and Disorders of Speech in Childhood.* Springfield, Charles C Thomas, 1965.
62. Kirk S, McCarthy J, Kirk W: *Illinois Test of Psycholinguistic Ability.* Revised ed. Urbana, IL, University of Illinois Press, 1968.
63. Knauf V: Language and speech training. In Katz J (ed): *Handbook of Clinical Audiology,* 3rd ed. Baltimore, Williams & Wilkins, 1985.
64. Kretschmer R, Kretschmer L: Communicative competence: Impact of the pragmatics revolution on education of hearing impaired students. *Topics Lang Dis* 9:4, 1989.
65. Lackner J: A developmental study of language behavior in retarded children. *Neuropsychologia* 6:301, 1968.
66. Lasky E, Cox L: Auditory processing and language interaction. In Lasky E, Katz J (eds): *Central Auditory Processing Disorders: Problems of Speech, Language and Learning.* Baltimore, University Park Press, 1983.
67. Lee L: *Developmental Sentence Analysis.* Evanston, IL, Northwestern University Press, 1970.
68. Lee L: *Northwestern Syntax Screening Test.* Evanston, IL, Northwestern University Press, 1971.
69. Lowe R: *Assessment Link Between Phonology and Articulation.* Moline, IL, Lingui-Systems, 1986.
70. McDonald E: Early identification and treatment of children at risk for speech development. In Schiefelbusch R (ed): *Nonspeech Language and Communication: Analysis and Intervention.* Baltimore, University Park Press, 1980.
71. McDonald J, Nichols M: *Environmental Language Inventory.* Columbus, OH, Charles E. Merrill, 1978.
72. McKinlay W: The short-term outcome of severe blunt injury as reported by relatives of the injured persons. *J Neurol Neurosurg Psychiatry* 44:527, 1981.
73. McNaughton S, Kates S: The application of Blissymbolics. In Schiefelbusch R (ed): *Nonspeech Language and Communication: Analysis and Intervention.* Baltimore, University Park Press, 1980.
74. Matkin N: The role of learning in language development. In Kavanaugh J (ed): *Otitis Media and Child Development.* Parkton, MD, York Press, 1986.

75. Menyuk P: *Sentences Children Use.* Cambridge, MA, The MIT Press, 1969.
76. Miller J: Assessing children's language behavior: A developmental process approach. In Schiefelbusch R (ed): *Bases of Language Intervention.* Baltimore, University Park Press, 1978.
77. Miller J: *Assessing Language Production in Children: Experimental Procedures.* Baltimore, University Park Press, 1981.
78. Miller J, Yoder D: The Miller-Yoder test of grammatical comprehension: Experimental Edition. University of Wisconsin, Madison, WI, 1975.
79. Moerk E: Verbal interaction between children and their mothers during the preschool years. *Dev Psych* 11:788, 1975.
80. Muller H: Facilitating feeding and prespeech. In Pearson P, Williams C (eds): *Physical Therapy Services in Developmental Disabilities.* Springfield, Charles C Thomas, 1971.
81. Myklebust H: Childhood aphasia: An evolving concept. In Travis L (ed): *Handbook of Speech Pathology and Audiology.* Englewood Cliffs, NJ, Prentice-Hall, 1971.
82. Mysak E: Cerebral palsy. In Shames G, Wiig E (eds): *Human Communication Disorders: An Introduction.* Columbus, OH, Charles E. Merrill, 1982.
83. Naremore R, Dever R: Performance of educable mentally retarded children and normal children at twelve age levels. *J Speech Hear Res* 18:18, 1975.
84. Nelson K: Structure in strategy in learning how to talk. *Monogr Soc Res Child Dev* 38:149, 1973.
85. Northern J, Downs M: *Hearing in Children,* 4th edition. Baltimore, Williams & Wilkins, 1991.
86. Oller D, Eilers R, Lynch M: Tactual artificial hearing as an aid to speech and language acquisition. *Topics Lang Dis* 9:4, 1989.
87. Platt L, Andrews G, Young M, Quinn P: Dysarthria of adult cerebral palsy: Intelligibility and articulation impairment. *J Speech Hear Res* 23:1, 1980.
88. Prather E, Hedrick D, Kern C: Articulation development in children aged two to four years. *J Speech Hear Dis* 40:179, 1975.
89. Proctor A: Stages of normal non-cry vocal development in infancy: A protocol for assessment. *Topics Lang Dis* 10:26, 1989.
90. Quigley SP, Kretschmer R: The education of deaf children. Baltimore, University Park Press, 1982.
91. Quigley S, Wilbur R, Power D, Montanelli D, Steenkamp M: Syntactic Structures in the Language of Deaf Children. Final Report Project No. 232175, U.S. Department of Health Education and Welfare, National Institute of Education. Urbana-Champaign Urbana, IL, University of Illinois, 1976.
92. Rankin J, Aram D, Horowitz S: Language ability in right and left hemiplegic children. *Brain Lang* 14:292, 1981.
93. Rapin I, Allen D: Developmental language, disorders. Nosologic considerations. In Kirk U (ed): *Neuropsychology of Language, Reading and Spelling.* New York, Academic Press, 1982.
94. Ray S: Context and the psychoeducational assessment of hearing impaired children. *Topics Lang Dis* 9:4, 1989.
95. Rees N: Pragmatics of language: Application to normal and disordered language development. In: Schiefelbusch R (ed), *Bases in Language Intervention.* Baltimore, University Park Press, 1978.
96. Reznick J, Goldsmith L: Multiple word form production checklist for assessing early language. *J Child Lang* 16:91, 1989.
97. Richard G, Hanner M: *Language Processing Test.* Moline, IL, LinguiSystems, 1985.
98. Robbins A: Facilitating language comprehension in young hearing-impaired children. *Topics Lang Dis* 6:3, 1986.
99. Rosen C, Carter R: *Head Trauma: Educational Re-integration.* San Diego, College Hill Press, 1986.

100. Ross M, Brackett D, Maxon A: *Hard of Hearing Children in Regular Schools.* Englewood Cliffs, NJ, Prentice-Hall, 1982.
101. Rowan L, Johnson C: Screening and Assessment. Paper presented at the June 1988 Infant and Toddler Communication Assessment and Intervention Workshop, Minneapolis, MN.
102. Ryan J: Mental subnormality in language development. In Lenneberg E, Lenneberg E (eds): *Foundations of Language Development.* New York, Academic Press, 1975.
103. Sacks H, Schlegloff E, Jefferson G: A simplest systemics for the organization of turn taking conversation. *Language* 50:696, 1974.
104. Sawyer D: *Test of Awareness of Language Segments.* Rockville, MD, Aspen Publishers, 1987.
105. Schwartz-Cowley R, Stephanik M: Communication disorders and treatment in the acute trauma center setting. *Topics Lang Dis* 9:1, 1989.
106. Schwartz E: Characteristics of speech and language development in the child with myelomeningocele and hydrocephalus. *J Speech Hear Disord* 39:465, 1974.
107. Schiefflin B: How Kaluli children learn what to say, what to do and how to feel: An ethnographic study of the development of communicative competence. Unpublished doctoral dissertation, Columbia University, 1979.
108. Shane H: Approaches to assessing the communication of non-oral persons. In Schiefelbusch R (ed): *Nonspeech Language and Communication: Analysis and Intervention.* Baltimore, University Park Press, 1980.
109. Silverman S: The education of deaf children. In Travis L (ed): *Handbook of Speech Pathology and Audiology.* New York, Appleton-Century-Crofts, 1971.
110. Sloan C: *Treating Auditory Processing Disorders in Children.* San Diego: College Hill Press, 1986.
111. Sparks S: Assessment and intervention with at-risk infants and toddlers: Guidelines for the speech-language pathologist. *Topics Lang Dis* 10:43, 1989.
112. Spinelli F, Terrell B: Remediation in context. *Topics Lang Dis* 5:1, 1984
113. Stein N, Glenn C: An analysis of story comprehension in elementary school children. In Freedle R (ed): *New Directions in Discourse Processing.* Norwood, NJ, Ablex, 1979.
114. Stocker B, Upsrich C: Stuttering in young children and the level of demand. *J Child Commun Disord* 1:116, 1976.
115. Swisher L, Pinsker E: The language characteristics of hyperverbal and hydrocephalic children. *Dev Med Child Neurol* 13:746, 1971.
116. Templin M: *Certain Linguistic Skills in Children.* University of Minnesota Press, Minneapolis, MN, 1957.
117. Templin M, Darley F: *The Templin-Darley Tests of Articulation.* The University of Iowa, Iowa City, IA, 1969.
118. Tough J: *The Development of Meaning.* New York, Halstead Press, 1977.
119. Travis L: *Handbook of Speech Pathology and Audiology.* New York, Appleton-Century Crofts, 1971.
120. Vanderheiden G, Yoder D. Overview. In Blackstone S (ed): *Augmentative Communication: An Introduction.* Rockville, MD, ASHA, 1986, p. 28.
121. Wechsler D: *Wechsler Intelligence Scale for Children-Revised.* New York, Psychological Corp, 1974.
122. Weiner F: *Phonological Process Analysis.* Baltimore, MD, University Park Press, 1979.
123. Wepman J: *Auditory Discrimination.* Chicago, The Language Research Association, 1958.
124. Wheatherby A, Prizant B: Early detection of communication problems in infants and toddlers. Paper presented at the annual convention of the American Speech Language Hearing Association, Boston, 1988.
125. Wiig E, Secord W: *Test of Language Competence.* Englewood Cliffs, NJ, Harcourt, Brace, Jovanovich, 1985.
126. Ylvisaker M: Language and communication disorders following pediatric head injury. *J Head Trauma Rehabil* 1:4, 1986.

127. Ylvisaker M (ed): *Head Injury Rehabilitation in Children and Adolescents.* San Diego, College Hill Press, 1985.
128. Ylvisaker M, Szekeres S: Metacognitive and executive impairments in head injured children and adults. *Topics Lang Dis* 9:34, 1989.
129. Yoder D, Miller J: What we may know and what we can do: Input toward a system. In McLean J, Yoder D, Schiefelbusch R (eds): *Language Intervention with the Retarded.* Baltimore, University Park Press, 1972.
130. Young E, Perachio J: *The Patterned Elicitation Syntax Screening Test.* Tuscon, AZ, Communication Skill Builders, 1981.
131. Zachman L, Huisingh R, Barrett M, Orman J, Blagden C: *The Adolescent Word Test.* Moline, IL, LinguiSystems, 1989.
132. Zimmerman I, Steiner V, Evatt R: *Preschool Language Scale.* Columbus, OH, Charles E. Merrill, 1969.

5

Psychosocial Issues

JESSIE K. M. EASTON

Handicapped children become handicapped adults and, as adults, they need to be able to function in society to the best of their ability. This includes not only physical abilities, but intellectual, psychological, and social skills needed to achieve the most normal life-style possible. The long-term future is sometimes neglected in the early stages of training and development, when most normal function is represented by physical achievements such as walking, eating, and toilet training. Intellectual, psychological, and social development are expected to follow naturally as physical goals are reached. Delayed accomplishment of physical goals may be followed by delayed, ineffective, or maladaptive learning of skills needed to help compensate for the physical disability. Parents and caregivers have to keep the child's total needs in mind as plans are made for management.

Legislation, such as the Americans with Disabilities Act, is intended to provide equal opportunity for all persons with handicaps, in employment, housing, transport, and recreation. Public Law 94–142 and more recent amendments deal with handicapped children's rights to free appropriate education. Mainstreaming and normalization have been popular ideas that needed careful implementation, adequate resources, and the recognition that not all handicapped people would be able to function in the mainstream all of the time. Rights are accompanied by responsibilities. The handicapped still have to obey the boss, maintain housing, be on time for transport, and follow the rules for comfortable enjoyment of recreational activities.

Rights and responsibilties are not part of the usual school curriculum. They are more likely to be learned as part of the culture, at home and play, through interaction, observation, and games. The "special" child may not have opportunity to interact, observe, or play in ways that allow learning how to get along in the world. Such children may feel that because they cannot do some things, they do not have to do others, and then they face a rude awakening when the world does not agree.

This chapter addresses psychosocial development in handicapped children, some common problems in the family and school, and some management strategies for optimum outcomes.

Developing Social Skills

Brazelton and Cramer (8) have discussed the need for parents to reconcile the reality of their new baby with the prenatal ideal fantasy infant each had in mind. With normal children, this is hard enough, with predictable milestones and expected care. When the baby has a handicap, initial bonding may not be accomplished if there is a delay in going home from the hospital. The achievement of separation, important to formation of identity and self-concept, may be delayed or abnormal if the baby is unable to learn self-control or self-comfort or is physically unable to move away from caregivers (7).

Delay in socialization may also occur if the parent is too depressed, tired, or preoccupied to interact with the baby in a consistent manner. Brazelton and Cramer describe "still face" studies in which the child's mother does not react to the baby with her usual facial expressions. The infant shows disappointment, frustration, and eventually gives up attempts to interact when the mother does not respond to his or her overtures (8). These normal babies remained wary of interacting with the mother for a time, until trust was re-established and expected responses once more were consistently present. The mother-baby interaction is based on smiles, frowns, noises, laughter, and mutual delight cycling along with short rests and repeats. If the delight is absent or if the child cannot see, or hear, or has inefficient motor responses, it is more difficult to achieve this kind of nurturing, growing interaction. The child's later ability to relate to others may be stunted (3).

Children develop at different rates, but milestones are achieved in a reasonably predictable order within ranges of time and age. Parents worry if their child is not walking or toilet trained as soon as a sibling, a cousin, a neighbor, or when the current authoritative book or grandmother says the baby should. Handicapped children's progress is not always predictable. They may do some things at the usual time and others much later or not at all, depending on the disability and how it is managed. Parents or teachers may react to this uncertainty by expecting too much while failing to accept or encourage what can be done; or by expecting too little and not encouraging performance that is possible (4, 20, 31).

Children's contacts influence their development as they move from the home into the world. These contacts begin with family; then peers as they play together; teachers and peers as they go to school; other role models and heroes in businesses, social activities, and the media, especially television. Medical personnel do not have much influence. The handicapped child has the same exposures, but in different proportions and degrees. In addition, there are doctors, nurses, psychologists, and various therapists, all with their own idea of what is important for the child to do, to know, and to accomplish (Figs. 5.1 and 5.2). Parents as the child's case managers may have difficulty maintaining a balance among the different influences.

Outside the family and its customs, the world of people and activities is to be mastered, with all the rules of right and wrong. Learning at home and elsewhere occurs by trial and error, by observation, by informal and formal teaching, depending on the subject and the situation.

Handicaps interfere with learning in different ways. Poor motor control or paralysis limits the opportunities for trial and error. Visual, auditory, perceptual, and reasoning deficits affect the accuracy of observation and its interpretation. Needed extra care takes time and effort that would normally go into informal teaching by parents, siblings, and other family members. Delays in development produce different priorities for formal teaching; for example, basic work on visual perception before reading begins. Lack of time or physical inability to participate in games and playtime will limit learning the rules of behavior with other children.

Parents and caretakers often focus on physical achievements, assuming other developmental skills will follow. This can lead to neglect of social and psychological accomplishments that are vital to successful function with

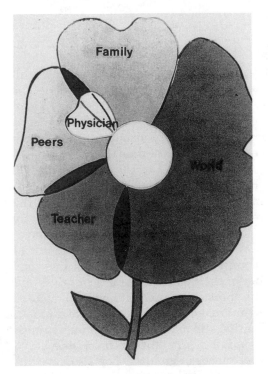

Figure 5.1. Relative influence of various factors in the social development of the normal child. The world outside has great influence; the physician has very little.

Figure 5.2. Relative influence of factors in social development of the handicapped child. Family is greater, world is much less, and medical factors, as represented by physician and therapists, are much greater than for a normal child.

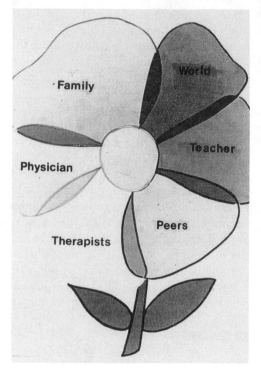

peers, in school, at work in later life, and in living with other people. Not all handicapped youngsters will achieve near-normal physical function. The fewer physical abilities they have, the more they need social skills to help them obtain physical assistance and companionship.

The lack of social skills may create a secondary disability that is more deterrent to eventual employment and social success than the original physical handicap (31, 35, 39).

The young child or teenager with a disability is isolated from social contact and learning with peers by limited motor skills and mobility and the need for time and energy-consuming therapy. This is not influenced greatly by the extent of traditional medical care (33). Children with less severe physical handicaps are more prone to develop chronic and severe psychosocial dysfunction (23), including nearly complete social withdrawal (6). This may be related to the higher standard they or their parents set for themselves and the difficulty of competing with nonhandicapped peers. It may also relate to uncompensated learning problems that make social function more difficult.

Experience with behavior modification and management techniques indicates that handicapped children often fail to generalize social skills learned in one setting spontaneously to other places or groups. They also have difficulty modifying learned behaviors to suit different situations (21, 35).

Physical disability alters opportunities for social interaction in frequency and variety. For example, adolescent paraplegics have more exposure to medical personnel than their nonhandicapped peers (33). Children who have had intensive therapy over a long period of time may absorb the adult conversational topics of the therapists (marriage, babies, dating, household problems) and then have difficulty relating to the "kidstuff" that is important to their peers. These differences in exposure influence social learning and the acquisition of skills in key areas of life, including family activities, education, work experience, sexual relations, leisure, and recreation. Nearly all the modes of social interaction that are important to the development of self-concept are affected.

The sense of identity and self-concept develop as a result of the child's social learning experience at home, in school, and in the world at large. Successful learning leads to better self-concept and a stronger sense of identity. Considering the differences in the learning environments of normal and handicapped children, it may be inappropriate to compare their accomplishments (23, 25). When a physically handicapped child is slow in acquiring knowledge and skills, it is important to make a clear distinction between delay due to diminished functional capabilities and that related to environmental limitations in opportunities to practice. It is essential for physicians and other professionals to keep this distinction in mind and to remember that secondary psychosocial handicaps may affect the handicapped child's overall adjustment and function.

"Normal" experiential learning models may not be effective for the handicapped child who needs to acquire social skills. The model's opportunities and abilities may be so different that what can be learned is not appropriate for many of the child's situations. This is more evident in the adolescent when normal peers are learning independence and making choices. The handicapped child must learn different ways of being independent and has a different array of right and wrong decisions to make. Parents and teachers have a difficult time letting their handicapped charges take the same risks as their normal peers; the children are allowed fewer choices.

It is easier for young children to establish relationships with peers as they all need some help to get together. Parents are involved in arranging play time and transport and everybody is supervised. Older children and teenagers are at an increasing disadvantage because their lack of mobility limits them from going where others do. They lack opportunities to practice age-appropriate social activities like phoning friends, making dates, having best friends and secrets, fighting and making up; such activities that help them develop feelings of self-worth and identity apart from the family.

In later teenage years and young adulthood, friends and siblings are big and strong enough to help the handicapped person physically and have access to cars for mobility. However, it is difficult for handicapped young persons to bridge the gap between childhood and adult behavior without a solid base of personal practice in the experiences of adolescent transition. The normal world may move on without them in spite of the fact that it is physically possible to be included.

Influence on the Family

Any new child in a family changes the balance and direction of relationships and distribution of effort. Changes occur as children grow and parents age. The stress of these adjustments can improve or damage the family as a unit. A handicapped child causes even more stress because his or her care takes more time and energy and the parents have different psychological adjustments to make. The discrepancy between the expected "ideal" child and the reality is greater. There may be guilt and blaming as to what might have caused the problem. Friends or members of the extended family may not understand the implications of the handicap or how the family is affected.

Individual relationships within the family are affected by the "differentness" of the child (11). The mother may be afraid to let anyone else handle the child, so siblings and father feel left out, or the demands of the child's care are such that her time is taken up and the family is left to manage for themselves. Siblings may be expected to help with care or to do housework at the expense of their own playtime and social development. Peers can tease them so they are reluctant to be seen in public with their handicapped sibling (25). They may be jealous of the attention the handicapped child gets and may be unable to cope with parental requests that they behave nicely to the sibling regardless of tantrums or unreasonable demands. One younger sister of a severely handicapped athetoid girl was heard to say, "I wish I had CP so mom would take me places." The father may feel inadequate in having produced a defective child, and reject or be unable to treat the disabled child as a real person. Not being able to brag about normal achievements may stunt the father's conversation at work and with his friends at the ball game or golf club. Enjoyment and, often, participation in these activities are lessened (40).

There are stages in the family's adaptation when they will need help to maintain realistic hopes and expectations. Slow physical development may be tolerated if normal intellectual function is expected. If learning deficits appear, a new adaptation is required. As school and social life proceed, new needs appear and must be met. Beyond school age, community and government supports are different. Plans need to be made for long-term living. Adaptation to having the child living out of the home forces a new adjustment of relationships within the family.

Professionals providing services individually or as part of a comprehensive program for handicapped children need to remember that long-term psychological development of the child depends on the parents and the home, regardless of available therapy and advice (32) (Fig. 5.3). Support for the family can be crucial to a successful outcome for the child.

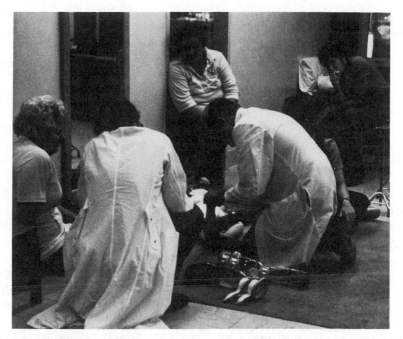

Figure 5.3. Caregivers may lose sight of the child's wishes, future as a potential adult, or the parent's needs when interacting as a team.

Management Strategies

Management begins as soon as the child is identified as being handicapped. This may be at birth, later when slow development is recognized, or after a period of normal development when there is a sudden loss of ability due to accident or illness.

For most children, the primary responsibility falls on the family. They must make the decisions and be the case manager and advocate in addition to providing physical care and general upbringing (27).

Management varies with the child's age and the family's adaptation and, to some extent, with the type and degree of disability, since physical and mental outcome is more predictable with some diagnoses than others. Timing of requirements for different kinds of support and help depends on when various aspects of the child's problem become evident.

The ultimate goal for the child is the highest feasible level of physical and social function. This will not always include independent living, employment, or marriage, but should achieve as normal a life-style as possible for the person's age and ability.

For the infant with a disability, the old advice "take him home and love him" is not all bad because it implies personhood and lovability. It is not enough for the family to know how to handle the physical aspects of care.

Where possible, they need to know the prognosis for long-term problems and where to turn for help. They also need to deal with the problems as they become evident. Extended family members will need information and support as well. Raising the child should be seen as a challenge rather than as a calamity (14).

The handicapped newborn infant's care is not much different from that of a normal baby, except when special equipment or feeding problems take extra time or training. Bonding between mother and child is facilitated by interaction. The same kind of vocal, visual, and tactile contact that all babies need is especially important when other kinds of care require more time. It will be more difficult for the parents when the baby is not able to respond with smiles, or cooing, or body movements. They will need encouragement and reassurance that their efforts are not wasted.

As the baby survives into the first year, early motor skills may be lacking, but the parents are controlled by the infant's needs and his or her behavior in the same way as for a normal child. Smiles reward them; crying makes them look for a cause and do something about it. They begin to recognize actual needs as distinguished from fussing for attention. They should be able to modify their responses to the baby and set some limits, so the infant may begin to develop the ability to control his or her own behavior.

The toddler years set the stage for the rest of development, as the child learns to communicate, control, act on his or her own, relate to others, and play.

Communication is the most important skill to establish early because it is the basis of learning and social relationships. If the child's handicap interferes with easy, practical, verbal communication, alternative means must be established. The child needs some way to indicate agreement, wants, and feelings; whether with words, by looking or pointing to a picture or symbol, or using a sophisticated communication device. More abstract ideas also are needed; right and wrong, reasons for happenings and limitations, and cultural customs and mores.

Choices are important if the child is to learn responsibility. Physical limitations may reduce the options for responding, as well as the consequences of any choice. The choice may be crying or accepting what the caretakers want. Since acceptance is rewarded and there is the risk that fussing will result in withdrawal of needed care, the severely handicapped child becomes the compliant, smiling small child in the wheelchair. Less handicapped children may have their choices limited by parents' fear of accidents and may be discouraged from experimenting with different responses (Fig. 5.4). This inhibition may be long-term, applied to other situations, and interfere with learning new skills appropriate for different social contexts (21).

Family members are not always able to encourage the child to attempt new skills. They may not know how or they may assume that the child will learn by observation. One young lady expressed this as "until I was about twelve

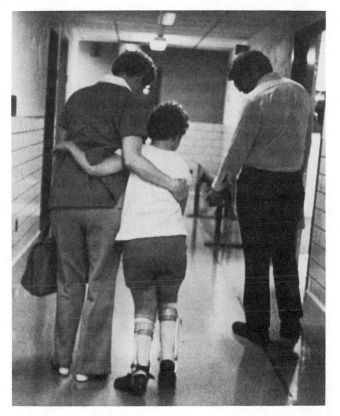

Figure 5.4. Overprotected; this child is able to walk with a walker but came to the clinic in a wheelchair and sat on mother's lap while waiting for doctor; denied opportunity.

I was a terrible kid, always in trouble. It was 'don't do that' or 'why did you do it' all the time. I finally began to figure out what it was they wanted me to do. It would've been so much easier if they had just told me the right way or showed me how they wanted it."

Parents may feel that some skills will not be needed; but whenever possible, the child should be taught to do things in the most socially acceptable way. A 5-yr-old should not be allowed to eat with his or her fingers unless it is also the only way to achieve independent eating, which is more important.

Manners are learned in preschool years, beginning with please and thank you, hello and goodbye, and progressing through ownership, taking turns, helping other children, and appropriate behavior in public and in private. Handicaps do not excuse children from having manners, although learning and expressing them may be more difficult.

Early play with other children is often limited by physical difficulty. It is important that the handicapped child have opportunities to interact with peers at age-appropriate levels in whatever way is feasible. This interaction is needed to establish a foundation for social skills needed later in school and work. It is also important in developing the sense of limits of behavior with other children, who may not be as tolerant as family members. Nursery school or preschool with normal or other handicapped children is a good opportunity. When finances or community resources are limited, neighborhood children can be included in the handicapped child's activities by invitation or by ploys such as attractive playground equipment in the back yard. Parents need to encourage interaction and to supervise the experiences to avoid the handicapped child becoming a passive spectator or another plaything.

Recognition and expression of emotion is a part of the small child's repertoire that may be difficult for the handicapped child. Anger or frustration may not be expressed for fear of loss of love or physical care. The resulting repression tends to use a lot of energy as the child presents the facade that seems to guarantee the provision of care and continued love. Parents need to be aware of this and recognize the child's right to be angry at times. They can let the child know that he or she can be angry or sad or happy and that they will still care for and help him or her. They may even be angry and still love him or her. Acceptable ways to express emotions can be taught, within the child's ability to communicate and do things physically.

Some behaviors that are accepted as cute in small children are not attractive in older ones. A handicap should not excuse the continuation of avoidable social annoyances, such as belching, whining, scratching, or masturbation in public.

Where professional staff are involved in a child's training, the social skills may be addressed at home and in the therapy setting. Family and staff need to agree on standards and consistency, so the child does not become confused or manipulative. Behavior taught by the therapist is not automatically used at home; sometimes because nobody insists; sometimes because the child fails to generalize from one situation to another. Professionals also need to understand and respect the family's preferences in matters of social orientation, manners, and mores.

Some children need to learn to initiate social interactions, whether or not they are able to do so independently (Fig. 5.5). They also need to learn that people are not always willing or able to respond when approached and that this is not a reflection on their worth.

Caretakers try to have the child succeed in order to avoid discouraging further effort or precipitating a depression. Failing and trying again are part of learning for normal children. Some of the reluctance to have the handicapped child fail may be rooted in the relatively large amount of effort required for the therapist or parent and the child to achieve anything, with limited opportunities to try again and again. With this attitude, there is a

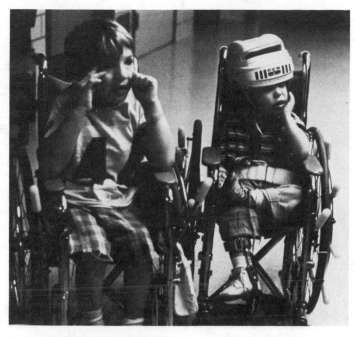

Figure 5.5 Learning disabilities contribute to relatively maladaptive, socially immature behavior in these two children who have good hand function and can see and hear; they could be playing together.

tendency to accept and praise substandard performance when the child is capable of working up to higher standards.

School-aged Children

Grade school tends to be a time of social isolation for the handicapped child, particularly in a mainstream situation (Fig. 5.6).

Socialization in grade school years occurs mostly in doing things with a best friend or buddy, in groups like Scouts, Sunday school, during recess, before- and after-school travel, or organized and supervised parties and excursions. Teams are chosen and games are played and won or lost. Sports skills are learned. Birthday and special occasion parties are a chance for the child to choose companions. Vacations are taken with the family. Sleepovers and camp-outs are practice for going away to camp in the summer. Parents are involved, supervising, driving, planning, and vetoing.

This is a difficult time for the handicapped child who is limited in ability to participate in the usual activities (Figs. 5.7 and 5.8) (1). Using a wheelchair and taking a special bus to school limit the casual contacts before and after school. There may be no one on the bus to relate to. Excursions may be

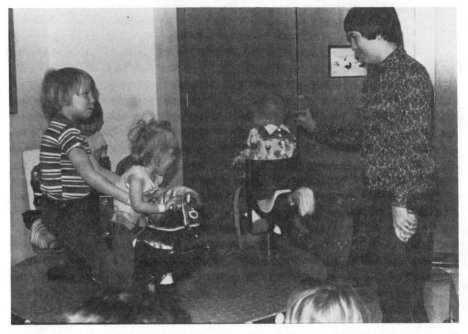

Figure 5.6. The child may be isolated, relating only to the teacher, or may be an accepted member of the class.

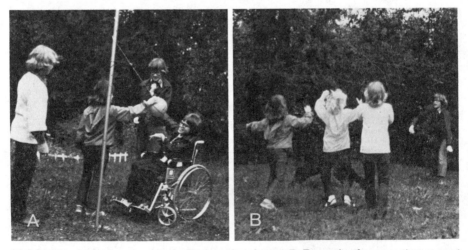

Figure 5.7. **A,** Example of game that can be shared. **B,** Example of a game that cannot be shared.

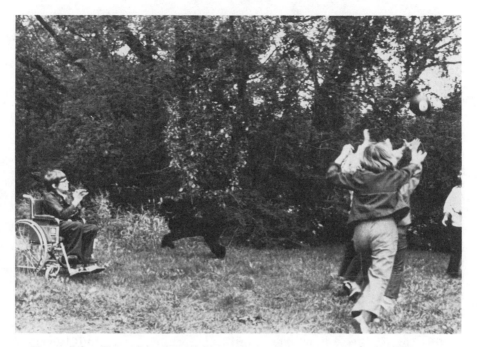

Figure 5.8. The child can participate as an active supporter of other's games.

missed because of lack of assistance in getting on the bus or fear of injury not covered by regular insurance. Sports participation may be limited to spectator or, with good friends and certain abilities, as timekeeper or mascot. Invitations to friends' parties may not come because there are steps into the house and the parent in charge has a bad back. The same is true of sleepovers and camping, which have the added problem of how the child manages bathing and toileting. Family vacations involve more planning and effort. Paths that are too rough or steep may limit access to sightseeing at the best view. Essential classes or after school clubs may be missed if time is spent in therapy or resource room to work on basic skills or remedial reading or improving hand control (31).

Activities specially designed for the handicapped do exist, such as Handiriders and the British Boating for the Handicapped (9), but they require a critical mass of participants and willing helpers. Parks provide accessible areas. With some adaptations, children can go fishing or swimming, play baseball, tennis, archery, or basketball from wheelchairs and can learn needed social skills with other handicapped children. Special Olympics gives some children an opportunity to compete for awards; practicing gives them physical activity with some motivation to improve their fitness level. Special camps for children with the same or different disabilities are also available.

For some children, contact with other handicapped children at a special camp can be helpful as they compare notes on problems and solutions, as they become aware that they are not alone, and as they make friends in a structured setting of activities that they are able to do without competing with more able children. The handicapped child's time at camp can also give the family a time to regroup and relate to each other.

Success in school is more dependent on intelligence and social skills than on the extent or kind of physical handicap. Plans for the child's educational program should begin in the preschool years and continue through all the grades, with careful assessment of abilities and problem areas, an appropriate Individual Educational Plan agreed to by all parties and realistic goal-setting, when possible including the child.

The Individual Educational Plan is for education. Physical and occupational therapy must be directly related to classroom requirements. Public Law 94–142 and its amendments does not mandate rehabilitation care or therapy. It is necessary to distinguish between therapy required for medical rehabilitative goals and that applicable to educational needs. Other terms relating to the law need clarification. "Least restrictive environment" may mean a resource room or separate classroom if the child is not able to learn in a regular class setting. "Mainstreaming" may include some special work in different settings, rather than a full-time regular classroom if the child has trouble in one or two areas. "Normalization" refers to life-style and does not imply that the handicap will resolve. In planning for handicapped children in school, the social implications of different placements should be considered, but the child's educational needs are most important and decisions should not be made solely on the basis of social impact. Since abilities and handicaps vary among diagnostic categories, planning should be based on the individual child rather than on the name of the disability (35, 36).

High School

High school can be a better time for the handicapped young person, as peers begin to develop some interests, such as language clubs or problem-solving contests, that do not require a lot of physical ability. Siblings and friends are learning to drive and can take the handicapped student along (26). The hard part is making sure that the handicapped student is interesting enough to be a desirable part of the group. Handicapped people tend to be boring because they have limited experience and interests and they tend to be rather egocentric. They need to learn about the topics that interest their peers and be able to join a discussion with information and opinions. For this purpose, communication skills are essential (30); such skills must be fast and easy enough to be used in a group without much effort for the sender or the receiver.

Handicapped young people often do not have reserve energy to pursue part-time work or extracurricular activities in high school. A lack of transportation also may limit activities. They miss some of the socialization and learning of workplace behavior that their peers get in the fast-food restaurant, carwash, or marching band. They also miss some of the contacts that lead to dating and comfortable relating to friends of both sexes (37).

Planning for life after school should start early and should be well under way in high school. When physical ability is limited, higher education is considered perhaps more often than usual with the thought that brains can substitute for brawn in the workplace (19). A careful realistic assessment of both physical and mental abilities in the high school years can help avoid wasted time and resources later. Most students have some difficulty adjusting to the greater freedom and responsibility of college life and, for the sheltered, handicapped youth, the transition can be very traumatic (2). Some time during high school should be spent learning to manage finite resources of money, time, and energy. Knowing how to do ordinary tasks, such as personal laundry, or organizing help so that the tasks get done, can lessen the stress of leaving home. If physical abilities permit, some handicapped youth would probably do better overall if they could have experience of working through work study or through a temporary full- or part-time job before starting a higher education program.

Some young people will need help in getting started with activities. Making friends is a skill that is learned by trial and error from preschool years. If missed in the early years, it may need to be taught in an informal or formal way. Family can help, by suggesting activities and people to include, by helping to find phone numbers so invitations can be made, by involving the young person in planning and organizing the activity, and, where possible, by allowing the same privileges and independence for the handicapped individual as for nonhandicapped siblings or peers (3).

Reaching out to invite others to do something can be very difficult. The invited person may decline because he or she has something else to do or is not interested in that activity. A refusal has no relation to like or dislike and is not an attack on the inviter's self-worth. This distinction needs to be understood. It may require direct discussion of how the inviter felt about the experience and how it might be handled next time. Acceptance of the invitation can be equally stressful because it commits the inviter to doing the activity and taking some responsibility for the guest's enjoyment. Once a one-on-one experience has been mastered, larger groups of two or more can be organized. Eventually, planning and managing a cooperative group event may be possible (24).

Exposure to the world means learning about different ways of doing things. The family may have to struggle harder to allow the handicapped youngster to follow the latest in hairstyles, clothing, or language, knowing that it will not make the child normal. The effect of current fashions in clothes and hair may be distorted by braces or an abnormal gait or wheel-chair. Within feasibility, if fashions made the handicapped child feel and, perhaps, be more easily accepted by peers and if they do not interfere with function, they should be tolerated, provided the family would have allowed the same behavior in a sibling.

Egocentricity, Manipulation, and Behavior Modification

Severe physical handicaps or communication deficits limit children's ability to reciprocate in social interactions. This leads to forced acceptance of a passive role in many relationships. It may also lead to an inability to appreciate the interactive nature of relationships between and among peo-ple. This leads to apparent egocentricity in the child or adolescent who can-not wait for attention, does not think of others' feelings, does not take responsibility for social interactions, or attempt to plan ahead for personal needs. Sometimes the egocentricity, which is normal at early ages, simply reflects the level of development of the handicapped child. In that case, it is expected to lessen with appropriate management over time. Where it per-sists into adolescence and early adulthood, with other development at higher levels, it may be necessary to institute planned intervention to help the young person acquire behaviors and skills that will allow comfortable social interaction. These skills are particularly important for severely hand-icapped individuals who have to be able to ask for help and to tell people, in a pleasant, assertive way, what they need.

A recreation therapist can be very helpful in dealing with the egocentric child (24). Starting with individual sessions to explain explicitly what is happening and how it affects the other person, the therapist and youngster can explore relating in different social situations. When the youngster begins to reciprocate by following through the greeting ritual to asking a question (how are you?) and can go on from there to an interested discussion of the reply, other topics of conversation can be introduced gradually. In this manner, the child builds up a repertoire of questions, comments, and infor-mation about the world. From individual sessions to sessions where a third person is introduced in the next step, the child learns to take turns in talk-ing. Activities, games, and expeditions can be used, with practice in remem-bering what happened so it can be discussed, approved, or criticized after-ward. Proceeding from small to larger groups and more difficult situations, with opportunities to analyze and discuss how the child and others felt, can help learning to appreciate how people relate to each other and to have some consideration for others' feelings. It is important to distinguish among dif-ferent kinds of relationships and emphasize when and how each is appro-priately expressed. Friends behave differently with each other than with acquaintances. Lovers have another set of behaviors with some properly kept for private settings. People at home and at work have different ways of relating to each other, since the tasks and the kinds of obligation are different. Since handicapped young people often do not learn well by observation and subtle hints from companions are unnoticed, a direct approach may be needed.

Some children are seen as manipulative because they cry and fuss, smile and laugh, withdraw or pay attention only to the adults in their lives. This behavior effectively blocks learning useful behaviors or the realization that treatment is needed. This may also reflect inconsistent handling by caretakers. Where inconsistent demands or rewards for behavior are the problem, parents and caretakers should agree on management. The child then feels more secure and the unwanted behavior fades. At other times, it may be the child's defense against demands for performance beyond real or perceived abilities. Where tasks have been too difficult, behavior can be improved by starting with activities the child can do and building up by small steps to achieve the goal for performance.

Behavior modification techniques have been helpful in dealing with relating socially and with learning physical tasks. Many parents are adept at using them without any formal training as they raise their children. However, they may be immobilized by fear of hurting the child, by guilt, or they may be persuaded that the handicap excuses the child from behaving in a socially acceptable manner. "It's so hard for him to do." Social life is much more difficult if the handicapped child has to overcome unnecessary discomfort in his or her companions before starting to relate to or work with them. An example is a child whose involuntary movements, as she sat in her wheelchair, pulled her legs up into flexion and abduction. Her pastor knew it was not voluntary but was still embarrassed. He found it difficult to relate to her family when she was with them, and to the child herself. An adjustment to the chair, to help control sitting position, while initially less comfortable and somewhat confining, would have helped not only her stability in the chair, but her social acceptance.

Psychosexual Issues

In *My Left Foot* (20) Christy Brown wrote "In time, indeed, and with the help of the Clinic, I might so overcome myself—that I would be enabled to lead a normal life, or at least a more ordinary, more independent one. But I knew, deep inside me, that there would always be something missing—. . . . No matter how well I might conquer my handicap, I would never be a normal individual leading a normal life. The old difference would always remain. I wanted so desperately to love and be loved, but. . . ."

The idea of loving and being loved in the sexual sense has not been a comfortable one when applied to the handicapped. This is changing slowly as the concept of sexuality has been distinguished from the sexual act itself and as societal attitudes toward intimacy are changing. Genetic knowledge of handicapping conditions has lessened the fear of producing disabled children. Increased employment and financial support for handicapped individuals have helped change attitudes about marriage and children. There is also greater tolerance of people who are different, with emphasis on the person rather than position, family, or race. The result is greater opportunity for disabled persons to develop intimate relationships, marry, and have children.

Opportunity does not automatically guarantee accomplishment and social skills are still needed. Before sexual intimacy can be satisfactorily achieved, it is necessary to have mature male-female relationships. This is more difficult for the handicapped, who often have to assist nondisabled in knowing how to relate to them; e.g., a blind person may have to initiate hand-shaking (7).

Parents have fears of rejection for their child in the complex social-sexual world. They need to realize that a lack of physical ability does not necessarily preclude maintaining a meaningful sexual relationship.

Adolescents with myelodysplasia reported less sexual experience than nondisabled peers and were less inclined to investigate contraception if they were sexually active. They also had somewhat different expectations with regard to marriage and having children (15).

Physical limitations to actual sexual performance need to be explored and information must be provided about possibilities for alternative methods of achieving satisfaction for the person or partner. Birth control needs to be discussed as part of responsible sexual behavior and, again, methods must be explored for possibilities compatible with the handicap. Sexually transmitted diseases are an essential area of education, particularly in view of AIDS, and the fact that some handicapped people seek sexual experience with prostitutes when the usual means of finding a partner do not seem to be available to them. The diagnosis of the handicapping condition needs to be defined and genetic information must be provided so that prognosis for future function and the possibility of an inheritable disorder are known; this allows intelligent decisions to be made about marriage and having children.

It is necessary to understand the medical aspects of disability as they relate to sexuality in order to provide realistic counseling. This applies to physicians as well as to guidance counselors and psychologists (13).

Whether or not full independence is anticipated for handicapped children when they reach adulthood, they are entitled to be treated and raised as sexual beings. As such, they need orientation to current roles of male and female in their society, assistance with identification of their own sexuality, and information about appropriate sexual behavior in different situations. This needs to be included in a context of social settings with emphasis on the social skills necessary to interest, attract, and become acquainted with someone who might be a sexual partner (16).

Counseling should include several essential notions. Intimacy begins with the eyes, ears, voice, or body. Substitution of a more effective use of voice or eyes for impaired body movements can communicate the intended message. Guilt is an inappropriate feeling. There are no legitimately imposed standards of behavior or performance and the family's attitudes should be respected.

Sexual information is obtained from parents, friends, enemies, and sometimes from schools teaching units with names like "Family Life." It may be accurate or not, depending upon the source and the recipient's level of understanding. Parents who are comfortable with their own sex lives and present a good model of family relations will find it easier to educate their children than those who find sex hard to talk about at any time and even harder to discuss with the handicapped child. They may fear rejection of the child in the social-sexual real world (2, 17, 18). All children need adequate, accurate information presented in a format appropriate for their age and experience, with a goal of allowing them to know and accept their sexuality in a healthy relaxed way. The handicapped child may not have access to street information and needs accurate education. There may also be difficulty appreciating the interpersonal relationships involved; help may be needed with reaching out before touching someone.

It is helpful if the adolescent can establish a relationship that allows frank and open discussion about intimacy, with a friend, counselor, or physician. Information needs to be accurate and in understandable language. Robinault (34) offers a list of precautions for counseling spinal cord-injured persons that applies equally well to other groups of disabled people. Where physical assistance is required for personal hygiene and preliminaries to sexual activity, some agreement is needed as to the role of the partner in providing the assistance. Some couples have a personal attendant do the mechanical preparation so they can focus on the relationship, while others consider it part of relating.

Whether or not to have children becomes "an emotionally charged subject." Considerations include the possibility of a heritable genetic defect and prenatal detection of some conditions; possible complications of pregnancy and their prevention; proper prenatal care; and how the prospective parents plan to cope with the task of parenting, both physically and financially. The need is for informed decision-making. Realistic possibilities for marriage vary greatly with particular physical disabilities and should be considered on an individual basis.

While the possibilities improve for a satisfying social-sexual life, those involved with the handicapped child still need to remember to include it in their thinking for the future. Like Christy Brown, they want "to know the joy of climbing a mountain on an early spring morning or of strolling home in the moonlight along rain-washed city streets with a beautiful girl by my side" (10).

Leisure and Work

After completing school, there should be a future for the handicapped child. Services are fewer and plans to use those that do exist should be made before the age of leaving school is reached. One of the difficulties for the young handicapped person moving into the world is that people without experience in dealing with disabilities are likely to react differently from the family he or she knows (12). The person whose family picked up things for him or her will be disappointed when friends do not feel that this is part of their duty in the relationship. Another problem lies in the lack of exposure to a normal workplace to help in the acquisition of social skills and standards for behavior. Nurses, therapists, teachers, and physicians behave in ways that are not usually encountered in social settings. Television offers cosmetically ideal models, with notions like the importance of sex and the influence of the right product on attractiveness. It does not realistically portray the sustained effort needed to begin, to develop, and to maintain a relationship. Appearance and behavior are important to comfort in the outside world. Clothing needs to suit the situation. As much as possible, drooling and involuntary movement need to be avoided. Stereotyped mannerisms, like the hand-flapping sometimes seen in blind children, have to be discourged. The ordinary body language movements of social attention need to be present, such as turning toward someone when listening or speaking (22, 24).

Independent living is a goal for handicapped and able-bodied young people. It may be defined differently in some circumstances, like the mentally handicapped living in apartments with a social worker supervising or a physically limited person requiring a personal attendant or housekeeper on a full- or part-time basis to live outside an institution. It is necessary to have a realistic appraisal of the person's abilities and resources and to inform the young person when his or her desired level of function is not realistically attainable, for whatever reasons. There is also the problem that others may not be comfortable with attempts to achieve activities that do not fit with stereotypes of disability.

Federal grants as well as state and local funding sources now support centers for independent living, with mandates to assist the handicapped to achieve the least restrictive life-style possible. Services and facilities vary from one center to another, but most include opportunities for social interaction and guidance in interpersonal relationships, money management, sexuality, and the administration of living space, including the management of household help and personal care attendants.

Choice of living arrangements will depend on abilities, needs, and finances. Accessible housing remains a problem because affordable apartments tend not to have elevators, wide doors, or large bathrooms. Other choices include living alone, with privacy but, perhaps, with a lack of company; in a group home, where shared space allows some privacy and there is still someone to relate to; or in a larger institution, where the pool of possible friends is larger but the exposure to nonhandicapped individuals in the community is less.

Isolation is common among handicapped adults with cerebral palsy. It relates to the nature of the physical handicap, lack of transport, inability to use the telephone, and other practical problems. It also relates to the inexperience or inability of some handicapped people to initiate activities or failure to appreciate the reciprocal nature of relationships. If egocentricity has been overcome, this should not be a problem, but if not, some education about initiating conversation and reaching out to others may be helpful. The idea of integration in work and social life is now being supplemented by the concept of inclusion, which implies a more active, equal role for the handicapped person (5).

For most people, normal life includes some sort of work activity, which is rewarded with money or other support and provides a part of their identity. For many, it also provides social life, as the place where they interact, begin friendships, go on to after-work activities, brag about their children or their golf game, and succeed or fail. They identify themselves as miners, writers, truck drivers, or waitresses; they adopt behaviors that are suitable for the personal interactions associated with the activities of the job site. Social life may be limited to the people met through work. It is generally considered healthier to have some social interests that are not dependent on the workplace. Relationships between workers can function without liking and it is better to have some good friends and activities that are separate and can lessen the effect of any unpleasant relationships on the job.

If work is not possible, the person who has other interests still has an identity and can go on in life with things to do and talk about.

Work may not be feasible, for whatever reason, and that aspect of identity has to be established in other ways. If it is feasible, then decisions must be made about what kind of and how much training is needed and how much help will be needed. Limited experience and observation of people at work may produce a student who does not appreciate the consistent effort and time needed to acquire the basic knowledge to get and keep a job. Handicapped young people, as well as older ones, have finite amounts of energy and time to spend during a day on activities of daily living, housework, getting to a job, and actually working. Counseling must consider this in helping with decisions about full-time work, as well as decisions concerning the client's financial situation and personal preferences for activities. Work may not be practical if the client receives Social Security benefits and medical insurance that will be cut off if work activity reaches a significant level and the person cannot afford equivalent private insurance. Transportation or building access may also preclude some employment, although there is a growing number of home-based, computer-based jobs available for those with the training, skills, and ability to work alone and without supervision. Quality of life must also be considered. If work takes all one's energy, leaving none for social activities or other enjoyment, then priorities must be established for what represents the client's best interests, regardless of societal norms and pressures to work.

Vocational counseling includes more than help in training for and finding a job (28). It also should address issues of social behavior at the workplace, proper dress and personal hygiene, work habits and timeliness. There is also the small matter of the boss's right to set the standards for behavior and productivity. Equal opportunity assumes that the worker is able to do the job regardless of handicap. The handicapped worker needs to appreciate the fact that the same standards of dress and behavior apply to able-bodied fellow-workers and that the boss is not being discriminatory when insisting on compliance. The vocational counselor now has options of supported employment with job coaches and close follow-up to be sure that the client can function in the workplace. This is in addition to the traditional job-finding help and money for training. Vocational counseling for the disabled is moving into the high schools, to help with planning while preparatory courses are still available. The independent living centers are also working with high school-aged youth to prepare them for living more or less independently after school, particularly if they are going to be away from home in college dormitories and apartments.

Reports of employment, marriage, and parenthood among the handicapped vary, with an employment rate of 30% in a group of young cerebral palsied adults reported by Bleck in 1987 (6); a rate of 19% for women and 34% for men was published in a 1983 report (41). More recently, in an older group with cerebral palsy, Murphy and Molnar reported that 50% are competitively employed at some time, 18% in sheltered workshops, 26% married at some time, and 9% have children (29). Tew, Lawrence, and Jenkins (38) report a 33% employment rate in a group of young adults with spina bifida and hydrocephalus, none of whom had severe physical or learning disabilities. While variables like transport and climate may be influential in the higher employment rates reported by Murphy and Molnar, their study is still a sign that the future may be better, given optimum circumstances.

Role of the Physiatrist

Physiatrists, with training in the management of the patient with disability, are uniquely qualified to assist handicapped children and their families, schools, and workplaces. They should be involved in assessing problems at different ages; providing counsel for the patient, the family, and others; prescribing and supervising specific therapy programs; advising about and prescribing adaptive equipment; providing information about the disability and its prognosis; helping with Individual Education Programs; and guiding the parents as they act as the child's principal case managers. They can refer the child for specific care, such as orthopaedic surgery. They will know if the therapies being provided are effective and can recommend other ways to accomplish the child's developmental goals. They should know how to find out about resources, such as respite care and summer camps, as necessary. They should be the ones to keep the child's long-term future in mind and to help keep plans and management realistic and balanced between physical and psychosocial needs and goals.

Conclusions

The developmental needs of the handicapped child are similar to those of the normal one. They include acquisition of skills in physical, mental, and social functions. The presence of a handicap may limit the child's acquisition of social skills in various ways: limited exposure, limited expectation, and limited ability to learn. The more severe the physical handicap, the more important it is that the child have good social ability to help with getting needed attention, company, and affection. The goal is as normal a life as possible within the limits of the handicap; employment is not always a necessary part and marriage and parenthood are increasingly viable options as community resources become available.

REFERENCES

1. Anderson EM: The disabled child at school: special needs and special provisions. In Bergsma D, Pulver A (eds): *Developmental Disabilities: Psychological and Social Implication.* New York, Allan R. Liss, Inc., 1976.
2. Athelstan GM: Psychosocial adjustment to chronic disease and disability. In Stolov WC, Clowers MR: *Handbook of Severe Disability.* U.S. Department of Education, Rehabilitation Services Administration, 1981, p 13.
3. Barth RP: *Social and Cognitive Treatment of Children and Adolescents.* San Francisco, Jossey Bass, 1986.
4. Battle CU: Disruptions in the socialization of a young severely handicapped child. *Rehabil Lit* 35:130, 1974.
5. Biklen D: Action for inclusion. *TASH Newsletter* 16:1, 1990.
6. Bleck EE: *Orthopedic Management in Cerebral Palsy.* Philadelphia, JB Lippincott, 1987, p 146.
7. Bloom-Feshbach J, Bloom-Feshbach S: *The Psychology of Separation and Loss.* San Francisco, Jossey Bass, 1987, p 136.
8. Brazelton TB, Cramer BG: *The Earliest Relationship.* New York, Addison-Wesley, 1990.
9. British Sports Association for the Disabled: *Water Sports for the Disabled.* Wakefield, England, EP Publisher, 1983.
10. Brown C: *The Story of Christy Brown (My Left Foot).* New York, Pocket Books, 1971.
11. Buscaglia L: *The Disabled and Their Parents: A Counselling Challenge.* Thorofare, NJ, Charles B. Slack, 1975.
12. Carrillo AC, Corgett K, Lewis, V: *No More Stares.* Disability Rights Education and Defense Fund, Berkeley, CA, 1982.
13. Cole TM, Cole SS: Sexual adjustment to chronic disease and disability. In Stolov WC, Clowers MR (eds): *Handbook of Severe Disability.* U.S. Department of Education, Rehabilitation Services Administration, 1981, p 279.
14. Coombs J: *Living with the Disabled: You Can Help.* New York, Sterling, 1984.
15. Cromer BA, Enrile B, McCoy K, Gerhardstein MJ, Fitzpatrick M, Judis J: Knowledge, attitudes and behavior related to sexuality in adolescents with chronic disability. *Dev Med Child Neurol* 32:602, 1990.
16. Diamond M: Sexuality and the handicapped. *Rehabil Lit* 35:34, 1974.
17. Downey JA, Low NL: *The Child with Disabling Illness. Principles of Rehabilitation,* 2nd ed. New York, Raven Press, 1982.
18. Dunham CS: Social-sexual relationships. In Goldenson RM (ed): *Disability and Rehabilitation Handbook.* New York, McGraw Hill, 1979.
19. Dunham CS: The role of the family. In Goldenson RM (ed): *Disability and Rehabilitation Handbook.* New York, McGraw Hill, 1979.

20. Furgang NT, Yerxa EJ: Expectations of teachers for handicapped and normal first grade students. *Am J Occup Ther* 33:697, 1979.
21. Harris FR, Wolf MM, Baer DM: The effects of adult social reinforcement on child behavior. *Young Child* 20:8, 1964.
22. Heller BW, Flohr LM, Zegans LS (eds): *Psychosocial Intervention with Physically Handicapped Persons.* New Brunswick, Rutgers University Press, 1989.
23. Jellinek MS, Murphy JM: Screening for psychosocial disorders in pediatric practice. *Am J Dis Child* 142:1153, 1988.
24. Jernberg AM: *Theraplay.* San Franciso, Jossey-Bass, 1979.
25. King SM, Rosenbaum P, Armstrong RW, Milner R: An epidemiological study of children's attitudes toward disability. *Dev Med Child Neurol* 31:237, 1989.
26. Lord J, Varzos N, Behrman B, Wicks J, Wicks D: Implications of mainstream classrooms for adolescents with spina bifida. *Dev Med Child Neurol* 32:20, 1990.
27. Meadow KP, Meadow L: Changing role perceptions for parents of handicapped children. *Except Child* 38:21, 1971.
28. Mosher J: Employment and job placement. In Goldenson RM (ed): *Disability and Rehabilitation Handbook.* New York, McGraw Hill, 1979.
29. Murphy K, Molnar GE: Employment and social issues in adults with cerebral palsy. *Arch Phys Med Rehabil* 70:1989.
30. Nicholas M: Communication and the multiply-handicapped child. *Teacher Deaf* 70:361, 1972.
31. Osman B, Blinder H: *No One to Play With: The Social Side of Learning Disabilities.* New York, Random House, 1982.
32. Pearlman, L Scott KA: *Raising the Handicapped Child.* Englewood Cliffs, NJ, Prentice Hall, 1981.
33. Perrin JCS, Reusch EL, Pray JL, Wright GF, Bartlett GS: Evaluation of a ten-year experience in a comprehensive care program for handicapped children. *Pediatrics* 50:793, 1972.
34. Robinault IP: *Sex, Society and the Disabled.* New York, Harper & Row, 1978.
35. Scherzer AL, Ilson JB, Mike V, Iandoli M: Educational and social development among intensively treated young patients having cerebral palsy. *Arch Phys Med Rehabil* 54:478, 1973.
36. Strain PS, Kerr MM: Treatment issues in the remediation of handicapped children's social isolation. *Educ Treat Child* 2:197, 1979.
37. Strax TE: Psychological problems of disabled adolescents and young adults. *Pediatr Ann* 17:756, 1988.
38. Tew B, Lawrence KM, Jenkins V: Factors affecting employability among young adults with spina bifida and hydrocephalus. *Zeitsch Kinderchir* (Suppl 1) 45:34–36, 1990.
39. Vining EPG, Accardo PJ, Rubenstein JE, Farrell SE, Roizen NJ: Cerebral palsy: A pediatric developmentalist's overview. *Am J Dis Child* 130:643, 1976.
40. Wallander JL, Varni JW, Babani L, DeHaan CB, Wilcox KT, Banis HT: The social environment and the adaptation of mothers of physically handicapped children. *J Pediatr Psychol* 14:371, 1989.
41. Yuker HE (ed): *Attitudes Toward Persons with Disabilities.* Berlin, Springer, 1988.

6

Electrodiagnosis

GLORIA D. ENG

Electrodiagnosis is a valuable extension of the neurological examination, particularly as it relates to the hypotonic infant and young child. As a diagnostic tool, it allows the examiner to differentiate the child who is hypotonic because of a cerebral, dysgenetic, or systemic cause from a child who is truly weak with a peripheral neuromuscular disorder. This information obtained from electrodiagnosis must be analyzed against a set of standards that vary with age and should be carefully interpreted in the light of the history, clinical examination, serum muscle enzyme and selected biochemical determinations, histochemical and electronmicroscopic results of an adequate muscle biopsy.

The examination requires infinite patience and consummate skill. It must be designed with care to be complete, yet not so extensive as to cause undue discomfort. The examination itself is easy in a weak and floppy infant who offers little resistance and the examination should be expeditiously done. At 18 months to 2 yr, children are readily distracted by sounds and lights on the oscillographic screen and the examination can be accomplished with minimal restraint. In the older child, gentle but firm restraint from an assistant may be necessary. The examiner should always be truthful about the probability of discomfort. This information should be given directly before the infliction of pain so that the anticipation of discomfort is not protracted. Certain parents are best separated from the child after an explanation of the procedure. In our experience, the interaction between a crying child and some parents often prevents a good complete study. In the event of a very agitated child, sedation of 50 to 75 mg/kg of chloral hydrate may be necessary. This facilitates nerve conduction velocity studies but is not preferred for EMG where active participation of the child is necessary for recruitment of motor unit action potentials (MUAP).

Instrumentation

Instrumentation requirements are similar to those used in adult electrodiagnosis (15, 42, 65). For nerve conduction velocity (NCV) studies, the stimulating electrodes should be separated by a space of 2 cm and the

143

recording electrodes can be small disc electrodes for convenient attachment to the infant or small child. For electromyography (EMG), the interpretation of amplitudes and duration of motor unit action potentials must be based on knowledge of the type of needle electrode used in the study.

The *monopolar needle* electrode is a steel needle covered with Teflon except at the tip. It can be used with a small skin surface reference electrode placed a short distance away, well secured with "just enough" electrode paste. To obviate baseline "noise," the needle electrode must be well inserted into the muscle with the reference electrode and ground electrode firmly attached to the skin. The needle must be examined for possible fraying or denudement of Teflon because if the needle is damaged, then the amplitude of the recorded potential will appear reduced.

The *concentric* needle electrode consists of a cannula with a central wire. The recorded potentials appear lower in amplitude and shorter in duration; however, there is less muscle and needle noise with this type of electrode.

In our experience in neonates, using monopolar needle electrodes of 26 to 28 gauge, with adequate depth to penetrate the subcutaneous tissue and fat, the amplitude of the MUAP ranges from 150 uV to 3 mV; duration is 2 to 5 msec depending on the muscle studied. Sacco et al. (58) found the duration of the MUAP shorter in young subjects but the amplitude was the same as in adults. DeCarmo (16) suggested that the mean amplitude is higher in infants than adults but the duration was 17% to 26% shorter compared to those in adults.

The use of a tape recorder or storage scope permits later retrieval of information for careful measurement and analysis. Temperature of the child should be monitored and controlled. Occasionally, it may be necessary to study an infant in an incubator. Adequate grounding is necessary but ground loops must be avoided if the infant is attached to other equipment.

Nerve Conduction Velocity Studies

These studies (32, 42, 44) are applicable to the child suspected of having a neuropathy. The problem may be an isolated disorder, as in facial palsy, or it may be diffuse, as in some of the hereditary or infectious neuropathies. Chronic lead intoxication and other toxins may cause neuropathy. Trauma to the brachial plexus, laceration, compression, or crush injuries of the peripheral nerves can be evaluated. There are neuropathies associated with central nervous system problems as in Krabbe's disease, metachromatic leukodystrophy, and/or neuroaxonal dystrophy. And finally, neuropathies must be considered associated with diabetes mellitus, other metabolic dysfunctions, and the relatively rare mucopolysaccharide disorders.

PLACEMENT OF ELECTRODES

The electrode placement must be precise with the recording electrode on the belly of the muscle and the reference electrode on the respective tendon, the ground placed between the stimulus electrode and the recording electrode. Because the surfaces are small, the electrical impulse at supramaximal stimulus can spread to the other nerves and the recording electrodes can pick up volume-conducted potentials from contiguous muscles. It is, therefore, necessary to study the configuration of the evoked potential proximally and distally to be sure that the major deflection is negative in polarity and that the evoked potential emanates from the particular nerve under study. The median and ulnar nerves can be easily studied with surface recording electrodes at the abductor pollicis brevis or at the abductor digiti quinti, respectively. The posterior tibial nerve is also readily available with the proximal stimulus applied at the popliteal fossa, the distal behind the medial malleolus, and the recording electrodes at the abductor digiti quinti. Stimulation of the peroneal nerve presents no problem at the head of the fibula. However, distally at the dorsum of the ankle, the response frequently gets "wiped out" because of the close proximity of stimulating and recording electrodes. The ground should be placed between the distal stimulus and the recording electrodes, which may not be possible in an infant. The use of a concentric needle electrode in the extensor digitorum brevis circumvents this problem.

The axillary, suprascapular, dorsal scapular, musculocutaneous, and radial nerves should be evaluated in brachial plexus injuries, brachial neuritis, and upper arm lacerations. Because distances are short, comparison of latencies of the involved nerve to that of the opposite arm as well as comparative analysis of the evoked potentials in terms of amplitude and duration can provide the desired information. Occasionally, it is necessary to study the phrenic nerves in cases of diaphragmatic paralysis or in high cervical cord injury in preparation for phrenic nerve pacing. The nerve is stimulated posterior to the sternocleidomastoid muscle above the clavicle and recording electrodes are positioned at the 4th or 5th intercostal space along the anterior axillary line (54). This study, performed under fluoroscopy, can define the vigor of the diaphragmatic contraction.

In the patient with severe muscle atrophy, as in spinal muscular atrophy or arthrogryposis, concentric needle electrode recording in whatever remaining trace muscle may give a reading. Choosing a bulkier muscle, such as the tibialis anterior for the peroneal nerve, may give information on the integrity of the proximal segment of that nerve.

Temperature control is important in babies who tend to cool rapidly thus affecting NCV. The exact decrease per degree of temperature fall has not been measured in children, but the presumption is that it is probably similar to the adult values of 2.4 M/sec/1° C drop.

Surface measurements between the stimulating electrodes proximally and distally are very short in infants. The distance between the head of the fibula and the dorsum of the ankle may range from 7.5 to 9 cm in a newborn. Inaccuracies in measurement will alter the conduction velocities by small increments but the shorter the distance, the larger the error.

The effect of age on velocity has to be considered in infants and children under the age of 5 yr. Motor conduction velocities rise with increasing age, as has been well documented by Gamstorp (31), Baer and Johnson (2), Cerra and Johnson (8), Ruppert and Johnson (57), Thomas and Lambert (68), Wagner and Buchthal (71), and, more recently, by Khater-Boidin and Duron (41). The conduction velocities can distinguish a short gestational age baby from a small-for-date baby. At birth, the velocities are approximately one-half of adult levels, and gradually reach adult levels between ages 3 and 5 yr. Wagner and Buchthal (71) determined velocities in children between 1 month and 4 yr of age; the scatter was 8 to 15 M/sec (2 SD). It, therefore, becomes apparent that it can be very difficult to decide if the velocities are within the normal range of if they are significantly slow in very young infants.

Since myelination is incomplete in very young infants, temporal dispersion may not be obvious and the evoked compound action potential may only remain low in amplitude. Edema of the limbs, as seen in hypothyroidism and some cases of diabetic acidosis, may cause difficulties in velocity determinations. The elicited responses may be very flat and hard to decipher on the oscilloscope.

There are certain parameters in the performance of motor NCV studies that must be considered in order to maintain accuracy of results. Setting the time indicator on the oscillographic rise time of the initial deflection of the "M" response remains the greatest source of error. If the rise time is slow and there exists an abnormal rounded, upward deflection, it is difficult to decide on the precise point of take off. Repositioning the recording electrode or changing filter settings may be indicated. Changing the sweep speed can also give a sharper take-off from the baseline.

SENSORY NERVE CONDUCTION VELOCITY

It is easy to elicit sensory nerve latencies in normal infants and children because the dermis and subcutaneous tissues are thin. Direct application of the stimulating electrodes to the fingers will give a crisp oscillographic response. Difficulties arise in tiny infants where the stimulating and recording electrodes are practically on top of each other and the electrode paste smears across anode and cathode. The grasp response is so strong in the normal infant's hand that it is sometimes impossible to have the fingers neatly extended for these studies. In suspected sensory neuropathies, it may be necessary to sedate the child, stabilize the test parts, and use direct needle stimulation to obtain results. A clue to the presense of sensory neuropathy may be the child's insensitivity to higher voltages of the stimulating current. The sensory nerve action potential may consist of a double peak in the infant indicative of the presence of rapid and slow conducting fibers within the incompletely myelinated nerve (53).

The H reflex (6) is easily elicited in infancy in almost any skeletal muscle on submaximal stimulation of the appropriate nerve. It is gradually suppressed by age 1 yr, with the exception of the muscles supplied by the tibial and the median nerves (29). Since the H reflex can be used to study NCV over a longer nerve segment, it may reveal a neuropathy in a child before the distal motor and sensory segments appear grossly abnormal. It is useful in studying the proximal segment in the Guillaine-Barré syndrome or in the root and trunk damage of brachial or sacral plexus involvement. The H reflex is easily elicited in all muscles in children who suffer upper motor neuron dysfunction as in some of the degenerating brain disorders, or in spinal cord lesions below the level of the pathology.

F WAVE

The F wave can be elicited by placing the recording electrode over the intrinsic muscles of the extremities while supramaximally stimulating the appropriate nerve (29, 47). It variably appears at approximately the same location as the H reflex. The stimulus ascends the motor fibers antidromically and impacts on the anterior horn cells to return orthodromically to cause muscle contraction. The F wave is not affected when the dorsal roots are disrupted. In children, it is not a particularly well-tolerated or useful determination.

Neuromuscular Transmission Studies (10, 27, 45, 52)

Myasthenia gravis is a disorder in which muscle weakness increases with exertion, but improves with rest and anticholinesterase medication. Reduced sensitivity of the postsynaptic membrane to acetylocholine accounts for the weakness. The defect can be elicited by repetitive nerve stimulation. According to Lambert (52), the optimal frequency of stimulation is 2 to 3/sec. The limb to be studied must be well immobilized with the stimulating and recording electrodes securely taped in place. The stimuli should be supramaximal, approximatley 50% over maximum. A train of three to five stimuli is applied. A smooth reproducible decrement of the evoked potentials of 8% to 10% may be significant. The muscle must be rested 15 sec between tests. The defect at the neuromuscular junction can be enhanced by exercise, which results in postactivation facilitation. About 2 to 4 minutes after the exercise, there is progressive decline during repetitive stimulation at 2 to 3/sec, which results in postactivation exhaustion.

It is important to keep in mind that there seems to be a difference between endplates of infants and adults. Repetitive stimulation in healthy premature and newborn infants at slow rates of speed shows good maintenance of evoked responses. However, at high rates of stimulation, there is rapid decrement and, in some normal infants, there is postactivation exhaustion (10, 50). These findings should be considered when an infant born to a myasthenic mother or with congenital myasthenia is studied.

It is necessary to keep the muscle warm at 35 to 37° C to facilitate the decremental response. Ischemia and exercise may also enhance the production of decrement. The decline of evoked potentials can be reversed by the injection of edrophonium chloride into the affected patient.

Children with ocular myasthenia frequently have normal peripheral muscle stimulation responses. Odzemir and Young (56) claim that when several proximal and distal muscles are tested to include facial muscles, decrement may be found in up to 95% of patients. This is usually not the case in the evaluation of a young child. Sometimes the dramatic clinical response to edrophonium chloride is still the best indication that the child indeed has the disorder.

Although the single fiber electromyography is useful in adult myasthenia patients where there is increased jitter and transmission block, the technique remains impractical in children under 7 yr of age (64).

Approximately 10% to 15% of infants born to myasthenic mothers have neonatal myasthenia. These infants should show decrement, even in distal muscles with slow repetitive stimulation, and prompt recovery with edrophonium chloride.

Congenital myasthenia occurs in infants of nonmyasthenic mothers and remains with the affected children through life. Although it accounts for 1% of all cases of myasthenia, it can be difficult to diagnose and manage. In unraveling this disorder, several different syndromes have been identified, each with a different mechanism of failure of neuromuscular transmission.

Engel and Lambert and associates (26, 27) have distinguished (a) a myasthenic syndrome with endplate acetylcholinesterase deficiency, small nerve terminals, and acetylcholine release; (b) familial congenital myasthenic syndrome with prolonged endplate potentials and normal acetylcholinesterase; and (c) familial congenital myasthenic syndrome, probably due to deficient synthesis of acetylcholine. Children affected show varying degrees of ophthalmoparesis and weakness of neck and peripheral muscles. In the last type, the neonatal course may be quite stormy with feeding and respiratory difficulties leading to possible early death. Juvenile myasthenia gravis affects older children and behaves more like the adult type. Although endocrinopathies were found in a number of their patients, a convulsive disorder was the most commonly associated problem.

The Eaton-Lambert syndrome usually found in adults with small cell carcinoma of the bronchus, has been described in children between 9 and 16 yr of age (9). The initial amplitude of the evoked responses on repetitive stimulation is low and, on slow stimulation, there is further decremental lowering of the amplitude (Fig. 6.1). After exercise or tetanic contractions, there is facilitation of the potentials by as much as 200%.

In infantile botulism (11), tic paralysis, antibiotic blockade, there is disturbance at the presynaptic membrane of the neuromuscular junction and repetitive stimulation may show features of the myasthenic syndrome (Figs. 6.2 and 6.3). In motor neuron disease, neuropathies, some of the metabolic myopathies, and myotonia, there may be a secondary effect on neuromus-

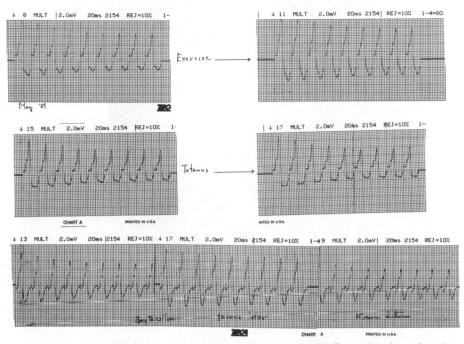

Figure 6.1. Neuromuscular transmission study in a boy with Eaton-Lambert disorder. Decrement in first five potentials on repetitive stimulation of 2/sec. Facilitation was more apparent after exercise than after tetanizing current. There was some improvement after Tensilon with evidence of minimal exhaustion 15 minutes later.

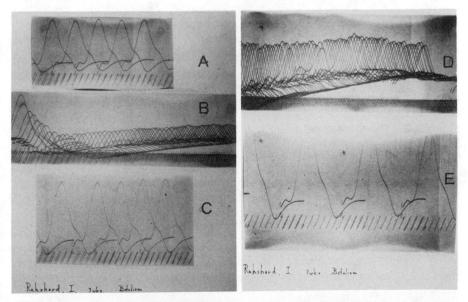

Figure 6.2. Neuromuscular transmission in a 7-week infant with botulism. **A,** repetitive stimulation at 2/sec; **B,** repetitive stimulation at 20/sec; **C,** facilitation seen after rapid stimulation without postactivation exhaustion on subsequent stimulation (**D** and **E**).

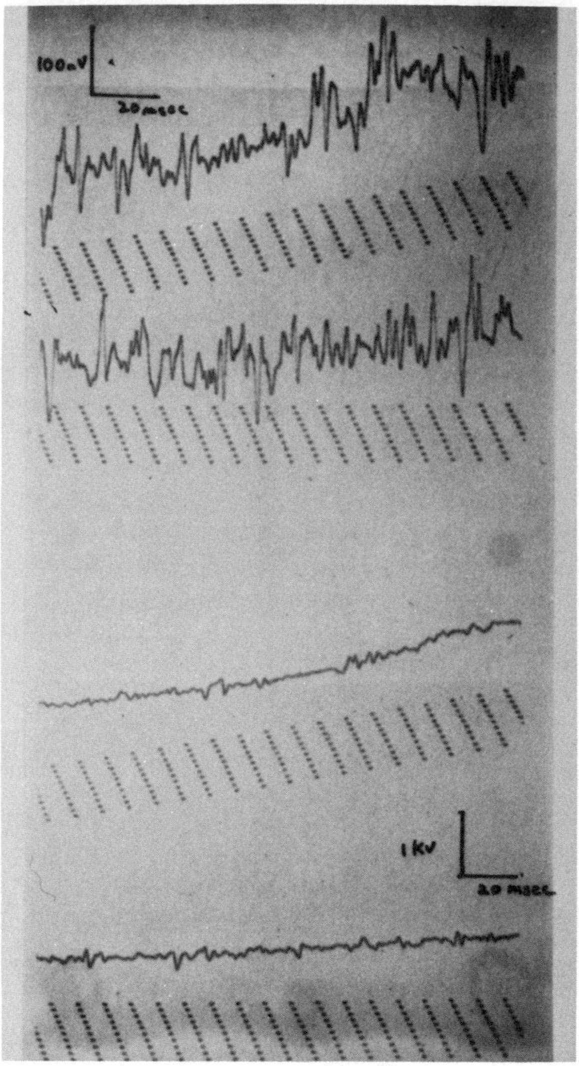

Figure 6.3. Seven-week-old infant with botulism. Note extremely low amplitude of MUAPs.

cular transmission manifested by abnormal stimulation studies and single fiber electromyography.

Electromyography

The design of an EMG study (7, 38, 39, 43) is based on why the study is being done in the first place. If the clinical lesion involves a plexus injury, then the affected extremity is methodically explored. If it is a spinal cord lesion, as in lumbosacral meningomyelocele, the lower extremities and available paraspinal muscles as well as rectal sphincter should be studied. If there is suspicion of a diffuse neuromuscular disorder, then the proximal and distal muscles in the lower extremity are sampled. In cases of facio-scapulohumeral dystrophy, facial, sternocleidomastoid muscle, trapezius, and tibialis anterior may be selected. When studying a child for a possible neuromuscular disorder, because of the hereditary nature of these diseases, the parents must be carefully assessed as well. Muscle selection to control for active contraction or relaxation is necessary in the uncooperative child to obtain adequate information. The biceps muscle is a good muscle to study for recruitment pattern, as is the tibialis anterior. The quadriceps and gastrocnemius are readily immobilized and allow for study of a relaxed muscle. A muscle should be placed at its shortest length from origin to insertion to obtain electrical silence (38, 40).

TECHNIQUE

Upon insertion of the needle electrode, the infant or child will contract the muscle immediately. This permits appreciation of the insertional activity, the recruitment pattern, and amplitude and duration of the MUAPs. The sweep speed of the oscilloscope should be set at 10 msec/cm, occasionally switching to 5 msec/cm to measure the duration of the MUAPs. The gain should be set at 100 μV, switching to 1 mV to observe the amplitude of the MUAPs. After the initial burst of activity, there is usually electrical silence. At this time, explore for spontaneous activity, such as fibrillation potentials and positive sharp waves. Avoid the endplate zones, which are frequently encountered in the small muscles of the infant. It may be necessary to switch to 50 μV/cm to "see" the fibrillation potentials.

Insertional Activity

Insertional activity results from movement of the needle electrode as it penetrates the muscle. This activity lasts for a fraction of a second. There is increased insertional activity in disorders of nerve and muscle when there is denervation, muscle membrane instability, and segmental isolation of muscle fibers. Examples include collagen-vascular disease, myotubular myopathy, glycogen-storage disorders. When there is severe atrophy or fibrosis of muscle the insertional activity is reduced and a "wooden feel" is appreciated on needle penetration.

MUAP Recruitment

As strength of voluntary contraction increases, there is orderly increase in MUAPs recruited. However, in very young infants and children, it is sometimes difficult to assess strength of voluntary contraction and determine when the interference pattern is a full one. The examiner has to gauge the strength of contraction as he or she views the recruitment pattern. The use of the Moro reflex, positioning the limb against gravity, can sometimes elicit a maximum contraction. In the extremely hypotonic infant, it is sometimes difficult to elicit recruitment. If small amounts of effort result in recruitment of many MUAPs, the possibility of a myopathic process has to be considered. If the infant in trying to contract a muscle against gravity or stretch only recruits a few MUAPs, then the possibility of a neuropathic process may be present.

Variation in amplitude of MUAPs may occur in neuromuscular transmission disorders; i.e., myasthenia gravis and infantile botulism, but may be seen in chronic myopathies where there is reinnervation of degenerating muscle fibers as well as in nerve damage with reinnervation.

Spontaneous Potentials

Muscles in neonates and children under 1 yr of age are quite small so that single insertion of the needle electrode with stellate exploration can cover an entire muscle. Neuromuscular junctions are numerous and readily encountered. High-frequency potentials and endplate noise—"sea shell sounds"—are abundant. Fibrillation potentials with an initial negative phase and firing patterns at a constant rate probably represent single fiber potentials and are secondary to spontaneous depolarization or after movement of the needle electrode. Fetal muscle, which is not innervated, has an oscillating membrane that can trigger an action potential along the muscle fiber, also resulting in fibrillation.

Positive sharp waves are biphasic, positive-negative potentials that fire at regular rate. They are thought to be the result of the needle electrode recording from the site of origin of the action potential and have the same significance as fibrillation potentials.

Complex repetitive discharges may represent synchronized firing of single fiber action potentials connected by ephaptic transmission between adjacent fibers. In infants, these potentials are seen in the glycogen-storage disorders, also in Type I hypotrophy with central nuclei (myotubular myopathy).

Myotonic discharges are the result of rhythmic repetitive discharges of single muscle fibers. They are usually biphasic spiked potentials with firing rates of 20 to 80 Hz and have amplitudes and frequencies that wax and wane.

Fasciculation potentials occur spontaneously at 2 to 20 Hz or continuously at 1 to 5 Hz and are found in neurogenic disorders.

SPECIFIC APPLICATIONS

Facial Palsy

Nerve excitability studies can be done within 72 hours comparing the intensity of the current required to elicit a response upon stimulation of one facial nerve versus the other (46). Nerve conduction latency studies can be performed 10 to 14 days after onset but the relative amplitude of the compound motor action potentials (CMAPs) at the 4th and 5th day is the best way to determine prognosis. Later degeneration may still occur, however. The blink reflex is difficult to elicit in infants and young children, especially the R_2 component, and has not been very useful in our hands. The children tend to move and cry, which creates baseline noise obliterating the evoked action potentials. EMG of the facial muscles is not well tolerated in young children. Surface EMGs avoiding the temporalis and masseter muscles as well as cross-over fibers from muscles on the unaffected side sometimes will give enough information about the underlying facial muscles even in a child who appears totally paralyzed.

Brachial Plexus Palsy

Traction injuries affecting the brachial plexus (24, 72) can occur during a difficult delivery. There may be stretching of trunks and even avulsion of the spinal roots. EMG and NCV studies can localize the site and extent of the lesion and can document recovery as reinnervation occurs. Specific nerves, such as the suprascapular, dorsal scapular, axillary, musculocutaneous, radial, ulnar, median, median sensory, radial sensory, ulnar sensory, as well as the phrenic nerve can be studied. Contrasting the nerve latency results obtained from the affected limb with the unaffected limb is necessary since no normative data of the proximal limb nerve latencies in infants and very young children exist. EMG should be performed at 14 to 21 days to determine the extent of paralysis. Absence of fibrillation potentials when there are no MUAPs recruited may signify neurapraxia. On the other hand, profuse fibrillation potentials may not indicate a complete lesion. The paraspinal muscles should be studied if root avulsion or an associated spinal cord lesion is suspected, especially in the child with bilateral plexus injuries. A second study should be done 6 to 8 weeks after the first examination. This will give information on relative recruitment of MUAPs, presence or absence of reinnervation indicated by increasing numbers of small polyphasic potentials. Later, surface EMG can determine recruitment patterns without the use of needle exploration.

Myelodysplasia

The level and extent of paralysis and the integrity of the sphincters can be determined by EMG in the child born with myelodysplasia (37). It is important to establish a spinal level in the neonatal period. The information can be predictive of future neuromuscular imbalance affecting the joints of the lower extremities and can suggest the level bracing required and the need for probable surgical intervention. More importantly, the EMG provides baseline information for later comparison should tethering or syrinx development in the cord change the initial level of paralysis.

THE HYPOTONIC INFANT (FLOPPY BABY)

In evaluating the hypotonic infant, the examiner has to differentiate between paralytic or nonparalytic causes (23). The most frequent reasons for nonparalytic hypotonia may be a dysgenetic or diffuse cerebral lesion that evolves into frank cerebral palsy, particularly of the dyskinetic form; mental retardation (MR) of obscure etiology; genetic disorders, such as Down or Prader-Willi syndromes; or systemic illness. The muscle strength reflexes are usually intact or hyperactive. Delayed assimilation of primitive reflexes may be obvious. A paralytic peripheral neuromuscular disorder must be suspected if the infant has real weakness and diminished or lost reflexes.

Spinal Muscular Atrophy (SMA)

Represented by a spectrum of disorders, SMA classified into an infantile form, a juvenile type, and a late-onset variety. The infantile form (Werdnig-Hoffman disease) is the most common peripheral neuromuscular disorder that affects infants. If paralysis occurs in utero, the baby can be born with arthrogrypotic changes. Otherwise, the infant may seem normal at birth and weakness may appear several weeks later. The infant develops sucking and swallowing problems and diminished respiratory capacity breathing primarily with the diaphragm; the typical posture of hips is abduction, arms in the "jug-handle" position, and the infant becomes increasingly limp and areflexic.

Motor and sensory NCVs are mostly within normal limits but the evoked CMAPs may be low in amplitude due to axonal loss.

There is decreased recruitment of MUAPs. Their configurations may be normal in amplitudes, but usually long in duration, exceeding 8 msec up to 20 msec. Some MUAPs are low in amplitude and may be only 2 to 3 msec in duration. Spontaneous activity in the form of rhythmic discharges occurring at 5 to 15 sec, even in the sleeping infant, have been noted. Fibrillation potentials may not be profuse (34) (Fig. 6.4).

In the more benign forms (34) of spinal muscular atrophy, the amplitude and duration of MUAPs increase. There are more spontaneous discharges in the form of fibrillations and positive sharp waves. Fasciculations are more prominent.

Myotonic Dystrophy. The fetal form is a relatively common disorder (40, 67). The infant usually suffers a complicated gestation and birth. Mothers frequently have a history of fetal wastage, develop polyhydramnios during the pregnancy, resulting in complicated deliveries, frequently by cesarean section. The infant presents with facial diplegia, a tented lip, ptosis of the eyelids, a weak suck and cry, cryptorchidism if a boy, and talipes equinovarus deformities. There may be bradycardia as well as sleep apnea. EMG study should focus on distal limb muscles (51). MUAP may be low in amplitude and short in duration. Myotonia is difficult to find and the runs of pos-

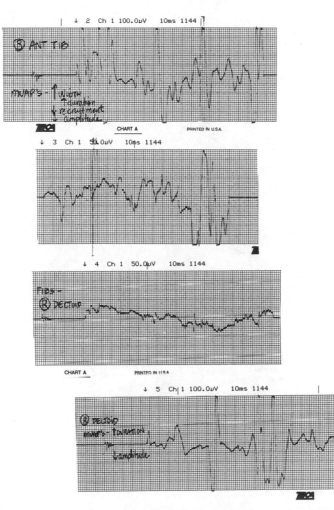

Figure 6.4. Spinal muscular atrophy, Type I. Diminishing recruitment of MUAP; long duration (>20 msec) MUAP, rare fibrillation potentials.

itive potentials may be brief without the obvious typical waxing and waning pattern. The parents, particularly the mother, should be studied to confirm the diagnostic impression. In myotonia congenita, the EMG shows the MUAPs to be normal. However, there is prolonged after-activity consisting of discharges of low voltage and short duration after the active contraction has stopped (Fig. 6.5).

Muscular Dystrophy. Infants may be born with congenital muscular dystrophy, the infantile form of facioscapulohumeral dystrophy, or limb-girdle dystrophy. The EMG usually shows increased recruitment patterns even with moderate effort (Fig. 6.6). Myotonia-like discharges, brief runs of pos-

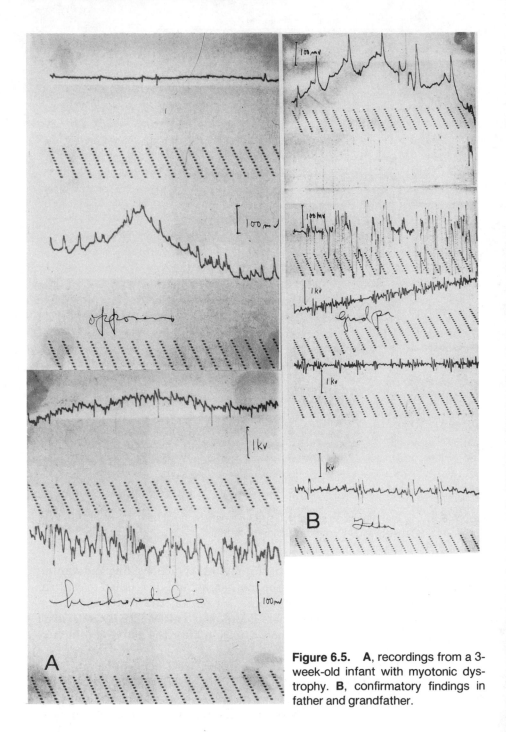

Figure 6.5. **A,** recordings from a 3-week-old infant with myotonic dystrophy. **B,** confirmatory findings in father and grandfather.

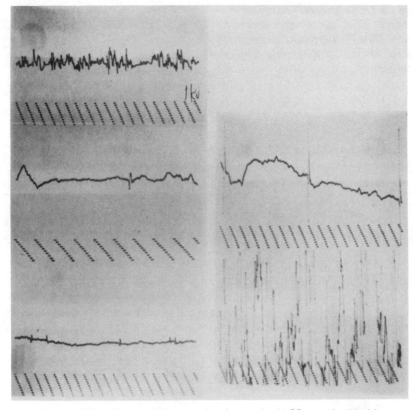

Figure 6.6. Congenital muscular dystrophy in 23-month-old girl.

itive potentials—probably reflecting membrane instability—may be seen. Because of segmental necrosis of muscle fibers, disruption of neural influence may allow some fibers to fibrillate. Increase in polyphasic potentials and parasite or satellite potentials may by evident (7, 17). Figures 6.7 and 6.8 show two EMG samples from Duchenne muscular dystrophy.

Congenital Myopathies. Congenital myopathies are a collection of muscle disorders of variable inheritance patterns, nonprogressive or slowly progressive, diagnosed best histologically and electron microscopically because the EMG findings are relatively nonspecific and may even be normal (19, 38, 40, 42) (Fig. 6.9). Only selected examples of more common congenital myopathies are described.

Myotubular Myopathy. Type 1 hyotrophy with central nuclei is a rare disorder whose genetic inheritance is variable (40). Physical examination reveals hypotonia, ptosis with ophthalmoplegia, and, if the affected infant survives the neonatal period, there is gradual improvement over the years.

The EMG reveals low amplitude, short duration MUAPs with increased

Figure 6.7. Duchenne muscular dystrophy. Low amplitude, short duration MUAP; increased recruitment for effort; Complex repetitive discharges.

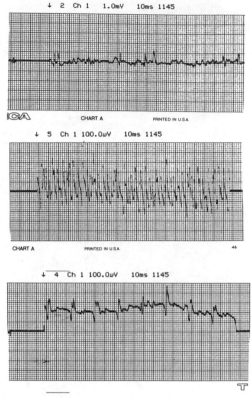

polyphasia, complex repetitive discharges, and profuse fibrillation potentials. It is the only myopathy "consistently" associated with spontaneous activity.

Nemaline Myopathy. This is an autosomal dominant disorder, with moderate hypotonia (55, 60). Respiratory complications sometimes necessitate early tracheostomy. The EMG is nonspecific. Low amplitude, short duration potentials or diminished recruitment of high amplitude, short duration potentials may be noted. Occasionally, fibrillation potentials, positive sharp waves, have been recorded.

Central Core or Multicore Disease. The affected infants may be mildly hypotonic (30, 61, 70). They may have dislocating hips and patellas; "lumpy" muscles as well as scoliosis have been noted in older children. These children are susecptible to MH (malignant hyperthemia) especially those with elevated creatine kinase (CK) (48). EMG is nonspecific. Low amplitude, "notched" potentials and some increase in polyphasic potentials have been seen.

Congenital Fiber Type Disproportion. Affected infants (3, 66) are hypotonic at birth and may be confused with SMA I. However, they may have a

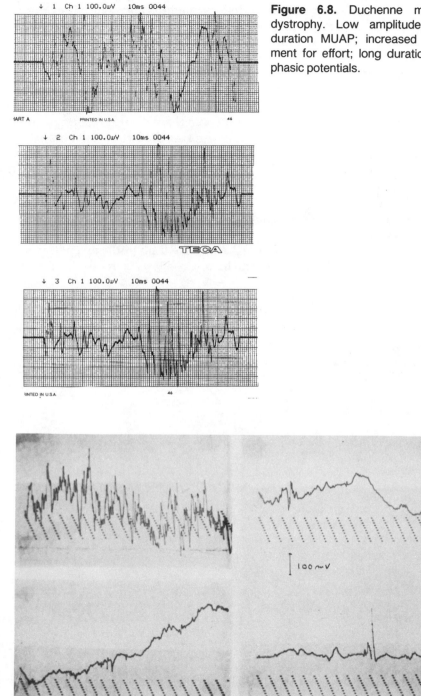

↓ 1 Ch 1 100.0µV 10ms 0044

HART A   PRINTED IN U.S.A.   46

↓ 2 Ch 1 100.0µV 10ms 0044

TECA

↓ 3 Ch 1 100.0µV 10ms 0044

RINTED IN U.S.A.   46

Figure 6.8. Duchenne muscular dystrophy. Low amplitude, short duration MUAP; increased recruitment for effort; long duration polyphasic potentials.

100 ~V

Figure 6.9. Recording from an infant with Type I hypotrophy with central nuclei.

dysmorphic facial appearance with dislocating hips and deformities of the feet. They may improve with time. EMG shows nonspecific changes compatible with myopathy and fibrillations, positive waves, and, occasionally, larger MUAPs.

Metabolic Myopathies. *Acid Maltase Deficiency (Glycogenosis).* An infant with profound weakness, cardiomegaly, and "rubbery" muscles should be suspect for glycogen storage disease (Pompe disease) (33, 36, 40). There is absence of lysosomal acid maltase in these disorders and the muscles are literally choked with glycogen disrupting the muscle membrane.

EMG shows increased insertional activity, repetitive discharges, low amplitude short duration potentials, myotonic discharges, profuse fibrillations, and positive sharp waves (Fig. 6.10).

Lipid Myopathies. Disorders of lipid metabolism (20, 25) include carnitine palmityl transferase deficiency, carnitine deficiency, and others awaiting definition.

Carnitine deficiency causes slowly progressive limb-girdle myopathy and episodic hepatic insufficiency. Muscle histology shows increased lipid droplets, especially in Type I fibers.

On EMG, there is increased recruitment, decreased amplitude, and increased duration of MUAPs. Fibrillations are occasionally present.

Carnitine palmityl transferase deficiency (20, 25) may result in muscle cramps and, in later childhood, in myoglobinuria. The child may not be weak between attacks. EMG may be normal.

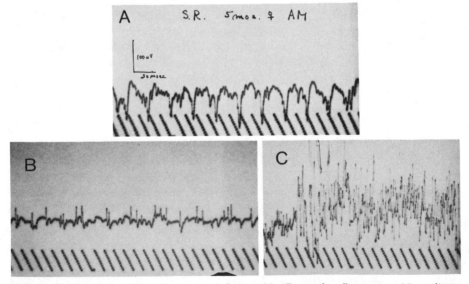

Figure 6.10. Recordings from an infant with Pompe's disease, acid maltase deficiency.

Polymyositis/Dermatomyositis. Polymyositis/dermatomyositis (40,69) has been described as early as 9 months of age. EMG reveals low amplitude, short duration MUAPs, increased polyphasic potentials with fibrillation potentials, and sharp waves. Complex repetitive discharges may be numerous.

Miscellaneous Studies. Vocal cord paralysis in children can be studied by monopolar EMG to determine partial or complete paralysis, whether truly paralytic secondary to denervation or due to structural adhesions (49).

Transmucosal EMG has been useful in the study of children suspected of having Hirschprung's disease (73). In the normal colon, the basic electrical rhythm consists of 4 to 6 waves/min with bursts of high frequency spikes, 3 to 4 sec, superimposed on the slow waves. In Hirschprung's disease, there is an irregular basic electrical rhythm with waves of variable duration and absence of high frequency potentials; the demarcation between normal and abnormal bowel is discrete.

EMG in kinesiologic studies has offered better insight to the pathomechanics of gait and movement, thus introducing a more reasonable approach to orthopaedic intervention in some patients (1). EMG has also been valuable in biofeedback techniques for muscle re-education and relaxation.

Brainstem and Somatosenory-evoked Potentials

Development in computer technology with averaging techniques has resulted in the ability to record auditory, visual, and somatosensory-evoked potentials in medical diagnosis. Because these techniques are noninvasive, they are particularly applicable to infants and young children. Over a decade of research (4, 5, 12, 18, 28, 59) has yielded information regarding the configurations of these potentials as they relate to maturation. The important fact to remember in these studies remains the need to develop well-controlled normative data in each laboratory, specific for different age groups. According to Desmedt et al. (18), conduction velocities in the median nerve in their laboratory reached the adult level by 12 to 18 months of age, whereas the central lemniscal pathways did not reach adult values until 5 to 7 yr of age. Segmental conduction velocities along the spinal cord in children are about half of those obtained in adults and attain adult values by age 5 yr (12).

Brainstem auditory-evoked responses are valuable in assessing infants under 6 months of age and in older noncooperative children with suspected hearing loss. The technique can be applied to infants with dysmorphic syndromes (visceral arch anomalies), premature infants with hypoxia, or infants with prolonged exposure to ototoxic drugs, congenital infections, meningitis, white matter degeneration, as well as those with brainstem abnormalities, including tumors or trauma. Brainstem auditory-evoked responses are also dependent on maturation: the younger the patient, the longer the component latency and the smaller the amplitude ratios (5, 35).

Visual-evoked potentials (62) are likewise useful in testing visual acuity affected by congenital defects, strabismus, or anisometropia. Optic nerve involvement, intrinsic, as in demyelinating disease, or extrinsic, secondary to increased pressure or tumor, can also be detected.

Somatosensory-evoked potentials allow a unique opportunity to study the entire neuraxis from the peripheral nerve to the cerebral cortex. Stimulation of the median nerve can suggest abnormalities of the peripheral nerve, brachial plexus, cervical root, and/or subcortical pathways to the somesthetic cortex. Stimulation of lower extremity nerves, either the tibial or peroneal, can identify lesions of the peripheral nerves and/or the spinal cord in demyelinating or degenerative diseases and space-occupying or traumatic lesions (13, 14). Caudal displacement or tethering of the cord may be detected by segmental conduction velocities of the spinal cord (12). The combined use of brainstem-evoked potentials and somatosensory-evoked potentials has been useful in the evaluation of brain function in severe head trauma in adults. The potentials have also been useful in intraoperative monitoring of spinal injury in surgery for scoliosis (63). These studies have to be done under stringent control because the effects of premedication and anesthesia may affect the cortical responses.

Summary

Careful electrodiagnostic evaluation, based on a complete history and physical examination and coupled with knowledge and experience in neuromuscular disorders, can suggest a diagnosis. The techniques can localize a lesion to nerve, neuromuscular junction, or muscle, with focal or diffuse involvement. They can distinguish between a neuropathic versus a myopathic disorder or transient membrane instability. However, even if the EMG is normal, certain congenital myopathies cannot be excluded. A technically well-prepared muscle biopsy should be performed to substantiate the diagnosis (21, 22).

REFERENCES

1. Adler N, Bleck EE, Rinsky LA: Gait electromyograms and surgical decisions for paralytic deformities of the foot. *Dev Med Child Neurol* 31:287–292, 1989.
2. Baer RD, Johnson EW: Motor nerve conduction velocities in normal children. *Arch Phys Med Rehabil* 46:698, 1965.
3. Banker BQ: Congenital fiber type disproportion in the congenital myopathies. In Engel AG, Banker BQ (eds): *Myology*. Chap. 51. New York, McGraw Hill, 1986, pp. 1550–1553.
4. Barnet AB, Friedman IP, Weiss IP, Ohlich ES, Shanks B, Lodge A: VEP development in infancy and early childhood. A longitudinal study. *Electroencephalog Clin Neurophysiol* 49:476, 1980.
5. Barnet AB, Ohlrich ES, Weiss IP, Shanks B: Auditory evoked potentials during sleep in normal children from ten days to three years of age. *Electroencephalog Clin Neurophysiol* 39:29, 1975.
6. Bryant P, Eng G: Normal values for the soleus H-reflex in newborn infants 31–45 weeks post-conceptional age. *Arch Phys Med Rehabil*, 71:811, 1990.
7. Buchthal F: An introduction to electromyography (EMG findings in myogenic paresis).

American Association of Electromyography and Electrodiagnosis. Custom Printing Inc., 1981.

8. Cerra D, Johnson EW: Motor conduction velocity in premature infants. *Arch Phys Med Rehabil* 43:160, 1962.
9. Chelmiska-Schorr E, Berstein LP, Zurbrugg EB, Huttenlocher PR: Eaton-Lambert Syndrome with a 9-year-old girl. *Arch Neurol* 36:572, 1979.
10. Cornblath DR: Disorders of neuromuscular transmission in infants and children. *Muscle Nerve* 9:606, 1986.
11. Cornblath DR, Sladky J, Sumner AJ: Clinical electrophysiology of infantile botulism. *Muscle Nerve* 6:448, 1983.
12. Cracco JB: Somatosensory evoked potentials in infants and children. *J Child Neurol* 4:70–72, 1989.
13. Cracco JB, Bosch VV, Cracco RQ: Cerebral and spinal somatosensory evoked potentials in children with CNS degenerative disease. *Electroencephalog Clin Neurophysiol* 49:437, 1980.
14. Cracco JB, Cracco RQ: Spinal somatosensory evoked potentials: maturational and clinical studies. *Ann NY Acad Sci* 388:526–537, 1982.
15. Daube J: Needle examination in electromyography. Mini-monograph #11. Rochester, MN, American Association of Electromyography & Electrodiagnosis, 1980.
16. Decarmo RJ: Motor unit action potential parameters in human newborn infants. *Arch Neurol* 3:136–140, 1960.
17. Desmedt JE, Borenstein S: Regeneration in Duchenne muscular dystrophy. Electromyographic evidence. *Arch Neurol* 33:642, 1976.
18. Desmedt JE, Brunko E, Debecker J: Maturation of the somatosensory evoked potentials in normal infants and children, with special reference to the early N_1 component. *Electroencephalog Clin Neurophysiol* 40:43, 1976.
19. DiMauro S, Bonilla E, Zevioni M, Nakagawa M, DeVino DC: Mitochondrial myopathies. *Ann Neurol* 17:521–538, 1985.
20. DiMauro S, Trevison C, Hays A: Disorders of lipid metabolism in muscle. *Muscle Nerve* 3:369, 1980.
21. Dubowitz V: *Muscle biopsy—a practical approach,* 2nd ed. London, Philadelphia, Baillère Tindall, 1985.
22. Dubowitz V: *Color Atlas of Muscle Disorders in Childhood.* Chicago, Year Book Medical Publishers Inc., 1989.
23. Dubowitz V: The floppy infant, ed. 2. *Clinics in Developmental Medicine,* No. 31, Spastics International/Heineman, 1980.
24. Eng G, Koch B, Smokvina M: Brachial plexus palsy in neonates and children. *Arch Phys Med Rehabil* 59:458, 1978.
25. Engel AG: Carnitine deficiency syndromes and lipid storage myopathies. In Engle AG, Banker BQ (eds): *Myology.* Chap 57. New York, McGraw-Hill, 1986, pp. 1663–1696.
26. Engel AG: Congenital myasthenic syndromes. *J Child Neurol* 3:233–246, 1988.
27. Engel AG, Fumagali G, Fukunaga H, Osame M: Clinical and morphologic approaches to disorders of neuromuscular transmission. In Serratrice G, Cros D, Desmuelle C, Gastant JL, Pelliser JF, Pouget J, Schigno A (eds): *Neuromuscular Diseases.* New York, Raven Press, 1984, p. 471.
28. Fagan ER, Taylor MJ, Logan WJ: Somatosensory evoked potentials: Part I. A review of neural generators and special considerations in pediatrics. *Pediatr Neurol* 3:189–196, 1987.
29. Fisher MA: The use of H reflexes and F responses in radiculopathies. Electrodiagnostic Approach to Common Clinical Problems. Mini Monograph American Association of Electromyography & Electrodiagnosis, Oct. 13, 1981.
30. Frank JP, Horati Y, Butler IJ, Nelson TE, Scott CI: Central core disease and malignant hyperthermia syndrome. *Ann Neurol* 7:11–17, 1980.

31. Gamstorp I: Normal conduction velocity of ulnar, median, and peroneal nerves in infancy, childhood, and adolescence. *Acta Paediatr Scand* 146:68, 1963.

32. Gilliatt RW: Electrophysiology of peripheral neuropathies—an overview. *Muscle Nerve* 5:S108–S116, 1982.

33. Gutman L, Hogan GR, Schmidt R: Electromyography and histology of Pompe's disease. *Bull Am Assoc Electromyography Electrodiag* 14:13, 1967.

34. Hausmanowa-Petrusewicz I, Karwanska A: Electromyographic findings in different forms of infantile and juvenile proximal spinal muscular atrophy. *Muscle Nerve* 9:37, 1986.

35. Hecox KE, Cone B, Blow ME: Brainstem auditory evoked responses in the diagnosis of pediatric neurologic diseases. *Neurology* 31:832, 1981.

36. Hogan GR, Gutmann L, Schmidt R, and Gilbert E: Pompe's disease. *Neurology* 19:894–900, 1969.

37. Ingberg HO, Johnson EW: Electromyography evaluation of infants with lumbar meningomyelocele. *Arch Phys Med Rehabil* 44:86, 1963.

38. Jablecki CK: Electromyography in infants and children: Review article. *J Child Neurol* 1:297, 1986.

39. Johnson EW: The EMG examination. In *Practical Electromyography,* 2nd ed. Chap. 1. Baltimore, Williams & Wilkins, 1988.

40. Jones HR Jr: EMG evaluation of the floppy infant: differential diagnosis and technical aspects. *Muscle Nerve* 13:338–347, 1990.

41. Khater-Boidin J, Duron B: Evaluation of motor, 1A and cutaneous nerve-fiber conduction velocities in premature and full-term newborns. *Dev Med Child Neurol* 31:47, 1989.

42. Kimura J: *Electrodiagnosis in Diseases of Nerve and Muscle. Principles and Practice,* 2nd ed. Chap. 25. Philadelphia, FA Davis Co, 1989, p. 535.

43. Kimura J: Electromyography—Techniques and normal findings. In *Electrodiagnosis in Diseases of Nerve and Muscle: Principles and Practice,* 2nd ed. Chap. 12. Philadelphia, FA Davis Co, 1989, pp. 227–243.

44. Kimura J: Principles of nerve conduction studies. In *Electrodiagnosis in Diseases of Nerve and Muscle: Principles and Practice,* 2nd ed. Chap. 5. Philadelphia, FA Davis Co, 1989, pp. 78–102.

45. Kimura J: Techniques of repetitive stimulation. In *Electrodiagnosis in Diseases of Nerve and Muscle: Principles and Practice,* 2nd ed. Chap. 9. Philadelphia, FA Davis Co, 1989, pp. 184–200.

46. Kimura J: The blink reflex. In *Electrodiagnosis in Diseases of Nerve and Muscle: Principles and Practice,* 2nd ed. Chap. 16. Philadelphia, FA Davis Co, 1989, pp. 307–331.

47. Kimura J: The F wave. In *Electrodiagnosis in Diseases of Nerve and Muscle: Principles and Practice,* 2nd ed. Chap. 17. Philadelphia, FA Davis Co, 1989, pp. 332–355.

48. Koch BM, Bertorini TE, Eng GD, Bochine R: Severe multicore disease associated with reaction of anesthesia. *Arch Neurol* 42:1204, 1985.

49. Koch BM, Milmoe G, Grundfast KM: Vocal cord paralysis in children studied by monopolar electromyography. *Pediatr Neurol* 3:288–293, 1987.

50. Koeningsberger MR, Pathen B, Lovelace RE: Studies of neuromuscular function in the newborn: A comparison of myoneural function in the full-term and the premature infant. *Neuropaediatrics* 4:350, 1973.

51. Kuntz NL, Daube JR: Electrophysiology of congenital myotonic dystrophy. *Abstract Electroencephalog Clin Neurophysiol* 56:S120, 1983.

52. Lambert EH: Neuromuscular transmission studies. Recent Advances in Clinical Electromyography. *Am Assoc Electromyogr Electrodiagnosis,* Sept. 1980.

53. Miller RG, Kuntz NL: Nerve conduction studies in infants and children. *J Child Neurol* 1:19, 1986.

54. Moosa A: Phrenic nerve conduction in children. *Dev Med Child Neurol* 23:434, 1981.

55. Norton P, Ellison P, Sulaiman AR, Hart J: Nemaline myopathy in the neonate. *Neurology* 33:351–356, 1983.

56. Odzemir C, Young R: The results to be expected from electrical testing in the diagnosis of myasthenia gravis. *Ann NY Acad Sci* 274:103, 1976.
57. Ruppert ES, Johnson EW: Motor nerve conduction velocities in low birth weight infants. *Pediatrics* 42:255, 1986.
58. Sacco G, Buchthal F, Rosenfalk P: Motor unit potentials at different ages. *Arch Neurol* 6:44, 1962.
59. Salamy A: Maturation of the auditory brainstem response from birth through early childhood. *J Clin Neurophysiol* July 1:293–329, 1984.
60. Shy GM, Engel WK, Somers JE, Wanko T: Nemaline myopathy; a new congenital myopathy. *Brain* 86:793, 1963.
61. Shy GM, Magee KR: A new congenital nonprogressive myopathy. *Brain* 79:610, 1956.
62. Sokol S: Pattern visually evoked potentials: Their use in pediatric ophthalmology. In Sokol S (ed): *Electrophysiology and Psychophysics: Their Use in Ophthalmic Diagnosis.* International Ophthalmology Clinics, Boston, Little, Brown, 1980.
63. Speilholz NI, Benjamin MV, Engler GL, Ransohoff J: Somatosensory evoked potentials during decompression and stabilization of the spine. *Spine* 4:500, 1979.
64. Stahlberg E: Single muscle fiber recording of the jitter phenomenon in patients with myasthenia gravis and in members of their families. *Ann NY Acad Sci* 274:189, 1976.
65. Stolov WC: Instrumentation and measurement of electrodiagnosis. Am Assoc of EMG and Electrodiagnosis. Mini monograph #16, Custom Printing, Inc. 1981.
66. Sulaiman AR, Swick HM, Kinder DS: Congenital fiber type disproportion with unusual clinicopathologic manifestations. *J Neurol Neurosurg Psychiatry* 46:175–182, 1983.
67. Swift TR, Ignacio OJ, Dyken TR: Neonatal dystrophia myotonia. Electrophysiologic studies. *Am J Dis Child* 129:734, 1975.
68. Thomas JE, Lambert EH: Ulnar nerve velocity and H reflex in infants and children. *J Appl Physiol* 15:1, 1960.
69. Thompson C: Infantile myositis. *Dev Med Child Neurol* 24:307, 1982
70. Torres CF, Griggs RC, Goetz JP: Severe neonatal centronuclear myopathy with autosomal dominant inheritance. *Arch Neurol* 42:1011–1014, 1985.
71. Wagner AL, Buchthal F: Motor and sensory conduction in infants and childhood. Reappraisal. *Dev Med Child Neurol* 14:189, 1972.
72. Wilbourn AJ: Electrodiagnosis of plexopathies. In Aminoff MJ (ed): *Neurologic Clinics.* Philadelphia, WB Saunders 3:3:511, 1985.
73. Yanagihara J, Tsuto T, Iwai N, Takahashi T: Anorectal electromyography in the diagnosis of Hirschprung's disease. *Z Kinderchir* 41:227–229, 1986.

7

Developmental Intervention and Therapeutic Exercise

PATRICIA J. TAGGART AND
DENNIS J. MATTHEWS

Rehabilitation management of the child with congenital or acquired motor dysfunction is complex and challenging. Planning an effective rehabilitation program requires a thorough understanding of the interaction of biologic, environmental, and developmental factors affecting each child. Because handicapped children often have multisystemic involvement, many professionals using a variety of training techniques and methods are necessarily involved in the program. The pediatric physiatrist, working with the child, family, and rehabilitation team and using the knowledge of interaction between structure and experience, seeks to foster an optimal developmental course so that the functional potential allowed by the organic deficits can be fully realized (47).

An accurate diagnosis, thorough assessment of the motor dysfunction and of the projected functional potential are necessary so that realistic rehabilitation goals can be established. An awareness of the life-long nature of the physical handicap is essential. Periodic reassessment and programmatic update assure that the functional goals correspond with the child's ability level.

Effective management of the child with motor dysfunction requires concern for both the child and the family. The ultimate prognosis for any handicapped child is as much dependent upon the functional effectiveness of the family in dealing with the problems as on the child's own capabilities (53). Involvement and cooperation of parents in the treatment program are essential. The family provides continuous and stable support, allowing the child to progress toward maturity and independence without loss of security (59).

The purpose of this chapter is to describe the general principles of therapeutic intervention for motor dysfunction. The potential efficacy of early intervention programs will be discussed and current research will be examined. Traditional and nontraditional theories of therapeutic exercise will be reviewed and their application to common neuromotor impairment will be discussed. A more comprehensive discussion of the application of techniques to specific disease entities and disabilities can be found in subsequent chapters.

Early Intervention Programs

There is an increasing emphasis on early recognition and referral to intervention programs of children with developmental disabilities, such as cerebral palsy, Down syndrome, other types of central nervous system dysfunction, and vision and hearing impairments. Children who do not currently demonstrate any of these disabilities, but are thought to be at high risk for developmental programs, are often recommended for enrollment in these programs (17).

Over the past decade, there have been a number of reviews that have highlighted both the risks and benefits of early infant intervention. The authors of these reviews emphasize the following points (4, 17, 33, 50, 54, 56, 58, 62):

1. Identification of infants who will do poorly is complicated and must include assessment of the infant, parent, and environment.
2. Early intervention programs are effective, particularly for those infants in whom biologic risk is coupled with environmental risk.
3. Initial gains in IQ scores may be transient, but other benefits, such as less need for special education services and repetition of grades in school, are evident in long-term follow up studies.
4. Structured curriculum, extensive parental involvement, family counseling and support services, and interventions involving the parent and child together are important factors in programs that demonstrate effectiveness.
5. Frequently, early intervention and preschool special educational programs need to be followed by further special education efforts once the child reaches elementary school.
6. Earlier referral seems to be more effective than later intervention.

An acceptable program for a developmentally disabled infant or one at high risk should be multi- or transdisciplinary in nature and closely allied with knowledgeable and supportive medical resources. A good program not only instructs and supports parents in carrying out a home exercise program, but also helps them to cope with irregularities of feeding, sleeping, crying, and other problems that lessen the chances of adequate family functioning (17).

The most extensive data available on long-term outcome in family-reared children are from preschool programs designed to prevent school failure in nonphysically handicapped children growing up in environmental risk situations (5, 6, 16, 17, 21). These programs place heavy emphasis on maternal involvement and regular home visits. All programs promoted normal development rather than being therapeutic.

Results of intervention programs in physically handicapped children and their families are less conclusive. In part, this is because there are greater difficulties in finding large homogeneous samples of children with matching and single disability. There is, however, a general consensus that these programs help improve the participants' functioning, particularly in terms of communication, social, and self-help skills, and provide considerable guidance and support to parents (13, 34). These programs tend to be more therapeutic in focus with multispecialist staff (17).

Premature and High-risk Infants

Several different schools of thought exist on the theoretical construct of intervention for preterm infants. One school argues that they should be viewed as extrauterine fetuses, with neonatal intervention aimed primarily at simulating the intrauterine environment. Peaceful, restful, womb-like activities along with vestibular, kinesthetic, and auditory stimulation characteristic of the intrauterine environment are emphasized.

The other school of thought vigorously asserts that since most body systems undergo profound physiologic changes at birth, it is quite reasonable to presume that the central nervous and sensory systems also change; therefore, the preterm infant differs substantially from the fetus and requires neonatal interventions simulating the extrauterine environment experienced by term infants. Advocates of this position tend to encourage more active, supplemental sensory stimulation with the infant awake, similar to what is done in a normal newborn nursery. Thus, the specific rationale guiding neonatal developmental intervention programs is not widely agreed upon and, in fact, continues to evolve over time (5).

The emphasis on intervention programs in the decade of the 1970s can be summarized as follows:

1. Attempt to normalize and humanize the disruptive effects of the neonatal intensive care nursery environment so that it more closely resembled the environment of term infants;
2. Correct for the presumed sensory deprivation endured by the preterm newborn treated in the neonatal intensive care nursery;
3. Compensate for intrauterine experiences lost as a result of a preterm birth (5).

Since the 1980s, there has been a shift of thinking away from efforts directed exclusively at the preterm infant toward more family-centered intervention emphasizing and facilitating parent-preterm infant interactions (4, 5, 17). These programs usually include parental instruction on infant readiness and preparedness for contact, methods to recognize and build on the infants' attempts to communicate, and instruction in the signs and symptoms of stimulation overload (gagging, vomiting, bradycardia, apnea, etc.). Parmalee (52) stresses the importance of carefully interpreting the individual infant's different behaviors as the key to the parents' understanding of preterm and term newborns' development.

Recommendations for onset, frequency, duration, and type of intervention vary from study to study. Providers also vary and include nurses, physical therapists, and occupational therapists. The reported results of intervention studies are as varied as the methodologies employed. Outcome patterns reveal great variability in terms of their nature, extent, significance, and duration (5). Positive outcomes most frequently reported include: increased state stabilization, improved neurobehavioral performance, particularly in visual and auditory orientation, higher performance on developmental scales, normalized muscle tone, decreased irritability, and increased positive affect. Medical improvements described are better feeding and subsequent weight gain, fewer apneic episodes, and more mature heart rate responses.

While most studies report at least some measurable benefit attributable to the specific intervention employed, many were not replicable in other investigations, which, in contrast, describe essentially negative findings. Because of these frequently contradictory results, only limited generalizations can be made from most of the efficacy studies.

Infants With Cognitive Deficits

Strong interest in the early evaluation of cognition is based on the idea that developmental intervention is most effective when started as early as possible. However, identification of the infant with cognitive deficit is difficult at best. Infant intelligence testing has been surrounded by controversy since its inception. Concerns about predictive value of infant tests, coupled with questions about the effect of detrimental labeling, place the value of such tests in question.

A number of medical events are known to place children at risk for cognitive impairment, including intrauterine growth retardation, severe perinatal asphyxia, extremely low birth weight, neonatal meningitis/encephalitis, intracranial hemorrhage, refractory neonatal seizures, and severe chronic lung disease with prolonged mechanical ventilation and oxygen requirements (5).

Children born with conditions accompanied by mental retardation may benefit from early intervention programs. Connolly and co-workers (19) compared developmental milestones and intellectual and adaptive functioning of 20 children with Down syndrome who participated in an early intervention program with 53 noninstitutionalized control subjects. Children in the intervention group showed earlier acquisition of motor and self-help skills and significantly higher intelligence and social quotients at 3 and 6 yr of age. Intervention consisted of 2½ hours weekly of center-based multidisciplinary program for two 10-week periods until age 3 yr.

Infants With Neuromuscular Dysfunction

Early diagnosis of motor dysfunction in the child at risk can be difficult. Knowledge of infantile motor development and movement patterns is expanding rapidly through the efforts of multidisciplinary studies (31, 36, 37, 49) as physicians, therapists, educators, and psychologists are developing better assessment tools (1, 23) and developmental examinations (2, 8) that permit earlier accurate identification.

Management in infancy includes careful positioning and alignment to prevent exaggeration of abnormal tone, reflexes, and postures. Proper handling techniques and selected sensorimotor experiences produce movement patterns and increase the child's experiences, thereby becoming the basis for learning and building blocks of future motor activity. Instruction of the parents in the therapeutic methods used to increase sensorimotor experience allows these techniques to be incorporated in the daily activities of the child (29, 43).

Most studies evaluating the effectiveness of early intervention for infants and children with motor dysfunction are anecdotal reports of personal experiences (8, 39, 41, 43). Kong (41) recommended early treatment with inhibition of tonic reflex activity, combined with facilitation of normal automatic movements provided as a center-based program for training parents. Of the 104 infants diagnosed as having cerebral palsy, 69 received intensive treatment for at least 1 yr. Of these children, 53 were reported to have minimal impairment and nine had slight involvement. No age-matched controls were used. The author postulated that early motor experience provided these children a chance to develop their normal potential, whereas those who were not treated developed subnormal skills. There are no objective data to support this proposition.

Wright and Nicholson studied the effect of physical therapy on 47 children with cerebral palsy under the age of 6 yr (66). They found no significant differences between treated and untreated groups. Their study has been criticized for flaws in design.

A more recent study by Palmer et al. (51) compared the effect of physical therapy on children with cerebral palsy. Forty-eight infants with mild to severe spastic diplegia were randomly assigned to receive either 12 months of physical therapy or 6 months of physical therapy preceded by 6 months of infant stimulation. Participants ranged in age from 12 to 19 months. In their study, differences in motor accomplishments after 12 months favored the group receiving infant stimulation. The authors suggest that the beneficial effects of infant stimulation may be due to better or broader parental understanding of the infant's development and capacities, which may have improved their ability to cope and interact (51).

Therapeutic Exercise

TRADITIONAL EXERCISES

Traditional exercises aimed at increasing strength, improving joint range of motion, and building endurance have a place in the treatment of children. However, the applicability of traditional methods may be limited in infants and preschool-aged children because of the need for cooperative participation in some forms of therapeutic exercise (42).

Activities aimed at increasing strength can take the form of progressive resistive exercises, isometric, and/or isokinetic training programs. The same purpose can be served in the younger child through the use of age-appropriate play, adaptive toys, and games.

Mobility of the joints and soft tissues is maintained by the normal movement of each part of the body. Limitation of range of motion is of greatest importance when it interferes with normal posture or activities. It is easier to prevent tightness by frequent repeated activities rather than to correct limitations after they develop. Movements should be performed through the full anatomic range several times daily (42). The child should actively perform mobility exercises after proper instructions involving the parents. Assisted active exercises may be necessary if there is weakness or pain.

Passive stretching to increase motion should be slow and gentle with the child completely relaxed. Stretching should stop just short of the point that produces pain in the joint. Although the child may experience some discomfort from the stretch of soft tissues, there should be no residual pain when the stretching is discontinued. Prolonged moderate stretching is more effective than intermittent vigorous stretch. The plastic "creeping" of connective tissue under moderate stretch increases with temperature up to the maximum of 43°C (42). Therapeutic heating through the use of hydrotherapy is well tolerated and enhances the effectiveness of therapy.

Instruction in joint protection by the occupational therapist is an integral part of treatment in children with inflammatory joint disease. Joint protection techniques should be incorporated into range of motion instruction provided to the child and parents.

Physical therapy is often needed after surgery and immobilization. Hydrotherapy has been found to be an effective modality to reduce stiffness and pain. Special attention must be provided to ensure that the child learns the new desired motor patterns. Casting and immobilization decreases sensory input and time will be needed to regain and learn the appropriate motor response based on a different sensory feedback. It often takes several months to achieve maximal motor performance and strength.

Children with motor disability have increased energy demands and must develop endurance and the ability to maintain static and dynamic muscle activity. Activities to increase endurance, such as bicycling, stair climbing, or rowing for upper extremities, can be easily added to a child's therapy program.

Occupational therapy to provide training in functional activities and, when necessary, in the use of adaptive methods or devices is an integral part of management (22, 47, 53). Goals are determined by the child's age and developmental status. The combination of fine and gross motor skills will determine the level of expected independence in activities of daily living. Hand activities are started very early, beginning with bimanual skills and progressing to fine motor control. Objects and toys should be designed and chosen to improve function and to expand motor, developmental, and sensory experiences of the child.

Feeding, dressing, and personal hygiene are basic skills of concern. The child should be expected to perform all skills or any part of a skill that he or she is capable of, not only in the course of a therapy session but also at home, in school, and all other situations. Consistent practice enhances physical independence and self-reliance and success will increase motivation for further development.

Therapeutic exercise in pediatrics must also address any disability from oral motor dysfunction. When a child or infant has difficulty with swallowing and chewing, feeding is not an enjoyable interaction and frequently becomes a source of major parental concern. Incoordination in the suck-swallow pattern can lead to feeding that requires hours to complete. Often, dramatic improvement can be made by teaching the mother to reduce abnormal tone and optimize oral motor function with adequate positioning and proper handling (29). Impairment of speech production is a later manifestation of oral motor dysfunction. A feeding program requires cooperative team efforts by the parents, nurse, occupational therapist, speech-language pathologist, psychologist, and physical therapist. A thorough understanding of oropharyngeal musculature, its control mechanisms, and possible ways of remediation is necessary (14, 23).

Many techniques have been described for alleviating oral motor dysfunction (2, 20, 24, 29, 48). A consistent feature is to enhance the basic function of oral exploration, coordination of respiration, phonation, and articulation, which develops in the prespeech period before the first true words are spoken (48). The newborn uses reflexive action for food intake. There is an organized, rhythmic suck-swallow reflex consisting of three sucks and an obligatory swallow (14). This nutritive reflex suck must be differentiated from the nonrhythmic, controllable sucking and oral play. The motor process of feeding helps differentiate oropharyngeal movements which are precursors of speech (48). It is also suggested that early oral exploration and the accompanying sensory input contribute to later language development.

Other Therapeutic Methods

Many methods of therapeutic exercise have been developed over the last 40 years. Most of these methods have evolved empirically from clinical observations and a theoretical framework was devised later to explain the possible neurophysiologic principles. This is true primarily for central nervous system dysfunction, such as cerebral palsy. To date, there are few controlled studies (51, 66) on the outcome of various treatment techniques despite the vigorous proclamations from various proponents. Controlling the extensive number of variables is most difficult and perplexing. The interaction of genetic, pathologic, psychologic, sociologic, and therapeutic factors produces a unique individual with unique problems. Matching subjects and selecting untreated controls is difficult and raises ethical considerations.

There is little good scientific evidence or clinical observation to indicate the superiority of one method over another. A review of the literature recommending each of these methods produces many questions. Basic assessment tools are lacking and, in many cases, may not be valid or reliable (23). Assessment of developmental progress does not separate the effect of treatment from maturation in individual cases. For these reasons, long-term follow-up into adulthood would be necessary to establish the ultimate influence of different treatment methods in childhood. The need for a control group of untreated children raises a separate set of issues for clinicians.

Neuromuscular Facilitation Methods

PROPRIOCEPTIVE NEUROMUSCULAR FACILITATION (PNF)

The method of PNF was developed by Kabat (38). Further work by Knott and Voss in the late 1950s and early 1960s refined this treatment method to its present-day usage. Based on the research of Sherrington, Coghill, McGraw, Gesell, Hellebrandt and Pavlov, this theory of treatment recommends a series of resistive exercises to facilitate movement by increased proprioceptive input. Additionally, sensory stimulation is used to facilitate movement. Various combinations of inhibitory techniques aimed at relaxation of the antagonists include contract-relax and hold-relax. Techniques aimed primarily at the agonists and considered facilitory include, among others, rhythmic stabilization and slow-reversal (40). These techniques have been most often applied to the older child or young adult. They have also been recommended for increasing joint motion in children with rheumatoid arthritis and hemophilia.

Rood

Margaret Rood's approach to muscular dysfunction places equal emphasis on both the sensory and motor aspects of movement (32, 55). She advocated the principle of activating muscles through sensory receptors, following a sequence of developmental patterns. Specific stimulation techniques are used to activate, facilitate, or inhibit motor response. The most effective methods of stimulus application, according to Rood, are brushing and icing. Therapy is aimed toward an awareness of normal pattern, rather than correction of an abnormal pattern. She recommends minimal conscious effort of the child and states that her method can be used well with infants and children of low intelligence, and those capable of full cooperation. She also suggests a training sequence for the motor function involved in respiration, sucking, swallowing, phonation, chewing, and speech.

Brunnstrom

Brunnstrom recommended facilitating a predictable synergistic pattern to produce purposeful motion by developing control of flexion and extension. In this technique of therapeutic exercise, means of facilitating the predictable activation of muscle groups within the synergy includes the use of responses progressing to isolated motion independent of reflex synergy and, finally, development of voluntary control (15). Training is directed first toward control of the head and trunk, then to proximal and distal movements. These methods most often have been applied to older children or adults with hemiplegia.

Neurodevelopmental Treatment Approach

This system of treatment, commonly referred to as neurodevelopmental treatment (NDT), was developed by the Bobaths. Their method is the most widely used for pediatric patients, particularly with cerebral palsy. Treatment is based on the premise that the chief obstacle to performance of normal movement is an impairment of postural mechanisms. Their hypothesis states that abnormal reflex activity produces abnormal distribution of muscle tone; therefore, tone should be influenced by inhibiting the patterns of abnormal reflex activity (8–10, 12).

The aim of treatment in the NDT approach is to alter abnormal postures, reduce or increase tone, improve balance in antigravity postures, and develop fundamental movement patterns following the normal developmental sequence. Movements are controlled through proximal joints, head, shoulders, and pelvis. Righting and equilibrium reactions are elicited through the use of aides, such as a large ball or bolster. Parents are enlisted and trained to handle the child in the same manner at home during daily activities (11).

Biofeedback Therapy

Biofeedback therapy has been reported to be an effective treatment modality for children with cerebral palsy. Based on the principle that patients can monitor their motor performance through the use of sensory modalities, auditory, visual, or EMG feedback are used to reinforce correct motor behavior (3). The immediate and continuous knowledge of one's own performance offers instantaneous detection and correction of error and reinforces accurate motor behavior (60). Seeger et al. reported that biofeedback successfully enhanced symmetrical gait in many hemiplegic children (60). A second study by Seeger and Caudrey (61) showed that gains made by biofeedback therapy were not maintained on long-term follow-up 18 to 24 months later. Others have reported improved head and trunk control in different types of cerebral palsy (57). It is theorized that, as the child learns correct motor action, the behaviors will generalize to other activities without the use of biofeedback.

Conductive Education

This method, as described by Peto, is an educational process aimed at maximal integration of the physically handicapped child. Activities are carried out by a "conductor" trained in education and movement therapy. The conductors use methods, such as rhythmic intention, which consists of verbal reinforcement of intended motor behavior. The child is taught to perform motor skills through sequence and rhythm, which will eventually lead to an unconscious control of the sequencing process of the movement (35). This method is used most widely in European countries.

Other Therapeutic Methods in Cerebral Palsy

DOMAN-DELACATO

Expanding on the ideas of Temple Fay (25–27), Doman and his associates recommended a program following the successive stages of locomotion adapted by animals ascending the phylogenetic scale. This highly controversial therapeutic method (18, 30, 63) uses a series of patterns repeated many times throughout the day, attempting to train cerebral dominance and normalization of function. Unlocking reflexes and positions are utilized to establish movements that are brought under volitional control. Continued performance is believed to result in improved function and strength of spastic muscles and in diminution of tone and postural disturbances.

The Doman-Delacato system also recommends periods of carbon dioxide rebreathing, ventilator-assisted breathing to increase cerebral oxygenation, and fluid restrictions.

VOJTA

Vojta describes a treatment method based on his clinical experience that shows that movements which can be provoked and observed in the cerebral-palsied child can be seen instantly in healthy newborns. He postulates the existence of a common neurogenic pattern in the subcortical area of the brain from which these originate. Thus, among a cerebral-palsied patient's motor abilities, there might be movement patterns from his newborn period that can be provoked and activated (65). Vojta suggests that by applying patterns of reflex locomotion to isolate different muscle functions in children with cerebral palsy, one can activate "postural ontogenesis" (65), the upright mechanism, and equilibrium reactions, with the assumption that there are normal neuron reserves in the central nervous system. Using the system of reflex locomotion, the child can develop postural and locomotion ontogenesis (65).

Other Methods

Several other nontraditional techniques initially developed for treating adult movement disorders, such as craniosacral therapy (64), myofascial release (44), and the Feldenkrais method (28) are now being applied to children with cerebral palsy. Controlled efficacy studies are not available in any population.

Developmental Considerations

There are a number of developmental considerations one must be aware of when planning an exercise program for an infant or child. These considerations include the child's age and mental ability, home and family environment, mobility level, and school placement.

In infancy, therapy to elicit active motion is delivered in the form of handling and by inducing spontaneous interaction. Range of motion exercises for maintaining or increasing joint mobility present little difficulty at this age. Infants frequently cry during vigorous stretching; parents need to be forewarned that the exercises are not hurting the baby.

Infancy is generally a period when the quality of the child's motor performance is most important. Many therapists feel that children will be best able to take advantage of their motor skills if "bad habits" are not allowed to develop.

Older infants and young preschoolers who can already recognize strangers may need time for adjusting to a therapeutic setting and to accept handling. A period of gradual weaning from the parents may be required when a child is enrolled in therapeutic preschool program. Continuing parental involvement in cooperative efforts with the therapists is important.

Motivation of the young child can be elicited through the use of developmentally appropriate toys, songs, and games. The noncooperative and rebellious child may respond better in a group setting. Social situations are frequently strong motivators for motor performance. When necessary, further incentives can be provided through the use of behavioral modification techniques. To be effective, the incentives must be meaningful and linked to the desired motor response.

The need for increased mobility becomes evident in the preschool child. The resulting expanded independence will enhance social interaction with peers and adults. As the child becomes older, the emphasis on therapy should be adjusted to complement rather than to interfere with education.

Choice of the most effective method of locomotion is based on kinesiologic aspects of motor dysfunction and developmental expectations. Training in basic self-care skills, such as feeding, dressing, and toileting, should begin at this age. The use of traditional exercises to increase strength, endurance, and skills generally becomes possible from late preschool age.

During the school-aged years, coordination of education and therapy is essential. At this stage, there is increased emphasis on the child's education and less on the supportive therapies. Exercise programs are more often indicated for maintenance of function with less emphasis on therapeutic attainment of new skills. In a school setting, therapists often function in a consulting role to enhance the child's educational experience and potential. The occupational therapist can be helpful in selecting appropriate adaptive devices and working with the teacher to alleviate potential perceptual motor difficulties. The physical therapist can assist with suggestions for mobility, sitting posture, and body alignment. Therapists can also assist the adaptive physical education teacher in selecting appropriate activities and developing realistic and attainable motor goals for the child during physical education.

Adolescence is an age of special concern because accelerated growth predisposes the child for the development of contractures and postural malalignment. Emotional problems, low self-esteem, and obesity may further compound the motor disability. These events frequently necessitate resumption of an active medical rehabilitation program, including direct therapeutic exercise and psychologic counseling. Training in advanced skills is often needed to assist in the achievement of vocational goals.

Sports as leisure activity or on a competitive basis offer significant physiologic and emotional benefits for handicapped children. Virtually all sports have been adapted for handicapped participants (45, 46). There are many local, national, and international sport organizations that provide a useful resource for helping establish a healthy, active life-style by children with different types of disabilities.

Conclusion

The treatment of motor dysfunction in children challenges the pediatric physiatrist, occupational therapist, and physical therapist. Appropriate program planning must take into account the child's developmental stage, the interaction of experience and dysfunction, physiologic trends in growth, and realistic long-term expectations. Only a reasonable and well-timed application of different nonoperative and operative therapeutic methods (7, 32) used in the framework of normal development can lead to accomplishment of optimal functional skills and quality of life.

REFERENCES

1. Ayres AJ: *The Development of Sensory Integration Theory and Practice.* Dubuque, IA, Kendall/Hunt Co., 1974.
2. Banus B: *The Developmental Therapist.* Thorofare, NJ, Charles B. Slack, Inc., 1971.
3. Basmajian J: Biofeedback in Therapeutic Exercise. In *Therapeutic Exercise.* Baltimore, Williams & Wilkins, 1984.
4. Bauchner H, Brown E, Peskin J: Premature graduates of the newborn intensive care unit: a guide to follow-up. *Pediatr Clin North Am* 35:4, 1988.
5. Bennett F: Neurodevelopmental outcome in low birthweight infants: The role of developmental intervention. In Guthrie R (ed). *Neonatal Intensive Care.* New York, Churchill Livingstone, 1988.
6. Berrueta-Clement J, Schweinhart W, Barnett S, et al: *Changed Lives: The Effects of the Perry Preschool Program on Youths through Age 19.* Ypsilanti, MI, The High/Scope Press, 1984.
7. Bleck EE: *Orthopedic Management of Cerebral Palsy.* Philadelphia, WB Saunders, 1979.
8. Bobath B: Motor development: Its effect on general development and application to the treatment of cerebral palsy. *Physiotherapy* 57:526, 1971.
9. Bobath B: The very early treatment of cerebral palsy. *Dev Med Child Neurol* 9:373, 1967.
10. Bobath B, Bobath K: *Motor Development in the Different Types of Cerebral Palsy.* London, Heinemann, 1975.
11. Bobath K: *A Neurophysiological Basis for the Treatment of Cerebral Palsy.* Clinics in Developmental Medicine no.75, Philadelphia, JB Lippincott, 1980.
12. Bobath K: The normal postural reflex mechanism and its derivation in children with cerebral palsy. *Physiotherapy* 57:515, 1971.
13. Bricker D: The effectiveness of early intervention with handicapped and medically at risk infants. In Frank M (ed): *Infant Intervention Programs.* New York, Haworth Press, 1985, pp. 51-65.
14. Bricker D, Dow M: Early intervention with the young severely handicapped child. *J Severe Handicap* 5:130, 1980.
15. Brunnstrom S: Walking preparation for adult patients with hemiplegia. J Am Phys Ther Assoc 45:17-29, 1965.
16. Bryant D, Ramey C: Prevention-oriented infant education programs. In Frank M (ed): *Infant Intervention Program Truths and Untruths.* New York, Haworth Press, 1985, pp. 17-35.
17. Chamberlin RW: Developmental assessment and early intervention programs for young children: Lessons learned from longitudinal research. *Pediatr Rev* 8:8, 1987.
18. Cohen HJ, Birch HG, Taft LT: Some considerations for evaluating the Doman-Delacato "patterning" method. *Pediatrics* 45:302, 1970.
19. Connolly B, Morgan D, Russell FF, Richardson B: Early intervention with Downs syndrome children. Phys Ther 60:1405, 1980.
20. Crickmay M: *Speech Therapy and the Bobath Approach to Cerebral Palsy.* Springfield, IL, Charles C Thomas, 1966.
21. Darlington R. Royee J, Snipper A, et al: Preschool programs and late school competence of children from low-income families. *Science* 208:202-208, 1980.
22. Deaver GG: Cerebral palsy—methods of treating the neuromuscular disorders. *Arch Phys Med Rehabil* 37:68, 1956.
23. Evans PR, Sachs Pehm MA: *Testing and Measurement in Occupational Therapy: A Review of Current Practice with Special Emphasis on Southern California Sensory Integration Test.* Monograph No. 15, Institute for Research on Learning Disabilities. University of Minnesota, Minneapolis, MC, 1981.
24. Farber SD: *Neurorehabilitation.* Philadelphia, WB Saunders, 1982.

25. Fay T: Basic considerations regarding neuromuscular and reflex therapy. *Spastic Quart* 29:327, 1954.
26. Fay T: Rehabilitation of patients with spastic paralysis. *J Int College Surg* 22:200, 1954.
27. Fay T: Use of pathological and unlocking reflexes in the rehabilitation of spastics. *Am J Phys Med* 33:347, 1954.
28. Feldenkrais M: *Awareness Through Movement.* New York, Harper & Row Inc., 1977.
29. Finnie N: *Handling the Young Cerebral Palsied Child at Home.* New York, EP Dutton, 1975.
30. Freeman RS: Controversy over "patterning" as a treatment for brain damaged children. *JAMA* 202:385, 1967.
31. Friedman SL, Sigman M: *Preterm Birth and Psychological Development.* New York, Academic Press, 1981.
32. Gillette HE: *Systems of Therapy in Cerebral Palsy.* Springfield, IL, Charles C Thomas, 1974.
33. Green M, Ferry P, Russman B, et al: Early intervention programs: Where do pediatricians fit in? *Contemp Pediatr* March: 92–118, 1987.
34. Greenspan S, White R: The efficacy of preventive intervention: A glass half full: Zero to three. *Bull Natl Ctr Clin Infant Program* 5:1–5, 1985.
35. Hari M, Tillemans T: Conductive Education. In Scrutton D (ed): *Management of the Motor Disorders of Children with Cerebral Palsy.* Clinics in Developmental Medicine no. 90, Philadelphia, JB Lippincott, 1984.
36. Holt KS: *Movement and Child Development.* London, Heinemann—Spastic International Medical Publications, 1975.
37. Horowitz FD: *Review of Child Development Research.* Chicago, University of Chicago Press, 1974.
38. Kabat H: *Proprioceptive Facilitation in Therapeutic Exercise.* In Licht S (ed). *Physical Medical Library III.* New Haven, E. Licht Publ, 1961.
39. Kendall PH: Evaluation of treatment in cerebral palsy. *Dev Med Child Neurol* 3:95, 1961.
40. Knott M, Voss D: *Proprioceptive Neuromuscular Facilitation.* New York, Harper & Row, 1968.
41. Kong E: Very early treatment of cerebral palsy. *Dev Med Child Neurol* 8:198, 1966
42. Kottke FJ, Lehmann JF (eds): *Krusen's Handbook of Physical Medicine and Rehabilitation.* Philadelphia, WB Saunders, 1990.
43. Levitt S: *Treatment of Cerebral Palsy and Motor Delay.* Oxford, Blackwell Scientific Publications, 1977.
44. Manheim C, Lavett D: *The Myofascial Release Manual.* New Jersey, Slack Inc., 1989.
45. Molnar GE: A developmental perspective for the rehabilitation of children with physical disability. *Pediatr Ann* 17:12, 1988.
46. Molnar GE: Rehabilitation benefits of sports for the handicapped *Conn Med* 45:574–577, 1981.
47. Molnar GE, Taft LT: Pediatric rehabilitation, part I: Cerebral palsy and spinal cord injury. *Curr Probl Pediatr* 7:1, 1977.
48. Morris SE: *Program Guidelines for Children with Feeding Problems.* Edison, NJ, Childcraft Education Corp, 1977.
49. Osofsky JD: *Handbook of Infant Development.* New York, John Wiley & Sons, 1979.
50. Palfrey J, Walker D, Sullivan M, et al: Targeted early childhood programming. *Am J Dis Child* 141:55–59, 1987.
51. Palmer F, Shapiro B, Wachtel R, et al: The effects of physical therapy on cerebral palsy. *N Engl J Med* 318:13, 1988.
52. Parmalee AH: Early Intervention for Preterm Infants. In Brown CC (ed): *Infants at Risk: Assessment and Intervention.* New Jersey, Johnson and Johnson Baby Products Co., 1981.
53. Pearson PH, Williams CE: *Physical Therapy Services in the Developmental Disabilities.* Springfield, IL, Charles C Thomas, 1972.

54. Purohit D, Ellison R, Zierler S, et al: Risk factors for retrolental fibroplasia: Experience with 3025 premature infants. *Pediatrics* 76:339–344, 1985.
55. Rood MS: Neurophysiological mechanisms utilized in the treatment of neuromuscular dysfunction. *Am J Occup Ther* 10:4 Part II, 1956.
56. Ross G: Home intervention for premature infants of low-income families. *Am J Orthopsychiatry* 54:263–270, 1985.
57. Russell G, Sharp E, Iles G: Clinical biofeedback applications in pediatric rehabilitation. *Interclin Informat Bull* 15:1–6, 1976.
58. Russman B: Early intervention for the biologically handicapped infant and young child. Is it of value? *Pediatr Rev* 5:51–55, 1983.
59. Schilling M, Siepp J, Patterson EG: *The First Three Years: Programming for Atypical Infants and Their Families.* A United Cerebral Palsy Nationally Organized Collaborative Project to Provide Comprehensive Services. New York, United Cerebral Palsy Association, 1974.
60. Seeger B, Caudry D, Scholes J: Biofeedback therapy to achieve symmetrical gait in hemiplegic cerebral palsied children. Arch *Phys Med Rehabil* 62:364–368, 1981.
61. Seeger B, Caudrey D: Biofeedback therapy to achieve symmetrical gait in children with hemiplegic cerebral palsy: Long-term efficacy Arch *Phys Med Rehabil* 64:160–162, 1983.
62. Simeonsson R, Cooper D, Scheiner A: A review and analysis of the effectiveness of early intervention programs. *Pediatrics* 69:635–640, 1982.
63. Sparrow S, Zigler E: Evaluation of a patterning treatment for retarded children. *Pediatrics* 62:137, 1978.
64. Upledger J, Vredevoogd J: *Craniosacral Therapy.* Seattle, WA, Eastland Press, 1983.
65. Vojta V: The basic elements of treatment according to Vojta. In Scrutton D (ed): *Management of the Motor Disorders of Children with Cerebral Palsy.* Clinics in Developmental Medicine no. 90, Philadelphia, J.B. Lippincott, 1984.
66. Wright T, Nicholson J: Physiotherapy for the spastic child: An evaluation. *Dev Med Child Neurol* 15:146–163, 1973.

8

Orthotics, Adapted Seating, and Assistive Devices

MICHAEL A. ALEXANDER,
MAUREEN R. NELSON, AND ANJALI SHAH

Orthoses, wheelchairs, and other assistive devices have long been used in rehabilitation to promote adaptive function. However, it is only in the last decade that adjustments and new designs have been developed to meet the special needs of children. Recent advances have been brought about in an era where scientific innovations led to the creation of new devices with both appearance and ergonometrics in mind.

General Considerations

Children have many of the same needs for adaptive devices that an adult has. These devices not only enhance function but play an integral role in their maturation (1). What makes children unique is that restricted mobility may have an effect on their personality, which may perpetuate dependence and emotional immaturity (38). As each person is shaped by previous experiences, the child who never knew the independence of standing and walking may not be the same as the one who has. Children who are not successful in exploring their environment may be less able to establish interaction with the world outside the immediate family. Humans learn to use movement to control themselves and their environment, to obtain pleasure and to reflect emotional state. In development, physical, emotional, social, and intellectual growth are interdependent so that progress in one influences the others. Motor activity links these developmental areas. If the opportunity to practice active motor activities is not given, then further development may be slowed (22). Thus, devices provided for children have to meet the experiential needs of various developmental stages. This consideration has led to the concept of the "wardrobe of devices" (41). The concept implies that children who are unable to crawl, stand, or walk need devices to assist in these activities. Some youngsters may require a succession of appliances to help them through the course of development. The approach of fitting a young child with a standing or walking device in spite of clinical certainty that this functional level would be lost in the future is based on the concept of developmental sequence.

Prescription of orthoses or other equipment for children requires thoughtful consideration of intended purpose and biomechanical principles. The child must be examined carefully by the physician. Information should be obtained from the family, therapists, and school as to what gains are expected from the device. After arriving at a tentative prescription based on what a device should and can accomplish, reflection must then turn to the possible limitations and potential unwanted effects that may be created by it. For example, a motorized wheelchair that provides independent mobility for a child with lower extremity weakness may present problems on transportation for the family.

All prescriptions should state details about desired features, model, and any special alterations. Weight, adjustability, durability, and cost are important factors in selecting a device. Accessibility and reliability of servicing and regional vendors must be considered. Social and financial information is important as funding may allow only limited pieces of equipment and revisions. One may have to consider prescribing a larger device and modifying it with inserts or other adjustable features to accommodate growth. It is the physician's responsibility to ensure that a careful clinical check-out is performed when a device is delivered.

Orthotics

Orthoses are devices that can provide support, apply dynamic forces, maintain weak body segments, substitute for absent movements, and control motion.

The purpose of this brief review is to highlight selected aspects of the application of orthotics to children. Only new designs and some frequently encountered and overlooked problems are included. For a detailed discussion of the principles of biomechanics and clinical considerations, the reader should consult the references that deal entirely with this subject (7). Furthermore, the use of orthoses in different disabilities is described in respective chapters of this volume and other publications (4, 35, 38).

The need for more extensive orthoses may arise during the years of growth to prevent skeletal abnormalities under the influence of weight-bearing forces. However, this consideration should be weighed in the context of function. A device that is too heavy, unwieldy, and uncomfortable can defeat the functional purpose for which it was intended or it may interfere with independence in other activities. A good example is a girl who was independent in toileting until the addition of a pelvic band to bilateral knee-ankle-foot orthoses made it impossible to pull down her underpants. Orthotic devices in the past sought control by blocking three planes of motion. There are now devices that are more selective and allow motion in two of three planes. An example is a hip guidance orthosis, which permits full extension and abduction but, at the same time, limits adduction and blocks hip rotation (49).

For stretching tight muscles and soft tissues, the orthotic device must control the alignment of all related anatomic structures. This is often overlooked when using thigh spreader bars to stretch spastic hip adductors in cerebral palsy. The device only results in abduction of the legs relative to each other. Without counterfixation against the trunk, one thigh may still remain in adduction relative to the pelvis while the other leg is in excessive abduction. A number of resting orthosis are available for this purpose (42). One device is shown in Chapter 10. Attention is essential to the kinesiology of two joint muscles, which tend to become shortened at the fastest rate in children. A contracted gastrocnemius cannot be stretched by an ankle-foot orthosis. Soft tissues with partial yield to passive stretch can be treated with success only if the device has adjustable or dynamic features. Spring-loaded ankle and knee joints can provide this type of action. Another example is the orthosis recommended for foot deformities, which allows sequential adjustment of straps to exert corrective forces not only in the direction of ankle dorsiflexion and plantar flexion but also of pronation and supination (7). Exact alignment of the corrective force with the axis of joint rotation is an essential requirement in these instances. Surgery should not be perceived as a final radical intervention but rather as an adjunct to rehabilitation. Without release of fixed contractures, children do not do well in a reciprocating walking brace.

Understanding the biomechanics of gait and the dynamic relationship between various lower extremity joints can be utilized sometimes to influence articular malalignment indirectly and thereby avoid the need for more extensive orthosis. Rosenthal and his associates (50) have studied children with diplegic cerebral palsy who had significant overactivity of the gastrocnemius without anatomic shortening and walked with considerable genu recurvatum. A rigid ankle brace set in a few degrees of dorsiflexion eliminated hyperextension of the knee. Conversely, ignoring this relationship between the major lower extremity joints may cause increased gait difficulties and articular malalignment. A rigid ankle orthosis to control foot drop enhances flexion moment at the knee in stance phase. As a result, instability of this joint increases when the quadriceps is weak and may lead to the development of compensatory genu recurvatum over time, particularly with associated hamstring weakness. Providing a hinge and a posterior stop in the plastic orthosis will improve stability of the foot on the floor, at the ankle, and vary the degree of plateau and dorsiflexion with built-in stops (Fig. 8.1).

Figure 8.1. Molded polypropylene hinged ankle-foot orthosis.

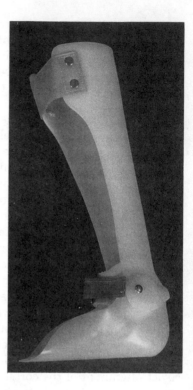

Inhibitory casts can be fabricated by both therapists and orthotists from a number of materials that take advantage of inhibitory and facilitatory foot reflexes (15, 20). These devices improve mobility (21) and with long-term use, significantly decrease both dynamic and static sensitivity of the foot in children with cerebral palsy (45).

Orthoses for walking, used exclusively in pediatrics, were originally designed for myelodysplasia. The parapodium (4, 32, 39), is a device that has found extensive application in many childhood disabilities. Examples of its use are elaborated in chapters 10, 14, and 18. Recent research has yielded a breakthrough in design of the basic parapodium, which significantly decreases the energy requirements for ambulation below that of bilateral knee-ankle-foot orthoses (KAFO) (43) or the parapodium (32). The ORLAU swivel walker (56) is propelled forward by special foot plates that, by a combination of initial torque forces, convert side to side motion to forward propulsion (Figs. 8.2 and 8.3). This device has allowed children with extensive motor dysfunction, including Duchenne muscular dystrophy to ambulate (55). When the purpose of an orthotic device is only standing, one can select the parapodium, which leaves the hands free; similarly, a rigid standing frame (7) allows standing without the need for support by the arms although the frame sacrifices hip and knee flexion necessary for sitting. The reciprocating hip-knee-ankle-foot orthosis (HKAFO) has a cable system that cou-

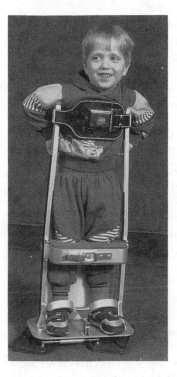

Figure 8.2. ORLAU swivel walker.

ples hip extension to flexion of the opposite hip. This device requires less energy than traditional HKAFO (Fig. 8.4).

There are many excellent discussions on upper extremity orthoses (3, 7, 28, 30). Children, even to a greater extent than adults, will rapidly and totally reject devices that are uncomfortable, interfere with sensory feedback, and do not significantly improve function. When splinting of both

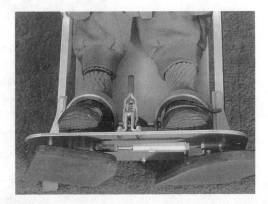

Figure 8.3. Torque converter on the underside of a swivel walker.

hands is unavoidable, one should be aware of the behavioral signs of rejection in very young children who cannot communicate verbally. Realizing that they cannot feel and grasp, the infants may become irritable or, even worse, ignore their hands. Alternately splinting the hands and minimizing the area of obliterated sensation alleviates these reactions. Bracing of the upper extremities to restrict uncontrolled movements in athetosis has met with limited success due to the difficulties with damping, weight, and cosmesis (28). Children with traumatic quadriplegia can learn and benefit from the use of various hand orthoses (Chapter 13). The need for a balanced forearm orthosis may arise in neuromuscular disabilities with severe proximal or generalized weakness and can be incorporated in a wheelchair insert, which is usually required in these cases (Fig. 8.5).

The efficacy of spinal orthoses in idiopathic scoliosis and kyphosis is well documented (7, 37). Spinal bracing has been used for myelomeningocele (13) and paralytic curves, including Duchenne muscular dystrophy (37). Physiatrists managing patients with scoliosis must be aware of the limitations of bracing and criteria for surgery and, unless they work closely with a surgeon, their role becomes one of detection and referral. The child with scoliosis, seating problems, and, possibly, pressure ulcerations may be a candidate for an orthotic seating device. The thoracic suspension orthosis offers limited success in the treatment of children with these problems. The child is encased in a thoracolumbosacral orthosis with side brackets that fit into struts attached to the back posts of the wheelchair; then the child is partially

Figure 8.4. Cable system on the reciprocating HKAFO.

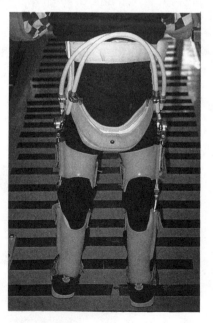

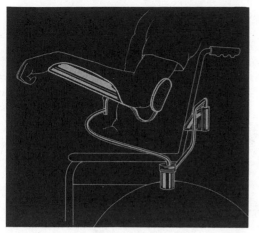

Figure 8.5. Balanced forearm orthosis (BFO).

suspended by the rib cage (14). The Milwaukee brace has found an unexpected application for children who have no head control (36). This brace was fitted tightly against the mandible for correction of spinal deformities and caused dental malocclusion with migration of molars (2). Long-term observations are needed to examine this aspect of growth when cervico-thoracolumbosacral orthoses are used for assisting head control because prolonged use may again prove to deform dental occlusion and even injure the temporomandibular joint.

Seating and Mobility Devices

In children, seating is as important in maintaining body alignment as an orthotic device and should receive the same careful consideration. As with all orthotic devices, one must keep in mind what is to be accomplished (64). Proper seating provides stability and support, decreases the likelihood of postural deformities, and enhances upper extremity control (34, 40). A well-constructed seating device allows a child, even one with the most severe physical handicap, to be out of bed. Alertness is heightened by the visual input on sitting erect rather than looking at the ceiling and enables the child to engage in more active social contact. Secretion is not pooled in the posterior pharynx and swallowing is facilitated. Mobility devices offer an interface for environmental exploration, opportunities to participate in activities at home, school, and community (41), and access to the world at large (22).

WHEELCHAIRS

The most common seating and mobility device prescribed for handicapped children is a wheelchair (24). Before considering specific clinical problems, one must examine the features of currently used models. From the viewpoint of the postural requirements of growing children, there is a basic flaw in the construction of traditional wheelchair seats that compromises proper alignment of the pelvis and femur. While sitting in the typical hammock seat of a wheelchair, the legs are adducted and internally rotated. This alignment, combined with hip flexion, places the femoral heads in a position to favor posterior superior subluxation. The concave supporting surface also results in asymmetrical sitting with pelvic obliquity, tilting the torso, and leaning on one arm (Fig. 8.6) (23). A firm, level seat should be the standard wheelchair modification for children in order to alleviate these postural deviations. Careful inspection of some commercial seats shows that these seats may still deform into a hammock (Fig. 8.7).

Cerebral Palsy

In the child with cerebral palsy, a major goal is to prevent contractures and reduce spastic reflex patterns, while maintaining appropriate body position (8, 16). In a study of patients with spastic cerebral palsy, it was shown that myoelectric activity of the extensor muscles of the lumbar spine was minimal at 0° seat surface inclination and 90° backrest inclination (44). Control of sitting posture depends on the stability of supporting base. A firm seat with appropriate contour decreases trunk instability. It should also maintain symmetrical pelvic alignment by controlling the wind-blown hip

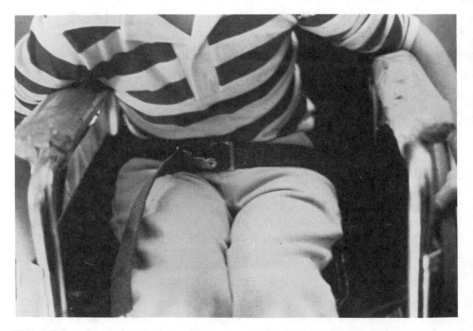

Figure 8.6. Sling seat in a standard wheelchair, legs adducted and internally rotated.

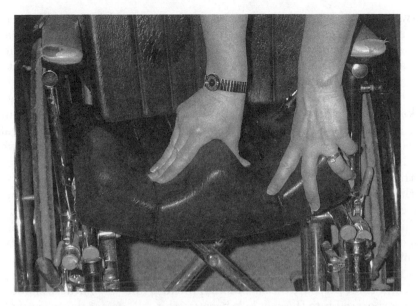

Figure 8.7. Over the counter seat, which still deforms without rigid base.

position and consequent spinal curvature (29). Stability can be also enhanced by three-point force; however, this principle is difficult to apply to a complex structure, such as the spine, or in a patient who moves a great deal. A seat that levels the pelvis in both the anteroposterior and lateral directions contributes to spinal support (8).

Seating children with cerebral palsy requires familiarity with primitive reflexes that contribute to pathologic postures and with the effect of position changes that can influence tone abnormalities (9, 26, 34). In some patients with persistent tonic neck reflexes, one must avoid pressure from the headrest on the occiput, atlas, and axis. A contoured neck rest may be more appropriate in these cases. Increased tone of leg extensors and arm flexors is thought to be mediated by labyrinthine reflexes. This posture becomes exaggerated when the head is reclined 15–20° from vertical (26). Tipping the chair backward in an attempt to keep the child with excessive trunk and lower limb extensor tone from slipping forward only exaggerates the labyrinthine posturing. It also leads to further increase of arm flexion and deterioration of hand function. Conversely, bringing the head forward suppresses the abnormal tone distribution and results in relaxation of arms and extensor hypertonicity of the back and legs (26).

In a growing child with cerebral palsy, increasing extensor tone and greater difficulties with sitting have been mistaken for neurologic deterioration. If these alterations of tone and function coincide with changing from infant chair to growing wheelchair, they may, in fact, be related to differences between the constructional features of the two models. In order to allow clearance between the casters and foot rests, which are now longer, the larger chair no longer maintains a 90° flexion alignment of the three major lower extremity joints. Reversal to the original postural alignment will correct this apparent neurological deterioration (Fig. 8.8).

Abduction pommels have been recommended to overcome scissoring and to keep a child with marked extensor spasticity in the chair. A large abductor pad should be avoided because it can press against the perineum (Fig. 8.9) causing traumatic urethritis with hematuria and vulvar irritation, which predispose to infections, in particular, monilial vaginitis. A better solution to this problem is to flex the hips slightly beyond 90° and elevate the front of the seat so that gravity will assist holding the child against the back of the chair (40). A lap belt brought at a 45° angle from under the seat will also significantly decrease the tendency to pull out of the chair by securing the upper torso. The so-called "H" harness is used, which provides anterior trunk support and fixation of the shoulders. This modification is preferable to a circumferential strap under the axilla, which may restrict chest expansion and exert pressure on the brachial plexus. The "H" harness should not be incorporated into the seat belt because this will defeat the 45° pull of the seat belt. A lap tray may be used as additional anterior support and to allow better use of the arms.

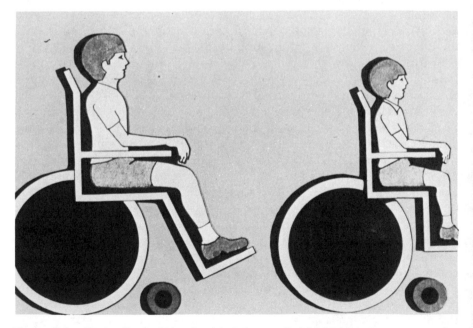

Figure 8.8. Body alignment in wheelchair for small child *(right)* and in growing chair *(left)*.

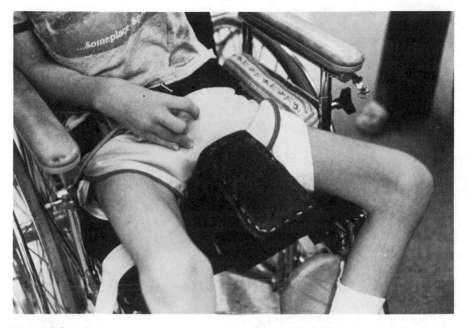

Figure 8.9. Abduction pommel used incorrectly to hold child in wheelchair, instead for separating knees.

Children with increased tone in all extremities and trunk frequently hold on to the chair with one hand to make their sitting more secure. Youngsters with a Moro reflex or startle response resort to the same habit because of their precarious postural control. An unstable trunk, particularly when it is combined with a tendency for sudden unexpected movements, makes it difficult if not impossible to utilize any hand function the child may have. Firm sitting surface, "H" harness, and, often, the addition of lateral supports provide greater trunk stability. Concomitantly, there is usually a diminution of overflow flexor posturing of the arms and, as the hands are lowered, the child may be able to perform midline activities. Trunk stabilization may also result in relaxation of facial features and a more cosmetic and socially acceptable appearance in cases with dyskinetic overflow of the muscles to the face.

Hypotonia

In children with diseases of the motor unit, one of the most significant problems is hypotonia. The sitting posture of an infant with hypotonia from birth or early age is, at first, an exaggerated kyphosis of the entire spine with protracted shoulders. When independent sitting is attained, the trunk is precariously balanced by passive mechanical alignment over a marked lumbar lordotic curvature. Asymmetrical sitting posture related to hand dominance and the habit of leaning on one arm to compensate for trunk instability (23), together with a lack of muscular support for the spine, inevitably lead to scoliosis. A firm seat and lateral supports are substitutes for trunk control. Stability of the torso and symmetrical posture are further enhanced by a lap tray, which also facilitates functional use of the weak upper extremities. The tray should be placed high enough to eliminate sagging of the shoulders and the upper trunk. Shoulder stabilization is an important component in proper seating for the weak child. Contact between the scapula and the back of the chair indicates that the shoulder girdle is adequately supported. Proximal stabilization of the upper extremity improves hand function. In some cases, a balanced forearm orthosis may be considered. A sufficiently rigid and properly aligned foot rest may retard progressive foot deformities.

Over the past 10 years, significant changes occurred in the treatment of scoliosis in Duchenne muscular dystrophy (63). Previously, attempts were made to control scoliosis by enhanced lumbar extension with spinal orthosis and custom-molded seat insert (62). This choice of support was based on the observation that scoliosis was less prone to develop in cases with increased lumbar lordosis during the stage of wheelchair use. However, more recent studies demonstrated that there was no significant difference in the severity of scoliosis among boys who used a lumbar extension support and those who did not (11, 47, 53). These studies recommend consideration of surgical stabilization of spinal curves of 30° or greater and a vital capacity of over 35% of predicted value in order to protect respiratory function and physical endurance (11, 27, 58). Contrary to previous studies, Lord et al. (31) found that there was no significant relationship between the development of scoliosis and wheelchair dependence within the first 2½ yr of this functional stage. Recent investigations have implicated asymmetry of the erector spine due to muscle fiber loss and fat replacement in the etiology of scoliosis (57).

When the aim is to maintain the lumbar spine in extension, elevating leg rests should not be used for stretching the tight hamstrings. Because of the two-joint action of this muscle, knee extension will produce decreased hip flexion and lumbar kyphosis (Fig. 8.10). The child should be allowed to sit with the knees flexed and a program of manual stretching should be given.

Other Considerations

A child with fixed skeletal deformities benefits from orthotic seating by having maximal comfort, support, and stability. Conforming seat inserts are the most useful and many innovative solutions have been used in individual cases.

For ambulatory children who use a wheelchair only part of the time, an important consideration is the proper height of the seat to enable getting into a standing position (24). To compensate for the added height of a firm seat insert, a lower chair than used for nonambulatory children may be required or the seat can be lowered by offset brackets below the usual height.

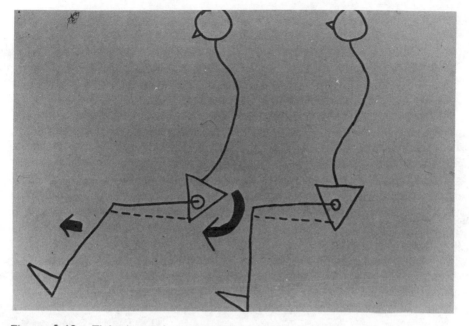

Figure 8.10. Tight hamstrings obliterating lumbar lordosis when the knees are extended.

Desk arms are a standard feature to allow play, work at school, and eating with the family at the table. Adjustable height arm rest should be ordered to compensate for the height of seat insert. As mentioned earlier, elevating leg rests promote kyphotic posture and forward sliding when the hamstrings are tight. In addition, they make it hard to maneuver in a limited space. There are now chairs available with a variety of adjustable features. However, the more complex the components, the more problems can arise adding costly maintenance to the already high initial expense.

Motorized chairs are prescribed with increasing frequency for children who have considerable upper extremity weakness or other problems making it impossible to propel a conventional wheelchair (6, 24). A child with good cognitive and perceptual ability should be able to learn safe operation of this device around 3-yr of age and successes have been achieved at even younger ages. Power chairs are available with power elevating seats that allow the child to go from floor level to sitting height and even to standing position (Fig. 8.11).

TRANSPORTATION CHAIRS

These devices are appropriate for very young children and for older ones with a combination of severe cognitive and physical deficits (34). They cannot be self-propelled. Traveling chairs have many features that allow opti-

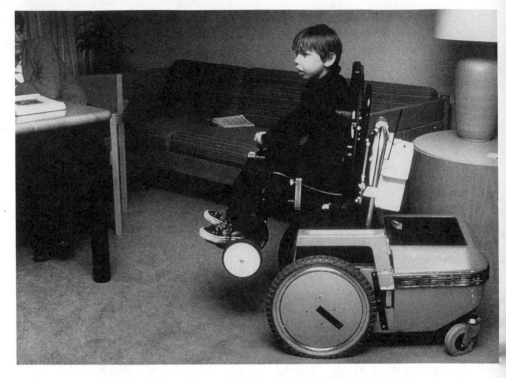

Figure 8.11. Power chair (Turbo) with adjustable height.

mal placement of the lower extremities, spinal stabilization, and head support. Most models are adjustable and can be used as car seats. Standard or folding commercial strollers and other similar devices can be adapted to the needs of handicapped children and serve as transportation devices. Car seats may be modified for therapeutic needs as well.

SEAT INSERTS

Inserts may be custom-made for an individual child using different materials and techniques (34). A relatively simple method is to fabricate an insert from plywood or foam with padding and naugahyde or other similar material for covering. This can be done virtually at any center although the appearance will vary from a homemade look to custom-manufactured furniture. Regardless of appearance, the components can be the same, including a proper seating surface, side wings for head and trunk support, and, if needed, hinges to permit sitting in different positions. Total contact inserts may be fabricated by a number of different methods. One technique (5) involves taking a positive mold of the child's body from which a vacuum-formed plastic or foam insert is made. Another technique is the foam in place, which has run into some difficulties because of fire hazard. For this method, the patient is placed on a rubber dam and the chemicals are mixed underneath for a total contact fit. A more recent approach is represented by the modular systems that use prefabricated components.

Inserts can be fitted for various wheelchair models, transportation chairs, or strollers. It is essential to make sure that the insert can be accommodated by the dimensions of the chair used or being prescribed.

Seats can incorporate cushions to redistribute pressure over the ischia and other bony prominences for protecting anesthetic skin areas. Foam cushioning materials with intercommunicating air cells (25) have been developed for this purpose. No particular padding material has proven to be better than another (19) and prevention of tissue trauma remains the best approach.

TRANSPORTATION SAFETY

An area of concern is transporting disabled children in automobiles and buses. There are child restraint systems that meet governmental safety standards on impact testing. Children are safer when secured in a restraint system, even when it is used inappropriately, than when they are in someone's lap, unrestrained, or sharing an adult belt (54). Commercially available car seats can be used for handicapped children weighing less than 50 lb. Additionally, there are seats tested for children up to 60 inches tall and over 50 lb, and without head and trunk control to use standard safety belts. These include The Special Seat and Orthopedic Positioning Seat. Several seats pass crash testing with the addition of special tethers, belts, and locks. Prestons Carry Car Seat, the Ortho Kinetic Travel Chair, and Safety Rehab Systems STC2900 series travel chairs are among these seating systems (52).

There are many new designs for securing wheelchairs. Some of these include using bolts on triangular plates, power lock-down systems, and steel bars. In using a frame anchor or other securing system, it is very important to assure that the material used is of adequate strength. Some recent testing has indicated that the primary weakness in many securement systems is actually the anchoring hardware (51).

To prevent serious injury in a motor vehicle accident, one must take steps to prevent the second impact of human collision striking the inside of the vehicle. To ensure that this does not occur, one must make sure that the occupant, as well as a wheelchair, are independently and securely fastened (51).

Although there are standards for general school bus safety, there are no federal requirements governing safety of transport of a child with disabilities (54, 58).

Principles recommended for transporting people with disabilities are facing the wheelchair forward or rearward, not to the side; broad padding head restraints; securing the wheelchair and occupants separately with occupant shoulder and lap belt; and using tie-down straps to tubing joints at the strongest point of the chair and with the proper hardware (52).

Basic guidelines of safety include prevention of impact with hard surfaces by use of adequate padding on all nearby surfaces. Additionally, this includes restraints over the skeletal region rather than over unprotected soft tissue areas, such as the abdomen. Rear head restraints can prevent excessive head and neck mobility that can result in whiplash and other more serious neck injuries. Velcro fasteners should not be used because of insufficient strength for possible force in a crash situation (51).

The Q-Straint, Aero-Quip, and Australian Safe-n-Sound restraint systems allow wheelchair and occupant restraint and have passed simulated 20-mph impact tests (54, 61). Their design does not require wheelchair modifications for safe use (17, 54). The Master-Loc is a different design, fitting only a standard wheelchair frame construction, and can only be used for transport of wheelchairs of almost identical design, but did show good test performance. A few wheelchairs have been dynamically impact tested. The Safety Travel Chair 2 passes testing at 30 mph (51).

Disabled children with mechanically assisted ventilation need separate, secure attachment of the ventilator and the child. A child who weighs less than 50 lb, should be in an approved car seat, as this offers more protection than a wheelchair. The car seat should not have a shield, to minimize the risk of occluding the tracheostomy tube (58). Tubing length should be adequate so that the battery can be secured on the floor of the vehicle.

OTHER MOBILITY DEVICES

Adaptive devices can assist disabled children in preambulatory stages of mobility (24). Scooter boards and inexpensive crawling devices available at toy stores will allow the child to lie prone, trunk and legs supported, while the arms are left free to pull along the floor. A special design made for handicapped children maintains the legs in abduction. These mobility aids are most useful for children who have sensory deficits and crawl beyond the expected age as the risk of traumatizing the skin increases with body weight. A low sitting device, which allows access to the floor for playing, is the caster cart designed for children with myelodysplasia (64). It consists of a low platform mounted on wheels and an optional back support; it can be wheeled by hand. Older children can use a hand-pedaled car (35) or a regular tricycle can be modified for this purpose (Fig. 8.12). For those who have adequate function of the legs, adjusted foot pedals and back rest may be sufficient. Toys, both electric and self-operated, should be considered from an early age on as means to mobility, keeping safety precautions in mind.

OTHER ADAPTIVE DEVICES

In the realm of equipment, one is only limited by technology and the imagination of those working with the children. The list of possible functional aids is virtually limitless (46, 48, 60).

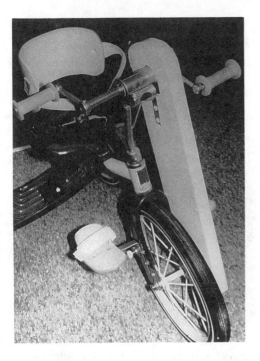

Figure 8.12. Standard tricycle modified to hand pedals, special foot rest, and backrest.

A standing table (38) can serve as a place of work or play. However, for children with cerebral palsy and excessive extensor spasticity, a prone board (16) is more appropriate.

Adapted clothing, feeding utensils, writing tools, and other implements should be considered at the appropriate stage of development when physical limitations impede the attainment of independence in daily activities.

In childhood, toys provide an outlet for imagination and experimentation. They serve as tools for learning and a way to exercise control over the world. Toys and games are therapeutic implements used in motor and developmental training of children. For selecting a suitable toy, one must consider the child's physical ability, cognitive and perceptual function, vision, hearing, special interests, and aptitudes, as well as the therapeutic, educational, or recreational goals. Most toys can be adapted with simple modifications, such as Velcro on doll's clothing or checker board. Battery-operated toys are particularly useful, although adaptation of switches may be needed (Fig. 8.13). Bioengineering centers are valuable resources but enlisting the help of a local ham radio operator, electrician, computer sales center, or television repairman can also produce very successful results. Despite their therapeutic and educational value, toys are not approved as equipment for funding. A talk to community service groups by the physician can help to obtain the needed funds.

The axiom the "less technology the better" is changing; however, children still do amazingly well with simple devices. A head pointer or a mouth stick

Figure 8.13. Water squirter modified to tongue switch.

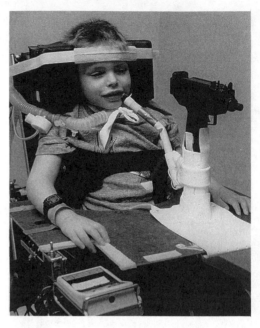

still represents a satisfying mode of direct selection (60). Pointers come with interchangeable tips for painting, writing, or turning pages. For a child's mouth stick, it is necessary to mount it on a custom-made mouth piece. Materson and Lotz (33) describe loosening of the teeth and periodontal ligaments with widening of spaces between the teeth in individuals using a mouth stick for a long time (10). They recommend that the oral prosthesis should extend beyond the anterior teeth and should not have a bite opening greater than the resting position of the jaw.

Technology and the use of keyboard emulators have allowed children to interact not only with nonverbal electronic communication aids (46, 59, 60) covered in chapter 4, but with environmental control systems (18, 60). Children readily take to computers and VCRs and can interface their equipment with single switches, joy sticks, pneumatic switches, electromyogram signals, and even by eye gaze. The advent of speech recognition systems will move toward the interface of robotics and rehabilitation in children.

Ultrasound technology has progressed to the point where wheelchairs can be equipped to detect walls, barriers, and curb drop offs and signal via different sounds the barrier type and its location.

In the next decade, robotics will become an important aid to the severely disabled child. A robotic arm system has already been shown to facilitate learning in very young disabled children (12).

Children will readily adapt to devices that enhance their function. For the clinician, the child's excitement is truly contagious.

REFERENCES

1. Alexander MA, Bauer RE: Cerebral palsy. In *Handbook of Developmental & Physical Disabilities.* Van Hasslet, VB, Strain PS, Hersen M (eds). New York, Pergamon Press, 1988.
2. Alexander RG: The effects of tooth position and maxillofacial vertical growth during treatment of scoliosis with the Milwaukee brace. *Am J Orthotics,* 52:86, 1966.
3. Bender LF: Upper extremity orthotics. In Kottke FJ, Lehman JF (eds): *Krusen's Handbook of Physical Medicine and Rehabilitation,* 4th ed. Philadelphia, WB Saunders, 1990, pp. 580–592.
4. Bowen JR: Orthotic management of the child with a myelomeningocele. *Inter-clinic Info Bull* 17:no. 10, 1981.
5. Bowker J: A vacuum formed plastic insert seat for neurologically handicapped wheelchair patients. *Inter-clinic Info Bull* 12:1, 10, 1973.
6. Breed AL, Ibler T: The motorized wheelchair: New freedom, new responsibilities and new problems. *Dev Med Child Neurol* 24:366, 1982.
7. Bunch WH: *Atlas of Orthotics,* AAOS 2nd ed. St. Louis, CV Mosby Co, 1985.
8. Carlson JM, Lonstein J, Beck KO, Wilkie DC: Seating for children and young adults with cerebral palsy. *Clin Prosthet Orthotics* 11:176–198, 1987.
9. Carrington EG: A seating position for the cerebral palsied child. *Am J Occup Ther* 32:179, 1978.
10. Cloran AJ: Oral telescoping orthoses: An aid to functional rehabilitation of quadriplegic patients. *J Am Dent Assoc* 100:876, 1980.
11. Colbert AP, Craig C: Scoliosis management and Duchenne muscular dystrophy: Prospective study of modified Jewett hyperextension brace. *Arch Phys Med Rehabil* 68:302–304, 1987.
12. Cook AM, Liu RY, Zenteno-Sanchez CM: Using a robotic arm system to facilitate learning in very young disabled children. *IEEE Trans Biomed Eng* 35:132–137, 1988.
13. Drennan J: Orthotic management of the myelomeningocele spine. *Dev Med Child Neurol (Suppl)* 37:97, 1976.
14. Drennan JC: The role of thoracic suspension orthosis in the management of myelomeningocele spinal deformities. *Inter-clinic Info Bull* 17:6, 1979.
15. Duncan WR, Mott DH: Foot reflexes and the use of the "Inhibitive Cast". *Foot Ankle* 4:145, 1983.
16. Finney N: *Handling the Cerebral Palsied Child at Home.* New York, EP Dutton, 1975.
17. Fisher WE, Seeger BR, Svensson NL: Development of an Australian standard for wheelchair occupant restraint: Assemblies for motor vehicles. *J Rehab Res Dev* 24:23–34, 1987.
18. Frankoff DJ, Alexander MA: The child and technology advances. in Eisenberg MG, Gerzesiak RC (eds): *Clinical Rehabilitation.* Vol 1. New York, Springer Publishing Co, 1983.
19. Garber SL, Drouskop TA, Carter ER: A system for clinically evaluating wheelchair pressure relief cushions. *Am J Occup Ther* 32:565, 1978.
20. Hanson CJ, Jones LJ: Gait abnormalities and inhibitive casts in cerebral palsy. *J Am Podiatric Medical Assoc* 79:53, 1989.
21. Hinderer KA, Harris SR, Purdy AH, Chew DE, Staheli LT, McLaughlin JF, Jaffe KM: Effects of 'tone-reducing' vs. standard plaster-casts on gait improvement of children with cerebral palsy. *Dev Med Child Neurol* 30:370–377, 1988.
22. Holt KS: How and why children move. *Clin Dev Med* 55:1–20, 1975.
23. Johnson EW, Yarnell S: Hand dominance and scoliosis in the Duchenne muscular dystrophy. *Arch Phys Med Rehab* 57:462, 1976.
24. Kamenetz HL: Wheelchairs and other indoor vehicles for the disabled. In Redford J (ed): *Orthotics Etc.,* ed. 3. Baltimore, Williams & Wilkins, 1986.
25. Koreska J, Albisser AM: A new foam for support of the physically handicapped. *Biomed Eng* 10:56, 1975.
26. Kottke FJ: The neurophysiology of motor function. In Kottke FJ, Lehman JF (eds): *Kru-*

sen's *Handbook of Physical Medicine and Rehabilitation,* 4th ed. Philadelphia, WB Saunders, 1990.

27. Kurz LT, Mubarak SJ, Schultz P, Parke SM, Leech J: Correlation of scoliosis and pulmonary function in Duchenne muscular dystrophy. *J Pediatr Orthot* 3:347–353, 1983.

28. Largent P, Waylett J: Follow-up study of upper extremity bracing of children with severe athetosis. *Am J Occup Ther* 32:56, 1978.

29. Letts M, Shapiro L, Mulder K, Klassen O: The windblown hip syndrome in total body cerebral palsy. *J Pediatr Orthot* 4:55–62, 1984.

30. Long C, Schutt A: Upper limb orthotics. In Redford J (ed): *Orthotics Etc.,* ed. 3. Baltimore, Williams & Wilkins, 1986.

31. Lord J, Behrman B, Varzos N, Cooper B, Leiberman J, Fowler W: Scoliosis associated with Duchenne muscular dystrophy. *Phys Med Rehabil Arch* 13–17, 1990.

32. Lough LK, Neilsen DH: Ambulation of children with myelomeningocele: Parapodium versus parapodium with ORLAU swivel modification. *Dev Med Child Neurol* 28:489, 1986.

33. Materson RS, Lotz J: Cloran telescoping oral orthosis. *Arch Phys Med Rehabil* 56:409, 1975.

34. Medhat MA, Trautman P: Seating devices for the disabled. In Redford J (ed): *Orthotics Etc.,* ed. 3. Baltimore, Williams & Wilkins, 1986.

35. Menelaus M: Orthosis and aids to mobility. In *The Orthopedic Management of Spina Bifida.* Edinburgh, Churchill Livingstone, 1980.

36. Mital MA, Belkin SC, Sullivan MA: An approach to head, neck and trunk stabilization and control in cerebral palsy by use of the Milwaukee brace. *Dev Med Child Neurol* 19:198, 1976.

37. Moe JH: *Scoliosis and Other Spinal Deformities.* Philadelphia, WB Saunders, 1978.

38. Molnar GE: Orthotic management of children. In Redford JB (ed): Orthotics Etcetera, 3rd ed. Baltimore, Williams & Wilkins, 1986.

39. Motloch WM: Device design in spina bifida. In Murdoch G (ed): *Advances in Orthotics.* Baltimore, Williams & Wilkins, 1976.

40. Motloch WM: Seating and positioning for the physically impaired. *Orthot Prosthet* 31:11, 1977.

41. Motloch WM: Wardrobe of devices. *Inter-clinic Info Bull* 12:8, 1974.

42. Nakamura T, Ohamu M: Hip abduction splint for use at night for scissor leg of cerebral palsy patients. *Orthot Prosthet* 34:13, 1980.

43. Nene AV, Orth D, Patrick JH: Energy cost of paraplegic locomotion with the ORLAU ParaWalker. *Paraplegia* 27:5, 1989.

44. Nwaobi OM, Brubaker CE, Cusick B, Sussman MD: Electromyographic investigation of extensor activity in cerebral palsied children in different seating positions. *Dev Med Child Neurol* 25:175–183, 1983.

45. Otis JC, Root L, Kroll MA: Measurement of plantar flexor spasticity during treatment with tone-reducing casts. *J Pediatr Orthop* 5:682, 1985.

46. Redford J (ed): Appendix I. Sources for More Information on Systems and Devices. *Orthotics Etc.,* ed. 3. Baltimore, Williams & Wilkins, 1986.

47. Rideau Y, Glorian B, Delaubier A, Tarle O, Bach J: The treatment of scoliosis in Duchenne muscular dystrophy. *Muscle Nerve* 7:281–286, 1984.

48. Robinault IP: *Functional Aids for the Multiply Handicapped,* 2nd ed. Hagerstown, Harper & Row, 1984.

49. Rose GK, Stallard J, Sankarankutty M: Clinical evaluation of spina bifida patients using hip guidance orthosis. *Dev Med Child Neurol* 23:30, 1981.

50. Rosenthal RK, Deutch SD, Miller W, Shumann W, Hall JE: A fixed ankle, below knee orthosis for the management of genu recurvatum. *J Bone Joint Surg* 57A:545, 1975.

51. Schneider LW: Protection for the severely disabled: A new challenge in occupant restraint. *Proceedings of the International Symposium on Occupant Restraint* 217–231, 1981.

52. Seeger BR, Caudrey DJ: Crash worthiness of restraints for physically disabled children in buses. *Rehabil Lit* 44:332–355, 1983.

53. Seeger BR, Sutherland AD, Clark MS: Orthotic management of scoliosis and Duchenne muscular dystrophy. *Arch Phys Med Rehabil* 65:83–86, 1984.
54. Shaw G: Vehicular transport safety for the child with disabilities. *Am J Occupat Ther* 35–42, 1987.
55. Sibert JR, Williams V, Burkinshaw R, Sibert S: Swivel walkers in Duchenne muscular dystrophy. *Arch Dis Child* 62:741, 1987.
56. Stallard J, Farmer IR, Poiner R, Major RE, Rose GK: Engineering design considerations of the ORLAU Swivel Walker. *Eng Med* 15:3, 1986.
57. Stern LM, Clark BE: Investigation of scoliosis in Duchenne dystrophy using computerized tomography. *Muscle Nerve* 11:775–783, 1988.
58. Stout JD, Boll MJ, Strup KB: Safe transportation for children with disabilities. *Am J Occupat Ther* 43:31–36, 1989.
59. Vanderheiden G, Yoder D. Augmentative communication: An introduction. *ASHA,* 1988.
60. Warren CG, Enders A: Introduction to systems and devices for the disabled. In Redford J (ed): *Orthotics Etc.,* ed. 3. Baltimore, Williams & Wilkins, 1986.
61. Wevers AW: Wheelchair and occupant restraint system for transportation of handicapped passengers. *Arch Phys Med Rehabil* 64:374–377, 1983.
62. Wilkins KE, Gibson DA: The patterns of spinal deformity in Duchenne muscular dystrophy. *J Bone Joint Surg* (AM) 24–32, 1958.
63. Winter RB: Spinal problems in pediatric orthopedics. In Morrissy RT (ed): *Lovell and Winter's Pediatric Orthopedics,* 3rd ed. Philadelphia, JB Lippincott Co., 1990.
64. Wooldridge CP: Purpose-designated patient vehicles. In Murdoch G (ed): *Advances in Orthotics.* Baltimore, Williams & Wilkins, 1976.

9

Pediatric Rehabilitation Nursing

SHIRLEY P. HOEMAN

Pediatric rehabilitation nursing has emerged as a unique, comprehensive approach to the assessment and care of children who have chronic or disabling disorders and their families. Nursing care plans address each child's cognitive, emotional, and social developmental needs, as well as physical and diagnostic problems (41).

Theoretical Base

One theoretical base is a systems model designed to incorporate multiple internal and external stressors and variables (46) and to encompass preinjury factors, acute and rehabilitation settings, and community re-entry. Within the model, the nursing process is conducted on primary, secondary, and tertiary levels of intervention.

Primary level intervention includes preventive measures, health promotion, and education. Secondary level intervention is treatment or strategies to limit disability. Tertiary level intervention targets optimal function, improved outcome, and develops lifelong coping and adaptation skills.

Open boundaries allow primary intervention during tertiary care, while rehabilitation becomes primary intervention in acute or emergency settings. For example, rehabilitation in the pediatric intensive care nursery is primary intervention; while in acute care units for a child with head injury, it entails prevention of pressure sores, contractures, or complications from immobility. Pediatric rehabilitation nurses coordinate transition among levels of intervention and the community.

Chronicity

Although the incidence rate of chronic conditions is relatively stable, the prevalence rate is changing (20). Today's "new pediatric survivors" live longer and are more visible in the community, forecasting an increase in chronically ill adults.

The impact of chronicity on family dynamics is often underestimated. Medically fragile children with severe or multiple disabilities require life-long technological support, assistive devices, and medical services (45). Their health care remains fragmented, costly, and complex, disintegrating the family system. Families become empowered and competent in caring for their children when they learn about human development, understand the natural history of the disease, and cope with uncertainty (33, 62).

Integrated Principles

The following principles are integral to the process and practice of pediatric rehabilitation nursing.

Each child is first a child who experiences, expresses, and perceives differently from an adult. The developing child is entitled to risk reduction and primary health care appropriate for his or her unique needs. Risk factors for many chronic conditions are developed in childhood (38). As for all other youngsters, a child with a spinal cord injury needs regular dental care; the child with a limb deficiency requires measles protection.

The family and child are one unit of service. They are co-managers with an interdisciplinary team, that may include siblings, extended family, and support groups. Families learn about promoting development, anticipatory guidance, and appropriate functional abilities alongside their children. Nevertheless, "chronic sorrow" occurs periodically as a natural response.

The long-term goal is effective transition to community-based health services and resources, such as specialized programs, support networks, education, recreation, work, and eventually, independent living. Educated, enabled, and empowered families seek effective transition through the life-long care of their children (13).

For these children, psychosocial, emotional, spiritual, and educational needs may be more related to the chronicity, deficits, and disablement than to the specific medical diagnosis. There is more variability within medical diagnostic groups than in the attendant psychosocial, emotional, educational, rehabilitative, and preventive issues raised by chronicity (58).

Assessments incorporate cultural relevance and sensitivity in both content and process (28). By the year 2030, Afro-American, Hispanic, and Native American children will compose more than 40% of the nation's pediatric population (14).

Advocacy supports teaching a child to perform self-care or to self-direct care assertively at developmentally appropriate times (29). The child who can perform self-care gains access to the least restrictive educational environment and may avoid complications from poor health habits and further functional loss.

Children with chronic or disabling disorders are at risk for behavioral problems, fragmented services, and may be arbitrarily placed in special education classes, independent of sociodemographic variables (21). Risk factors include: sick role, learned helplessness, body image, self-esteem, stigma, maladaptive coping mechanisms, learning, and attention deficit disorders.

Framework for Practice

Pediatric rehabilitation nursing process is collecting data, assessing long- and short-term goals related to specific nursing diagnoses, planning therapeutic interventions, and evaluating outcome within a family-focused interdisciplinary team context (4). Caring (60) and basic needs (11, 50) are frameworks consistent with the scope of practice. The following samples are not inclusive, but relate to topics encountered in this book.

SKIN

Assess the color, temperature, turgor, hydration, and texture of the skin. Inspect for lesions or secretions, circulation, edema, lubrication, and redness or other signs of pressure. Take advantage of many opportunities to check skin during bathing, dressing, or play. Injuries, especially burns, may indicate child abuse. While feeding or performing oral care, assess the condition of the lips, tongue, mucosa, teeth, and gums; check for malocclusion, injuries, including those self-inflicted from biting, and other lesions.

Prevention of pressure areas is the best intervention. Eliminate mechanical and chemical irritants, such as pressure on bony prominences, urine, feces, continually wet clothing, ill-fitted urine collection or ostomy devices, and friction or shearing movements. Active children may pound splints against objects, store food inside casts, and chew or suck on edges of dressings. A child wearing a corrective orthotic device may incur skin damage as increased muscle tone or spasticity causes skin pressure against the device.

Prevent covert skin damage by monitoring circulation in an extremity fitted with a cast or appliance; check residual limbs for irritation or pressure along the suture line and bony prominences. Consider a child who walks with an altered gait pattern as simply responding to irritation from chafed skin. Compensate for the increased vulnerability of a child who has lost sensation by anticipating injuries and being vigilant to prevent burns from hot liquids, frostbite or sunburn, insect stings, and other skin damage. Closely monitor special dressings or garment wraps a child with burns may wear to prevent scarring and keep grafts intact.

Prevention is linked with life-style. Self-initiated skin inspections assisted by an adaptive mirror, self-monitored positioning and alignment of extremities, and half-hourly weight shifts are part of the routine for children with neurological impairments and sensory loss. When in bed, a child is turned at least every 2 hours; schedule turns so that the child faces the correct direction to participate in activities, socialization, or meals. Nutrition and hydration are essential to healthy skin and tissue repair. Preventive skin care includes good hygiene and use of lubricants and skin barriers, special mattresses, flotation or gel cushions, and sheepskins.

BREATHING

Assess the rate, depth, and quality of respiration, use of accessory muscles, and respiratory sounds. Respiratory assessment includes: dyspnea, apnea, cyanosis, mucus congestion or sputum production, and ability to cough. Oxygen level, blood gases, vital capacity, and respiratory infections are commonly monitored.

Prevent the spread of respiratory infections. A properly humidified dust-free environment, adjusted fluid intake, and selected diet can be adjuncts to improved breathing and lower the viscosity of mucus. Whenever mechanical ventilators or other respiratory equipment is used, ascertain the meaning the child and family attach to its use. Monitor the child as well as the machinery. For example, adolescents with spinal cord injury have developed stress ulcers in response to ventilator dependency.

Teaching families to care for their children demystifies technology. Instruct families in the care of tracheostomy, including suctioning when appropriate; have the child learn glossopharyngeal breathing techniques. Teach preventive and self-care measures, such as postural drainage, positioning, exercises for breathing, strengthening the diaphragm and abdominal tone, spirometer use, and seating postures that aid pulmonary function.

MOBILITY

Assess mobility from three views: movement based on expectations for the child's corrected age, functional mobility based on the level and type of disability, and neurologically influenced movements. Identify developmentally appropriate fine and gross motor function. Note any movement that is inappropriate, such as hyperextension of joints, movement where there should be none, immobility, and abnormal patterns, such as spasticity. Assess the range of joint motion, voluntary and involuntary muscle action, functional abilities to transfer, bear weight, ambulate, and move about in bed. Assess coordination, balance, and ability to move or transfer safely.

Hazards resulting from immobility, such as pressure areas, thrombophlebitis, contractures, congestion, disorientation, or confusion can be prevented with positioning, turning, and weight shifts (47). Consistent 24-hour nursing intervention may positively influence outcome for children who have surgical intervention to improve mobility and prevent contractures.

Children learn through play and interactions and, therefore, are encouraged to assume an upright position as much as possible during the day. For example, placing a child in a prone stander may increase bone strength and improve weight bearing as well as improve cognitive attention. Reinforce correct procedures for moving children. For example, teach families that a child with cerebral palsy is not to be lifted from under the arms or tossed and caught in the air during play (56).

Work closely to reinforce physical and occupational therapy activities that use a variety of devices, such as posture chairs, customized wheelchairs, bracing for scoliosis, or serial orthoses. During daily activities, such as eating or play, ensure that children use the assistive devices provided for them (5). Night splints to prevent contractures and deformities are labor intensive, but they are useful long-term preventive measures, including for those children with progressive neuromuscular conditions who may eventually become ventilator dependent (18, 53).

Capitalize on one benefit of spasticity, knee stability when coming to a standing position, to increase mobility. Evaluate whether a child will encounter potential problems with safety, seating, transfers, continence, and activities of daily living (35). Children with cerebral palsy must be monitored, even during rest or play, so that they do not assume positions that lead to contractures or deformities that are detrimental to mobility.

NUTRITION, FLUIDS, AND EATING

Assess and analyze the intake and output of fluids and nutrients adjusted for age and specific needs. Obtain a dietary history or log and document meal patterns, food allergies, and favorites. Evaluate a child's means of getting food into his or her mouth and observe the mechanics of sucking, chewing, and swallowing. If the child has a device such as a gastrostomy tube, assess it for proper insertion, patency, and stoma irritation.

Work collaboratively with speech therapists and occupational therapists to assist children who have eating and swallowing disorders. A child who has a tendency to choke or regurgitate, will do better in an environment with minimal distractions. Select foods prepared in a texture that the child can manage to swallow; a mashed potato consistency often works well, while liquids may be difficult.

Sit the child upright, flexing the head slightly forward to eat while providing support for the trunk to keep alignment. Place food in the back of the child's mouth or toward the cheek on one side, as directed. The child should be positioned to sit upright for 30-40 minutes after eating. Safety precautions and emergency responses in case of choking or aspiration should be pre-established. These children require excellent oral hygiene. When possible, introduce assistive devices to older children so they can perform their own brushing and flossing.

Concentrate on children's food preferences, provide finger foods, and add color or texture when selecting a nutritional program for conditions such as constipation, flatus, diarrhea, an ostomy, or dietary restrictions. Teach parents that fluids are needed to replace those lost through upper respiratory infections, fever, diarrhea, vomiting, or perspiration from increased activity.

Attention to the role of nutrition in healing and the nutritional status of children is important in hospitals (32) and, later, at home. The effects of early nutritional deficits are apparent in the long-term neurosensory or neuromuscular deficits that become problems for 10–25% of infants who survive with very low birth weights (7). Unfortunately, these infants may develop oral feeding aversions in response to the suctioning and intubation during their intensive care experiences.

Balancing and calculating nutrition and fluids may be complex. Infants with bronchopulmonary dysplasia have increased caloric requirements, but need restricted fluid intake. Following traumatic brain injury, fluids are closely monitored to prevent increasing cerebral edema. Children who have burns and other injuries require high caloric and high protein diets to promote a positive nitrogen balance. Children with spina bifida and muscular dystrophy who are in wheelchair have a tendency toward obesity. A child with juvenile rheumatoid arthritis is encouraged to maintain ideal weight to relieve pain and assist mobility.

Gastrostomy tubes are used when oral feeding is no longer possible or becomes inefficient for nourishment and to supplement the diet. For children who are candidates, a gastrostomy "button" may lessen the perception of changes in body image (31). Pediatric rehabilitation nurses prepare the child, family, and school personnel to manage a gastrostomy.

SLEEP AND REST

Assess patterns and quality of sleep and rest, periods of apnea, sleeping arrangements and environment, and investigate causes of sleep disturbances.

Sleep and nap schedules are adjusted for each child's age and development. Regular sleep and rest contributes to healing, reality orientation, and promotes metabolism and bowel regularity. Furthermore, naps may be the only respite times parents can claim for their own rest. Recurrent sleep difficulties may signal emotional stressors as well as physical problems.

Children do not associate the sources of pain or distress in the same manner as adults. Families may not perceive a relationship between a sleep disturbance and a health problem, such as sleep disturbances associated with gastroesophageal reflux. Infants with shunts may sleep longer and nap more often; however, an early warning shunt malfunction may be expressed by sudden awakening with irritability and crying. Children with juvenile rheumatoid arthritis benefit from increased rest prior to and between activities; they require more sleep during exacerbations.

SENSORY EVALUATION

Assess sensory function of vision, hearing, touch, smell, taste, sense of direction, and coordination. For example, children with cerebral palsy may have more auditory and visual deficits, but should not be designated retarded based solely on diminished sensory functions.

Senses are a child's link to his or her environment so that even with deficits, the child can benefit from intervention to increase stimulation and orientation on all sensory fronts and greater awareness of the environment. Use toys with adaptive switches and toys that create sounds or movement, encourage fine motor movements, stimulate reaching, or require hand-eye coordination. Adaptive and assistive equipment specifically designed for visual and auditory deficits is available.

The plan for hyperactive, restless children is to reduce excessive external stimulation and stressors. Whenever a child becomes agitated or argumentative, do not confront him or her or insist that the child do something; instead, seek a quiet environment and wait awhile. Cover the child's eyes, close the room, and offer one food choice, creating a controlled environment for an acutely agitated child, such as in a child who has suffered traumatic brain injury (61).

COMMUNICATION

Assess the quality and clarity of age-appropriate communication using a developmental communication guide. A child uses a variety of skills to communicate, especially through play and exploration of the environment. Evaluate expressive and receptive skills, precursors to language communication, and differentiate between speech and language production at different developmental stages. Delayed communication skills may be related to sensory dysfunction.

Support the speech-language therapy program as a team. If a child cannot or will not respond verbally, work with the family to develop consistent signals or use picture language boards, computer software, and other augmentative communication devices. Familiar photographs, toys, or music can reduce anxiety and cue communication. Pay special attention to a child's ability to communicate with others for comfort and safety and to enhance cognitive development.

The nonverbal child requires a consistent system of augmented communication and early implementation of communication strategies, such as sign language (24). Do not discuss children or their conditions in their presence; absence of response or expression is not an indicator of hearing loss or lack of understanding.

BOWEL FUNCTION

Assess peristalsis, bowel habits, amount, consistency, color, odor, and appearance. Incontinence is caused by neurological damage, other complications, psychosocial factors, or lack of training. Assess dietary fiber and fluid intake, activity level, medication regimen, and muscle tone. When ostomy is used, assess the appliance, skin barrier or seal, and the child's toileting technique.

Incorporate data about the child's unique needs into the bowel retraining program. For example, a child retaining stool due to behavioral encopresis, may develop a dried, painful impaction. Liquid stool soiling around the impaction confounds the assessment (15). Determine whether digital stimulation, medications, or the Valsalva maneuver are medically safe for a bowel retraining program. Children with spinal cord injuries above the level of T6 may risk autonomic dysreflexia if the bowel becomes distended or in response to rectal stimulation, suppositories, or enemas.

Bowel programs in early morning or 30 minutes following a meal capitalize on the natural stimulation of the gastrocolic reflex. Choose a private relaxed environment where the child can be positioned comfortably. If the child can safely sit and balance on the commode seat, offer a book or other distraction.

Keep a log to evaluate the toileting schedule, but do not change the program too frequently. It takes time to adjust to the retraining and frequent program changes will not be beneficial. Concentrate on the child learning to associate signals that will help self-monitoring of the bowel program. Review skin care, hygiene, exercise, diet, and fluids. Be patient.

A child who has an ostomy needs a similar bowel retraining program consistent with his or her ability. An anatomically correct doll may assist a child in learning irrigation techniques in a nonthreatening manner. Begin by teaching good handwashing and regular self-monitoring for irritated skin or scar tissue, leakage around the appliance, dietary controls, and personal hygiene (1). Use appliances sized for children. Children will not injure the stoma during normal play, but cover stoma to deter bruising or picking (42).

BLADDER FUNCTION

Assess the amount, color, odor, pH, and clarity of urine. Assess urinary frequency, force of stream, complete emptying of the bladder, signs of urinary tract infection, and control, including dribbling, seepage, and nighttime control. Determine whether the bladder is flaccid, spastic, or mixed. Prior to beginning a bladder training program, review data from urodynamic studies and urine cultures. Assure frequent and complete bladder emptying to prevent urinary track infections and reflux; do not *routinely* withhold fluids. Simple measures prevent renal failure, the most common cause of death for children with spinal bifida (43).

Give developmentally correct bladder training instructions. Consider toileting as a social skill rather than as a medical procedure. Assist children who have difficulty managing their clothing or who wear casts, braces, or orthotics; some appliances can be modified. Family, professionals, and the child must work together to achieve continence but, whenever possible, children are taught to perform their own clean intermittent catheterizations(55). (Table 9.1.) Stressors, irritable bowel syndrome, recurrent gastrointestinal infections, dietary changes, or indulgence may sabotage a program unless all concerned are dedicated. Offer rewards, not shame or punishment.

Table 9.1.
Home-Based Tracheostomy Care[a]

KNOW
Universal precautions and aseptic technique
Anatomy and physiology of the respiratory tract
How and when to suction
Parts and style of tracheostomy tube
Mechanical ventilator procedures, if needed
Oxygen or AmbuBag procedures
How to change tracheostomy ties
Specific safety precautions
Signs/symptoms of complications or distress
Alternate communication and nonverbal expressions
Prearranged emergency plan
Spare supplies and assistant are available

DO
Keep the tracheostomy stoma patent
Observe for fluid or blood leakage around the tube
Assess skin integrity
Clean around the stoma q.i.d. with a cotton-tipped applicator dipped in half-strength hydrogen
    peroxide and distilled water; rinse with water and pat dry
Check that ties are dry and in place
Maintain a dust-free, humidified environment
Consider the child's needs and comfort

DO NOT
Allow the stoma to close
Leave the child alone
Allow anything, food or water, to enter
Use Vaseline-type lubricants
Give shower baths
Prop bottles
Cover the stoma with clothes or bedding
Choose toys and bedding with furry material

PREPARATION
Wash your hands, (wear gloves, when ordered)
Assemble equipment
Assess child's breathing and need to suction
Position the child correctly; use a small pillow or towel under the shoulders to expose stoma or
    a small neck roll; mummy wrap an infant or carefully restrain a small child for safety only
If needed, suction the child; allow time to recover
When ordered, give an oxygen boost or use AmbuBag
Explain what you are going to do; ask children if they are ready to participate
Assemble all supplies, equipment, and spare setup *before removing* the old tube

EQUIPMENT
Pediatric-sized tracheostomy tubes and cannulas with connectors clean or sterilized as
    ordered.
Tracheostomy ties
Hydrogen peroxide
Suction equipment
Dressings or Telfa pads
Blunt-edged scissors
Oxygen or AmbuBag
Bedside or Worktable
Stethoscope
Saline or distilled water
Flashlight
Cotton-tipped applicators

Table 9.1.
Home-Based Tracheostomy Care—*Continued*

EQUIPMENT (cont.)

    Water-soluble lubricant
    Spare setup
    Basin
    Follow specific instructions for cuffed tracheostomy tubes used with mechanical ventilators; a
        portable ventilator system with humidifier and alarms is used for wheelchairs and other
        mobility devices

PROCEDURE

    Wash hands (gloves if ordered)
    Use aseptic technique
    Open tube setup, keeping a sterile tube in the package; still in the package, fit the tie through a
        flange on one side of the tube, then secure it in place
    Holding the old tube in place, cut ties with a scissor; when necessary to change ties, get
        assistance
    Remove old tube; use a smooth, coordinated motion
    Grasp only the flanges, not the tube, lift the new tube from the package
    Cleanse skin and stoma now or after procedure, depending on the stoma remaining patent
        and the child's tolerance
    Lubricate the tube and obturator (water-soluble lubricant)
    Insert the obturator and gently, but securely hold it in place with a thumb
    Insert the tube into the stoma; use a gentle, coordinated upward motion, then rotate to curve
        downward, following the tracheal anatomy
    Remove the obturator and place in a container with a lid
    Hold onto the tracheostomy tube until ties are fastened
    Place any dressings or pads underneath ties; fasten ties securely, but allow a fingerbreadth
        between ties and neck, rotate sites where ties are knotted against the child's neck
    Insert inner cannula, if used
    Wash hands
    Reposition the child and assess chest and breathing
    Reassure the child, touch or hold him or her, perhaps use a play activity to encourage
        communication about the procedure
    Clean (hydrogen peroxide and water) or sterilize reusable tubes before storing; discard soiled
        items and disposables properly; wash hands (26)

[a]Tracheostomy care can be successfully accomplished by family members in the home once they have learned and demonstrated the ability to perform techniques safely and comfortably.

PAIN

Pain is a complex multidimensional phenomenon that exists as it is defined by an individual child. The assessment, relief, management, and ongoing evaluation of chronic pain in children is a relatively new challenge. Until recently, the prevailing theories stated that infants and young children with incompletely developed nervous systems did not feel or experience pain (51).

Chronic pain in children must be assessed on physiological, psychological, and experiential levels. Experiential assessment is further divided into the expression and the experience of pain. Currently, assessment tools developed for children in acute pain are used to asess chronic pain as well. Children may not transmit or communicate information about their pain in accurate or reliable communications; changes in behavior, sleep patterns, appetite, and activity may indicate pain. Children may invest in play or activity to detract from pain, to shield their pain from others, or to avoid pain management measures. For example, a child may perceive an injection as more negative than the pain itself (27).

Children who have had surgery, incurred burns or had other injuries are usually undermedicated for their pain. This may be true for phantom pain following amputations (54), recurrent pain in juvenile rheumatoid arthritis, and reflex sympathetic dystrophy syndrome (RSDS) (22). Pain management and relief for children with burns or juvenile rheumatoid arthritis may enable them to achieve increased participation in physical activities and attend school successfully (23, 48).

A child may become socially isolated when unable to participate in activities with peers or when he or she becomes irritable simply because of feeling poorly. The child may assume positions or acquire habits that evade pain, thereby causing secondary problems, such as deformities, poor posture, or contractures. Assistive devices, appliances, or equipment enable children to cope by working around their pain, thereby gaining function. For example, a child with severe joint pain may not be able to hold a pencil for writing or flex the hips to position himself or herself on a regular toilet seat. An enlarged pencil or computer mouse and an elevated toilet seat may improve functional abilities when used in conjunction with rest, heat, exercises, medication, and positioning.

REGULATORY MECHANISMS

Body regulatory mechanisms are not refined in infants and young children; rapid fluctuations or undetected changes quickly lead to critical events. Assess for signs and symptoms of hypothermia or hyperthermia, such as perspiration, chills, fever, heat cramps, changes in respirations, heart rate, or blood pressure, and irritability with confusion.

Investigate external stressors, such as dehydration, infection, hot and cold objects or weather, allergies, medications or treatments, responses to burns, severe diaper rash, and injury or trauma. Irritants may induce seizures, asthmatic crisis, or autonomic dysreflexia.

Planned alterations in regulatory mechanisms include those to increase function, relieve discomfort, or administer treatments. A child with joint pain should take a warm bath prior to activity or perform range of motion exercises underwater during pool therapy. Induced hypothermia may be used with proper precautions and monitoring to decrease cerebral metabolism following head injury; however, the extremities must be monitored to avoid edema. A similar challenge is to prevent heat loss and regulate temperature following burns while avoiding overhydration. Procedures should be reconciled with specific manufacturer instructions when using equipment from several vendors. Regulatory technology is frequently used for signaling shunt malfunctions, monitoring sleep apnea, assisting respiration, and providing temperature regulation, such as cooling blankets or environmental control units.

When the child has paresis with sensory or proprioceptive loss, evaluate his or her awareness of alterations in comfort or temperature coupled with the individual's unique means of expressing or signaling concern and discomfort. Pay attention to the environment, dressing the child appropriately for the temperature, providing nutrients and fluids, monitoring regulatory functions and electrolytes, and preventing pressure areas.

SAFETY

Safety, an ongoing assessment, relies on anticipation and understanding of a child's changing development. Review specific safety concerns with the family prior to each developmental stage. Environmental safety issues differ as the child's area of freedom and range of activity enlarge. At the same time, family members who lift, turn, and carry need to be trained to do so properly, without injuring themselves. Safety-checked equipment requires regular maintenance. A variety of safety-tested products are available including toys, fireproof sleepwear, lead-free environments, and hypoallergenic formulas. Protective helmets, seat belts, transfer belts, bedrails and grab bars, padded equipment, locking wheels, and adaptive seating contribute to safe activities.

Safety issues differ with the severity of the child's condition and his or her reliance on technology for survival. General guidelines for families at home are to: learn emergency procedures, such as CPR for infants and children; arrange for emergency backup with rescue squad, local power companies, and an emergency response system; have access to a telephone, store spare batteries, a generator, tracheostomy setups, or other equipment; and post the Poison Control Center number. Prepare safety plans for home, school, and other community places.

Safety issues may be specifically related to the child's condition, such as concerns about choking or aspiration for the child with cerebral palsy or injury during a seizure. Too often, attempted or intended suicide, substance abuse, child abuse, or neglect are safety issues ignored until an incident occurs.

Future Directions

Future directions for pediatric rehabilitation nursing include: utilizing research, developing transdisciplinary practice models, coordinating transition among levels of intervention, examining outcomes of care and cost benefits of technology, and identifying practice for issues such as substance abuse, early intervention, pediatric AIDS or hospice, and continuing advocacy for the unique and special needs of children within culturally relevant, family-focused, community-based programs.

Community-Based Rehabilitation

The following section discusses two community-based rehabilitation procedures, family-administered tracheostomy care, and child self-care for clean intermittent catheterization. For either procedure, both home and school situations are monitored regularly (49). The family's ability to cope with increased stressors and the child's opportunities to achieve developmental and social growth, as well as technologically correct care, must be evaluated (12).

The impact of technology on medically fragile children begins with survival and continues as technological advances support improved quality of life and independent community living. A lengthy literature debates complex issues surrounding home-based technology (59). Candidates selected for home mechanical ventilation meet specific criteria including stable medical condition, emergency response networks, backup equipment, and family acceptance.

Family-Administered Tracheostomy Care

Prior to community-based care, the nurse teaches the family about the natural history of the child's condition; offers anticipatory guidance related to deficits (52), stresses, signs and symptoms of respiratory distress and other emergencies; teaches procedures such as suctioning and tracheostomy care; evaluates the family's return demonstrations; and coordinates the transition to home, school, and community (3, 9, 39). A contract to clarify agreements and delineate responsibilities among the child, family, and team is useful when they hold conflicting expectations about the outcome of care, such as whether weaning is a long-term goal for the child (30). The procedure of tracheostomy care is described in Table 9.1.

Clean Intermittent Catheterization for Children

Many children with neurogenic dysfunction are able to achieve self-management. Medical goals are complete emptying of the bladder without infection, bladder distension, incontinence, or reflux. Research results indicate that children at risk for deteriorating bladder problems benefit from prophylactic clean intermittent catheterization (CIC) (16). CIC is simple, harmless, and effective both for protection of the upper urinary tract and for control of urinary incontinence during long-term use (40). Families with infants and young children can perform CIC without added stress (34). Successful CIC allows many children to be clean, dry, uninhibited by urinary devices, free from urinary tract infections, and socially continent (2, 36).

Interpretations of PL 94–142 consider CIC both as a related service and as an assurance that a child attends school in the least restrictive environment (6, 19). CIC may increase independence and heighten self-esteem for a child who personalizes incontinence, devaluing self-worth and limiting functional ability (37). On the other hand, children and their families should be screened for psychological and psychomotor readiness prior to learning self-catheterization. A child with inadequate coping mechanisms may develop a fear of failure and resist learning this and other self-care procedures (17).

In general, children with higher level neurological lesions can be expected to have delays beyond peers when learning personal care and hygiene skills; these delays may be unrelated to neurological dysfunction or hand-eye coordination skills (57). Motor developmental skills and hand-eye coordination necessary to complete the task and cognitive ability precede problem-solving or self-directing the procedure (8). However, teaching and learning must be evaluated on each child's achievement of developmental tasks, not only chronological age, neurological function, or hand-eye coordination skills, Table 9.2 shows the procedure of teaching CIC.

Table 9.2.
Self-Catheterization with CIC for Children[a]

TEACHING CIC TO CHILDREN

Ideally, a child is taught to perform or direct his or her own care (25). The following list of suggestions applies to teaching procedures to children.

Provide developmentally correct information about the child's condition; anatomically correct dolls and toys (44), books, videocassettes, computer-assisted learning programs are available

Choose a time conducive to learning, not nap time or mealtime

Schedule a session appropriate for the child's attention span

Use principles of sequential task learning (10)

Provide privacy and minimize distractions; arrange assistance for managing clothing or positioning, develop cues to remind the child confidentially about performing CIC and socially acceptable ways to answer questions; share these with teachers and extended family members

Consider the meaning of the procedure to the child at his or her developmental stage; anticipate concerns or fears that may arise

Teach handwashing and other infection-control measures

Assemble an unobtrusive travel kit containing catheters and disposable towelettes in plastic ziptop bags; store clean and soiled catheters separately

Keep dry clothing on hand at school

Be patient and allow time for learning; the child may need several months to a year to retrain the bladder; encourage the child through error, accidents, or setbacks due to illness or other causes

Develop performance or memory aids that the child can refer to when away from home; include him or her in recording intake and output, testing urinary pH, and recognizing the signs of infection or complications

Regularly monitor the child's procedure and psychosocial response

Use behavior modification and other rewards; encourage the child

PROCEDURE

Wash hands

Assemble equipment

Clean straight catheter of selected size

Storage or carrying containers for clean and soiled catheters

Sterile water-soluble lubricant for males

Packettes of wipes or towels

Table 9.2.
Self-Catheterization with CIC for Children—*Continued*

PROCEDURE (cont.)

Move to a safe, comfortable position for catheterization, choose a private location where the child can use as natural a position for urination as function permits; encourage girls to sit on the toilet and boys to stand in front

Arrange clothing to keep dry and out of the way

Use sequential learning tasks; if assisted, the child does whatever steps he or she is able to do, such as positioning the catheter or helping to push on insertion

GIRLS

Wash hands

Cleanse the urethral area with water and wipe front to back with a disposable towelette

Hold the catheter in one hand with the open end draining into the toilet

Separate the labia, locate the urethral meatus; use a mirror to visualize the urethra

BOYS

Wash hands

Cleanse the penile meatus, with water or wipe with a disposable towelette

Lubricate the catheter tip with water-soluble lubricant

Grasp the penis on two sides, holding it upward and outward from the body during the entire process

Hold the catheter in one hand with the open end draining into the toilet

BOTH GIRLS AND BOYS

Insert the catheter

Hold the catheter in place until all urine has completely drained

Remove the catheter

Wash the catheter with water, rinse and dry or store soiled catheters in a container to wash later

Wash hands

PRECAUTIONS

Maladaptive psychosocial responses

Incorrect technique

Unsafe balance or positioning abilities

Soreness of urethra, or other pain

Discharge or other signs of infection

Bleeding, skin tears, or injuries

Difficulty passing the catheter

Changes in color, odor, character, or amount of urine

Unique complications, such as autonomic dysreflexia

*a*Children who are proper candidates can perform clean intermittent catheterization safely and simply in home and school settings; sterile techniques are reserved for hospitals and institutions. Guidelines for bladder volume by age are in Table 1.1.

Conclusions

Resolutions of issues for children of the 1990s will impact future generations of adults. Quality of life, advanced or computer-assisted technology, lifelong care planning, and family-focused, community-based programs form concepts and raise ethical questions in the same phrases. A core contributor to interdisciplinary rehabilitation, pediatric rehabilitation nursing uses theory bases to form frameworks for practice. Clinical practice addresses children and families; body, mind, and spirit.

Acknowledgment: Thanks to Maryann Solimine, RN, MLS, for assistance with the literature search.

REFERENCES

1. Adams DA, Selekof JL: Children with ostomies: Comprehensive care planning. *Pediatr Nursing* 12:429–433, 1986.
2. Altshuler A, Meyer J, Butz MKJ: Even children can learn to do clean self-catheterization. *Am J Nursing* 97–101, 1977.
3. Andrews MM, Nielson, DW: Technology dependent children in the home. *Pediatr Nursing* 14:111–114, 151, 1988.
4. Association of Rehabilitation Nurses & American Nurses' Association Joint Committee on Rehabilitation Nursing Practice: *Rehabilitation Nursing: Scope of Practice: Process and Outcome Criteria for Selected Diagnoses.* ANA, Kansas City, MO, 1988.
5. Atkins DJ, Meier RH: *Comprehensive Management of the Upper Limb Amputee.* Springer-Verlag, New York, 1989.
6. Ballard J, Ramirez B, Zantal-Wiener K: PL 94–142, Sect 504 & PL 99457: Understanding what they are and are not. Reston, VA, Council for Exceptional Children, 1987, pp. 1–16.
7. Bennett FC: Recent advances in developmental intervention for biologically vulnerable infants. *Infants Young Children* 3:33–40, 1990.
8. Brown JP, Reichenbach MAB: Screening children with myelodysplasia for readiness to learn self-catheterization. *Rehabil Nursing* 14:334–337, 1989.
9. Burkett KW: Trends in pediatric rehabilitation. *Nursing Clin North Am* 24:239–255, 1989.
10. Clarkson JD: Self catheterization training of a child with myelomeningocele. *Am J Occupat Ther* 36:95–98, 1982.
11. Dittmar S: *Rehabilitation Nursing.* St. Louis, CV Mosby Co., 1989.
12. Donar ME: Community care: Pediatric home mechanical ventilation. *Holistic Nursing Practice* 2:68–80, 1988.
13. Dunst C, Trivette A, Deal A: *Enabling and Empowering Families, Principles and Guidelines for Practice.* Cambridge, MA, Brookline Books, 1988.
14. Edelman MW: Perspective—broadening the view: Hopes and responsibilities. *Infants Young Children* 3:vi–viii, 1990.
15. Ellett ML: Constipation/encopresis: A nursing perspective. *J Pediatr Health Care* 4:141–146, 1990.
16. Geraniotis E, Koff SA, Amile B: Prophylactic use of clean intermittent catheterization in treatment of infants and young children with myelomeningocele and neurogenic bladder dysfunction. *J Urol* 139:85, 1988.
17. Gil KM, Perry G, King LR: The use of biofeedback in a behavior program designed to teach an anxious child self-catheterization. *Biofeedback Self-Regul* 13:347–355, 1988.
18. Gilgoff I, Prentice W, Bayden A. Patient and family participation in management of respiratory failure in Duchenne muscular dystrophy. *Chest* 95:519, 1989.
19. Glucksman J: Clean intermittent catheterization—the law. *Spina Bifida Spotlight:* August 1985.
20. Gortmaker SL: Demography of chronic childhood diseases. In Hobbs N, Perrin JM (eds): *Issues in the Care of Children with Chronic Illness.* San Francisco, Jossey-Bass Publishers, 1985, pp. 135–154.
21. Gortmaker SL, Walker D, Weitzman M, Sobol A: Chronic conditions, socio-economic status and behavioral problems in children and adolescents. *Pediatrics* 85:267–276, 1990.
22. Greipp ME, Thomas AF: Reflex sympathetic dystrophy syndrome: A nursing challenge. *Orthop Nursing* 6:32–36, 72, 1987.

23. Grindley JF: The handicapped child in school: Considerations for health care. *Holistic Nursing Practice* 2:11–19, 1988.
24. Hall SS, Weatherly KS: Using Sign Language with Tracheotomotized Infants and Children. *Ped Nurs.* 15(4):362–370, 1989.
25. Hannigan K, Elder JS: Teaching catheterization to children. In Resnick MI, Elder MD (eds): *The Urologic Clinics of North America.* Philadelphia, W.B. Saunders Co., 15:653–660, 1988.
26. Hazinski MF: Pediatric home tracheostomy care: A parent's guide. *Pediatric Nursing* 12:41–48, 223, 225, 1986.
27. Hoeman SP: Childhood pain: Raising the accountability/question for rehabilitation nursing. Paper presented at the *Association of Rehabilitation Nurses Annual Educational Conference,* Nov 2, 1989. Nashville, TN.
28. Hoeman SP: Cultural assessment in rehabilitation nursing practice. *Nursing Clin North Am* 24:277–289, 1989.
29. Hoeman SP: *Rehabilitation/Restorative Care in the Community.* St. Louis, CV Mosby Co., 1990.
30. Hoeman SP, Winters DM: Case management for clients with high cervical spinal cord injuries. *Quality Review Bulletin: Special Publication: Case Management: Guiding Patients Through the Health Care Maze.* Chicago, JCAHO, 1988.
31. Huth MM, O'Brien ME: The gastrostomy feeding button. *Pediatr Nursing* 13:241–245, 1987.
32. Jaffe KM, Hays RM: Pediatric head injury: Rehabilitative medical management. *J Head Trauma Rehabil* 1:30–40, 1986.
33. Jessop DJ, Stein REK: Uncertainty and its relation to the psychological and social correlates of chronic illness in children. *Soc Sci Med* 20:993–999, 1985.
34. Joseph DB, Bauer SB, Colodny AH, Mandell J, Retik AB: Clean intermittent catheterization of infants with neurogenic bladder. *Pediatrics* 84:78–82, 1989.
35. Katz RT: Management of spasticity. *Arch Phys Med Rehabil* 67:108–116, 1988.
36. Lapides J: Clean intermittent self-catheterization in the treatment of urinary tract disease. *Urology* 107:458, 1972.
37. Lozen MH: Bladder and bowel management for children with myelomeningocele. *Infants and Young Children* 1:52–62, 1988.
38. Margolis LH, Sparrow AW, Swanson GM: Growing into healthy adults: Pediatric antecedents of adult disease. Health Monogram Series #3. Lansing, MI, Dept. of Public Health, 1989.
39. McCarthy MF: A home discharge program for ventilator-assisted children. *Pediatric Nursing* 12:331–335, 380, 1986.
40. Mollard P, Basset T, Gounot E, Hernandez, Viguier JL: Results of intermittent catheterization in neurogenic bladder in children and adolescents. *Chir Pediatr* 28:269–275, 1987.
41. Molnar GE: A developmental perspective for the rehabilitation of children with physical disability. *Pediatr Ann* 17:766–776, 1988.
42. Motta GJ: Life span changes: Implications for ostomy care. *Nurs Clin North Am* 22:333–339, 1987.
43. Myers G: Myelomeningocele: The medical aspects. *Pediatr Clin North Am* 31:165–175, 1984.
44. Neef NA, Parrish JM, Hannigan KF, Page TJ, Iwata BA: Teaching self-catheterization skills to children with neurogenic bladder complications. *J Appl Behav Anal* 22:237–243, 1989.
45. Nelkin V (ed): *Family Centered Care for Medically Fragile Children. Principles and Practices.* National Center for Networking, Community Based Services, Georgetown University Child Development Center, 1987.
46. Neuman B: *The Neuman Systems Model, Application to Nursing Education and Practice.* New York, Appleton-Century-Crofts, 1982.

47. Olson EV: The hazards of immobility. *Am J Nursing* 1990; March: 43–48.
48. Page-Goertz SS: Even children have arthritis. *Pediatr Nursing* 15:11–16, 1989.
49. Peters SG, Viggiano RW: Home mechanical ventilation. *Mayo Clin Proc* 63:1208–1213, 1988.
50. Roper N, Logan WW, Tierney AJ: *Using a Model for Nursing.* Edinburgh, Churchill-Livingstone, 1983.
51. Ross DM, Ross SA: *Childhood Pain: Current Issues, Research and Management.* Baltimore, Urban Schwarzenberg, 1988.
52. Rubin IL: Etiology of developmental disabilities. *Infants Young Children* 3:25–32, 1990.
53. Russman BS: Rehabilitation of the pediatric patient with a neuromuscular disease. *Neurol Clin* 8:727–740, 1990.
54. Sherman RA: Stump and phantom limb pain. *Neurol Clin* 7:249–264, 1989.
55. Smith, KA: Bowel and bladder management of the child with myelomeningocele in the school setting. *J Pediatr Health Care* 4:175–180, 1990.
56. Steele S: Young children with cerebral palsy: Practical guidelines for care. *Pediatr Nursing* July/August: 259–267, 1985.
57. Sullivan-Bobyai, Swanson SM: Toilet training the child with neurogenic impairment of bowel and bladder function. *Issue Compr Pediatr Nurs* 7:33–43, 1984.
58. Stein RE, Jessop DJ: What diagnosis does not tell: The case for a noncategorical approach to chronic illness in childhood. *Soc Sci Med* 29:769–778, 1989.
59. U.S. Congress, Office of Technology Assessment: *Technology Dependent Children: Hospital v. Home Care—A Technical Memorandum.* Washington, DC, U.S. Govt. Printing Office, OTA-TM-H-38, 1987.
60. Watson J: *Nursing: Human Science and Human Care. A Theory of Nursing.* Norwalk, CT, Appleton-Century-Crofts, 1985.
61. Yanko J, Barovitch E, Kozik JL, O'Donnell J: Nursing and the continuum of recovery. In Ylvisaker M (ed): *Head Injury Rehabilitation: Children and Adolescents.* Boston, College Hill Press, Little Brown & Co., 1985, pp 141–163.
62. Yoos L: Chronic childhood illness—developmental issues. *Pediatr Nursing* 13:25–28, 1987.

Rehabilitation of Childhood Disabilities

10

Myelodysplasia

ANGELES BADELL

The term spina bifida was used first by Nicholas Tulp (129) in 1652 to describe a group of defects with a common feature of separation of the posterior elements of the vertebral column. Morgagni (86), in 1761, noted the relationship of spina bifida with hydrocephalus. In 1894, Arnold (3) and, in 1891, Chiari (23) contributed their studies of the brainstem malformations associated with hydrocephalus.

Survival and Quality of Life

Before the advent of antibiotics, most infants born with spina bifida died within the first year of life. Medical advances in infection control improved survival and, after the disappearance of poliomyelitis, those children began to receive increasing attention for rehabilitation and orthopaedic care (8, 109). The availability of neurosurgical techniques for the treatment of hydrocephalus (94, 100) started another era of heightened interest in the treatment of this condition and led to further decrease in mortality. Sharrard and associates at Sheffield Children's Hospital reported in 1963 (110) that early closure of the spinal defect greatly decreased the rate of mortality. Survival rates of patients treated with early unselected closure were reported, in 1983, to be 62% to age 12 yr and 54% to age 19 yr (48). In 1971, Lorber (64) presented an analysis of the condition of surviving children from the Sheffield Hospital early closure cohort and concluded that there was a need for selective treatment. He suggested that medical and surgical intervention be withheld when the extent of defects at birth is considered severe enough to result in poor quality of life.

These recommendations created an ethical controversy (78). Comparisons between populations that were selected or unselected for early closure indicate that higher intellectual function is more likely in the selected group (65), but there are no significant differences reported for survival, renal function deficits, and ambulation independence (80).

Lorber's reports define poor quality of life among the surviving children and adolescents as having gross deformities in the legs, wheelchair dependence, socially unacceptable incontinence, obesity, and decubitus ulcers.

They note that no persons with such severe handicaps are likely to be able to earn a living in competitive employment unless they have an IQ score of at least 100 (64). Poor outlook is compounded by the difficulties that the families experience (37, 52) and by the social and financial burden that the long-term care of these handicapped individuals represents (68).

It should be noted that the problems identified as characteristics of the perceived poor quality of life are mostly the sequelae of inadequate prevention. To define the expected quality of life among the surviving children, one should clearly identify the origin of different factors that contribute to the ultimate outcome. There are, in fact, two sources of physical disability: (a) primary organic deficits caused by and related to the extent of birth defects; and (b) secondary complications that evolve progressively during the child's development and increase the functional limitations and disability of the individual.

Long-term follow-up studies of the quality of life of adults born with spina bifida indicate that anticipatory care should address not only progressive physical musculoskeletal deformities but also attend to the prevention of deficits arising from poor attention to the social, emotional growth of the child and the family and to inadequate social, educational, and vocational support services (19, 125). A most relevant issue to physiatric management is to distinguish between these factors. Understanding the nature of progressive secondary disabilities is the basis of proper intervention. The task of preventing or correcting these complications is not easy and, at times, it may not be successful. However, this argument does not justify inaction on the part of the physician or, even worse, a lack of clear understanding of the pathogenesis of the potential acquired disabilities that can affect the long-term quality of life for these children.

Familiarity with new concepts of pathogenesis, embryogenesisc, etiology, prevalence, and prevention is necessary for adequate physiatric assessment of the anticipated disability. This knowledge will enable the physician to provide adequate management for individual children and offer effective guidance and counseling for their parents.

Spina Bifida Syndrome

Spina bifida is a term accepted by usage. It serves to describe a syndrome consisting of multiple structural anomalies as an expression of the abnormal embryonic development of the neural tube and its surrounding structures. The characteristic paraplegia in the spina bifida syndrome is caused by myelodysplasia, a term that denotes variable degrees of a spinal cord malformation (14).

PATHOGENESIS/EMBRYOGENESIS

The teratogenic events causing these anomalies are still a subject of debate (40). The unresolved question is whether the neural tube fails to close around the 28th day of embryonic development (96) or it opens later due to focal necrosis, thus, initiating the process of malformation (105).

ETIOLOGY

Epidemiological studies have documented familial predilection and suggest that genetic factors interacting with multiple unknown environmental agents lead to the occurrence of neural tube defects in human embryos (59). Recent studies propose that at least part of the genetic predisposition to neural tube defects could reside in an abnormality associated with vitamin B_{12} production, transport, or metabolism (41).

INCIDENCE

The incidence of neural tube defects in the United States is approximately 0.5/1000 live births. It is one of the leading causes of disability in children. Overall incidence correlates with many factors well documented in extensive epidemiological studies (26, 92). In some geographic areas, especially in the British Isles, the incidence is as high as 4.5/1000 births. An increased rate is also observed in females, midspring conceptions, and in families of low socioeconomic class. Of particular significance is the recurrence rate among siblings with an estimated 5% higher risk after the first affected child rising to 10% after two affected siblings (85). The use of valproic acid during pregnancy results in an absolute 1% to 2% risk of spina bifida (57).

PREVENTION

Studies that suggested that periconceptual vitamin supplementation could prevent the occurrence of this congenital malformations (93) are controversial (116, 119). The birth of infants with neural tube defects can be prevented by early intrauterine detection followed by intervention to terminate the pregnancy. Because of the increased incidence in families with one affected member, genetic counseling is offered. Monitoring of subsequent pregnancies is recommended for prenatal detection of neural tube defects which can be demonstrated by elevated α-fetoprotein (AFP) in the amniotic fluid (25). A less invasive method for prenatal screening of all pregnancies regardless of familial history is determination of AFP in the maternal serum (13). Increased serum AFP at 16–18 weeks of pregnancy was found to be a reliable test, although definitive diagnosis is based on amniotic fluid examination for high levels of AFP and acetylcholinesterase as well as ultrasound studies (70). Prenatal detection offers the options of terminating the pregnancy or prelabor cesarean section can be planned to facilitate care during birth (113).

Clinical Correlates of Fetal Malformations

The teratogenic processes causing maldevelopment of the caudal posterior neural tube lead to variable extent of myelodysplasia with corresponding levels of paraplegia. A distinction between neural tube defects into those that arise during the process of neurulation from those related to postneurulation helps in understanding the clinical presentations (60). Neurulation defects include anencephaly, craniorachischisis, and spina bifida aperta. Neurulation defects are not skin covered and are amenable to prenatal detection. Skin-covered lesions, for example, lumbo-sacral lipomas and teratomas, arise from the continued development of the neural tube after closure of the posterior neuropore. This postneurulation process is also associated with frequent malformations of the conus and filum terminale and is important in the genesis of a variety of tumors in the area (43). Abnormal development of the cephalic anterior neuropore gives rise to anomalies, such as the Arnold-Chiari malformations, which impede the flow and absorption of cerebrospinal fluid. The result is hydrocephalus, which occurs in over 90% of infants with neural tube defect. Other brain anomalies, such as micropolygyria, are frequent. Arnold-Chiari malformation, in particular, is associated with hypotrophic lobes, loss of neuron cells, heterotopia, and dysplasia of the cerebellum (14). Mesodermal structures surrounding the neural tube may be also malformed, including the vertebrae, ribs, and the cranial vault. Vertebral and rib anomalies have particular clinical significance because they lead to early development of severe kyphotic and scoliotic deformities. The ectodermal covering may be absent over the malformed cord segments or it may develop a dysplastic continuity with the cystic meningeal sac in case of meningomyelocele. Pigmentation, hair tufts, or dermal sinus generally signal the presence of an underlying occult myelodysplasia. There is a high incidence of urinary tract anomalies, such as solitary kidney or malformed ureters, which contribute to increased morbidity in the presence of neurogenic bladder dysfunction.

Clinical Correlates of Abnormal Prenatal Development

An important clinical aspect of abnormal development in utero is the occurrence of arthrogryposis-like deformities of the lower limbs, most frequently different types of club feet (109). Congenital hip flexion and knee extension contractures as well as hip dislocation are encountered. These deformities represent intrauterine muscle imbalance due to denervation and the resultant contractures are consistent with the action of those muscles that have been preserved. It is surprising that, despite the early embryonic onset of denervation, the majority of infants are born without deformities. A significant implication of prenatally acquired deformities is that they usually fail to respond to corrective surgical intervention.

Intrauterine hydrocephalus is reflected by radiologically demonstrable craniolacunae at birth and the progressive ventricular dilation produces distortion of the cortex and other cerebral and cerebellar structures.

Pathomechanism of Changing Early Postnatal Course

The trauma of birth and subsequent exposure to extrauterine environment leads to progressive degeneration of the myelodysplastic tissues; infection may rapidly ensue. For this reason, urgent neonatal closure has been advocated; however, the delay needed to allow for informed parental decision-making has been noted not to affect the infant negatively (22). Early surgery permits dissection and isolation of viable spinal cord and nerve roots and reconstruction of a continuous dural sac (102). The level of neurologic dysfunction observed after a carefully performed early closure is frequently asymmetrical with mixed lower and upper motor neuron signs reflecting the structurally disorganized spinal cord.

Prior to the 1950s, delayed closure was the accepted practice. Surgery was performed at 12 months of age or later because by that time spontaneous epithelization made the closure easier. Furthermore, it was assumed that earlier closure would aggravate the hydrocephalus. Adult survivors of this approach show flaccid paraplegia with symmetrical neurological levels. These types of lesions are consistent with the classical description of spina bifida syndrome and resulted from local trauma, infection, and the surgical technique of delayed closure, which, in combination, created a virtual cordectomy.

If the child survives, hydrocephalus tends to become arrested during the first few years of life (58). Arrest is assumed to occur as increased absorption of the cerebrospinal fluid over the expanding surface of dilated ventricles reestablishes an equilibrium between production and absorption (112). Although ventricular dilatation is not incompatible with reasonable cognitive function, intellectual impairment is a clinical correlate of significant hydrocephalus (6). These children exhibit specific types of cognitive impairment and defective language function; the excessive inappropriate chatter and poor linguistic content are characteristic (31).

It is difficult to predict the intellectual outcome in a newborn known to have hydrocephalus. Statistically, significant cognitive dysfunction predominates among children with central nervous system infections, those with signs of craniolacunae, and among those with high levels of paralysis. Intellectual prediction in the neonate with hydrocephalus is made even more uncertain by the availability of neurosurgical treatment. The outcome may improve beyond expectations with successful shunting whereas the reverse occurs when infection and blockage complicate a shunted hydrocephalus (71, 79).

Infants with a poorly functioning shunt as well as those with decompensated nonshunted hydrocephalus present characteristic signs and symptoms, including lethargy, irritability, stridor, ocular motor incoordination, hyperreflexia in the upper extremities, and overall developmental delay (46).

Pathomechanism of Late Progressive Neurological Course

It is recognized that the course of the spina bifida syndrome is a dynamic process. During growth, progressive neurological involvement may appear. Deterioration related to spinal cord pathology may be attributed to tethered conus or filum terminale, lipomeningocele, or diastomatomyelia; tethered cord is suspected in all patients who had immediate closure of the myelodysplastic defect (131). Surgery to relieve tethering may prevent further functional loss if deterioration is detected (123). Spinal computerized tomography (CT), particularly metrizamide CT, myelography, and, most recently, magnetic resonance imaging (MRI) (50, 117) provide precise depiction of the anatomic derangements that characterize these entities (91). The efficacy and timing of neurosurgical intervention is a matter of controversy because many findings in neuroradiological imaging interpreted as tethered cord syndrome may exist without evidence of progressive neurological impairment (49).

Syringohydromyelia associated with unshunted or clinically compensated hydrocephalus was found to cause progressive scoliosis, spasticity, and increasing weakness of the extremities. Clinical and radiological examinations of the spine demonstrate a rapidly progressive high or midthoracic scoliosis (107). Appearance of stridor (46), gastroesophageal reflux, oculomotor incoordination, and respiratory irregularities indicate progressive brainstem compression due to Arnold-Chiari malformation that may occur despite an adequately functioning shunt and controlled hydrocephalus (17).

The causes of progressive neurological deficits of delayed onset are poorly understood. At times, it is difficult to ascertain an insidious deterioration. However, early detection and treatment of the documented underlying pathology may be successful in preventing further functional loss.

NATURAL HISTORY OF THE SPINA BIFIDA SYNDROME

The natural history of spina bifida reflects the interactive consequences of primary functional deficits and acquired secondary disabilities as shown in Figure 10.1.

Primary Functional Deficits

Paraplegia with motor and sensory impairment, mental retardation, and neurogenic sphincter dysfunction are the primary functional deficits produced by the neurological lesion. Neonatal prediction of the degree of disability should be approached with caution considering the variable outcome as a result of changing neurological status, effect of environment, and therapeutic intervention. An important factor, which compounds the disability, is that the defect is apparent at birth. Information given to the parents and the manner in which it is conveyed will influence their reaction at this most vulnerable time and will affect the future of the child and the family. Separation of the newborn from the mother interferes with early bonding (54). Fear of death and death wishes create feelings of confusion in the parents (30). Thus, an emotional atmosphere may evolve that is inadequate for fostering the child's development and stable family life (89). Many studies

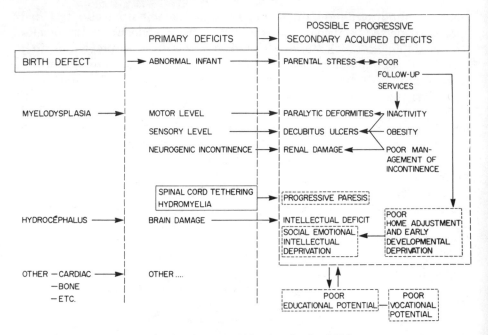

Figure 10.1. Natural history of spina bifida.

demonstrated the vulnerability of these families (127) and the subsequent poor social, educational, and vocational adjustment of the children upon reaching adolescence and adulthood (64, 77).

Acquired Secondary Disabilties

Progressive development of musculoskeletal complications and the nature of deformities can be anticipated from the distribution of paralysis at birth (5, 83, 109, 122). Although not always successful, prevention of these complications calls for a well-coordinated plan of physical therapy, orthotic intervention, orthopaedic procedures, and a most conscientious collaboration of the family in implementing this plan. The parents must have a clear understanding of the mechanism that can eventually lead to complications to be able to implement measures that must be strictly followed to avoid them. Prevention of renal damage due to neurogenic bladder dysfunction requires care long before parents would become concerned about the social aspects of bladder and bowel incontinence (69).

Severely stressed families create a less than adequate environment for nurturing the child's early development. Frequent separations for necessary hospitalizations and the resulting emotional, social, and intellectual deprivation may enhance a primary cognitive deficit and the likelihood of poor educational vocational achievements (7).

PHYSIATRIC ASSESSMENT AND MANAGEMENT

Individual Habilitation Plan

The potential outcome for a child with spina bifida syndrome is directly related to the primary organic deficits and long-term achievements can be improved by averting secondary organic or functional deficits (8).

Physiatric management is based on a clearly formulated individual habilitation plan considering all aspects of dysfunction. Anticipatory intervention for the prevention of secondary disabilities is an essential ingredient in this plan and requires considerable attention. A second broad aspect of management is adaptive functional training as needed by the extent of the disability and the developmental stage of the child. The objectives of an individual habilitation plan may need revision if secondary complications, such as hip dislocation, scoliosis, progressive deterioration of renal function, or significant emotional maladjustment, develop. A recent review by Carroll of his extensive experience in the orthopaedic management of spina bifida affirms this approach to management (20).

Parental Guidance

There is a crucial role for the parents in the successful implementation of the individual habilitation plan. It is important to start expanding their knowledge early about all aspects of care and about the impact of many interrelated factors that determine the level of ultimate accomplishments. For example, an adolescent may stop ambulating because of excessive weight gain, recurrent ulcers of the feet, and concurrent development of foot deformities. Early intensive guidance in nutritional needs and other contributing factors may prevent this cycle of events. Parents of a young child tend to be concerned most about eventual locomotor function and, not infrequently, the orthopaedic care of the lower extremities is the only objective pursued instead of a more comprehensive management directed to the achievement of full functional capacity (121).

Early and accurate parental guidance by well-informed physicians is an often neglected aspect of the care of children with myelodysplasia. Publications for parents introduce general information but cannot address individual needs. Physiatrists should ensure that the long-range plan is well defined, clearly explained, and repeatedly discussed with the family. It is necessary to clarify the child's disability but it is more important for the parents to gain an understanding of the child's potential function and the role of anticipatory care. To provide effective counseling, the physician must have a knowledge of the child's functional outlook and the skills to handle the emotional reactions of the parents so that information presented will lead to constructive adjustment on the part of the family (108). Medical and other commitments, at times, place excessive burdens upon these families.

Professional caretakers' concerns about lack of follow-up at home should be replaced by plans to assist the family in coping with the demands placed on their physical and emotional stamina (77). Parents who receive constructive support and understand the objectives of management can adjust to "lead" the professional team toward the goal of improving the outcome of the child and family.

MANAGEMENT OF PHYSICAL DISABILITY

Observing the newborn's postural attitude and spontaneous movements renders valuable information to assess the level of motor paralysis and preserved muscle function. An objective detailed muscle testing is not possible at this age; however, targeting on major muscle groups that are innervated by different spinal segments permits an assessment of the level of paraplegia (Table 10.1). The key movements to observe are hip flexion and adduction, knee flexion and extension, dorsiflexion, and plantar flexion at the ankle.

Sensory stimuli and moving the infant in various positions may be used to elicit voluntary or reflex postural movements. These movements can be distinguished from reflex motion related to isolated spinal function. Deformities should be noted and their range of flexibility measured on passive joint motion.

In *thoracic paralysis,* the legs appear flaccid; in supine lying, the posture is external rotation, abduction and flexion at the hips, knees are in semiflexion with external tibial rotation, and the feet in plantar flexion. Although there are no spontaneous movements, partial or total withdrawal of the legs may be elicited by pinprick without facial or emotional reactions to pain. This is a spinal reflex activity originating from preserved cord elements distal to the clinically evident level of lesion. The repetitive patterned nature of response that can be also evoked by pinching the buttocks is an indication of reflex activity in distinction from volitional movements.

The infant with a *high or midlumbar paralysis* lies in an attitude of hip flexion and adduction, the latter posture becoming more marked in midlumbar lesions. When L3 segment is preserved, a restless baby will show some kicking movements with intermittent knee extension and flexion combined with internal tibial torsion indicating innervation of the quadriceps and gracilis muscles. Medial hamstrings are likely to be active at mid to low lumbar levels and become a strong deforming force in the absence of lateral hamstring function (122).

In *low lumbar lesions,* the infant's postural attitude in the supine position is hip flexion adduction. An upset baby may show kicking movements with feeble hip abduction and extension. The most characteristic posture, however, is ankle dorsiflexion, which intensifies when the baby is restless. It indicates active function of the tibialis anterior muscle unopposed by weak plantar flexors.

Electromyographic studies can demonstrate denervation potentials in

Table 10.1.
Clinical Evaluation in Myelodysplasia

No.	Name		B.D.	Exam Date	Signature

Rt.	MUSCLE POWER	SENSATION (pain)	GROUP	SENSATION (pain)	MUSCLE POWER	Lt.
T12			I			T12
L1						L1
L2	Iliopsoas / Adductors / Quadriceps / Ant. Tibial / Hamstrings / Peroneals / Triceps Surae / Gluteus Maximus / Intrinsic Feet Musc. / Perineal & Sphincter		II		Perineal & Sphincter / Intrinsic Feet Musc. / Gluteus Maximus / Triceps Surae / Peroneals / Hamstrings / Ant. Tibial / Quadriceps / Adductors / Iliopsoas		L2
L3						L3
L4			III			L4
L5						L5
S1			IV			S1
S2						S2
S3			V			S3
S4						S4

OBSERVATIONS	Rt.	DEEP TENDON REFLEXES	Lt.	MUSCLE POWER RATING	
		Patellar		Normal	
		Achilles		Good	
		Ankle Clonus		Fair	
		SUPERFICIAL REFLEXES		Poor	
		Abdominals-upper		Zero	
		Abdominals-lower		SENSORY RATING	
		Plantar Responses		Normal	
		Cutaneous-Anal		Hypoesthesia	
	Anal sphincter tone			Anesthesia	
	Anal sphincter tension			Paraesthesia	

various muscles. However, the presence of normal motor units does not rule out a coexisting upper motor neuron lesion, a consideration that limits the usefulness of this diagnostic tool for clinical purposes. The technique of somatosensory-evoked potentials may be of value to assess the extent of spinal cord lesion (103). This method was found to be useful in older children suspected of having neurological deterioration (45).

EARLY ANTICIPATORY CARE

Early and repeated assessment of motor function constitutes the basis for an appropriate prevention program. Measures to avert soft tissue contractures should be instituted in the neonatal period. This is the time to plan for the coordination of long-range orthopaedic, orthotic, and physical therapy intervention.

Acquired soft tissue contractures develop as a result of several factors: (a) Muscle imbalance leads to paralytic deformities that are consistent with the action of the unopposed or stronger muscle (11); for example, hip flexion contracture in the absence of hip extension in L2 lesion. (b) Deformities may appear under the effect of gravity and positioning; an example is plantar flexion contracture of a flail ankle. (c) Spinal reflex activity may contribute to the development of certain deformities, as in the case of flexion-abduction contracture of the hip in high thoracic paralysis. It should be noted that deformities are less severe and easier to prevent around a completely flail joint than in the presence of paralytic muscle imbalance or reflex activity.

As the threat of contractures exists from birth, passive range of motion exercises and stretching should be started within the first few weeks of life. Short periods of exercises several times daily are sufficient and can be quite successful if the soft tissues yield to stretch. The parents should be involved early. At first, they perform the exercises under supervision and, eventually, at home on a regular daily basis. Aside from its benefits to the infant, this program also helps the parents to understand the objectives of management and gives a sense of confidence in their ability to take care of the child. Orthotic positioning devices are indicated in some cases as an additional preventive measure and are discussed later.

FUNCTIONAL TRAINING

An infant with myelodysplasia should be followed regularly to assess the quality and quantity of motor function and the development of postural control. With significant hydrocephalus, there will be a delay in attaining head control. Thoracic and lumbar levels of motor paralysis interfere with sitting. Head and trunk control are necessary for upper extremity stabilization and dexterous hand use. Therefore, it is important to develop the postural mechanism for these gross motor milestones or substitute passive support, when needed, in order to promote eye-hand coordination and manipulatory skills. Some children have mild neurological impairments of the upper extremities indicated by hypotonicity, weakness, or hyperactive deep tendon reflexes (15, 73). Training to compensate for these deficits should start early and progress along the developmental sequence as attainment of new skills becomes feasible. Preschool and school-aged paraplegic children are instructed in the use of alternative methods for self-care and other activities of daily living. Carry-over of these skills to the home and school environment should be stressed.

AMBULATION TRAINING

The prognosis for walking varies according to the extent of paralysis. However, due to medical complications, intellectual, emotional, and other factors, not every child will accomplish the maximal level of ambulation expected for a particular segmental lesion. The ability to walk may also regress during the years of growth if obesity or progressive postural malalignment develops (4). Furthermore, the high energy cost of paraplegic ambulation becomes more apparent and limiting in the adolescent who needs to travel longer distances than a younger child (36, 39, 47).

Regardless of the long-term outlook and even in those cases where upright mobility is expected only for the purpose of exercises, ambulation training should be instituted. Prerequisites of crutch walking are head control, the ability to maintain erect posture with balance aids, adequate strength, and coordination of the shoulder girdles and arms. Erect posture and locomotion are the best methods to maintain good alignment of the growing body.

Improved gross motor control leads to better sitting balance with symmetrical weight distribution and contributes to ischial decubitus prevention, proficiency in wheelchair mobility, and self-care skills. Weight-bearing decreases osteoporosis and the incidence of neuropathic fractures. The experience of standing and walking is important for the developing self-image of growing children and for their need to establish some control over their body and environment (74). However, ambulation is not a measure of the quality of life. Independent mobility can be achieved from a wheelchair and is often more functional than limited walking at the cost of physical exhaustion. Under these circumstances, the choice of wheelchair locomotion permits more appropriate concentration of energy on educational and vocational goals and social and recreational interests. Adolescents should be supported in their decision-making about the most preferred mode of locomotion even though it may counter parental desires. Training to achieve competence in all aspects of wheelchair mobility is an essential phase of rehabilitation.

There are many reasons for recommending passive standing to paraplegics (29), but the practice of passive standing becomes impractical if it requires the use of cumbersome orthotics, standing frames, and the aid of others for transfers. The development of motorized mobility (12) and wheelchairs with automatic standing mechanisms are promising trends for the paraplegic when this equipment becomes accessible economically (Figs. 10.2 and 10.3).

When ambulation training is initiated, the level of expected function should be clearly defined. This must be discussed with the parents from the outset and repeatedly thereafter. The possibility of regression as the child grows must be pointed out. When realistic goals are achieved and further functional gains cannot be expected, formal therapy is no longer indicated. However, the child must carry on at home and in school an appropriate level of daily activities to maintain and improve endurance. It is important to encourage a life-style with adequate level of physical activities, including housework, self-care, adaptive physical education, and sports.

ORTHOPAEDIC SURGERY: GENERAL GUIDELINES

In functional terms, the aim is to provide proper musculoskeletal alignment for stable sitting and stance (82). The postural requirements to meet this goal include symmetrical spine and hips, absence of significant limitation of motion at the hip and knee joints, and plantigrade feet (20, 83).

There are a number of general indications for surgical intervention:

1. Restoration of muscle balance to prevent paralytic deformities that occur most often around the hip and ankle joints (109);

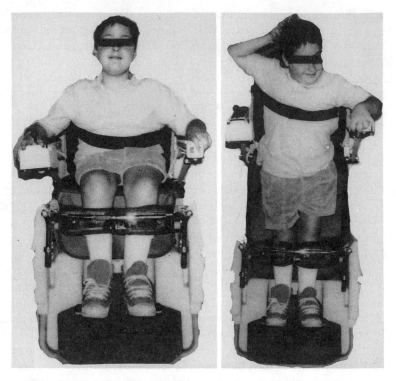

Figure 10.2. *Left,* Motorized automatic standing chair, sitting.
Figure 10.3. *Right,* Motorized automatic standing chair, standing.

2. Release of soft tissue contractures that do not yield to stretching and can produce secondary postural deformities with growth; for example, unilateral hip abduction and flexion contracture leading to pelvic obliquity, contralateral hip dislocation, and scoliosis (122);
3. Bone deformity present at birth, such as club foot, or developing during growth as a result of unbalanced muscle action; for example, internal tibial torsion caused by an active medial hamstring when its lateral portion is denervated (122);
4. Correction of any deformity may be considered with the understanding that recurrence is preventable only by a vigorous postoperative mobilization that entails a realistically implementable plan; for example, hip and knee flexion contractures inevitably recur in a child who continues to sit, without receiving a conscientious maintenance program (122).

Careful planning of surgical intervention is most important. Timing plays a significant role, particularly in case of paralytic muscle imbalance around the hip. The success of iliopsoas transfer decreases considerably when the secondary femoral and acetabular abnormalities are already present (44). If multiple procedures are planned, it is desirable to perform as many as possible during one hospitalization (83). The anxiety-producing disruptive effect of many hospitalizations on the child and family are obvious. Prolonged postoperative immobilization is to be avoided for it increases the risk of neuropathic fractures (109), epiphyseal separation (55), urinary stasis with infection and calculus formation, and regression of bowel regulation. Tachdjian advises 2 weeks of immobilization in plaster cast after soft tissue surgery with several hours a day of weight-bearing while in cast (122). Postoperative rehabilitation must be planned in advance so that delay in obtaining the necessary orthosis and in starting physical therapy will not jeopardize the result of surgery and the expected functional gains.

MANAGEMENT IN DIFFERENT LEVELS OF SPINAL CORD DYSFUNCTION

It is well to remember that the motor paralysis may be asymmetrical, that it may be a combination of upper and lower motor neuron lesions, and that, in some cases, it may show a changing course. Also of note is the frequent discordance between motor and sensory levels because absence or presence of proprioceptive sensation affects postural function. In spite of these considerations, it is helpful to distinguish four major groups of segmental neurological deficits that are accompanied by characteristic musculoskeletal deformities (Table 10.2). The challenge of preventing these complications is especially difficult and is not met with uniform success. It requires timely control of multiple factors related to medical, psychosocial, and economic problems.

T6 to T12 Lesions

Congenital subluxation or dislocation of the hips may occur in this level of paralysis. If the joints remain lax and mobile, surgical correction may be unnecessary since symmetry of the suprapelvic structures and a satisfactory sitting posture can be usually maintained. Although surgery may lead to a pleasing radiological appearance of the hips, clinical results are difficult to predict and reduced joint mobility can compromise the child's ability for sitting and passive standing (38, 122). Hip flexion and abduction contractures, especially when they are asymmetrical, should be released surgically.

Positioning orthoses should be applied as early as possible to avoid contractures induced by gravity. The habitual posture in this level of lesion is flexion, abduction, and external rotation of the hips and plantar flexion of the ankles. The device usually applied is a hip positioning brace (Fig. 10.4) with a ratchet joint that can be set at any degree of flexion or extension. Hip abduction is adjusted by bending the lateral thigh bars and is usually aligned at 15°. The "frog leg position" splintage of congenital nonparalytic hip dysplasia should not be used (122); it would cause severe contractures of the iliotibial band. Hip positioning splints need a spinal extension to control simultaneously the pelvic and trunk posture, thereby maintaining sym-

Table 10.2.
Neurological Levels, Complications, and Ambulation in Myelodysplasia

Groups	Musculoskeletal deformities (most frequent)	Orthosis and Crutches			Range of Locomotion	
		Preambulation (Positioners)	Ambulation Training	Efficient Ambulation	Minimal	Maximal
I						
T6	Kyphoscoliosis	Hip extension with 15°–15° hip abduction and Denis Browne bar	Parapodium Gait swivel and drag	HKAFO, but may need to attach trunk support	Gait: none	Gait: drag, swing Endurance: exercise or household
T12	Hip dislocation, usually bilateral					
	Hip flexion and abduction, external rotation	Early surgery	Crutch: underarm	Gait: drag, swing Crutch: underarm Lofstrand	Wheelchair use, dependent	Wheelchair use, independent
II						
L1	Hip flexion and adduction with dislocation	Presurgical (to prevent hip flexion contractures)	Postsurgical (to prevent hip dislocation)	May need HKAFO and hip extension assist	Gait: none	Gait: four-point Endurance: household or community
L2	Contralateral hip abduction, flexion	Hip extension with 15°–15° hip abduction and Denis Browne bar	HKAFO; and may need hip extension assist	AFO		
L3	Scoliosis	Parapodium	Gait: four point	Gait: four-point	Wheelchair use, dependent	Wheelchair use, independent
	Calcaneo-valgus		Crutch: Lofstrand	Crutch: Lofstrand		
III						
L4	Slow progression of hip flexion and lumbar lordosis; late hip dislocation	90° AFO or high-top shoes	Presurgical (to prevent calcaneus deformities)	Postsurgical	Gait: fourpoint Endurance: household or community	Independent ambulation Endurance: community
L5	Calcaneo-valgus, varus		AFO Gait: four-point Crutch: Lofstrand	High-top shoes Plantigrade inserts May need crutches	Wheelchair use, independent	
IV						
S1	Calcaneo-varus	None	Presurgical (to obtain plantigrade feet)	Postsurgical	Independent ambulation	Independent ambulation Endurance: normal
S2	Toe clawing	None	High-top shoes	Low shoes May need inserts	Wheelchair use while treating foot ulcers	
S3	None	None	None	None	Normal	Normal

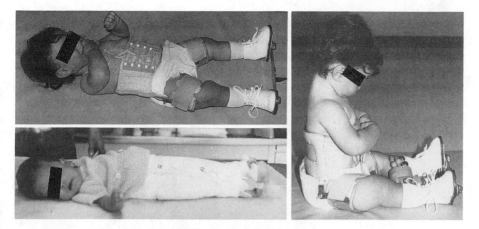

Figure 10.4. *Top left,* Hip positioning orthosis in extension.
Figure 10.5. *Right,* Hip positioning orthosis in sitting.
Figure 10.6. *Bottom left,* Towel wrapping in young infant to maintain hip extension.

metrical alignment of the hips. When the child has secure head control, this orthosis can be used for sitting with the hip joints set in flexion. The spinal extension provides trunk support (Fig. 10.5). Addition of a Dennis-Browne bar controls hip rotation and holds the feet in plantigrade position. Positioning braces should be used for 12 hours daily, preferably while the child is sleeping. Their application should be continued after surgery to maintain correction. In a very young infant or while awaiting the orthosis, a towel wrapping can be applied to maintain the legs in the desired position (Fig. 10.6).

Around 1 year of age, the parapodium (87) (Fig. 10.7) provides positioning and crutchless standing for the child who has good head control and stable shoulder girdle. Because of the safe balance provided by the base plate, gait training can be started earlier than it is possible with conventional orthosis. Initially, the child holds on to the hands of the therapist using a swivel motion to progress. Many children learn independent swivel locomotion and have functional household mobility at an early age. As strength and coordination of the shoulder girdle and arms develop, the child is ready to learn a drag of swing-type ambulation with walkerette or crutches. Increase in height or the need to provide 15° to 20° of hip abduction requires a larger base plate. Eventually, the size of this component interferes with mobility and cannot be properly accommodated for sitting in a wheelchair. For the tall preadolescent and the adolescent who has good endurance for crutch walking, thoracic-hip-knee-ankle-foot orthosis (THKAFO) makes it easier to clear the ground. The Orlau swivel modification type of parapodium orthosis may be a useful alternative for the older child. This device is reported to reduce the metabolic cost of ambulation compared with parapodium (67).

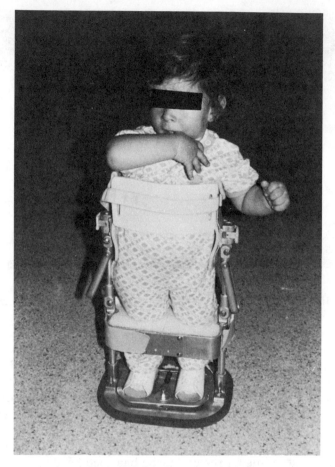

Figure 10.7. The parapodium.

Maximal ambulatory function with this level of paralysis remains limited to household ambulation even with good musculoskeletal alignment because of the extremely high energy cost. Foot deformities and hip and knee flexion contractures can interfere with maintaining erect stance. For functional mobility, a wheelchair is required. Symmetrical posture with mobile hips and good spinal alignment ensures balanced sitting and endurance for independent wheelchair function.

L1 to L3 Lesions

Children with high and especially with midlumbar paralysis are at the highest risk for progressive paralytic hip dislocation and have the most to gain from well-timed surgical intervention (11).

Since paralytic muscle imbalance is significant around the hip joints, a program to prevent flexion and adduction contractures must start early. Application of the hip positioning brace described in thoracic paralysis and daily passive range of motion exercises intend to serve this purpose. The orthosis is used on sitting at the age when this milestone is expected, since it provides stability to compensate for lack of hip extension and prevents excessive flexion during sitting. As long as the hips are stable, the infant is allowed time out of the brace for crawling. Frequent evaluations are needed to ascertain that no gradual reduction occurs in the range of passive hip movements when these gross motor activities are achieved. A parapodium can be prescribed around 1 yr of age for standing and as an initial walking device. After orthopaedic intervention to decrease hip flexion extension power imbalance, fitting the child with a hip-knee-ankle-foot orthosis (HKAFO) allows a reciprocal gait using a walkarette or crutches.

With some exceptions (27), there is general agreement about the advisability of preventing hip dislocation in L1 to L3 lesions. There is, however, a difference of opinion as to which procedure is most effective. Iliopsoas transfer was advocated as a unique solution to re-establish muscle balance but long-term results were less satisfactory than it was initially hoped (21, 34). The procedure is advised for its benefit of decreasing the unopposed deforming forces of hip flexion rather than as an effective replacement for abduction and extension (82). Femoral varus derotation osteotomy has been reported as successful in providing hip stability (134). A follow-up study of ilipsoas transfer indicated that hip dislocation had been prevented in most patients; however, there was a high proportion of "nonwalkers" among those children who had surgery during the first year of life or who had questionable iliopsoas power preoperatively (118).

Postsurgical orthotic training should stress maintenance of proper erect posture without excessive lumbar lordosis. The reciprocating gait orthosis (RGO) attempts to decrease hip flexion on stance (Fig. 10.8) (76).

Use of the RGO with strong hip flexors frequently stretches and breaks the extension cables and the child assumes a flexed hip position. If the hip flexion power is assymetrical, a pelvic rotation tilt develops. These considerations may help to explain the following contradictory reports. The LSU (Louisiana State University) RGO is recommended only after preparing the patient with correction of hip flexion contractures (75), but others suggest that the RGO is most successful when strong hip flexor power is available (135).

Assymetrical mid to upper lumbar neurological dysfunction leads to unequal deformities that enhance the possibility of rapid unilateral hip dislocation. A combination of abduction, flexion contracture in L1, L2 lesions, and flexion adduction deformity with contralateral L3 segmental innervation is a case in point (Fig. 10.9). Formation of the joint may be disturbed in utero and continue to deteriorate postnatally resulting in femoral anteversion, coxa valga, and defective acetabulum. In these cases, the need for

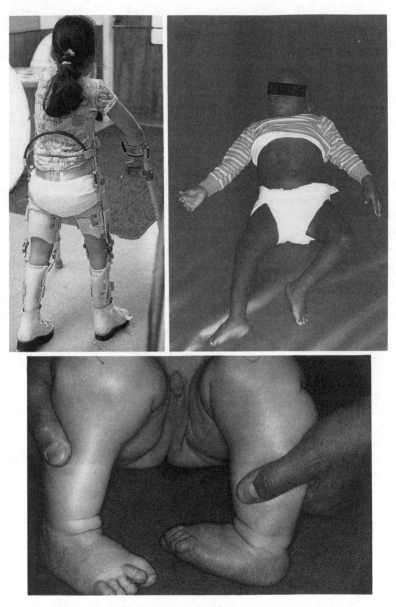

Figure 10.8. *Top left,* Reciprocal gait orthosis (RGO).
Figure 10.9. *Top right,* Right hip flexion, adduction with dislocation; left hip flexion abduction contracture.
Figure 10.10. Internal tibial torsion in midlumbar lesion.

appropriate femoral osteotomy and acetabular reconstruction must be considered because soft tissue surgery does not deter the progression of already existing bony abnormalities (44).

Surgical reduction of hip dislocation, has to be considered, particularly in unilateral abnormalities. However, restoration of joint mobility is often incomplete and loss of motion may interfere with sitting and standing.

At the knee, valgus attitude may develop with iliotibial band contracture and tibial external rotation. The appearance of medial torsion deformity of the tibia is related to an imbalance between the medial and lateral knee flexors, specifically to a preponderant action of the gracilis (Fig. 10.10). A secondary valgus attitude of the flail ankle compensates for the internal tibial rotation. Tibial osteotomy will correct the tibial deformity and prevents the development of a consequent foot abnormality.

Congenital club foot requires surgical treatment. As in all prenatally acquired arthrogrypotic deformities, correction is difficult to obtain and preserve. Combination of soft tissue and bony procedures, including talectomy (83) may be necessary. Bracing will be advisable to maintain proper foot alignment postoperatively. Orthosis is ineffective prior to surgery and may lead to decubiti.

Passive exercise is usually a satisfactory preventive measure when the ankle is flail but foot positioning orthoses should be considered if loss of motion is noted. An unstable flail ankle assumes a valgus attitude on weight-bearing and needs orthotic support. Extra-articular arthrodesis prior to the closure of growth centers in the foot, or triple arthrodesis thereafter, are surgical measures to contain this deformity.

When mediolateral malalignment of the ankle joint is severe, supramalleolar tibial osteotomy may be required to restore plantigrade foot alignment (83, 109, 122).

Children with L3 segmental innervation have a good chance to develop adequate pelvic alignment and good knee stability so that orthotic support can be reduced to ankle braces.

Although they have a waddling gait, some attain limited community ambulation with crutches but need a wheelchair for long distances. Household or exercise ambulation is the usual level of achievement in high lumbar lesion. Worsening hip flexion deformity with lumbar lordosis decreases endurance for ambulation and excessive lumbar lordosis makes stance and gait difficult.

The postural deviations caused by scoliosis and unilateral or bilateral hip dislocation curtail the child's ability for ambulation and may interfere with trunk stability needed for independent wheelchair function.

L4, L5 Lesions

At this level of paralysis, the hip abductors and extensors are partially innervated. However, the strong opposing muscles continue to create unbalanced forces around the hip joint with the possibility of slowly progressive hip flexion deformity and dislocation by late childhood or adolescence. Progressive neurological loss may contribute to these changes. The integrity of the hip joint must be monitored and preventive surgery as discussed in upper lumbar paralysis may be indicated.

Foot deformities as a result of active dorsiflexion and weak plantar flexion become a major concern in low lumbar lesions because nonplantigrade weight-bearing generates decubiti. When both plantar flexors and inverters are weak, there is progressive calcaneovalgus associated with external tibial torsion, fibular shortening, and tilting of the ankle mortise (122). A conventional short leg brace with limited ankle motion eliminates excessive dorsiflexion and provides stability on standing. It should be attached to high top shoes with soft cushion heel, midsole rocker bar, and a Y strap added for mediolateral support. Molded plastic ankle foot orthosis with limited hinged ankle motion offers the additional advantages of light weight and some hindfoot control. Tenotomy or transfer of the tibialis anterior decreases the paralytic muscle imbalance. Muscle transfer is usually deferred until the child is walking but surgery is recommended before significant deformity of the growing bone occurs (16). It is advisable to continue postoperative protective bracing until skeletal maturity. If ankle instability persists, triple arthrodesis may be performed. Neuropathic joint changes may compromise the result of surgery and subsequent ambulation (95, 106).

If the clinical course is uncomplicated, children with low lumbar myelodysplasia are expected to become community ambulators, mostly without crutches. Gait deviations, consisting of gluteus medius lurch and gastrocnemius limp result in decreased endurance.

S1-S2 Lesions

Foot deformities prevail as a result of intrinsic-extrinsic muscle imbalance and partial weakness of eversion and plantar flexion. Cavus foot and clawtoes are quite characteristic, sometimes combined with calcaneous and/or varus deformities. There is no limitation in ambulation but ulcerations are prone to develop over the insensitive plantar surface of a nonplantigrade foot.

Surgical correction of the foot deformities may be indicated (109, 122). For a young child, high top shoes are recommended. Shoe modifications in the older child depend on the foot abnormalities and should provide plantigrade weight-bearing and protection of the insensitive skin areas.

SPINAL DEFORMITIES

Radiological examination of the entire vertebral column and ribs should be performed on all children with myelodysplasia. The deficit of posterior elements at the site of myelodysplasia contributes to spinal instability.

There may be malformations of the vertebral bodies and ribs in locations other than the neurological lesion. Hemivertebrae, fixed bifurcated ribs, and bony ridges cause relentlessly and rapidly progressing scoliosis.

Kyphosis can be related to congenital vertebral malformation or it is a manifestation of collapsing spine in high thoracic paraplegia. Severe lumbar kyphosis has been surgically treated in patients with high thoracic levels of myelodysplasia. After spinal stabilization, children with high paraplegia do not need to use their arms for sitting support and can reach skeletal maturity with decreased propensity to develop pressure ulcerations from postural malalignment on sitting (81).

Scoliosis may accompany paralysis at any level but the underlying mechanisms are different (98). Asymmetrical muscle forces originating from infrapelvic or suprapelvic structures affect spinal stability already weakened by the bifid defect. Unilateral hip dislocation is notorious for initiating this course of events leading to pelvic obliquity and scoliosis with primary lumbar and secondary thoracic curvatures (51). A rapidly progressive primary upper or midthoracic curve is a highly suspicious sign of syringohydromyelia of the cervical and upper thoracic spinal cord (97, 107). A low profile thoraco-lumbo-sacral-orthosis (TLSO) or, in case of upper thoracic curve or kyphosis, a Milwaukee brace, are devices currently used in the conservative management of scoliosis. Although the need for surgical treatment of scoliosis and kyphosis often arises, orthotic intervention may serve as a temporizing measure (56).

Progressive scoliosis is one of the most severe complications of myelodysplasia. It leads to a decline of ambulation, endurance for sitting, wheelchair mobility, and even basic self-care skills. A most serious medical consequence is compromise of cardiopulmonary function.

NEUROPATHIC FRACTURES

Osteoporosis associated with lower motor neuron paralysis, lack of weight-bearing, and inactivity are responsible for neuropathic fractures that occur after minor unnoticed trauma. Children with thoracic paralysis are particularly prone to develop this complication. However, it is also encountered in youngsters with lumbar lesions especially after postsurgical immobilization or prolonged recumbency for decubiti (33, 62). There is swelling and redness at the fracture site that mimics the clinical appearance of cellulitis or osteomyelitis. Due to a lack of sensation, the child does not complain of pain. Fractures are treated with splinting and heal rapidly. Resumption of weight-bearing as early as possible is important since immobilization will further aggravate the underlying osteoporosis. Bone deformities following a displaced fracture and growth disturbances after epiphyseal injury or separation may complicate the already existing skeletal abnormalities (1, 55).

SENSORY DEFICIT-DECUBITUS ULCERS

The parents must be made aware of the areas of defective or absent sensation and the necessary precautions. A thorough inspection of the skin should be part of the child's routine daily care. Exposure of the insensate skin to extreme heat or cold should be avoided. Apparently innocuous circumstances, such as sitting in a swing heated by the sun or standing in hot sand, can cause burns in a few minutes.

Pressure necrosis of soft tissues is a preventable complication. Ill-fitting shoes and orthoses must be immediately adjusted. If pressure marks retain their reddish discoloration overnight, the brace should not be reapplied until modifications have been made. Casts require generous padding. Asymmetrical weight-bearing on sitting or standing is a well known cause of decubiti over the ischial area and in foot deformities. Healing can be expected only if the precipitating mechanical factors are eliminated and surgical correction of the postural abnormality should be considered if ulcerations recur. As height and weight increase, recurrent decubiti can lead to prolonged morbidity and the necessary immobilization or hospitalizations contribute to the functional disability. Recurrent decubitus ulcers are reported to affect 73% of the young adults with spina bifida (128). Medical and surgical methods of decubitus care are discussed in the chapter on spinal cord injury. In patients with mid to low lumbar levels of paralysis, an innervated tensor fascia lata flap may decrease the likelihood of recurrences (99).

NEUROGENIC BLADDER DYSFUNCTION

The objectives of urological management are prevention of renal damage (104) and the establishment of a socially acceptable control of incontinence. It is essential for the family to have a clear understanding of the problem, goals, and their role in handling the urinary dysfunction. Poorly managed incontinence is a most serious functional disability and becomes an insurmountable obstacle to the social adjustment of the child.

Repeated urological evaluations are a necessity. It is advisable to perform urological evaluation in the first 2 weeks of life, at 6 months, and yearly thereafter or as often as indicated by the course and results of the urological examination. Regular monitoring is paramount to rule out a high pressure bladder, which can induce significant, rapid renal damage (24).

Regulation of bladder capacity and outlet resistance with pharmacological agents is based on influencing detrusor and sphincter activity or their dyssynergistic action. Anticholinergic drugs can improve storage capacity of a small spastic bladder. Bladder outlet resistance is increased by α-adrenergic agents. The reader is referred to Chapter 13 for a more detailed listing of pharmacological agents and their indications. Drug treatment of bladder dysfunction is directed by the urologist who regularly follows the child (9, 88).

Combination of pharmacological regulation and intermittent clean catherization (ICC) can eliminate residual urine retention with a decrease in the incidence of infections. It also provides a means of enhancing social continence. Early use of ICC may be recommended for very young children with high pressure bladder and incipient signs of renal deterioration. For the purpose of social continence, the age of beginning to use this method is at the time when bladder continence is usually achieved. At first, the parents are trained to perform the technique of ICC. When cognitive and emotional maturity allows, the child can learn self-catheterization and eventually take over this responsibility (35, 130). It has been reported that bladder training programs that include the use of ICC and regulation of detrusor activity achieve better "continence" if started before the age of 3 yr (10). Some studies suggest that biofeedback conditioning improves self-regulation of detrusor and sphincter function (53).

Long-term follow-up studies have demonstrated that urinary diversion, particularly ileal conduit, has many complications and is not as successful in preventing renal damage as it was previously thought (28). When upper urinary tract damage requires obstacle-free drainage vesicostomy is considered a better alternative. Reconversion of ileal conduit is considered if the capacity of the defunctioned bladder is adequate (84) or augmentation cystoplasty may be performed (42).

Various types of artificial sphincters are perfected and used more frequently in adolescents and adults. Results are encouraging but the patient must maintain a proper schedule of bladder emptying (61).

NEUROGENIC BOWEL DYSFUNCTION

Absent sensation of rectal fullness, lack of anorectal sphincter control, and dyssynergy with intestinal peristalsis are the underlying mechanisms of neurogenic bowel incontinence (72). Social continence is achieved by establishing bowel habits so that rectal emptying will occur regularly and at predictable times. Successful bowel management requires soft, but good consistency stools, avoidance of constipation, and scheduled rectal elimination (132). Appropriate diet and stimulation of intestinal and rectal reflex emptying by external sphincter distension, suppositories, or enemas are the means to achieve this end.

Biofeedback has been recently suggested for enhancing the awareness of rectal fullness (133). A study of rectosphincteric responses found some degree of rectal sensation in many patients and reports a high level of satisfactory fecal continence with the use of biofeedback conditioning (111). Studies of the anorectal motility of spina bifida individuals note findings ranging from normal to partially abnormal rectoanal inhibitory reflexes or complete hypotonia (2).

Constipation with fecal stasis, increasing distension, and atonia of the intestinal wall during infancy generate difficulties for later bowel management. Diet modification and cautious use of small doses of laxatives at regular intervals are usually effective to avert this course of events. A difficult problem to overcome is increased intestinal peristalsis that may be present in some cases and impede the establishment of regularity.

Instruction of the parents in the handling of bowel dysfunction is a gradual process. Observation and dietary regulation of emptying habits, stool consistency, and prevention of constipation should begin during infancy. The actual technique to establish regularity and reflex emptying will be taught when the child reaches the expected age of bowel continence.

COGNITIVE AND LANGUAGE FUNCTION

Many reports noted low IQ scores in children with myelodysplasia, particularly among those with hydrocephalus (6) and with higher levels of paralysis. Follow-up studies of patients born after the introduction of selective neonatal closure indicate that normal range of intelligence is more likely in the selected group; however, one fifth of those given delayed treatment, because of adverse criteria, were also found to have normal levels of intelligence (124). Visuomotor perceptual integration deficits and a discrepancy between performance and verbal scores were observed in several studies (6). The level of clinically tested perceptual dysfunction may underestimate the ability to learn in real-life situations (115). A study of learner drivers with spina bifida confirmed greater driving skill performance than expected from tested perceptual skills (114).

Language characteristics are described as irrelevant content and excessive chatter (120), but with good vocabulary and grammatic construction that are above the level of actual comprehension (31). Screening of a large group of these children showed that 10% had speech deficits and the incidence of hearing loss due to conductive or sensorineural impairment was as high as 13.4% (101).

SOCIAL AND EMOTIONAL ADJUSTMENT AND EDUCATION

The degree of expected social integration depends largely on the extent of organic disability but its full realization is also contingent on emotional strength and stability. The development of these personality traits is influenced by the ability of the parents to accept the child's disability, to provide loving support, and, yet, to set limits and encourage independence.

Identification of changing concerns during the years of development define the issues for counseling the family and child. Whereas problems related to physical management are in the foreground during early childhood, educational needs and social experiences become priorities for the older child (128).

Special school attendance is one of the factors that correlates with poor academic achievement (18, 126). The majority of "postselection" spina bifida children are capable of integrating into "ordinary" schools (32).

Changes in educational laws also offer better opportunities for mainstreaming into regular school classes. Preschool programs offer a combination of training in physical and social skills and prepare the child for entry into elementary school. Day programs fulfill a real need for the parents as they provide a respite from the practical realities that are created by the prolonged dependence of a disabled child. Preadolescents and adolescents should be supported in their adjustment to growing up with a disability (66). Sexual counseling should be offered, but it is frequently omitted. Of a group of 115 spina bifida adults, 66% reported not having had opportunities to discuss marriage and sexual relationships (63).

SERVICE DELIVERY SYSTEMS

After the neonatal neurosurgical treatment, a major part of management entails preventive intervention for musculoskeletal, urinary, and other potential complications. It is also during the first few weeks and months that a tentative long-range individual rehabilitation program is formulated and discussed with the parents. The expertise and specialized care that a team of specialists can provide at a medical center is required for this early phase of management. Coordination and continuity of care are essential although social and economic factors may interfere with the best laid plans.

Periodic assessment during the first year makes prognostication of physical, adaptive, and intellectual function more accurate. The medical center involved in the initial care should continue its role of supervising the child's management and guiding the parents. However, a proprietary attachment to "spina bifida clinics" stigmatize the child and, in the long run, this may be detrimental to the integration of the child and family in their community. Instead, the rehabilitation team should assume the responsibility of helping the family to explore and utilize services close to their home.

Working in concert with the medical center, local facilities and the child's primary care physician (90) can become significant support systems in implementing many aspects of care, "normalizing" the child's development, and the family's adjustment.

Under optimal circumstances, intensive medical intervention and rehabilitation should be completed by the time the child is enrolled in elementary school. "Normalization" and a good quality of life are best achieved if health care professionals can remain as invisible as possible after that age.

REFERENCES

1. Anschuetz RH, Freehafer AA, Schaffer JW, Dixon MS Jr: Severe fracture complications in myelodysplasia. *J Pediatr Orthop* 4:22, 1984.
2. Arhau P, Faverdin C, Devroede G, et al: Anorectal motility after surgery for spina bifida. *Dis Colon Rectum* 27:159, 1984.
3. Arnold J: Myelocyste, Transposition von Gewebskeimen und Sympodie. *Beitr Pathol Anat Allgemeinen Pathol* 16:1, 1894.

4. Asher M, Olson J: Factors affecting the ambulatory status of patients with spina bifida cystica. *J Bone Joint Surg* 65-A:350, 1983.
5. Badell A, Binder H, Dikstra D, et al: Pediatric rehabilitation disorders of the spinal cord: Spinal cord injury, myelodysplasia. *Arch Phys Med Rehabil* 70:S170, 1989.
6. Badell-Ribera A, Shulman R, Paddock N: The relationship of nonprogressive hydrocephalus to intellectual functioning in children with spina bifida cystica. *Pediatrics* 37:787, 1966.
7. Badell-Ribera A, Siegel MS, Swinyard C: Vocational rehabilitation caseload and potential of patients with spina bifida and myelomeningocele. In Swinyard C (ed): *Comprehensive Care of the Child with Spina Bifida Manifesta.* New York University Medical Center, Rehabilitation Monograph No. 31, 1966.
8. Badell-Ribera A, Swinyard GA, Greenspan L, Deaver GG: Spina bifida with myelomeningocele: Evaluation of rehabilitation potential. *Arch Phys Med Rehabil* 45:443, 1964.
9. Bauer SB, Colodny AH, Retik AB: The management of vesiculoreteral reflux in children with myelodysplasia. *J Urol* 128:102, 1982.
10. Bille B, Erikson B, Gierup J: Early bladder training in patients with spina bifida. *Acta Paediatr Scand* 73:60, 1984.
11. Breed AL, Healy PM: The midlumbar myelomeningocele hip: mechanisms of dislocation and treatment. *J Pediatr Orthop* 2:15, 1982.
12. Breed AL, Ibler I, Etlauger P: The motorized wheelchair: New freedom, new responsibility, new problems in transportation. *Dev Med Child Neurol* 23:113, 1981.
13. Brock DJH, Scrimgeour JB, Steven J, Barron L, Watt M: Maternal plasma alphafetoprotein screening for neural-tube defects. *Br J Obstet Gynecol* 85:575, 1978.
14. Brocklehurst G: The pathology of spina bifida. In Spina Bifida for the Clinician. *Clinics in Developmental Medicine,* no. 57, Philadelphia, JB Lippincott Co, 1974.
15. Brunt D: Characteristics of upper limb movements in a sample of meningomyelocele children. *Percept Motor Skills* 51:431, 1980.
16. Burkus JK, Moore DW, Raycroft JF: Valgus deformity of the ankle in myelodysplastic patients. Correction by stapling of the medial part of the distal tibial physis. *J Bone Joint Surg* 65-A:1157, 1983.
17. Carmel PW: The Arnold Chiari malformation. In McLaurin RL, Epstein F (eds): *Pediatric Neurosurgery: Surgery of the Developing Nervous System.* New York, Grune & Stratton, 1982.
18. Carr J, Halliwell M, Pearson A: The relationship of disability and school type to everyday life. *Z Kinderchir* 39:(Suppl) 2, 135, 1984.
19. Carr J, Pearson A, Halliwell M: The effect of disability on family life: *Z Kinderchir* 38:(Suppl)103, 1983.
20. Carroll NC: Assessment and management of the lower extremity in myelodysplasia. *Orthop Clin North Am* 18:709, 1987.
21. Carroll NC, Sharrard WJW: Long term follow-up of posterior iliopsoas transplantation for paralytic dislocation of the hip. *J Bone Joint Surg* 54A:551, 1972.
22. Charney EB, Weller SC, Sutton LN, et al: Management of the newborn with myelomeningocele: Time for a decision making process. *Pediatrics* 74:58, 1985.
23. Chiari H: Uber Veranderungen des Kleinhirns in folge von Hydrocephalie des Grosshirns. *Dtsch Med Wochenschr* 17:1172, 1891.
24. Chiaromonte RM, Horowitz EM, Kaplan GM, Brook WA: Implications of hydronephrosis in the newborn with myelodysplasia. *J Urol* 136:427, 1986.
25. Cowchock FS, Jackson LG: The use of alpha-fetoprotein for diagnosis of neural-tube and other defects. *Clin Obstet Gynecol* 7:83, 1980.
26. Cowchock S, Ainbender E, Prescott G, Crandall B, Lau L, Heller R, Muir WA, Kloza E, Feigelson M, Mennuti M, Cederquist L: The recurrence risk for neural-tube defects in the United States. A collaborative study. *Am J Med Genet* 5:309, 1980.

27. Crandall RC, Birkeback CR, Wintor BR: The role of hip location and dislocation in the functional status of the myelodysplastic patient. A review of 100 patients. *Orthopaedics* 12:675, 1989.
28. Crooks KK, Enrile BG: Comparison of the ileal conduit and clean intermittent catheterization for myelomeningocele. *Pediatrics* 72:203, 1983.
29. Cybulski GR, Jaeger RJ: Standing performance of persons with paraplegia. *Arch. Phys Med Rehabil* 67:103, 1986.
30. Delight E, Goodal J: Love and Loss, Conversations with Parents of Babies with Spina Bifida Managed Without Surgery, 1971–1981. *Dev Med Child Neurol* (Suppl 61) 1990.
31. Diller L, Paddock N, Badell-Ribera A, Swinyard C: Verbal behavior in children with spina bifida. In Swinyard C (ed): *Comprehensive Care of the Child with Spina Bifida Manifesta.* New York University Medical Center, Rehabilitation Monograph No. 31, 1966.
32. Dodd KD: Where should spina bifida children go to school? *Z Kinderchir* 39 (Suppl 2):129, 1984.
33. Drummond DS, Moreau M, Cruess RL: Post operative neuropathic fractures in patients with myelomeningocele. *Dev Med Child Neurol* 23:147, 1981.
34. Drummond DS, Moreau M, Cruess RL: The results and complications of surgery for the paralytic hip and spine in myelomeningocele. *J Bone Joint Surg* 62-B:49, 1980.
35. Enrile BG, Crooks KK: Clean intermittent catheterization for home management in children with myelomeningocele. *Clin Pediatr* 19:743, 1980.
36. Evans EP, Tew B: The energy expenditure of spina bifida children during walking and wheelchair ambulation. *Z Kinderchir* 34:425, 1981.
37. Evans O, Tew B, Lawrence KM: The fathers of children with spina bifida. *Z Kinderchir* 41 (Suppl 1):42, 1986.
38. Feiwell E: Surgery of the hip in myelomeningocele as related to adult goals. *Clin Orthop* 148:87, 1980.
39. Findley TW, Agre JC: Ambulation in the adolescent with spina bifida II. Oxygen cost of mobility. *Arch Phys Med Rehabil* 69:855, 1988.
40. French BN: The embryology of spinal dysraphism. *Clin Neurosurg* 30:295, 1983.
41. Gardiki-Kouidou P, Seller MJ: Amniotic fluid folate vitamin B12 and transcobalamins in neural tube defects. *Clin Genet* 33:441, 1988.
42. Gearhart JP, Albertsen PC, Marshall FF, et al: Pediatric applications of augmentation cystoplasty: The Hopkins experience. *J Urol* 136:430, 1986.
43. Gregarious GB, Green B, Page L, Thompson S, Monforte H: Spinal cord tumors presenting with neural tube defects. *Neurosurgery* 6:962, 1986.
44. Gugenheim JJ, Gerson LP, Sadler C, Tullos HS: Pathologic morphology of the acetabulum in paralytic and congenital hip instability. *J Pediatr Orthop* 2:397, 1982.
45. Heinz ER, Rosenbaum AE, Scarff TB, Reigel DH, Drayer BP: Tethered spinal cord following meningomyelocele repair. *Radiology* 131:153, 1979.
46. Hesz N, Wolraich M: Vocal cord paralysis and brainstem dysfunction in children with spina bifida. *Dev Med Child Neurol* 27:529, 1985.
47. Hoffer MM, Feiwell E, Perry R, Perry J, Bonnett C: Functional ambulation in patients with myelomeningocele. *J Bone Joint Surg* 55A:137, 1973.
48. Hunt GM: A study of death and handicap in a consecutive series of spina bifida treated unselectively from birth. *Z Kinderchir* 38 (Suppl 2):100, 1983.
49. Just M, Ernest J, Higer HP, et al: Magnetic resonance imaging of post repair myelomeningocele findings in 31 children and adolescents. *Neurosurg Rev* 10:45, 1987.
50. Just M, Schwartz M, Ernest J, et al: Magnetic resonance imaging of dystrophic myelodysplasia. Findings in 56 children and adolescents with posterior meningomyelocele. *Childs Nervous System* 4:149, 1988.
51. Kahanovitz N, Duncan JW: The role of scoliosis and pelvic obliquity on functional disability in myelomeningocele. *Spine* 6:494, 1981.

52. Kazak AE, Clark MW: Stress in families of children with myelomeningocele. *Dev Med Child Neurol* 28:220, 1986.
53. Killani PE, Jeffries JS, Varni JW: Urodynamic biofeedback treatment of urinary incontinence in children with myelomeningocele. *Biofeedback Self-Regul* 10:161, 1985.
54. Klaus MH, Kennell JH: Infant Bonding, 2nd ed. St. Louis, CV Mosby, 1982.
55. Kumar SJ, Cowell HR, Townsend P: Physeal, metaphyseal and diaphyseal injuries of the lower extremities in children with myelomeningocele. *J Pediatr Orthop* 4:25, 1984.
56. Kumar SJ, Townsend P: Posterolateral spinal fusion for the treatment of scoliosis in myelodysplasia. *J Pediatr Orthop* 2:514, 1982.
57. Lammer EJ, Sever LE, Oakley GP Jr: Teratogen update: valproic acid. *Teratology* 35:465, 1987.
58. Laurence KM: The natural history of hydrocephalus. *Lancet* 2:1152, 1958.
59. Leck I: Causation of neural-tube defects: Clues from epidemiology. *Br Med Bull* 30:158, 1974.
60. Lemire Ronald J: Neural tube defects: Clinical correlations. *Clin Neurosurg* 30:165, 1983.
61. Light JK, Pietro T: Alteration in detrusor behavior and the effect on renal function following insertion of the artificial urinary sphincter. *J Urol* 136:632, 1986.
62. Lock TR, Aronson DD: Fractures in patients who have myelomeningocele. *J Bone Joint Surg* 71-A:1153, 1989.
63. Lonton AP, O'Sullivan AM, Loughlin AM: Spina bifida adults. *Z Kinderchir* 38 (Suppl 2):110, 1983.
64. Lorber J: Results of treatment of myelomeningocele. An analysis of 524 unselected cases with special references to possible selection for treatment. *Dev Med Child Neurol* 13:279, 1971.
65. Lorber J, Saifiedl S: Results of selective treatment of spina bifida cystica. *Arch Dis Child* 56:822, 1981.
66. Lord DJ, Varzos N, Behrman B, Wicks B, Wicks D: Implications of mainstream classrooms for adolescents with spina bifida. *Dev Med Child Neurol* 32:20, 1990.
67. Lough LK, Nielson DH: Ambulation of children with myelomeningocele: parapodium versus Orlau swivel modification. *Dev Med Child Neurol* 28:489, 1986.
68. Macias R: Surgical considerations in the management of myelomeningocele. *Childs Nervous Syst* 2:10, 1986.
69. Magnus RV: Vesicoureteral reflux in babies with myelomeningocele. *J Urol* 114:122, 1975.
70. Main DM, Menutti MT: Neural tube defects: Issues in prenatal diagnosis and counselling. *Obstet Gynecol* 67:1, 1986.
71. Mapstone TB, Rekate HL, Nielsen FE, Dixon MS, Glaser N, Jaffe M: Relationship of CSF shunting and IQ in children with myelomeningocele. A retrospective analysis. *Child Brain* 11:112, 1984.
72. Mare M, Sakaniwa M, Takahashi H, Iwai J: Management of defecation in spina bifida. *Prog Pediatr Surg* 24:97, 1989.
73. Mazur JM, Menelaus MB, Hudson I, et al: Hand function in patients with spina bifida cystica. *J Pediatr Orthop* 6:442, 1986.
74. Mazur JM, Schurtleff D, Menelaus MB, et al: Orthopedic management of high level spina bifida. Early walking compared with early use of wheelchair. *J Bone Joint Surg* 71A:56, 1989.
75. McCall RE, Douglas R, Rightor N: Surgical treatment in patients with myelodysplasia before using the LSU Reciprocating Gait System. *Orthopaedics* 6:843, 1983.
76. McCall RE, Schmidt WT: Clinical experience with reciprocal gait orthosis in myelodysplasia: *J Pediatr Orthop* 6(2):157, 1986.
77. McCormick MC, Charney EB, Stemular MM: Assessing the impact of a child with spina bifida on the family. *Dev Med Child Neurol* 28:53, 1986.
78. McLaughlin JF, Schurtleff DB, Lamers JY, Stutz JT, Hayden PW, Kropp RJ: Influence

of prognosis in decisions regarding the care of newborns with myelodysplasia. *N Engl J Med* 312:1589, 1985.

79. McLone DG, Czyzewski D, Raimondi A, Sommers R: Central nervous system infections as a limiting factor in the intelligence of children with myelomeningocele. *Pediatrics* 70:338, 1982.

80. McLone DG, Dias L, Kaplan W, Sommers M: Concepts in the management of spina bifida. Proceedings of the American Society for Pediatric Neurosurgery. Concepts in Pediatric Neurosurgery. Basel, S. Karger, 1984.

81. McMaster MJ: The long term results of kyphectomy and spinal stabilization in children with myelomeningocele: *Spine* 13:417, 1988.

82. Menelaus M: Progress in the management of the paralytic hip in myelomeningocele. *Orthop Clin North Am* 11:17, 1980.

83. Menelaus M: *The Orthopedic Management of Spina Bifida Cystica*, 2nd ed. Edinburgh, Churchill Livingstone, 1980.

84. Menon M, Elder JS, Mauley CB, Jeffs RD: Undiverting the ileal conduit. *J Urol* 128:998, 1979.

85. Milhan S: Increased incidence of anencephalus and spina bifida in siblings of affected cases. *Science* 138:593, 1962.

86. Morgagni JB: *The Seats and Causes of Diseases Investigated by Anatomy*. Translation by William Cooke. London, Longman, 1822.

87. Motloch WM: The parapodium. An orthotic device for neuromuscular disorders. *Artif Limbs* 15:36, 1971.

88. Mulcahy JJ, James HE: Management of neurogenic bladder in infancy and childhood. *Urology* 13:235, 1979.

89. Murch RL, Cohen LH: Relationship among life stress, perceived family environment and the psychological distress of spina bifida adolescents. *J Pediatr Psychol* 14:193, 1989.

90. Myers GJ: Myelomeningocele: The medical aspects. *Pediatr Clin North Am* 31:165, 1984.

91. Naidich TP, Hardwood-Nash DC, McLone DG: Radiology of spinal dysraphism. *Clin Neurosurg* 5:341, 1983.

92. Nevin NC, Johnston WP, Merrett JD: Influence of social class on the risk of recurrence of anencephalus and spina bifida. *Dev Med Child Neurol* 23:155, 1981.

93. Noetzel MJ: Myelomeningocele: current concepts of management. *Clin Perinatol* 16:311, 1989.

94. Nulsen FE, Spitz EG: Treatment of hydrocephalus by direct shunt from ventricle to jugular vein. *Surg Forum* 2:399, 1952.

95. Olney BW, Menelaus MB: Triple arthrodesis of the foot in spina bifida patients. *J Bone Joint Surg* 70B:234, 1988.

96. Padget DH: Neuroschisis and human embryogenic maldevelopment. *Neuropathol Exp Neurol* 29:192, 1970.

97. Park TS, Cail WS, Maggio WM, et al: Progressive spasticity and scoliosis in children with myelomeningocele. Radiological investigation and surgical treatment. *J Neurosurg* 62:367, 1985.

98. Piggott H: The natural history of scoliosis in myelodysplasia. *J Bone Joint Surg* 62-B:54, 1980.

99. Posma AN: The innervated tensor fascia latae flap in patients with meningomyelocele. *Ann Plast Surg* 21:594, 1988.

100. Pudenz RH, Russell FE, Hurd AH, Shelden CH: Ventriculo-auriculostomy: A technique for shunting cerebrospinal fluid into the right auricle. Preliminary report. *J Neurosurg* 14:171, 1957.

101. Radke J, Gosky GA: Hearing and speech screening in a hydrocephalus myelodysplasia population. *Spina Bifida Ther* 3:25, 1981.

102. Ramirez OM, Ramasastry SS, Pang D, Putrell JW: A new surgical approach to closure of large lumbosacral meningomyelocele defects. *Plast Reconstr Surg* 80:799, 1987.

103. Reigel DH, Dallman DE, Scarff TB, Woodford J: Intra-operative evoked potentials studies of new born infants with myelomeningocele. *Dev Med Child Neurol* 37 (Suppl):42, 1976.

104. Rickwood, AMK, Grundy DJ, Thomas DG: Danger of inadequate urological supervision of patients with congenital neuropathic bladder. *Br Med J* 228:1677, 1984.

105. Rokos J, Knowles J: Experimental contribution to the pathogenesis of spina bifida. *J Pathol* 118:21, 1976.

106. Ruderman RJ, Goldner JL, Hardaker WT: Pantalar fusion in myelodysplasia: A procedure too hastily rejected? *Orthop Trans* 4:152, 1980.

107. Samuelson L, Bergstrom K, Thomas KA, Harringsson A, Wallensten R: MR imaging of syringohydromyelia and Chiari malformations in myelomeningocele patients with scoliosis. *AJNR* 8:539, 1989.

108. Scheers MM, Beeker TW, Hertogh CM: Spina Bifida: feelings, opinions and expectations of parents. *Z Kinderchir* 39(Suppl 2):120, 1984.

109. Sharrard WJW: *Pediatric Orthopedics and Fractures,* 3rd ed. Oxford, Blackwell Scientific Publications, 1980.

110. Sharrard WJW, Zachary RB, Lorber J, Bruce AMA: Controlled trial of immediate and delayed closure of spina bifida cystica. *Arch Dis Child* 38:18, 1963.

111. Shepherd K, Hickstein R, Shepherd R: Neurogenic fecal incontinence in children with spina bifida: Rectosphincteric responses and evaluation of a physiological rationale for management including biofeedback conditioning. *Aust Paediatr J* 19:97, 1983.

112. Shulman K, Marmarou A: Pressure volume considerations in infantile hydrocephalus. *Dev Med Child Neurol* 25 (Suppl):90, 1971.

113. Schurtleff DB: Meningomyelocele: A new or a vanishing disease? *Z Kinderchir* 36(Suppl 2):16, 1986.

114. Simms B: Learner drivers with spina bifida and hydrocephalus: The relationshiop between perceptual cognitive deficits and driving performance. *Z Kinderchir* 41 (Suppl 1):51, 1986.

115. Simms B: The rote learning ability of young people with spina bifida and hydrocephalus and their able bodied peers. *Z Kinderchir* 42 (Suppl 1):53, 1987.

116. Smithells RW, Sheppard S, Schorah CJ: Possible prevention of neural tube defects by periconceptional vitamin supplementation. *Lancet* 1:339, 1980.

117. Stanley P, Senec MO Jr, Segall HD, et al: Syringohydromyelia following meningomyelocele surgery, role of metrizamide myelography and computer tomography. *Pediatr Radiol* 14:278, 1984.

118. Stilwell A, Menelaus MB: Walking ability after transplantation of the iliopsoas. A long term follow-up. *J Bone Joint Surg* 66B:656, 1989.

119. Stone HD: Periconceptual vitamin suplementation (letter). *Lancet* 1:647, 1980.

120. Swisher L, Pinscher E: The language characteristics of hyperverbal hydrocephalic children. *Dev Med Neurol* 13:746, 1981.

121. Szalay EA: Orthopedic management of the lower extremities in spina bifida. *AAOS Instr Course Lect* 36:275, 1987.

122. Tachdjian MO: *Pediatric Orthopedics,* 2nd ed. Philadelphia, WB Saunders, 1990.

123. Tamaki N, Shirataki F, Kojomo N, et al: Tethered cord syndrome of delayed onset following repair of myelomeninogele. *J Neurosurg* 69:393, 1988.

124. Tew B, Evans R, Thomas M, et al: The results of selective surgical policy on the cognitive abilities of children with spina bifida. *Dev Med Child Neurol* 27:606, 1985.

125. Tew B, Laurence KM: Possible personality problems among 10 year old spina bifida children. *Child Care Health Dev* 11:375, 1985.

126. Tew B, Laurence KM: The relationship between intelligence and academic achievement in spina bifida adolescents. *Z Kinderchir* 39 (Suppl 2):122, 1984.

127. Tew BJ, Payne H, Laurence KM: Must a family with a handicapped child be a handicapped family. *Dev Med Child Neurol* 32 (Suppl):95, 1974.
128. Thomas AP, Bax MCO, Smith DPL: The health and social needs of young adults with physical disabilities. *Clinics in Developmental Medicine* no. 106 Philadelphia, JB Lippincott Co, 1989.
129. Tulp N: *"Observationes Medicae."* Medicarum Librum III, Amsterdam, 1652.
130. Uelung Smith J, Meyer J, Bruskewitz R: Impact of an intermittent catheterization program on children with myelomeningocele. *Pediatrics* 76:892, 1985.
131. Venes JL: Surgical considerations in the initial repair of meningomyelocele and the introduction of a technical modification. *Neurosurgery* 17:111, 1985.
132. Vigliarolo D: Managing bowel incontinence in children with meningomyelocele. *Am J Nursing* 80:105, 1980.
133. Wald H: Use of biofeedback in treatment of fecal incontinence in patients with meningomyelocele. *Pediatrics* 68:45, 1981.
134. Weisl H, Fairclough JA, Jones DG: Stabilization of the hip in myelomeningocele. Comparison of posterior iliopsoas transfer and varus derotation osteotomy. *J Bone Joint Surg* 70B:29, 1988.
135. Yngve DA, Doulas R, Roberts JM: The reciprocating gait orthosis in myelomeningocele. *J Pediatr Orthop* 4:304, 1984.

11

Head Injury

GABRIELLA E. MOLNAR AND JANE C. S. PERRIN

During the last decade, concerted efforts of the National Head Injury Foundation and the professional community have brought into sharp focus the magnitude and complexity of problems resulting from head trauma (41, 212). Childhood injury to the brain and the central nervous system has unique and often disastrous consequences. Critical developmental processes are arrested or altered, learning ability may suffer radical constriction, and a youth of promise may be destroyed before adulthood is achieved. Pediatric rehabilitation promotes and supports the efforts to regain the developmental tract.

Discussion in this chapter is limited to management of the consequences of head trauma occurring after the neonatal period from infancy through adolescence.

Epidemiology

The overall risk of traumatic brain injury in children is estimated at 4% in boys and 2.5% in girls (192). Age-specific rates for severe head trauma increase from under 5 yr of age reaching a peak in adolescence and are higher for boys at all ages as shown in Table 11.1. The estimated number of children who require hospital admission is around 200,000 cases/yr; of these, about 15,000 need a prolonged stay (130, 190–192, 206, 221).

Major causes in pediatric age group are: falls (42%), motor vehicle accidents as car occupants or victims of road collisons (34%), and a variety of other accidental circumstances (24%) (23, 87, 106, 135, 149, 160, 206). Some epidemiological surveys suggested a trend in the relative frequency of causes by geographic location, socioeconomic class, and ethnicity (110, 235). Motor vehicle-related accidents account for the vast majority of *severe* head injuries with multiple trauma and for about 70% of those associated with coma in all age groups (149, 179, 206).

A head injury of unknown prevalence in infants and young children is abuse (90, 191, 192, 206). On hospital admissions, head trauma was present

Table 11.1.
Age Specific Rates of Head Injury In
Children[a,b]

	In 100,000 Population/Yr	
Age	Boys	Girls
Below 5 yr	150–200	100–170
5–15 yr	<400	200–300

[a]Data from references 87, 128, 130, 190, 192, and 206.
[b]Average incidence rate 220/100,000 population/yr for both sexes.

in 25% to 40% of cases (191, 192). However, it is suggested that, in children under 12 months of age, as much as 65% to 80% of head injuries may be nonaccidental (25, 191, 206). In one study, 50% of the surviving children suffered permanent neurological and cognitive deficits (206).

Head trauma is the leading cause of mortality among all childhood injuries and is responsible for 43% of accidental deaths from 5 to 9 yr of age in the United States (128, 220, 232). Mortality among children rendered comatose is at least 10 times that of the overall death rate for pediatric injuries. Motor vehicle accidents are the most common cause of accidental deaths in the United States under 14 yr of age (12, 35). From 1980 to 1985, motor vehicle accidents resulted in a mortality rate of 37% compared to a 2.2% rate associated with falls (12, 232). A Maryland study of children under 15 yr old killed as motor vehicle occupants revealed an alarmingly high mortality rate especially in children under age 2 yr; this group constituted only 9% of the crash victims but 24% of the fatalities (118). Head trauma is also the most frequent cause of death in child abuse (206).

That head injury is a major worldwide threat to health and life among children is also illustrated by surveys from other countries (106, 113, 126, 129, 187, 206). However, due to lack of information from some parts of the world, the true international scope of the problem cannot be assessed on a global scale.

Pathomechanism

Disproportionately large head and brain weight supported on a weak neck are visible structural differences between young children and adults. Other anatomic variations may modify the effect of injury in children under 2 yr of age but have no significant influence thereafter (126, 206, 244). Head trauma is classified by several aspects of the injury that affect neuropathological sequelae and clinical outcome.

In penetrating or open injuries, an object entering the cranium initially inflicts lacerations, bleedings, followed by reactive edema, cellular swelling, and the risk of infection. Tissue necrosis, scarring, and, unless all imbedded particles are removed, localized foreign body reactions ensue (206). Far more common are blunt or closed head injuries where differences in the biomechanics of trauma have a significant role.

Based on biomechanical considerations one can distinguish: (a) impression injury when the impact is received by a stationary head or (b) acceleration injury caused by impact to a moving head (206, 244). Regardless of age, the mechanism of trauma is acceleration injury in the majority of cases. Impression injury produces a typical coup lesion at the site of impact due to indentation and/or depressed fracture of the skull; countercoup damage is rare. On the other hand, acceleration injury results in differential displacement of the skull and cranial contents (244). Linear or angular rotational forces generate shearing and lead to multiple distant lesions; countercoup is characteristic (244).

A further classification of head trauma is: (a) primary injury caused directly and immediately by the impact; and (b) secondary injury, which evolves as a result of pathophysiological changes initiated by the primary trauma (206, 244). While in the majority of cases no specific treatment exists for the primary mechanical effects of injury, neurosurgical and intensive care can prevent the progressive events of secondary injury.

Clinical correlations indicate that diffuse white matter damage of shearing injuries is the most important factor governing the eventual outcome of persistent vegetative state (87, 206, 244). However, in children, subcortical myelin sheath damage without axonal disruption may be reversible and consistent with more favorable prognosis after the transient physiological disruption of function resolves (87, 206). Diffuse brain swelling attributed to impaired cerebral vasomotor regulation occurs particularly in children (37, 38, 87, 105, 206). In a series of 286 cases, one third of them being in the pediatric age group, 25% of the children demonstrated acute diffuse cerebral swelling (246). Hypoxic brain damage correlates with clinical episodes of hypotension and increased intracranial pressure, which result in reduced cerebral perfusion. In whiplash injury of abuse, the infant suffers tears of bridging veins, subdural, subarachnoid, and retinal hemorrhages (5, 60, 123, 206, 238). Other external signs of trauma are often absent but multiple fractures at different stages of healing may confirm suspected abuse (123, 191, 206). Table 11.2 shows the most frequent pathological sequelae of head injury. A detailed discussion is available in several reviews (126, 206, 244).

Cerebral perfusion of 50 ml/100 g/min is necessary to meet the brain metabolic demands of 45–50 ml/min O_2 and 60 mg/min glucose (113). Cerebral metabolic rate increases during seizures and possibly in the first 12 to 24 hours of coma (87, 113). Energy metabolism falls after complete brain ischemia with loss of consciousness after 20 sec and extensive neuronal damage after 60 min (113). Hypoxemia ($PaO_2 < 50$ mm Hg) suppresses cerebral metabolism, causing impaired learning and judgment, coma, and, finally, at $PaO_2 < 10$ mm Hg, permanent neuronal damage (113). Since cerebral per-

Table 11.2.
Pathology and Pathogenesis[a]

Primary Head Injury	Secondary Head Injury	Other Consequences
Immediate impact with or without skull fracture	Increased intracranial pressure Focal or vascular	Fat embolism—long bone fractures Infection—basal skull fractures
Intracranial hemorrhage Epidural, subdural, subarachnoid, intracerebral, burst lobes	compromise infarcts, parahippocampal gyral necrosis Brain shift, herniation	Cerebral atrophy Posttraumatic hydrocephalus Scarring and cyst formation Growing skull fracture
Cerebral contusions/ lacerations—mostly temporal/frontal lobes, coup and countercoup	Cerebral hypoperfusion Ischemic/hypoxic damage, cortical artery boundary zones, basal ganglia, cerebellum	Posttraumatic hypopituitarism
Central brain damage Diffuse subcortical white matter, corpus callosum, rostral brain stem	Cerebral edema Vasogenic or cytotoxic Acute brain swelling Loss of cerebral vasoregulation	
Impact injury to other structures Cranial nerves		

[a]Data from references 87, 206, and 244.

fusion pressure (CPP) is the difference between systemic arterial pressure (SAP) and intracranial pressure (ICP), the latter is a determinant of perfusion contingent cerebral oxygenation. The physiological formula of this relationship is: SAP of 60 to 90 mm Hg − ICP <20 mm Hg = CPP > 50 mm Hg (113). Cerebral blood flow falls when ICP is within 40 to 50 mm Hg of arterial pressure either from elevated ICP or arterial hypotension or both (113). When cerebral blood flow is less than one third of normal, somatosensory-evoked potentials are extinguished.

EARLY POSTTRAUMATIC STAGE

Assessment

Pioneers in the management of head injury, Glasgow neurosurgeons Teasdale and Jennett (217) developed a coma assessment scale that became a basic tool for patient care and international communication (Table 11.3). Coma is defined as an unarousable state in which the child does not open his or her eyes, obey commands, or speak. Coma depth score is one of the outcome predictors. Injuries are considered severe if the coma lasts longer than 24 hours or the state of post-traumatic amnesia (PTA) is more than 7 days. PTA is defined as the interval between injury and regaining continuous day-to-day memory, a parameter difficult to assess in children. The Glasgow Coma Scale (GCS) (87, 206) is not useful for children under 12 months. Its application is modified in children up to 2 to 2½ yr because ver-

Table 11.3.
Glasgow Coma Scale[a]

Choose One Response in Each Category	Score
Eye opening	
Spontaneous	4
To speech	3
To pain	2
None	1
Best motor response upper extremity	
Obeys command	6
Localizes pain[b]—hand above chin	5
Flexor withdrawal to pain[b]	4
Abnormal spastic stereotyped flexion posture	3
Extensor response at elbow	2
No movement	1
Verbal response[c]	
Oriented conversation	5
Confused conversation	4
Inappropriate words	3
Incomprehensible sounds	2
No vocalization	1
Total score possible	3 to 15

[a]From Teasdale G, Jennett B: Assessment of coma and impaired consciousness: A practical scale. *Lancet* 2:81–84, 1974.
[b]Painful stimuli, supraorbital pressure, nail bed pressure with pencil.
[c]Not applicable in children less than 2 yr of age.

bal responses cannot be graded in the very young child. Because crying does not occur in coma, Bruce (87) recommends to substitute this behavior for verbal responses with a score of 4 if present and 1 if it is not.

Recognizing the shortcomings of GCS for very young age groups, a number of other coma scales were developed for children (34, 169, 181, 208). Among these, the Simpson-Reilly scale provides adjusted aggregate scores for different ages (208). Yager et al. (242) found that the rate of interobserver agreement was highest for the Simpson and Reilly, Jacobi, and O-IV scales.

Associated skeletal and other systemic injuries indicate not only the severity of trauma but may also affect the outcome of head injury as a result of bleeding, shock, and other attendant complications (119, 221). The Injury Severity Scale (ISS) (61, 119) was designed with these considerations in mind and provides a highest possible score of 75 for the most severe multisystemic injuries. A pediatric trauma score is available (61).

Initial medical evaluation includes assessment of vital signs; general examination for multisystemic injuries and depressed skull fracture; neurological examination for anterior fontanelle tension, pupillary responses, and reflex eye movements (83, 87, 206). Funduscopic examination for papilledema or retinal hemorrhages is essential. Radiological examination of the skull, complete spine, pelvis, and extremities should be obtained in a comatose child to rule out fractures, even though children can develop intra-cranial hematoma and spinal cord injury without associated fractures (173). Level of consciousness, parameters of Glasgow or pediatric coma scales, should be assessed together with tone and muscle weakness.

Computerized axial tomography (CAT) scan permits immediate detection of surgical hematoma, intracerebral hemorrhage, brain shift, or herniation (38, 87, 189, 206, 246). Diffuse shearing injury of the cerebral white matter presents as hemorrhagic corpus callosum (87, 246). CAT scan differentiates cerebral edema from diffuse cerebral swelling. Slit ventricle but mainte-nance of normal brain density are characteristic signs of the latter on CAT scan (37, 87, 246). For magnetic resonance imaging (MRI), resuscitation equipment poses practical problems immediately after the injury. However, in later stages, this method can demonstrate small contusions not detected on a CAT scan (87, 111, 139). Positron emission tomography (PET) (136, 157, 177, 222) and single photon emission computerized tomography (SPECT) (1, 156) measure cerebral metabolism and can demonstrate abnor-malities in specific areas of the brain not visualized on other imaging tech-niques. Wider availability of these methods should lead to better under-standing of clinicopathological correlations in the future.

Intracranial pressure monitoring is a technique for management of coma-tose children (87, 206, 244). ICP levels of greater than 20 to 25 mm Hg (torr) are considered elevated.

Auditory, visual, and somatosensory evoked cerebral potential studies can provide information about the site of the lesion and the prognosis as well as have significant application in pediatric head trauma. Under normal cir-cumstances, evoked potential latencies show maturational decreases and reach adult values at about 18 weeks of age in visual-evoked potentials (VEP) (14), by 8 yr in somatosensory-evoked potentials (SSEP) (236, 237), and by 3 yr in auditory-evoked potentials (BAERS) (100, 166, 201). In chil-dren with head injury, VEP abnormalities occur with lesions of the optic nerve, central visual system, and hypoxia. Because of the eight peaks rep-resenting different levels of the auditory pathways, BAERS are especially useful to test brainstem integrity during coma (100). Persistent loss of peaks or gross abnormality 1 week after coma indicates irreversible brainstem damage and is used as a brain death criterion (201). SSEPs by median or peroneal nerve stimulation are sensitive means to determine somesthetic perceptual loss with hemiparesis, to ascertain an associated spinal cord injury, and to prognosticate the outcome of coma (104, 185, 236, 237). Another bedside technique to evaluate brainstem function is the blink reflex. Absence of both R1 and R2 responses indicates severe brainstem disorder.

EEG confirms, although it does not necessarily exclude, seizures. As a tool to localize hematomas, it has been replaced by radiological imaging meth-ods. A flat EEG is used as a criterion of brain death but is not considered obligatory for the diagnosis. Event-related potentials (ERP) of computer-averaged EEG correlate with perceptual and cognitive processes on tasks that require recognition, attention, and other aspects of information processing (188). This method is currently used as a research tool and, eventually, may prove to be useful in late stages of head injury.

Acute Care

Immediate efforts are directed at the control of systemic abnormalities that would lead to secondary insults by hypoxia, hypotension, hypercarbia, anemia, and to counter intracranial hypertension (87, 206). Management of children arriving in the emergency room with severe head injury is vigorous. It includes endotracheal intubation with assisted ventilation; when indicated, pancuronium paralysis, attention to bleeding, circulatory status, multisystemic injuries, and uninterrupted urinary output. These procedures are followed by prompt surgical evacuation of intracranial hematomas (204) and placement of ICP monitor in the presence of brain swelling. Techniques to control elevated ICP (87, 206) include sitting position, hyperventilation to regulate cerebral blood flow and oxygenation, and administration of mannitol, furosemide, and dexamethasone. Induction of hypothermia and barbiturate coma may be elected.

Neurogenic pulmonary edema in childhood is an early complication of traumatic increased ICP with secondary systemic and pulmonary hypertension (163). Treatment is containment of elevated ICP. Aspiration atelectasis, pneumonitis, and lung abscess are potential causes of fever in comatose patients. Pulmonary embolism may be secondary to thrombophlebitis or fat emboli from long bone fractures. The child with head injury and on steroid treatment is subject to gastrointestinal erosion and bleeding. Prophylaxis with antacids and/or histamine H_2-receptor antagonists does not prevent a lesion but reduces the incidence of bleeding (93).

In a comatose child, serum electrolyte and fluid intake and output levels must be monitored and calculated to body weight or surface area and to replace losses for elevated temperature and muscle activity. Nutritional needs are delivered by nasogastric tube, gastrostomy, or central venous line, if necessary. Protein intake should consider age-appropriate requirements and catabolic state as a result of injury (114, 244). Urine collection is managed to prevent wetting and skin macerations. A postural drainage program is instituted and the eyes are kept moist with methylcellulose.

Skeletal fractures are treated by the orthopaedic surgeon (28, 31). Associated internal injuries, such as ruptured spleen, torn urethra, or kidney laceration, require surgical care. Acute tubular necrosis and infection are additional potential complications of the urinary system.

Early Preventive Rehabilitation

Intervention to prevent musculoskeletal complications should be started in the intensive care unit. A contracture and decubitus prevention program is established by proper positioning, range of motion exercises, and splinting (87, 206, 244). Observation of abnormal postures assumed by the child is a guide to anticipate potential deformities.

In the early comatose or obtunded stage, tone abnormalities are the most frequent neuromuscular findings. Severe hypertonicity with rigid dystonic extension of all extremities or flexion of both arms is designated as decerebrate or decorticate posturing. Severe generalized flaccidity is considered a poor prognostic sign associated with high mortality (206). Flaccid paralysis may be an indication of spinal cord injury. Selective decrease of extremity movements, in response to pain or spontaneously, suggests evolving paresis, such as hemiplegia, when it is unilateral or spinal cord injury SCI when it involves both legs.

Extensor dystonia of the decerebrate posturing may be suppressed in supine hips and knees flexed in semi-Fowler position or in sitting with neck flexion (206, 244). In the absence of tracheostomy, prone lying with the ankles maintained at plantigrade will discourage contractures when flexion posture predominates. Passive range of motion exercises are made difficult by the extreme extensor and flexor tone associated with decerebrate or decorticate posturing. Neck flexion or rotation suppresses the disinhibited tonic neck and labyrinthine reflexes that underlie these postures. The resultant tone reduction in respective extremities allows passive movements with greater ease and range (206). Passive exercises should be applied to all limbs during coma in the presence or absence of abnormal tone and progress to active assistive exercises when movements emerge in response to sensory stimuli or spontaneously.

Splints are most frequently needed to control abnormal ankle, wrist, or hand postures (87, 206, 244). Progressive cylinder or bivalve cast may be needed for large joints, such as the knee. Splints or casts are neither tolerated nor are they successful to overcome the severe dystonic extensor rigidity in decerebrate state. In all cases, they should be used judiciously by weighing reasonably expected gains, applied by intermittent on/off schedule, and with precautions for excessive skin pressure.

Decubiti are less prone to develop in young children because of their lighter body weight. However, a relatively heavy head makes the occiput a site of predilection compared to propensity for ischial, trochanteric, and heel decubiti in adolescents and adults (210). Prevention by expert nursing care is the optimal method of "treating" decubiti. Frequent position changes and water or air mattresses are helpful adjuncts.

Multisensory stimulation is advocated to heighten the state of arousal during prolonged coma and especially in persistent vegetative state. The rationale is to increase input into the reticular activating system through all senses, including tactile, taste, smell, visual, and auditory modalities. Multisensory stimulation is not advisable in early stages of coma while ICP is elevated or unstable because it may precipitate increased pressure waves (206). In prolonged coma or persistent vegetative state, repeated brief sessions, selected stimuli, preferably with emotional significance, such as recordings of parents' voice, are recommended. In a study of the presumed effect of coma stimulation involving three cases, which served as their own controls, EEG demonstrated decreased low voltage Δ waves and increased α activity during stimulation. Although these changes were not consistent, Weber (234) suggested that they may be signs of heightened awareness. There are no controlled studies on the efficacy of coma stimulation programs.

REHABILITATION STAGE

On transfer to a pediatric rehabilitation service, medical problems and functional intervention must be concurrently addressed (109).

Medical Treatment

Weaning from endotracheal intubation or tracheostomy may take place during the early phase by a gradual process of using smaller size cannulas and increased time of obliteration before permanent closure is allowed. Stridor, hoarseness, and aphonia are signs of laryngotracheal granuloma or stricture, which occurs in children at a frequency related to the length of intubation. Endoscopy will differentiate anatomic abnormalities from the less frequent laryngeal nerve pressure paralysis and determine whether surgical treatment of granuloma or stricture is needed. Chest percussion, postural drainage, and suctioning are administered prophylactically or for atelectasis when the child has difficulties with handling airway secretions.

Introduction of oral alimentation proceeds with gradual reduction of supplemental nasogastric or gastrostomy feeding as oral intake increases. Fluid and caloric requirements must be monitored (109, 244) and maintained for age as shown in Table 1.1. Dysphagia is a virtually universal complication in severe head injury as a result of supranuclear palsy with bilateral neurological lesions or injury to cranial nerves IX, X, XI. Coexistent oral motor apraxia may enhance the feeding dysfunction. A child with dysphagia should be evaluated by a feeding team including an occupational therapist, a speech pathologist, a rehabilitation nurse, and a nutritionist (87, 244, 245). Videofluoroscopy of oral motor function and swallowing is indicated in severe cases to rule out aspiration. Esophageal pH probes may be also necessary to rule out gastroesophageal reflux, another potential source of aspiration (87, 182, 226). In the presence of tracheostomy, the blue dye test will demonstrate tracheal aspiration (244). The basic principles of treating dysphagia are to overcome abnormal tone and reflexes, to facilitate oral motor function, and to select food with appropriate consistency. For details of feeding techniques, the reader is referred to the extensive literature on this subject (51, 71, 87, 114, 147, 244, 245).

In severe unrelenting dysphagia and prolonged coma, gastrostomy or jejunostomy by percutaneous or other types of surgical procedures is required for adequate nutritional maintenance. Stoma irritation may develop and infection can be a source of fever. The technique of gastrostomy button decreases mechanical tissue irritation from the indwelling cannula, eliminates accidental dislodgment, and makes daily care easier. Gastroesophageal reflux is an indication for Nissen fundoplication (182, 226).

Weight monitoring is fundamental information for children with head injury (87, 109, 244). Malnutrition may occur in the postinjury catabolic state, or due to decreased appetite resulting from lesion to the olfactory nerve with anosmia, from damage to the hypothalamic appetite regulatory center, or from emotional depression. At the other extreme, obesity may develop from organic or behavioral hyperphagia caused by hypothalamic injury (193, 244) or perseverative behavior. Roberts reported a 9% frequency of hyperphagia of apparently hypothalamic origin (193). Controlled food intake and offering only an allocated portion are management techniques for hyperphagia. Parents should be advised about both causes and handling particularly when the problem persists.

The risk of gastrointestinal stress ulceration exists after the acute stage of head injury (109, 206, 244). Stool monitoring for occult blood should be continued. Treatment options are antacids or histamine H_2-receptor antagonists. Cimetidine produces significant elevation of plasma phenytoin and, less frequently, of carbamazepine levels, a consideration in patients on anticonvulsant treatment (102). Some children on high caloric supplements may develop diarrhea, a problem that responds to changing the formula, but may lead to interim decreased intestinal absorption of medications, including reduced anticonvulsant levels. Constipation due to intestinal stasis after abdominal injuries or from bedrest should be treated with mild laxatives. Training to regain bowel control is by scheduled toileting reinforced with behavior modification and is usually accomplished within a reasonable time period in alert children of appropriate age.

Hypothalamic/pituitary injuries may accompany moderate to severe head trauma and lead to a variety of syndromes (17, 30, 87, 109, 244). Hyperphagia and anorexia have been mentioned earlier. Child abuse has been reported as a cause of hypopituitarism (162). The syndrome of inappropriate antidiuretic hormone secretion (SIAHDS) (30) attributed to posterior pituitary dysfunction is usually manifested by otherwise unexplainable hyponatremia and is treated with judicious fluid restriction guided by serum electrolyte monitoring. Another hypopituitary syndrome is diabetes insipidus. In a series of 149 patients aged 5 to 25 yr, Roberts ascertained a 3.5% frequency (193). Desmopressin, a vasopression analogue has been used successfully to treat children. Both syndromes appear within a few weeks after head injury and are generally transient. In diabetes insipidus, other aspects of anterior pituitary function should be investigated as signs of deficiency of growth, adrenocortical and thyroid-stimulating hormones as well as precocious puberty may become evident over time (207). Serial growth measurements are mandatory in all children after head injury.

Persistent systemic hypertension ascribed to hyperadrenergic state or hypothalamic dysfunction may follow severe head injury (109, 117, 194). At times, it is associated with other signs of autonomic disturbance and hyperthermia (53). Severe hypertension, particularly when accompanied by left ventricular hypertrophy, should be treated with antihypertensive medications keeping in mind their potential neuropsychological side effects. The diagnosis of central hyperthermia is based on exclusion of all other potential sources of infection. The most frequent causes are infections of the respiratory system, urinary tract, traumatic or surgical wounds, meningitis complicating CSF leak through basal skull fracture, intracranial abscess, or empyema (87, 109). Tracheostomy, nasogastric tube, or other medical equipment may be the focus of infection. A complete medical examination should be performed to rule out intercurrent infections, such as viral disease or otitis media, not unusual in children. Radiological imaging of the cranium will clarify whether surgically treatable intracranial pathology or perhaps sinusitis, a potential complication of nasogastric cannula, is present. After blood, urine, tracheostomy, and, if indicated, CSF cultures were obtained along with appropriate consultations, antibiotics should be started. Treating the primary cause is essential while tepid sponge baths or a cooling mattress contribute to controlling high temperatures.

Up to one third of children sustaining severe head trauma also have skeletal fractures; most commonly, long bones, clavicle, and, occasionally, the spine (28, 31, 221). Complications of nonunion or osteomyelitis prolong the rehabilitation process. Basal skull fractures may escape radiological detection and carry a high risk of meningitis. Orbital hematoma with racoon eyes and CSF rhinorrhea are present when the anterior fossa is involved. Mastoid hematoma, Battle sign, and bloody CSF otorrhea occur when the middle fossa is affected. Middle ear injury with rupture of the tympanic membrane and dislocation of the ossicles accompany longitudinal fractures of the petrous temporal bone (82) but discontinuity of the ossicular chain may also occur from impact without fracture. Both instances require reconstructive surgery to restore anatomic integrity and conductive hearing. Inner ear injury is a complication of transverse temporal fractures (82). Damage to the cochlea can cause permanent profound sensory hearing loss. Injuries of the semicircular canal lead to vertigo and vestibular nystagmus (65, 228). Endolymphatic fistula is amenable to reconstructive surgery and may alleviate these symptoms. Electronystagmogram (ENG) detects vestibular dysfunction (13, 65). A late complication that occurs several months after injury in children under 3 yr of age is growing skull fracture. It presents as a soft pulsating calvarial mass that contains a CSF-filled arachnoid cyst and, occasionally, herniated brain tissue (206).

Periarticular new bone information is a well-described entity occurring 1 to 6 months after head trauma with propensity among patients in long-term coma and spasticity (57, 165). It is manifested by pain, swelling, and decreased joint motion. Frequently involved joints are hip, shoulder, elbow, and knee, in that order, with the highest incidence of ankylosis at the elbow. In the presence of fractures, elevated alkaline phosphatase is not pathognomonic. Radionuclide bone scan is positive 2 to 3 weeks before x-ray. The frequency of heterotopic ossification is lower in young children but seems to approach the adult rate around adolescence. Cristofaro and his associates (57) reported a rate of 5% to 20% in several series of severe pediatric head injuries, all with spasticity. Mild hypercalcemia without evidence of hyperparathyroidism was present in some cases. The incidence of ankylosis in children is not known, but occasional patients require excision after the ossification matures as indicated by serial bone scan, mature trabeculated bone on x-ray, and normal alkaline phosphatase. Disodium etidronate, which blocks formation of crystal hydroxyapatite, has been found to be prophylactic in spinal cord injured adults (214). However, in growing children, interference with bone metabolism is a concern (52). Recently, Mital et al. (165) reported favorable results by oral ASA administration combined with surgery. Indomethacin or NSAIDs are used with some success for prophylaxis and treatment. Contrary to some reservations expressed in the past, Stover et al. (214) concluded from a controlled study that passive exercises increase joint range of motion and lead to fragmentation of ossification.

Abdominal pain, nausea, cramps, and constipation are clinical signs of immobilization hypercalcemia in a child (57). Although this complication is more frequent in spinal cord injury, it should be considered in the differential diagnosis of abdominal symptoms in head trauma. Laboratory studies for calcium/phosphorus balance and parathormone levels should be conducted. Furosemide or calcitonin treatment is discussed in the chapter on spinal cord injury.

Adequacy of urinary output is recorded together with specific gravity as a measure of hydration (87, 109, 244). For well-known reasons, intermittent catheterization is the choice over indwelling catheters in the child with incontinence. An uninhibited bladder is the usual cause of incontinence but unexpected detrusor outlet dyssynergy should be ruled out (94). Continence training begins with scheduled toileting and can be reinforced by behavior modification in the child able to cooperate.

Posttraumatic hydrocephalus ex vacuo is common in severe head trauma with cerebral atrophy and becomes demonstrable on brain imaging several months to within 1 yr after the injury (43, 127). Posttraumatic hydrocephalus with increased pressure is rare but should be suspected in a child who develops unexplained deterioration of behavior or other neurological signs, most notably, ataxia. CSF flow studies can differentiate the nature of hydrocephalus and indicate whether shunting is needed. Subdural fluid collections and hygromas (87, 206) are apt to accumulate in infants and young children, and, if untreated, may cause clinical deterioration.

Early seizures, so designated if they occur within 1 to 2 weeks after head trauma, may be focal or generalized (124). An overall incidence of 2.6% to 9% is reported under 16 yr of age. However, the frequency ranges from 30% in severe injuries to 1% in mild cases. Propensity for early seizures among infants and toddlers accounts primarily for the increased seizure rate in children compared to adults (124). On the other hand, late posttraumatic seizures, defined as the first episode occurring more than 2 weeks after injury, are less frequent than in adults. The peak onset is within 3 months and 90% develop within 4 yr. Prediction of late posttraumatic epilepsy is uncertain. Studies of correlation with early seizures have not produced uniform conclusions. Annegers et al. (8) found a frequency ranging from 0.2% in mild injuries to 7.4% in severe cases. McQueen et al. (159) in a study of severe pediatric head trauma, reported a rate of 2.3%. Some factors suggested to increase the risk of late seizures are depressed skull fracture, intracranial hematoma, and cortical laceration. EEG is not a reliable predictor since it is abnormal in approximately 50% of cases after head injury, even in the absence of late seizures; conversely, it may be normal between seizure episodes (124). Because temporal lobe, partial complex, or other atypical seizures may be the first manifestation, unexplained episodes of peculiar or confused behavior should be viewed with suspicion and indicate referral to a pediatric neurologist. Clinical seizure manifestations may change over time and generalized seizures evolve in two thirds of cases.

In early seizures, fast-acting phenytoin or clonazepam is the generally preferred treatment (124); intravenous diazepam is the usual choice to control status epilepticus, for which young children are at the greatest risk (124). Persistent late seizures require anticonvulsant therapy (124). Prophylactic treatment following early seizures but no recurrence after 2 weeks is controversial (99, 124). There is no agreement whether medication should be discontinued before discharge or tapered over 1 to 2 yr or by 4 yr after the injury. Low risk of posttraumatic epilepsy in childhood and lack of prophylactic effect are arguments in favor of abandoning long-term therapy (124, 219). Anticonvulsants, especially phenobarbital, affect alertness and learning ability (124, 229). These and other side effects should be considered in selecting the medication when persistent seizures with two or more late episodes necessitate treatment. Carbamazepine, which does not seem to have significant behavioral effects, is a frequent choice; bone marrow and liver function should be monitored (124). Valproic acid is used for complex absent seizures with precaution for adverse reactions.

Cranial nerve injuries were assumed to be less frequent in children than in adults. However, surveying 741 pediatric cases, Jacobi et al. (107)

described 35% cumulative frequency of postraumatic abnormalities, about one third persisting after 6 months. Permanent sequelae can interfere with rehabilitation, development, and schooling. Olfactory nerve damage and its consequence have been mentioned earlier. The optic nerve, firmly fixed by the dura in the optic canal, is subject to shearing injury causing optic atrophy, monocular or binocular blindness, field defects, or decreased visual acuity (7, 87, 206). Chiasmal trauma causes bitemporal hemianopsia or "split chiasm," resulting in an incapacitating reading disability, and is often associated with diabetes insipidus (7). Homonymous hemianopsia accompanies damage to the optic radiation. Often associated with hemiparesis and cortical sensory deficit, it enhances neglect of the affected side and contributes to spatial orientation difficulties. Cortical blindness is uncommon and usually transient in children (4). However, permanent impairment has been associated with other signs of severe brain damage in battered infants. Visual-evoked potential studies aid in diagnosis. In the series of Jacobi et al. (107), injuries to the oculomotor, trochlear, and abducens nerves occured most often at 20% frequency, a finding consistent with our experience. Extraocular muscle paralysis with dysconjugate gaze and diplopia further complicate impaired central visual motor processing. The majority of ocular nerve palsies resolve; interim treatment of diplopia is eye patching, although it is not well tolerated by young children. Surgical correction is warranted for persistent extraocular muscle paralysis after 1 yr. The high incidence of injuries to the visual system make ophthalmological consultation mandatory for head-injured children. Late facial nerve palsy associated with longitudinal fractures of the petrous temporal bone has a good prognosis as it represents compression from edema rather than axonal injury (82). Transverse temporal fractures, which constitute about one third of all cases are more likely to disrupt the facial nerve with immediate paralysis and often occur with VIIIth nerve lesion (82).

A few severely injured children sustain concomitant spinal cord or brachial plexus injury. The incidence of these complications was 4% and 2%, respectively, in a series of Hoffer et al. (103). Notoriously, spinal cord injury can occur in children without radiological signs of vertebral fracture or dislocation (173). An SSEP study confirms clinical suspicion. Brachial plexus injury will be most apparent by distribution of lower motor neuron weakness and EMG changes. Plexus root avulsion, most common in motorcycle accidents, results in a permanent flail extremity and may be associated with clavicular fracture. In rare instances, the lumbosacral plexus or other intrapelvic nerves are injured in conjunction with pelvic fracture. A variety of peripheral nerve injuries may accompany long bone fractures, dislocations, or severe trauma of surrounding soft tissues. An exceptional and preventable cause is positional pressure neuropathy during immobilization.

Rehabilitation Care

Remediation of motor dysfunction and cognitive deficits are the two major concerns of functional rehabilitation and proceed in parallel with the treatment of above-outlined medical complications.

Motor Dysfunction

Persistent neuromuscular deficits may present with diverse clinical signs predominantly or in combination (33, 34, 87, 206, 244). The most common patterns are: (a) spastic hemiparesis from unilateral cortical or pyramidal tract damage; (b) bilateral spasticity from hemispheric lesions, frequently asymmetrical; (c) ataxia of cerebellar and/or vestibular origin with or without spasticity; (d) rarely dyskinetic movement disorder due to lesions of the basal ganglia (152), at times associated with spasticity; and (e) decerebrate rigidity, which is usually transient but when long lasting may herald persistent vegetative state.

The frequency of hemiparesis is 30% to 45% (33, 34, 206). The initial motor deficit may range from dense paralysis without useful function to mild impairment of fine coordination. Gradual improvement of volitional control is the usual course in all but the most severe cases. Mildly affected children may show a virtual resolution of functional limitations despite persistent hyperreflexia. Children with hemiparesis become independent ambulators within a few weeks or months. Coexistent parietal lobe syndrome with cortical sensory deficit and, even to a greater extent, severe cognitive dysfunction prolong the achievement of walking. Upper extremity paresis creates more significant functional curtailment due to the complexity of fine motor control. When motor dysfunction is severe, or when mild but associated with cortical sensory deficit, spontaneous hand use is quite limited. Some children with relatively slight motor deficit will change hand dominance. Independence in activities of daily living (ADL) consistent with age and mental abilities is expected since children are very adept at developing compensatory solutions.

In bilateral spasticity, both ambulation and ADL function are contingent on the degree of preserved volitional control (33, 34, 206, 244). Cognitive impairment will influence ADL independence to a greater extent than ambulation. Bilateral spasticity does not exclude unassisted ambulation but some children need assistive devices or a wheelchair. While neuromuscular dysfunction is the primary determinant of walking, mental retardation modifies expectations based solely on the physical disability.

Ataxia by itself or with spasticity is the most frequent neuromuscular deficit in children with 60% or greater frequency (33, 34, 206, 244). The true extent of this neurological sign is often not evident until the child achieves some degree of independent function, such as sitting. In the early course of recovery, ataxia significantly prolongs attainment of gross motor milestones.

Intention tremor of the hands can impose severe limitations in daily activities. In a long-range perspective, ataxia has a good prognosis and recovery can continue for several years with minimal or no ultimate functional impediment. Children who initially need a wheelchair for severely ataxic gait may become community ambulatory after 1 yr or longer. In some cases, surprisingly little residual impairment is evident only on advanced gross motor skills that require intact balance. Clarification of the origin of ataxia, whether it is cerebellar or vestibular (13, 65), is essential since vestibular dysfunction due to endolymphatic fistula is surgically correctible.

Rarely, a dyskinetic movement disorder follows basal ganglion insult from anoxia or vascular compromise of the perforating middle cerebral artery branches (152). Associated spasticity is quite common.

Decerebrate rigidity in children is not necessarily as ominous a prognostic sign as in adults. Bruce (87, 206) proposes that this phenomenon may reflect a disruption of physiological function rather than white matter shearing injury in children. For reasons unexplained, this striking motor dysfunction does not seem to lead to contractures as often as early spasticity. Long-lasting decerebrate posturing may be an antecedent of persistent vegetative state with gradual relaxation of tone but no return of purposeful function.

An integrated team approach of treatment proceeds sequentially to re-educate the child for regaining past developmental milestones and to learn new skills in compensation for deficient function (87, 91, 206, 244). Motor experiences are needed and mesh with maturation of all other skills. Since no single system of motor training proved to be more effective than others, various physical and occupational therapy techniques are utilized to alleviate residual neuromuscular dysfunction.

The principal goals of physical therapy are prevention of deformities and training in gross motor skills. Occupational therapy concentrates on upper extremity function and on both physical and cognitive aspects of daily living skills. An appropriate program combines therapeutic exercises for the neuromuscular deficit with direct practice of functional activities. Age, the nature of motor dysfunction, level of physical regression, alertness, behavior, and neuropsychological cognitive deficits determine the selection of activities and methods of treatment. As an example, in severely affected children, head control or partial self-feeding may be the first step; whereas a less physically impaired child may practice ambulation but require training in the most elementary self-care skills on account of significantly regressed mental abilities or behavior. The treatment program is adjusted as recovery and improvement evolve. Considerations in designing therapeutic intervention for children are discussed in Chapter 7. Technical details of traditional and neuromuscular facilitation exercise methods are the subjects of standard textbooks.

The physically impaired child needs provision for assisted or substituted means of mobility, skills of daily life, and exploring the environment. The spectrum of mobility devices extends from scooter board to motorized wheelchairs (Chapter 8). The principles of adapted seating apply to head injury as well. Walkerette or crutches may be needed temporarily or, in some cases, permanently for ambulation. Added weights are, at times, helpful in ataxia. The indications for orthotic correction of gait abnormalities are identical with other physical disabilities (167). In view of the often remarkable improvement in motor function, splints are used as early temporizing measures; decrease or discontinuation of initially needed orthoses is a possibility when improvement continues over long time. Functional electrical stimulation (FES) may be tried for muscle re-education in selected cases. Training in compensatory techniques for upper extremity dysfunction is an important aspect in the repertory of skilled occupational therapists. Adaptive devices encompass a wide range of choices, such as adaptive feeding utensils; Velcro straps for buttoning or fastening; or electronic equipment for writing, environmental control, and other purposes when physical limitations are severe (Chapter 8).

Methods for prevention or management of spastic deformities are splints and progressive serial casting (122, 244). Phenol blocks of motor nerves or motor points offer transient relief (77, 122). Surgical tendon lengthening or transfer effectively corrects progressive or fixed contactures (122). As in all other childhood physical disabilities with severe neurogenic muscle imbalance around the hip joint, progressive subluxation is a possibility that calls for radiological monitoring. Early hip adductor and flexor release prevents painful dislocation for which children with severe spasticity and in a wheelchair are particularly prone (122). In this group of children, scoliosis is another complication of early onset neuromuscular dysfunction, although not as frequent as after spinal cord injury. Significant progressive deformity requires spinal fusion.

The drug of choice for cerebral spasticity is dantrolene sodium, which acts on muscle excitation-contraction coupling (77). Transient liver enzyme abnormalities may occur and need to be monitored, although liver toxicity has not been reported in children. In severe spasticity, particularly when it is combined with extensor hypertonia, simultaneous administration of dantrolene sodium and baclofen, a γ-aminobutyric acid antagonist, may yield greater relaxation. Diazepam affects brain and spinal cord interneuron activity. A sedative side effect limits the use of this drug to cases where alertness is not a consideration.

Dorsal spinal cord and cerebellar stimulation implants for control of cerebral spasticity have been abandoned. Selective posterior rhizotomy used for spasticity in cerebral palsy may find application to head injury.

Neuropsychological Deficits

The literature on the neuropsychological effects of head injury is extensive (70, 137, 141, 198, 199, 206, 216, 241). Cognitive and communication sequelae are discussed also in preceding chapters. Nevertheless, a brief summary is included here since recognition and treatment of these deficits have obvious importance in all phases of rehabilitation, educational planning, and community reintegration.

BEHAVIOR AND PERSONALITY CHANGES

Confusion and disorientation are typical in the early stage of recovery from coma (87, 114, 164, 206, 244). A structured, calm environment, continuity of nurses and therapists, repeated information about place, time, and daily schedule, favorite toys and other familiar objects from home, and the presence of family members help to reassure the child and re-establish a sense of reality.

Behavior and personality changes are one of the most consistent and distressing findings after head injury and cannot be measured by traditional testing (36, 137, 141, 175). Termed the posttraumatic syndrome of children (27), behavior disorders are manifested by two extremes: disinhibition or passivity. Variations exist in the severity of symptoms at both ends of the spectrum. Uninhibited aggressive behavior, agitation, hyperactivity or hyperkinesis, emotional lability, and lack of impulse control represent one mode of behavior dysfunction (36). Rarely, frank psychosis may develop. In a prospective study of children with mild and severe head trauma, Brown et al. (36) found an increased rate of psychiatric disorders compared to uninjured controls. Disinhibition and socially inappropriate behavior were the predominant pattern in the severely injured group. At the other extreme of behavior disorders is marked inertia, apathy, excessive placidity, flat affect, slow mental processing, low level of mental and physical energy, reduced self-directed inner drive, withdrawal, and depression. Severe withdrawal in the early stage of recovery has been called "feigned death" or "sleeping beauty syndrome" (224). Causal relationships are not always established. However, frontal lobe lesions tend to manifest with disinhibited behavior whereas passivity and inertia are more likely to occur in nondominant hemispheric injury resembling the affective component of adult strokes with left hemiparesis (200, 211). The hypothalamus, limbic system, and the reticular activating system have been implicated as the origin of different behavior disorders. Brown et al. (36) demonstrated a correlation between the severity of injury and the frequency of posttraumatic behavior disorders. They noted that dysfunctional symptoms often reflect an exaggeration of premorbid personality traits. Other potential contributory factors are sensory/perceptual impairments, physical limitations, the child's increasing awareness of these deficits, and adverse pretraumatic social and environmental circumstances (87, 155, 206).

In the immediate posttraumatic period, the child or adolescent in a prolonged agitated state is an especially difficult problem for nursing and staff.

Management techniques are removal of all possible causes of discomfort, confrontations, overstimulation, and potential sources of injury (87, 244). The child should be provided with structured stimuli and consistent supervision by family members or other reliable volunteers. Behavior modification is ineffective when recent memory is impaired or disorganized. When it becomes appropriate, behavior modification should be implemented by applying consistent specific expectations and limits, and objective measurements of improvement. If a reward system using privileges or tokens is set up, it should be practical and meaningful for the child.

Medication is used sparingly. For agitation, the most useful drugs are propranolol (239) or a short-acting benzodiazepine. The cerebral stimulant drugs, dextroamphetamine and methylphenidate, are helpful in some learning disabled children to improve inhibitory control, decrease hyperactivity, and enhance concentration and attention span (203); they may alleviate similar symptoms in some cases of posttraumatic behavior disorder as well. Therapeutic trial of any medication requires dose adjustments for optimal behavioral effect and minimal adverse reactions (42, 239). Consultations with a child psychiatrist are helpful. The treatment program relies heavily on the social worker who is the family counselor throughout the rehabilitation and whose skills in individual and group therapy are particularly important to guide the family in coping with frustrating behavior problems (114, 230, 244).

MEMORY DEFICITS

The complex neuropsychology of memory disorders in head injury is described in many reviews (6, 164, 213, 223, 240). The hippocampus, thalamus, limbic, and reticular activating systems with their extensive thalamic and cortical connections have been implicated (10). Memory, as a collective term, entails several processes. Functionally, it can be construed as acquisition and retrieval of memory traces. Retrograde amnesia is a loss of memory for information stored prior to the injury and is considered a disorder of retrieval. Deficit in remembering new information represents a disorder of acquisition and is designated anterograde amnesia. Learning is contingent also on alertness and attention, particularly selective attention, which is frequently affected in head injury and interferes with the acquisition of new memories. In relation to time, short-term memory or immediate recall is distinguished from long-term storage and retrieval (87, 164, 168, 206, 244).

Head injury is accompanied by retrograde and anterograde amnesia. Duration and severity of both correlate with the severity of trauma (87, 142, 244). In many cases, retrograde amnesia gradually abates or resolves over time ranging from days to months or years. Anterograde amnesia is the most common persistent neuropsychological dysfunction in pediatric head injury. Visual or auditory memory can be affected to different degrees; the latter is selectively or more significantly impaired in focal left temporal lobe lesion. Both short- and long-term memory deficits are encountered. Although improvement is the usual course, some degree of residual dysfunction is typical of severe trauma.

The Children's Orientation and Amnesia Test (COAT) (67) consists of a brief scale appropriate for daily administration to assess recovery from amnesia. An evaluation instrument designed specifically to assess verbal memory function is the Selective Reminding Test (40), which was also standardized for children. Hannay et al. (95) devised the Continuous Recognition Memory Test, which also taps attentional function. Levin and associates (142) demonstrated that children and adolescents with severe head injury had persistent impairment at 1-yr follow-up on both tests. Among the standard Psychological tests discussed in Chapter 3, the WPPSI-R, WISC-R, and the McCarthy Scales of Children's Abilities contain memory subtests applicable from preschool to adolescence.

Informal memory training occurs at all therapeutic encounters the child is exposed to during the rehabilitation process. Simple, step-by-step instructions focused on the task at hand, exclusion of distracting extraneous verbal or other stimulus modalities, repeated reminders, and cueing are a common sense approach dictated by understanding memory and attention deficits. Although in the last decade formal memory training has become a major interest, the efficacy of different methods remains controversial or equivocal (79, 87, 177, 240, 244). Memory remediation methods use three basic principles: (a) practice and exercise drill by rote repetition; (b) learning mnemonic strategies with visual imagery or verbal cues; and (c) external memory aids or memory prostheses including diaries, lists, or so-called active devices such as alarm watch or pocket buzzer (164, 240). Studies indicate that the first method may help in learning specific limited information but generalization from one set of information or task to another fails to occur. Training by computer does not improve the results. Mnemonics can help remember a list of names or other similar sets of data but the wide range of demands in daily life restrict their practical value. External memory aids are mostly used for cueing prospective memory, i.e., to perform future action. Experience shows that patients rarely utilize lists or diaries, but that active reminders are helpful if provided within close time proximity. Glisky and Schacter (79) describe limited trials of a new approach, the acquisition of domain-specific knowledge. The method combines repetitive practice, a teaching technique of vanishing cues, and training in requisite skills for a specific task.

Neuropharmacological studies suggest that cholinergic agents, catecholamines, vasopressin, naloxone, and the new class of nootropic drugs facilitate memory processes (55). There are no pediatric trials with memory-enhancing drugs. As noted earlier, dextroamphetamine may be helpful when attention deficits play a significant role in learning and memory dysfunction. In selecting drugs for behavior or seizure disorder, their adverse effect on alertness and learning should be always considered.

COMMUNICATION DISORDERS

The differential diagnosis of absent or impaired communication falls in two broad categories: speech production deficits and language dysfunction. A combination of both may occur.

Mutism of the early stage may merely reflect depressed mentation and recover, unless there are other underlying communication impairments (143, 170). After intubation, aphonia or dysphonia is a temporary complication that resolves in a relatively short time in the absence of laryngeal nerve palsy. Dysarthria or, in severe cases, anarthria accompanies supranuclear palsy in bilateral lesions of the motor system with spasticity, ataxia, or basal ganglion syndrome. Because swallowing and speech production share many of the same muscles for volitional control, dysphagia is an associated finding (9, 244). Dysarthria can persist in various degrees of severity after dysphagia has improved or recovered attesting to the greater complexity of volitional motor control required for speech. Oral motor dyspraxia (161), defined in neurological terms as impairment of central planning and execution of speech in the absence of motor and sensory dysfunction, may contribute to dysarthria. The diagnosis is difficult to establish since the stipulated neurological criteria are rarely met in head injury.

Language is connected with hemispheric specialization of the human brain (26). Although not absolute, it commits linguistic abilities as well as analytical and arithmetic function to the left side. Integration of spatial, pictorial, and geometric perception, tactile discrimination, musical and time concepts are delegated to the right hemisphere. Anatomic asymmetry of cerebral hemispheres is evident by 29 weeks of gestation. Left hemispheric specialization for language is complete by 5 yr. That childhood language development proceeds despite severe dominant hemispheric lesion is an often-quoted example of the apparently greater plasticity of the young brain (137). However, several studies showed subtle signs of inferior language competence in children with congenital or early onset right hemiparesis and after left hemidecortication in infancy (59, 115, 183, 227).

In children, aphasia due to left hemispheric injury may be mixed with receptive and expressive components although the latter type predominates (68, 115, 137). Prognosis is most favorable in injuries sustained under 5 yr but good recovery up to 9 to 11 years is known to occur from childhood-acquired aphasia. Improvement is fastest within 12 months but can continue for several years. However, dysnomia, impairment of language-mediated memory and reasoning, often persists despite apparent verbal fluency (67, 68, 115, 137, 244).

Aprosody is a central disorder in nondominant hemispheric injury (197). The monotonous speech that lacks inflection and emotional intonation mirrors the flat affect and decreased facial expressions in this syndrome.

Reduced speed of responsive and conversational speech occur with aprosody or result from the general posttraumatic slowing of mental processes, intellectual deficit, or word finding difficulties. Posttraumatic intellectual impairment leads to overall regression of language function.

Specific deficits of written communication described in adult aphasic syndromes are rarely seen in children; however, dysgraphia, and particularly, dyslexia occur in visuomotor/intersensory integration disorders although other aspects of language dysfunction may be comparatively mild or occasionally absent. Children injured before 8 yr of age and comatose for 3 days or longer have a higher incidence of severe reading disability defined as performance 2 yr or more below expectations for chronological age (205).

After the resolution of posttraumatic amnesia, hearing, language, and speech evaluations are mandatory. Since hearing deficits enhance any communication disorder, audiogram, tympanogram, and auditory-evoked potential responses should be included. Assessment of oral and speech musculature is performed as indicated. Linguistic testing, complemented by appropriate psychological assessment, will analyze the nature of language deficit as described in preceding chapters. Sarno (202) found that visual naming, sentence repetition, word fluency, and the Token Test are particularly sensitive to detect subclinical aphasia and dysarthria after head injury.

The treatment of communication disorders depends on their type and severity, as well as on the age and cooperation of the child (87, 137, 244). A variety of strategies may be used for language deficits to take advantage of preserved function, as melodic intonation through the right hemisphere, and increasing complexity of tasks meant to retrain impaired abilities in auditory memory or reading. In severe oral motor dysfunction, feeding and speech training start simultaneously and proceed to remediation of phonation, articulation, and other aspects of speech production (87, 244). Simple nonverbal communication devices, for example, signing or a pointing board, may be needed temporarily until oral speech improves. For persistent severe dysarthria, the choice of electronic augmentative communication devices is virtually unlimited (58). Vocal cord paralysis and velopharyngeal incompetence are amenable to surgical treatment. Surgical correction of middle ear disruption, hearing aids, lip reading, and/or sign language are remedial measures when specific auditory deficits contribute to impaired communication.

INTELLECTUAL DEFICITS

Recovery of cognition or, conversely, residual intellectual impairment is the primary factor determining the quality of life for the child and family after severe head injury. Children have the advantage over adults of greater plasticity or extensive learning capacity of the immature brain in the broadest sense. The neurological mechanisms of plasticity are the subject of extensive reviews (73, 86, 114, 137, 154).

On the other hand, the age-related developmental stage before the injury is also a contributing factor. Studies of long-term outcome of intellectual functioning have not confirmed the previously held view that children have a better prognosis than adults (21, 56, 116, 135, 231). On the contrary, the emerging trend seems to be that, in childhood, there is an inverse relationship with age at the time of the injury (56, 72, 134, 231). Early disruption of the normal developmental process of cognition and learning has a more adverse effect; the earlier in life the brain damage occurs, the less experience and skills have been acquired prior to destruction of participating neural structures. Another important consideration in the context of development is that when some aspects of intellectual function that are expected to emerge at a later age fail to occur, deficits may become more apparent. Abstract reasoning, which emerges after 10 to 12 yr of age, is one example.

Brink and associates (33) reported a series of head-injured children with 60% rate of mental retardation in the younger age group, under 8 yr, compared to a 14% rate in those individuals injured between 10 and 18 yr of age. The overall rate of IQ scores below 70 was 37% in the entire group. Klonoff et al. (129) estimated that cognitive function is usually reduced by 10 to 30 IQ points but did not find differences on neuropsychological tests 5 yr later between children injured before or after age 9 yr. Levin and associates (141) found that intellectual prognosis is less favorable when the injury occurs under 10 yr of age and that diffuse brain damage leads to more severe cognitive deficit in the young child. A series of children who were injured during infancy or before they were 5 yr old showed persistent significant intellectual deficits on follow-up 6 to 14 yr later. Posttraumatic amnesia and the depth and duration of coma are suggested as predictive guidelines for cognitive outcome. However, Chadwick and associates (47-50) concluded that, in children, there is a stronger correlation with length of coma lasting 24 h or longer than with GCS scores. Improvement of intellectual functioning is fastest during the first year after injury but may continue up to 5 yr at a slower pace (48, 129). Performance IQ scores are more affected and show less improvement than verbal scores (19, 66). The discrepancy is attributed to a general slowness of information processing, deficits in manual dexterity, in visual motor and visual spatial function, and to impaired problem-solving skills since these abilities have a greater influence on performance scores (66).

Psychological assessment at intervals after the posttraumatic amnesia includes evaluation of general cognitive ability using traditional intelligence and achievement tests (Chapter 3) (70, 137). Deficits in specific areas of neuropsychological function can be more accurately identified on the Halstead-Reitan (186) and Luria-Nebraska Neuropsychological Test batteries (80, 178), which have been revised for different pediatric age groups. Evaluation procedures have also been developed to assess motor speed, visual motor, visual spatial, and somatosensory perception in children with head injury (95).

Cognitive training starts in the acute rehabilitation setting and, to some extent, pervades all modalities of treatment regardless of their primary aim (87, 137, 244). Psychologists and, at an appropriate time, educators create a systematic structured framework for this aspect of intervention. Remediation of deficits and enhancement of preserved abilities are the leading principles of training. Cognitive function as the main determinant of educational placement is a central concern in discharge planning (39, 74).

Community Reintegration

Preparation for discharge is one of the most complex aspects of the rehabilitation process. Coordinated planning must involve the family, school system or other community facilities, and the rehabilitation team (87, 184, 244). Discharge options depend on neuropsychological and physical recovery.

Plans for educational placement are completed before discharge with assurance that the child is enrolled in a suitable structured school program (44, 137, 244). The Education For All Children Act, PL 94–142 mandates free appropriate public education for handicapped children. Principles of the act are schooling in the least restrictive environment, parental consent to placement, and an Individualized Educational Plan (IEP) of goals and services for the child. PL 99–457 is an extension to preschool education for disabled or at-risk children from 3 yr of age. School placement of children with significant physical disability usually requires a setting that provides physical, occupational, and communication therapy (244).

Often, a sequential educational reintegration is necessary progressing from home instruction to part-time or full-time school attendance in special education or in regular classes with adjusted curriculum or a resource teacher (81, 196). Ewing-Cobbs et al. use recovery of long-term memory as a guide for selecting the academic subjects of education (66). Sometimes, tenacious persistence is in order by a professional child advocate to ensure procurement of learning disability class or special tutoring for the adolescent who returns to school without visible handicap, but who is, indeed, a different person (22, 24, 108). Understanding on the part of the parents and teachers of the educational and behavioral peculiarities following head injury is important for successful learning and to prevent secondary behavior problems and low self-esteem of the child (20, 39, 54, 66, 98). The National Head Injury Foundation provides a most useful guide for teaching children with head injury (171). Anticipatory guidance, monitoring progress, and maintaining contact with the school are essential aspects of the rehabilitation process after discharge. Some children may require a therapeutic cognitive training program prior to or supplementing return to school (98, 218). Problems that may need to be addressed include not only learning ability and memory but also behavior (137, 244). A child with selective attention deficit may find it overwhelming to cope with the impact of multiple distracting stimuli in a group (114). Poor impulse control and impaired social judgment may interfere with class attendance and peer interaction (125, 158). In concept, cognitive rehabilitation strategies for the pediatric age group are similar to adults, targeting on defective skills, compensatory alternatives, and generalization outside the learning situation (18, 84, 87, 137, 244). Developmental considerations enter into planning defined goals and the content of training. Computer games as a tool for cognitive rehabilitation have special appeal to children but superiority of results have not been demonstrated with this method (18). The controversy as to which strategy of cognitive rehabilitation is most effective for children and adolescents remains unresolved because of the extreme scarcity of well-designed studies conducted at this age. Educational and cognitive intervention programs have increased recently and are reported in the literature of pediatric head trauma (11, 146).

Rehabilitation of a child with head injury must also focus on the parents who remain primarily responsible for bringing up their child (114, 137, 244). The relatively few studies of families suggest that their emotional responses show a range similar to those experienced by parents of children with other disabilities and is influenced by their own personalities (230). However, the emotional stress is compounded by anxiety surrounding the initial trauma and, subsequently, by the need to adjust their previous child-rearing style. Among the siblings, grief is often enhanced by guilt if they were present at the accident or emotional difficulties may ensue for perceived unequal share of parental attention following the accident. In children recovering from head injury, loss of previous friends is a source of sadness and depression and heightens their awareness that they are different from what they were prior to the accident (87, 137, 244). The pediatric physiatrist must be sensitive to these issues, provide adequate information for the families to understand and manage changes in the child's behavior and functioning in daily life situations, and initiate referral for counseling. Family support groups and contacts with local facilities of the National Head Injury Foundation are invaluable help for parents (62).

Minor Head Injury

The usual criteria for minor or mild head injury are Glasgow Coma Scale of 13 to 15, loss of consciousness for less than 20 minutes, and no intracranial pathology or skull fracture (76). Additional symptoms include confusion, transient posttraumatic amnesia, dysesthesias, and incoordination. Cerebral concussion, the medical diagnostic term for these symptoms, is used to imply that stress forces from a blow or sudden head movement, altered axonal excitability but no organic lesions occurred. Recent studies suggest that depending on the severity of cerebral strain there may be minute structural changes, even disruption of some axons, so called axonotomy, which escape detection on current brain imaging methods (180).

The postconcussion syndrome of adults consists of persistent headache, nausea, tinnitus, dizziness, poor concentration, memory disturbances, and, at times, hearing difficulties, diplopia, weakness, and numbness of various extent and length of time (15, 76, 120). Transient cortical blindness is a most striking symptom (63, 121, 243). Children, particularly young ones, generally cannot identify these symptoms, which may explain why the effect of minor pediatric head injuries became recognized only recently (29, 32, 45, 46, 97, 138). More typical manifestations in childhood fall into two categories: (a) behavior, consisting of irritability, hyperactivity, and personality changes that may create difficulties with handling a previously easy-going child; and (b) learning ability presenting as a decline in scholastic achievements among school-aged children (137, 140). Gulbrandsen (88) studied 56 children aged 9 to 13 yr with mild head injury and with less than 15 minutes loss of consciousness. All had the diagnosis of cerebral concussion on arrival to the emergency room. Compared to a control group, they showed deficits on virtually all neuropsychological subtests 6 months after the injury. Other neuropsychological studies, which included children with a spectrum of severe to mild head trauma, demonstrated impairments in cognitive and school performance in the mildly injured group with resolution over time (137, 140). Figure 11.1 shows two samples of a 6-yr-old child's drawing before and after two consecutive mild head injuries without loss of consciousness.

Estimates suggest that as much as 80% of childhood head injuries are mild and that, around home and on playgrounds, several million minor accidents of this nature may occur annually in the United States (97). However, the exact scope of the problem arising from minor pediatric head injuries is not known since many children sustain mild head trauma without apparent or detected residual impairment. Discernible neuropsychological changes occur in an undefined proportion of cases. Large-scale long-term studies are not available.

Outcome

Since the 1970s, intensive efforts were directed at prognosticating and assessing the outcome of head trauma. Great variations in the nature and severity of injuries, age, range and extent of residual deficits, and differences in premorbid function and social circumstances make analyses of outcome a most difficult and complex task. In children, these problems are further complicated by the fact that development is not completed. A study of accomplishments in adulthood, which would be the true measure of outcome, are not available at present.

Measurement of outcome requires reliable and reproducible assessment methods. Most recovery and assessment scales were developed for adults and require adaptation, particularly when applied to preschool age. Jennett and Bond (112) proposed the first systematic measure, the Glasgow Outcome Scale (GOS) (Table 11.4). Another frequently used and somewhat sim-

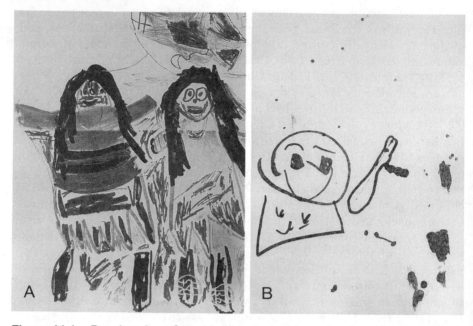

Figure 11.1. Drawings by a 6-yr-old child who had two minor head injuries without loss of consciousness; 6 months after the accident persistent irritable behavior and decline in school performance; *A*, creative drawing of native Indian dancers prior to injury. *B*, drawing of a man 6 months following her injury illustrates regressed visuomotor performance.

ilar approach is the Levels of Cognitive Functioning developed at Rancho Los Amigos Hospital (Table 11.5) (89). The scale is applicable to school-aged children and, with adjustment, to children under 5 yr old. Alexander described a behavioral recovery scale that also includes treatment guidelines for each level (137). The Disability Rating Scale provides quantitative scores for eight aspects of function. Validity of this assessment tool was demonstrated in adults but it would need modifications for children (85). Wee FIM, an adaptation of the functional independence measure from 6 months to 6 yr is in the stage of development and field testing (92). The Tufts Assessment of Motor Performance (TAMP) is a 32-item standardized test that has a pediatric version and includes a wide range of skills with qualitative grading (92). The foregoing assessment methods are useful for delineating the course of recovery and outcome in terms of broad functional categories. Neuropsychological, developmental, scholastic achievement, language, and other formalized tests are necessary to identify outcome in specific areas of cognitive function as discussed earlier in this book and elsewhere in the literature (69, 90, 101, 137, 141, 172).

Table 11.4.
Glasgow Outcome Scale[a]

Death (D)
Persistent vegetative state (VS)
No cortical function, eye opening with sleep/wake cycles, subcortical postural reflexes
Severe disability (DS)
Conscious but dependent, severe physical and/or mental impairment requiring care and supervision
Moderate disability (MD)
Independent but disabled; capable of activities of daily living, travel, and some school or work but persistent mental and/or physical impairment
Good recovery (GR)
Returns to normal life although all normal functions may not be fully restored

[a]From Jennett B, Bond M: Assessment of outcome after severe brain damage. A practical scale. *Lancet* 1:480–484, 1975.

Major predictive criteria for recovery from severe head injury with coma reflect previous developmental stage, severity of brain damage, and recovery pattern (3, 16, 64, 87, 131, 151, 164, 181). *Age* at injury, *depth of coma,* and *duration of coma* emerged as the most significant outcome correlates.

Patients under 15 to 18 yr have a better prognosis. Of children under 15 yr old, 60% to 90% progressed to good recovery/moderate disability level irrespective of other factors (69, 87, 206). Although a German study of comatose children indicated a lower survival rate in the under 10-yr age group compared to the 10- to 20-yr age group (75), this finding was not confirmed by Luerssen et al. (148).

Neuropsychological studies suggest more profound cognitive deficits when injuries occur before 9 to 10 yr of age, and especially in preschool aged children (3, 21, 72, 132, 134, 137). Persistent vegetative state is rare in children, even after severe head injury, and is more likely to follow coma from hypoxic/ischemic insult than from trauma (3, 78, 153). Electrophysiological and cerebral metabolic studies predict the evolution of persistent vegetative state (144, 225, 231).

Table 11.5.
Levels of Cognitive Function[a]

I. No response to stimulation
II. Generalized response to stimulation
III. Localized response to stimulation
IV. Confused, agitated behavior
V. Confused, inappropriate, nonagitated behavior
VI. Confused, appropriate behavior
VII. Automatic, appropriate behavior
VIII. Purposeful, appropriate behavior

[a]From Hagen C, Malkmus D, Durham P: *Levels of Cognitive Functioning.* Downey, CA, Rancho Los Amigos Hospital, 1979.

The Glasgow Coma Scale is considered an indication of the severity of injury. Because of the tendency for acute brain swelling, deep coma in childhood injuries does not necessarily indicate parenchymal injury as in adults (87, 206). Outlook for children seems to be better than for adults with identical GCS. Unlike in adults, there is also a significant recovery rate from coma with GCS score of 4. High morbidity and mortality are associated with a score of 3. Persistent vegetative state is most frequent with this score among the survivors and flaccid coma has a particularly poor prognosis for survival. The critical predictive score at 24 hours in children may be 5 instead of 8 or above as in adults, taking into account the inability or reluctance of young children to speak.

Comatose state of less than 3 months augurs a prognosis ranging from good recovery to moderate disability by 1 year (215). In a series of 344 patients under 18 yr of age managed by Brink and associates (34), 94% regained independence in ambulation and self-care from coma lasting 6 weeks or less and 78% recovered with various degrees of limitaions after being comatose for up to 12 weeks. Chadwick et al. found a closer relationship between cognitive deficits and duration rather than depth of coma (50). The length of posttraumatic amnesia has an inverse correlation with cognitive outcome in adolescents and adults but this variable is difficult to test in young children.

Lewin and Roberts (145) note that recovery in children may continue on occasion up to 5 yr. A similar trend in cognitive recovery was suggested by Klonoff (129). Other neuropsychological studies demonstrated increase in I.Q. scores at 1 yr after injury with slower improvement thereafter (67).

Bruce suggests that certain features of the initial CAT scan consistent with specific injuries have prognostic usefulness (37, 38, 87). Decreased ventricular size and compressed cisterns with normal or increased brain density represent diffuse cerebral swelling with good prognosis. Low supratentorial brain density with loss of gray-white matter interface is consistent with severe ischemia and extremely high mortality. Corpus callosum, thalamus, or midbrain hemorrhages are signs of diffuse axonal injury with high mortality or most severe disability. Significant brain atrophy on CAT scans after 2 months is a poor prognostic sign (133). Rivara et al. (189) demonstrated that CAT scans may be abnormal even though clinical signs are absent or deceivingly mild.

Unfavorable prognostic factors include intracranial hematoma requiring surgical evacuation (3, 203), systemic hypertension for more than 6 weeks (34), intracranial pressure over 40 mm Hg (87, 206), abnormal brainstem auditory-evoked potentials after 1 week (100, 150), and serum CPK isoenzyme BB abnormalities (96). The overall trend emerging from outcome studies is that children have a greater potential to recover from neuromuscular dysfunction and from deficits caused by focal lesions, such as aphasia, than from the cognitive and behavioral consequences of head injury.

Research and Prevention

Traumatic brain injury is recognized as an international problem of enormous proportions. In the United States, it is the leading cause of accidental death among children. While advances in critical care are reducing mortality and morbidity, head injury remains the most common reason for inpatient admission to pediatric rehabilitation facilities. Further research and collaborative studies are needed to elucidate many aspects of treatment and prognosis.

By far, the most important attack on head injuries is prevention (190, 192, 195). Any child restraint system reduces motor vehicle fatalities as much as 90% (2). Effective preventive measures are legally mandated use of seat belt, car seats for young children, cycle helmets (176, 233), construction of bicycle lanes, education against drunk driving, early detection of child abuse, proper supervision and equipment for contact sports, and restriction of all terrain and unstable recreational vehicles.

REFERENCES

1. Abdel-Dayem HM, Sadek SA, Kouris K, et al: Changes in cerebral perfusion after acute head injury: Comparison of CT with T 99 m HM-PAO SPECT. *Radiology* 165:221-226, 1987.
2. Agran P, Castillo D, Winn D: Childhood motor vehicle occupant injuries. *Am J Dis Child* 144:653-662, 1990.
3. Alberico AM, Ward JD, et al: Outcome after severe head injury. Relationship to mass lesions, diffuse injury, and ICP course in pediatric and adult patients. *J Neurosurg* 67:648-656, 1987.
4. Aldrich MS, Alessi AG, Beck RW, Gilman S: Cortical blindness: Etiology, diagnosis and prognosis. *Ann Neurol* 21:149-158, 1987.
5. Alexander RC, Schor DP, Smith WL: Magnetic resonance imaging of intracranial injuries from child abuse. *J Pediatr* 109:975-979, 1986.
6. Alkon DL: *Memory Traces in the Brain*. Cambridge University Press, 1988.
7. Anderson RL, Panje WR, Gross CE: Optic nerve blindness following blunt forehead trauma. *Ophthalmology* 89:445-455, 1982.
8. Annegers JF, Grabow JD, Groover RV, et al: Seizures after head trauma: A population study. *Neurology* 30:683-689, 1986.
9. Aten JL: Spastic dysarthria: Revising understanding of the disorder and speech treatment procedures. *J Head Trauma Rehabil* 3:63-73, 1988.
10. Auerbach SH: Neuroanatomical correlates of attention and memory disorders in traumatic brain injury: An application of neurobehavioral subtypes. *J Head Trauma Rehabil* 1:1-12, 1986.
11. Bagnato SJ, Mayes SD, et al: An interdisciplinary neurodevelopmental assessment model for brain-injured infants and preschool children. *J Head Trauma Rehabil* 3:75-86, 1988.
12. Baker SP, Waller AE: Childhood Injury. State by State Mortality Facts. Baltimore, The Johns Hopkins Injury Prevention Center, 1989.
13. Baloh RW, Furman JMR: Modern vestibular function testing. *West J Med* 150:59-67, 1989.
14. Barnet AB, Friedman IP, Weiss IP, Ohlrich ES, Shanks B, Lodge A: VEP development in infancy and early childhood. A longitudinal study. *Electroenceph Clin Neurophysiol* 49:476, 1980.

15. Barth JT, Macciochi SN, Giordani B: Neuropsychologic sequelae of minor head injury. *Neurosurgery* 13:529–533, 1983.
16. Barzilay Z, Augarten A, et al: Variables affecting outcome from severe brain injury in children. *Intensive Care Med* 14:417–421, 1988.
17. Barzilay Z, Somekh E: Diabetes insipidus in severely brain damaged children. *J Med Clin Exper Theor* 19(1):47–64, 1988.
18. Batchelor J, Shores EA, et al: Cognitive rehabilitation of severely closed-head-injured patients using computer-assisted and noncomputerized treatment techniques. *J Head Trauma Rehabil* 3:78–85, 1988.
19. Bawden HN, Knights RM, Winogron W: Speeded performance following head injury in children. *J Clin Exper Neuropsychol* 7:39–54, 1985.
20. Begali V: *Head Injury in Children and Adolescents: Resource and Review for Schools and Allied Professionals.* Brandon, VT, Clinical Psychology Publishing, 1978.
21. Berger MS, Pitts LM, Lovely M, et al: Outcome from severe head injury in children and adolescents. *J Neurosurg* 62:194–199, 1985.
22. Berger-Gross P, Shackelford M: Closed head injury in children: neuropsychological and scholastic outcomes. *Percept Motor Skills* 61:254–258, 1985.
23. Bergner L, Mayer S, Harris D: Falls from heights: A childhood epidemic in an urban area. *Am J Public Health* 61:90, 1971.
24. Bigler ED: Acquired cerebral trauma: epidemiology, neuropsychological assessment and academic/educational deficits. *J Learn Disabil* 20:516–517, 1987.
25. Billmire ME, Myers PA: Head injury in infants. *Pediatrics* 75:340, 1985.
26. Bishop DV: Plasticity and specificity of language localization in the developing brain. *Dev Med Child Neurol* 251–254, 1981.
27. Black P, et al: The post-traumatic syndrome in children. In Walker AE, Caveness WF, Critchley M (eds): *The Late Effects of Head Injury.* Springfield, Charles C Thomas, 1969.
28. Blasier D, Letts M: The orthopaedic manifestations of head injury in children. *Orthop Rev* 18:350–358, 1989.
29. Boll T: Minor head injury in children: Out of sight, but not out of mind. *J Clin Child Psychol* 12:74–80, 1983.
30. Born JD, Hans P, Smitz S, et al: Syndrome of inappropriate secretion of antidiuretic hormone after severe head injury. *Surg Neurol* 23:383–387, 1984.
31. Botte JM, Moore TJ: The orthopedic management of extremity injuries in head trauma. *J Head Trauma Rehabil* 2:13–27, 1987.
32. Boyce BB, Gaspard NJ: *Effects of Major and Minor Head Injury in Children.* Southborough MA, National Head Injury Foundation, 1986.
33. Brink JD, Garrett AL, Hale WR, et al: Recovery of motor and intellectual function in children sustaining severe head injuries. *Dev Med Child Neurol* 12:565–571, 1970.
34. Brink JD, Imbus C, Woo-Sam J: Physical recovery after severe closed head trauma in children and adolescents. *J Pediatr* 97:721–727, 1980.
35. Brison RJ, Wicklund K, Mueller BA: Fatal pedestrian injuries to young children: A different pattern of injury. *Am J Public Health* 78:793–795, 1988.
36. Brown G, Chadwick O, Shaffer D, et al: A prospective study of children with head injuries, III. Psychiatric sequelae. *Psychol Med* 11:63–78, 1981.
37. Bruce DA, Alavi A, Bilaniuk L, Colinskas C, Obrist W, Uzzell B: Diffuse cerebral swelling following head injuries in children—the syndrome of malignant brain edema. *J Neurosurg* 54:170–178, 1981.
38. Bruce DA, Schut L: The value of CAT scanning following pediatric head injury. *Clin Pediatr* 19:719–725, 1986.
39. Burns PG, Gianutsos R: Reentry of the head injured survivor into the educational system: First steps. *J Commun Health Nurs* 4:145–152, 1987.
40. Buschke H: Components of verbal learning in children: Analysis by selective reminding. *J Exp Child Psychol* 18:488–496, 1974.

41. Bush GW: The National Head Injury Foundation: Eight years of challenge and growth. *J Head Trauma Rehabil* 4:73–77, 1988.

42. Campbell M, Spencer EK: Psychopharmacology in child and adolescent psychiatry: A review of the past five years. *J Am Acad Child Adolesc Psychiat* 27:269–275, 1988.

43. Cardoso ER, Galbraith S: Post-traumatic hydrocephalus—a retrospective review. *Surg Neurol* 23:261–264, 1985.

44. Carter RR, Savage RC: Education and the traumatically brain injured: Rights, protections and responsibilities. *Cognitive Rehabil* 3:14–17, 1985.

45. Casey R, Ludwig S, McCormick MC: Minor head trauma in children: An intervention to decrease functional morbidity. *Pediatrics* 80:159–162, 1987.

46. Casey R, Ludwig S, McCormick MC: Morbidity following minor head trauma in children. *Pediatrics* 78:497–502, 1986.

47. Chadwick O: Psychological sequelae of head injury in children. *Dev Med Child Neurol* 27:72–75, 1985.

48. Chadwick O, Rutter M, Brown G, et al: A prospective study of children with head injuries: II. Cognitive sequelae. *Psychol Med* 11:49–61, 1981.

49. Chadwick O, Rutter M, et al: Intellectual performance and reading skills after localized head injury in childhood. *J Child Psychol Psychiat* 22:117–139, 1981.

50. Chadwick O, Rutter M, Shaffer D, Shrout PE: A prospective study of children with head injuries: IV Specific cognitive deficits. *J Clin Neuropsych* 3:101–120, 1981.

51. Cherney LR, Cantieri CA, Pannell JJ: *Clinical Evaluation of Dysphagia.* Frederick, MD, Aspen Publishers, 1985.

52. Chiodo A, Nelson V: Rickets associated with etidronate use in a head injured pediatric patient. *Arch Phys Med Rehabil* 68:645, 1987.

53. Clar H: Disturbance of hypothalamic thermoregulation. *Acta Neurochir* 1985:75:106–112.

54. Cohen SB: Educational reintegration and programming for children with head injuries. *J Head Trauma Rehabil* 1:22–29, 1986.

55. Cope DN: The pharmacology of attention and memory. *J Head Trauma Rehabil* 1:34–42, 1986.

56. Costeff H, Abraham E, et al: Late neuropsychologic status after childhood head trauma. *Brain Dev* 10:371–374, 1988.

57. Cristofaro RL, Brink JD: Hypercalcemia of immobilization in neurologically injured children: A prospective study. *Orthopedics* 2:485–491, 1979.

58. De Ruyter F, Becker MR: Augmentative communication: Assessment, system selection and usage. *J Head Trauma Rehabil* 3:35–44, 1988.

59. Dennis M, Lovett M, Wiegel-Crump C: Written language acquisition after left or right hemidecortication in infancy. *Brain Lang* 12:54–91, 1981.

60. Duhaime A, Gennarelli TA, Thibault LE, Bruce DA, Margulies SS, Wiser R: The shaken baby syndrome: A clinical, pathological and biomedical study. *J Neurosurg* 66:409–415, 1987.

61. Eichelberger MR, Gotschall CS et al: A comparison of trauma score, revised trauma score, and the pediatric trauma score. *Ann Emerg Med* 18:1053–1058, 1989.

62. Eisner J, Kreutzer JS: A family information system for education following traumatic brain injury. *Brain Injury* 3:79–90, 1989.

63. Eldridge PR, Punt JAG: Transient traumatic cortical blindness in children. *Lancet* 1:815–816, 1988.

64. Esparza J, Portillo J, et al: Outcome in children with severe head injuries. *Childs Nerv Syst* 1:109–114, 1985.

65. Eviatar L, Bergtraum M, Randel RM: Post-traumatic vertigo in children: a diagnostic approach. *Pediatr Neurol* 2:61–66, 1986.

66. Ewing-Cobbs L, Fletcher JM, Levin HS: Neurobehavioral sequelae following head injury in children: Educational implications. *J Head Trauma Rehabil* 1:57–65, 1986.

67. Ewing-Cobbs L, Levin HS, Fletcher JM, Miner ME, Eisenberg HM: Post-traumatic

amnesia in head-injured children: Assessment and outcome. *J Clin Exper Neuropsych* 11:58–61, 1989.

68. Ewing-Cobbs L, Miner JM, Fletcher JM, Levin HS: Intellectual, motor and language sequelae following closed head injury in infants and preschoolers. *J Pediatr Psychol* 14:531–547, 1989.

69. Facco E, Zuccarello M, et al: Early outcome prediction in severe head injury: Comparison between children and adults. *Childs Nerv Syst* 2:67–71, 1986.

70. Fay G, Janesheski J: Neuropsychological assessment of head injured children. *J Head Trauma Rehabil* 1:16–21, 1986.

71. Field LH, Weiss CJ: Dysphagia with head injury. *Brain Injury* 3:19–26, 1989.

72. Filley CM, Cranberg LD, Alexander MP, Hart EJ: Neurobehavioral outcome after closed head injury in childhood and adolescence. *Arch Neurol* 44:194–198, 1987.

73. Finger S, Stein DG: *Brain Damage and Recovery.* New York, Academic Press, 1982.

74. Friedman SL, Klivington KA, Peterson RW: *The Brain, Cognition and Education.* New York, Academic Press, 1986.

75. Frowein RA: Prognostic assessment of coma in relation to age. *Acta Neurochir* 28:3–12, 1979.

76. Gennarelli TA: Mechanisms and pathophysiology of cerebral concussion. *J Head Trauma Rehabil* 2:23–29, 1986.

77. Glenn MB, Whyte J (eds): *The Practical Management of Spasticity in Children and Adults.* Philadelphia, Lea & Febiger, 1990.

78. Gilles JD, Seshia SS: Vegetative state following coma in childhood: Evaluation and outcome. *Dev Med Child Neurol* 22:642–648, 1980.

79. Glisky E, Schachter DL: Remediation of organic memory disorders: current status and future prospects. *J Head Trauma Rehabil* 1:54–63, 1986.

80. Golden CJ: The Luria-Nebraska Children's Battery: Theory and formulation. In Hynd GW, Orbzut JE (eds): *Neuropsychological Assessment and the School-Age Child: Issues and Procedures.* New York, Grune & Stratton, 1981.

81. Goldstein FC, Levin HS: Intellectual and academic outcome following closed head injury in children and adolescents: Research strategies and empirical findings. *Dev Neuropsych* 1:195–214, 1985.

82. Goodwin WJ: Temporal bone fractures. *Otolaryngol Clin North Am* 16:651–659, 1983.

83. Gordon NS, Fois A, Jacobi G, et al: Consensus statement: the management of the comatose child. *Neuropediatrics* 14:3–5, 1983.

84. Gordon WA, Hibbard MR, Kreutzer JS: Cognitive rehabilitation: Issues in research and practice. *J Head Trauma Rehabil* 4:76–84, 1989.

85. Gouvier WD, Blanton PD, LaPorte KK, Nepomuceno C: Reliability and validity of the Disability Rating Scale and the Levels of Cognitive Functioning Scale in monitoring recovery from severe head injury. *Arch Phys Med Rehabil* 68:94–97, 1987.

86. Greenough WE, Juraska JM: *Developmental Neuropsychobiology.* New York, Academic Press, 1986.

87. Griffith ER, Rosenthal M, Bond MR, Miller JD (eds): *Rehabilitation of the Child and Adult with Traumatic Brain Injury,* ed 2. Philadelphia, FA Davis, 1990.

88. Gulbrandsen GB: Neuropsychological sequelae of light head injuries in children 6 months after trauma. *J Clin Neuropsych* 3:257–268, 1984.

89. Hagen C, Malkmus D, Durham P: *Levels of Cognitive Functioning.* Downey, CA, Rancho Los Amigos Hospital, 1979.

90. Hahn YS, Chyung C, et al: Head injuries in children under 36 months of age. Demography and outcome. *Childs Nerv Syst* 4:34–40, 1988.

91. Haley SM, Cioffi MI, et al: Motor dysfunction in children and adolescents after traumatic brain injury. *J Head Trauma Rehabil* 5:77–90, 1990.

92. Haley SM, Hallenborg SC, Gans BM: Functional assessment in young with neurologic impairments. *Topics in Early Childhood Education* 9:106–126, 1989.

93. Halloran LD, Zfass AM, Gayle WE, Wheeler CB, Miller JD: Prevention of acute gastrointestinal complications after severe head injury: a controlled trial of cimetidine prophylaxis. *Am J Surg* 139:44–48, 1980.

94. Hannah MK, Scipio W, Suh K, et al: Urodynamics in children. Part II. The pseudoneurogenic bladder. *J Urol* 125:534–537, 1981.

95. Hannay HJ, Levin HS, Grossman RG: Impaired recognition memory after head injury. *Cortex* 15:269–283, 1979.

96. Hans P, Albert A, Franssen D, Born J: Improved outcome prediction based on CSF extrapolated creatine kinase BB isoenzyme activity and other risk factors in severe head injury. *J Neurosurg* 71:54–58, 1989.

97. Harris B, Schwaitzberg S, et al: The hidden morbidity of pediatric trauma. *J Pediatr Surg* 24:103–106, 1989.

98. Hartlage LC, Telzron CR: The neuropsychological basis of educational intervention. *J Learn Disabil* 16:521–528, 1983.

99. Hauser WA: Prevention of post-traumatic epilepsy. *N Engl J Med* 323:540–541, 1990.

100. Hecox KE, Cone B, Blaw ME: Brainstem auditory evoked response in the diagnosis of pediatric neurologic disease. *Neurology* 31:832–840, 1981.

101. Heilman KM, Valenstein E (eds): *Clinical Neuropsychology,* ed 2. New York, Oxford University Press, 1985.

102. Hetzel DJ, Bochner F, Hallpike JF, Shearman DJ: Cimetidine interaction with phenytoin. *Br Med J* 282:1512, 1981.

103. Hoffer M, Garrett A et al: The orthopedic management of brain-injured children. *J Bone Joint Surg* 53A:567–577, 1971.

104. Hume AL, et al: Central somatosensory conduction time in comatose patients. *Ann Neurol* 5:379–384, 1979.

105. Ito V, et al: Brain swelling and brain edema in acute head injury. *Acta Neurochir* 79:120–125, 1986.

106. Ivan LP, Choo SH, Ventureyra EC: Head injuries in childhood: A two year study. *Can Med Assoc J* 128:281–284, 1983.

107. Jacobi G, Ritz A, Emrich R: Cranial nerve damage after pediatric head trauma: A long term follow-up study of 741 cases. *Acta Pediatr Hung* 27:173–187, 1986.

108. Jacobson HS, Rubenstein EM, Bohannon WE, et al: Follow-up of adolescent trauma victims: A new model of care. *Pediatrics* 77:236–241, 1986.

109. Jaffe KM, Hays RM: Pediatric head injury rehabilitative medical management. *J Head Trauma Rehabil* 1:30–40, 1986.

110. Jagger J, Levine JT, Jane JA, et al: Epidemiologic features of head injury in a predominantly rural population. *J Trauma* 24:40–44, 1984.

111. Jenkins A: MRI scan after head trauma. *Lancet* 2:445–448, 1986.

112. Jennett B, Bond M: Assessment of outcome after severe brain damage. A practical scale. *Lancet* 1:480–484, 1975.

113. Jennett B, Teasdale G: *Management of Head Injuries.* Philadelphia, FA Davis, 1981.

114. Johnson DA, Uttley D, Wyke M (eds): *Children's Head Injury, Who Cares?* New York, Taylor and Francis, 1989.

115. Jordan FM, Ozanne AE, Murdoch BE: Long-term speech and language disorders subsequent to closed head injury in children. *Brain Injury* 2:179–185, 1988.

116. Kaiser G, Rudenberg A, et al: Rehabilitation medicine following severe head injury in infants and children. In Raimondi AJ, Choux M, Di Rocco C (ed): *Head Injuries in the Newborn and Infant.* New York, Springer Verlag, 1986.

117. Kanter RK, Carroll JB, Post EM: Association of arterial hypertension with poor outcome in children with acute brain injury. *Clin Pediatr* 24:320–323, 1985.

118. Karwacki JJ, Baker S: Children in motor vehicles: Never too young to die. *JAMA* 242:2848–2851, 1979.

119. Kaufmann CR, Maier RV, et al: Evaluation of pediatric trauma score. *JAMA* 263:69–72, 1990.

120. Kay T: *The Unseen Injury: Minor Head Trauma.* Southboro MA, National Head Injury Foundation.

121. Kaye EM, Herskowitz J: Transient post-traumatic blindness: brief vs prolonged syndromes in childhood. *J Child Neurol* 1:206–210, 1986.

122. Keenan MAE: The orthopedic management of spasticity. *J Head Trauma Rehabil* 2:62–71, 1987.

123. Kempe CH, Silverman FN, et al: The battered child syndrome. *JAMA* 251:3288–3294, 1984.

124. Kennedy CR, Freeman JM: Post-traumatic seizures and post-traumatic epilepsy in children. *J Head Trauma Rehabil* 1:66–73, 1986.

125. Kerr MM, Nelson CM: *Strategies for Managing Behavior Problems in the Classroom.* Columbus OH, Charles E. Merrill, 1983.

126. Kissoon N, Dreyer J, Walian: Pediatric trauma: Differences in pathophysiology, injury patterns and treatment compared with adult trauma. *Can Med Assoc J* 142:27–34, 1990.

127. Kishore PR, Lipper MH, et al: Post-traumatic hydrocephalus in patients with severe head injury. *Neuroradiology* 16:261–265, 1978.

128. Klauber MR, Barrett-Conner E, Marshall LF, et al: The epidemiology of head trauma: A prospective study of an entire community—San Diego County, California. *Am J Epidemiol* 113:500–509, 1981.

129. Klonoff H, Low M, Clark C: Head injuries in children: A prospective five year follow-up. *J Neurol Neurosurg Psychiat* 40:1211–1219, 1977.

130. Kraus JF, Fife D, Conroy C: Pediatric brain injuries: the nature, clinical course and early outcomes in a defined United States population. *Pediatrics* 79:501–507, 1987.

131. Kraus JF, Rock A, Hemyari P: Brain injuries among infants, children, adolescents and young adults. *Am J Dis Child* 144:684–691, 1990.

132. Kretschmer H: Prognosis of severe head injury in childhood and adolescence. *Neuropediatrics* 14:176–181, 1983.

133. Kriel RL, Krach LE, Sheehan M: Outcome of profound traumatic head injuries in children: unconsciousness longer than 90 days. *Arch Phys Med Rehabil* 69:678–681, 1988.

134. Kriel RLK, Krach LE, Panser LA: Closed head injury: Comparison of children younger and older than 6 years of age. *Pediatr Neurol* 5:296–300, 1989.

135. Lange-Cosack H, Wider B, Schlesner HJ, et al: Prognosis of brain injuries in young children (one until five years of age). *Neuropaediatria* 10:105–127, 1979.

136. Langfitt TW, Obrist WD, Alavi A, et al: Computerized tomography, magnetic resonance imaging, and positron emission tomography in the study of brain trauma. Preliminary observations. *J Neurosurg* 64:760–767, 1986.

137. Lehr E: *Psychological Management of Traumatic Brain Injuries in Children and Adolescents.* Rockville Md, Aspen Publishers, 1990.

138. Leonidas JC, Ting W, et al: Mild head trauma in children: When is a roentgenogram necessary? *Pediatrics* 69:139–143, 1982.

139. Levin HS, Amparo EG, et al: Magnetic resonance imaging after closed head injury in children. *Neurosurgery* 24:223–227, 1989.

140. Levin HS, Eisenberg HM, Benton AL (eds): *Mild Head Injury.* New York, Oxford University Press, 1989.

141. Levin HS, Grafman J, Eisenberg HM (eds): *Neurobehavioral Recovery from Head Injury.* New York, Oxford University Press, 1987.

142. Levin HS, High WM, Ewing-Cobbs L, et al: Memory functioning during the first year after closed head injury in children and adolescents. *Neurosurgery* 22:1043–1052, 1988.

143. Levin HS, Madison CF, Bailey CB, et al: Mutism after closed head injury. *Arch Neurol* 40:601–606, 1983.

144. Levy DE, Sidtis JJ, Rottenberg DA, et al: Differences in cerebral flow and glucose utilization in vegetative versus locked in patients. *Ann Neurol* 22:673–682, 1987.
145. Lewin W, Roberts AM: Long term prognosis after severe head injury. *Acta Neurochir* S28:128–133, 1979.
146. Light R, Neumann E, Lewis R, et al: An evaluation of a neuropsychologically based reeducation project for the head-injured child. *J Head Trauma Rehabil* 2:11–25, 1987.
147. Logeman J: *Evaluation and Treatment of Swallowing Disorders.* San Diego, College Hill Press, 1983.
148. Luerssen TG, Klauber MR, Marshall LF: Outcome from head injury related to age. *J Neurosurg* 68:409–416, 1988.
149. Lundar T, Nestvold K: Pediatric head injuries caused by traffic accidents: A prospective study with 5 year follow-up. *Childs Nerv Syst* 1:24–28, 1985.
150. Lutschg J, Pfenniger J, et al: Brainstem auditory evoked potentials and early somatosensory evoked potentials in neurointensively treated comatose children. *Am J Dis Child* 137:421–426, 1983.
151. Mahoney WJ, D'Souza BJ, Haller JA, et al: Long term outcome of children with severe trauma and prolonged coma. *Pediatrics* 71:756–762, 1983.
152. Maki Y, Akimoto H, Enomoto T: Injuries of basal ganglia following head trauma in children. *Child Brain* 7:113–123, 1980.
153. Margolis LS, Shaywitz BA: The outcome of prolonged coma in children. *Pediatrics* 65:477–481, 1980.
154. Marshall JF: Neural plasticity and recovery of function after brain injury. *Internat Rev Neurobiol* 26:201–247, 1985.
155. Matheny AP, Fisher EJ: Behavioral perspectives on children's accidents. *Adv Dev Behav Pediatr* 5:221–264, 1984.
156. Maurer AH: Nuclear medicine: SPECT comparison to PET. *Radiol Clin North Am* 26:1059–1074, 1988.
157. Mazziotta JC, Phelps ME, Miller J, Kuhl DE: Tomographic mapping of human cerebral metabolism: Normal unstimulated state. *Neurology* 31:503–516, 1981.
158. McGuire TL, Rothenberg MB: Behavioral and psychosocial sequelae of pediatric head injury. *J Head Trauma Rehabil* 1:1–6, 1986.
159. McQueen JK, Blackwood DHR, et al: Low risk of late post-traumatic seizures following severe head injury: Implications for clinical trials of prophylaxis. *J Neurol Neurosurg Psychiatry* 46:899–904, 1983.
160. Meller JL, Shermata DW: Falls in urban children: A problem revisted. *Am J Dis Child* 141:1271, 1987.
161. Miller N: *Dyspraxia and Its Management.* Frederick, MD, Aspen Publications, 1986.
162. Miller WL, Kaplan SL, Grumbach MM: Child abuse: a cause of post-traumatic hypopituitarism. *N Engl J Med* 302:724–728, 1980.
163. Milley JR, Nugent SK, Rogers MC: Neurogenic pulmonary edema in childhood. *J Pediatr* 94:706–709, 1979.
164. Miner M, Wagner KA (eds): *Neural Trauma: Monitoring and Rehabilitation Issues.* Boston, Butterworths, 1986.
165. Mital MA, Garber JE, Stinson JT: Ectopic bone formation in children and adolescents with head injuries: Its management. *J Pediatr Orthop* 7:83–90, 1987.
166. Mochizuki Y, et al: Developmental changes of brain stem auditory evoked potentials (BAEPs) in normal human subjects from infants to young adults. *Brain Dev* 4:127–133, 1982.
167. Molnar GE: Orthotic management of children. In Redford J (ed): *Orthotics Etc.* Baltimore, Williams & Wilkins, ed. 2. 1986.
168. Morgan SF: Measuring long-term memory storage and retrieval in children. *J Clin Neuropsychol* 4:77–85, 1982.

169. Morray JP, Tyler DC, et al: Coma scale for use in brain-injured children. *Crit Care Med* 12:1018–1020, 1984.
170. Murdoch BE, Chenery HJ, Kennedy M: Aphemia associated with bilateral striato-capsular lesions subsequent to cerebral anoxia. *Brain Trauma* 3:41–49, 1989.
171. National Head Injury Foundation, Special Education Task Force: *An Educator's Manual: What Educators Need to Know about Students with Traumatic Brain Injury.* Revised Edition. Framingham, MA, National Head Injury Foundation, 1988.
172. Obrzut E, Hynd GW: Cognitive dysfunction and psychoeducational assessment in individuals with acquired brain injury. *J Learn Disabil* 20:596–602, 1987.
173. Pang D, Wilberger JE: Spinal cord injury without radiographic abnormalities in children. *J Neurosurg* 57:114–119, 1982.
174. Parente R, Anderson-Parente JK: Retraining memory: Theory and application. *J Head Trauma Rehabil* 4:55–65, 1989.
175. Parmelee DX: Neuropsychiatric sequelae of traumatic brain injury in children and adolescents. *Psychiatr Med* 7:11–16, 1989.
176. Paulson JA: The case for mandatory seat restraint laws. *Clin Pediatr* 20:285–290, 1981.
177. Phelps ME, Mazziotta JC: Positron emission tomography: human brain function and biochemistry. *Science* 128:799–809, 1985.
178. Plaisted JR, Gustavson JL, et al: The Luria-Nebraska Neuropsychological Battery—Children's Revision: Theory and current research findings. *J Clin Child Psychol* 12:13–21, 1983.
179. Pless BI, Verreault R, Arsenault L, Frappier J, Stulginskas J: The epidemiology of road accidents in childhood. *Am J Public Health* 77:358–360, 1987.
180. Povlischock JT, Becker DP, Cheng CLY, et al: Axonal damage in minor head injury. *J Neuropath Exp Neurol* 42:225–252, 1983.
181. Raimondi AJ, Choux M, Di Rocco C (eds): *Head Injuries in the Newborn and Infant.* New York, Springer Verlag, 1986.
182. Ramenofsky ML, Powell RW, Curreri RW: Gastroesophageal reflux: pH probe directed therapy. *Ann Surg* 203:531–534, 1986.
183. Rankin J, Aram D, Horowitz S: Language ability in right and left hemiplegic children. *Brain Lang* 14:292–294, 1981.
184. Rapp D: *Brain Injury Casebook: Methods for Reintegration into the Home, School and Community.* Springfield, IL, Charles C Thomas, 1986.
185. Rappaport M: Brain evoked potentials in coma and the vegetative state. *J Head Trauma Rehabil* 1:15–29, 1986.
186. Reitan RM, Wolfson D: *The Halstead-Reitan Neuropsychological Test Battery: Theory and Clinical Interpretation.* Tucson, Neuropsychology Press, 1985.
187. Ring IT, Berry G, et al: Epidemiology and clinical outcomes of neurotrauma in New South Wales. *Aust NZ J Surg* 56:557–566, 1986.
188. Ritter W, Ford JM, Gaillard AWK, et al: Cognition and event related potentials: I. The relation of negative potentials and cognitive processes. *Ann NY Acad Sci* 425:24–38, 1989.
189. Rivara F, Tanaguchi D, et al: Poor prediction of positive computed tomography scans by clinical criteria in symptomatic pediatric head trauma. *Pediatrics* 80:579–584, 1987.
190. Rivara FP: Child pedestrian injuries in the United States. *Am J Dis Child* 144:692–696, 1990.
191. Rivara FP, Kamitsuka MD, Quan L: Injuries to children younger than 1 year of age. *Pediatrics* 81:93–97, 1988.
192. Rivara FP, Mueller BA: The epidemiology and prevention of pediatric head injury. *J Head Trauma Rehabil* 1:7–15, 1986.
193. Roberts AH: *Severe Accidental Head Injury.* London, McMillan Press LTD, 1979.
194. Robertson CS, Clifton GL, Taylor AA, et al: Treatment of hypertension associated with head injury. *J Neurosurg* 59:455–460, 1983.

195. Rodriquez J, Brown S: Childhood injuries in the United States. *Am J Dis Child* 144:627–646, 1990.
196. Rosen C, Gerring J: *Head Trauma: Educational Reintegration.* San Diego, College Hill Press, 1986.
197. Ross ED: The aprosodias: Functional organization of the affective components of language in the right hemisphere. *Arch Neurol* 38:561–589, 1981.
198. Rourke BP, Fisk JL, Strang JD: *Neuropsychological Assessment of Children: A Treatment Oriented Approach.* New York, The Guilford Press, 1986.
199. Rutter M (ed): *Developmental Neuropsychiatry.* New York, Guilford Press, 1983.
200. Sackeim HA, Greenberg MA, et al: Hemispheric asymmetry in the expression of positive or negative emotions. *Arch Neurol* 39:210–218, 1982.
201. Salamy A: Maturation of the auditory brainstem response from birth through early childhood. *J Clin Neurophysiol* 1:293–329, 1984.
202. Sarno MT: The nature of verbal impairment after closed head injury. *J Nerv Ment Dis* 168:685–692, 1980.
203. Schain RJ: *Medications in Learning Disorders: Neurology of Childhood Learning Disorders.* Baltimore, Williams & Wilkins, 1977.
204. Seelig JM, Becker DP, Miller JD, Greenberg RP, Ward JD, Choi SC: Traumatic acute subdural hematoma: Major mortality reduction in comatose patients treated within 4 hours. *N Engl J Med* 304:1511–1518, 1981.
205. Shaffer D, Bijur P, Chadwick OF, Rutter M: Head injury and later reading disability. *J Am Acad Child Psychiat* 19:592–10, 1980.
206. Shapiro K (ed): *Pediatric Head Trauma.* Mount Kisco, NY, Futura Publishing Co, 1983.
207. Shaul PW, Towbin RB, Chernausek SD: Precocious puberty following severe head trauma. *Am J Dis Child* 139:467–469, 1985.
208. Simpson D, Reilly P: Pediatric coma scale. *Lancet* 2:450–454, 1982.
209. Slater EJ, Bassett SS: Adolescents with closed head injuries. *Am J Dis Child* 142:1048–1051, 1988.
210. Solis J, Krouskop T, Trainer N, Marburger R: Supine interface pressure in children. *Arch Phys Med Rehabil* 69:524–526, 1988.
211. Sollee ND, Kindlon DJ: Lateralized brain injury and behavior problems in children. *J Abnorm Child Psychol* 15:479–491, 1987.
212. Spivack MP: Advocacy and legislative action for head-injured children and their families. *J Head Trauma Rehabil* 1:41–47, 1986.
213. Squire L, Butters N (eds): *Neuropsychology of Memory.* New York, Guilford Press, 1984.
214. Stover SL, Niemann KM, Miller JM: Disodium etidronate in the prevention of post-operative occurrence of heterotopic ossification in spinal cord injury patients. *J Bone Joint Surg* 58A:683–688, 1976.
215. Stover SL, Zieger HE: Head injury in children and teenagers: Functional recovery correlated with the duration of coma. *Arch Phys Med Rehabil* 57:201–205, 1976.
216. Tarter RE, Goldstein G (eds): *Advances in Clinical Neuropsychology.* Vol. 2. New York, Plenum Press, 1984.
217. Teasdale G, Jennett B: Assessment of coma and impaired consciousness: A practical scale. *Lancet* 2:81–84, 1976.
218. Telzrow CF: Management of academic and educational problems in head injury. *J Learn Disabil* 20:536–545, 1987.
219. Temkin NR, Dimken SS, Wilensky A, et al: A randomized double-blind study of phenytoin for the prevention of post-traumatic seizures. *N Engl J Med* 323:497–502, 1990.
220. Tepas JJ, Ramenofsky ML, Barlow B, Gans BM, Di Scala C: Mortality in head injury: The pediatric perspective. *J Pediatr Surg* 25:92–96, 1990.
221. Tepas JJ, Ramenofsky ML, et al: The pediatric trauma score as a predictor of injury severity: An objective assessment. *J Trauma* 28:425–429, 1988.

222. Ter-Pogossian MM, Raichle ME, Sobel BE: Positron emmission tomography. *Scientif Am* 243:170–181, 1980.
223. Thompson RF: The neurobiology of learning and memory. *Science* 233:941–946, 1986.
224. Todorow S: Recovery of children after severe head injury: Psychoreactive superimpositions. *Scand J Rehabil Med* 7:93–96, 1975.
225. Tsubokawa T, Yamamoto T, Katayama Y: Prediction of outcome of prolonged coma caused by brain damage. *Brain Injury* 4:329–337, 1990.
226. Vane DW, Shiffler M, Grossfield JL, et al: Reduced lower esophageal sphincter (LES) pressure after acute and chronic brain injury. *J Pediatr Surg* 17:960–964, 1982.
227. Varga-Khadem F, O'Gorman AM, Watters GV: Aphasia and handedness in relation to hemispheric side, age at injury and severity of cerebral lesion during childhood. *Brain* 108:677–696, 1985.
228. Vartiainen E, Karjalainen S, Karja J: Auditory disorders following head injury in children. *Acta Otolaryngol* 99:529–536, 1985.
229. Vining EPG, et al: Effects of phenobarbital and sodium valproate on neuropsychologic function and behavior. *Ann Neurol* 14:360–364, 1983.
230. Waaland PK, Kreutzer JS: Family response to childhood traumatic injury. *J Head Trauma Rehabil* 3:51–63, 1988.
231. Wagstyle J, Sutcliffe AJ, Alpar EK: Early prediction of outcome following head injury in children. *J Pediatr Surg* 22:127–129, 1987.
232. Waller AE, Baker SP, Szocka A: Childhood injury deaths: National analysis and geographic variation. *Am J Publ Health* 79:310–315, 1989.
233. Watson GS, Zador PL, Wilks A: The repeal of helmet use laws and increased motorcyclist mortality in the United States, 1975–1978. *Am J Publ Health* 70:579–585, 1980.
234. Weber PL: Sensorimotor therapy: Its effect on electroencephalograms of acute comatose patients. *Arch Phys Med Rehabil* 65:457–462, 1982.
235. Whitman S, Cooley-Hoganson R, Desai BT: Comparative head trauma experience in two socioeconomically different Chicago-area communities: A population study. *Am J Epidemiol* 119:570–580, 1984.
236. Whittle IR, Johnston IH, Besser M: Short latency somatosensory evoked potentials in children. Part I. Normative data. *Surg Neurol* 27:9–18, 1987.
237. Whittle IR, Johnston IH, Besser M: Short latency somatosensory evoked potentials in children. Part 3. Findings following head injury. *Surg Neurol* 27:29–36, 1987.
238. Wilkinson WS, Han DP, Rappley MD, Owings CL: Retinal hemorrhage predicts neurologic injury in the shaken baby syndrome. *Arch Ophthalmol* 107:1472–1474, 1989.
239. Williams DT, Mehl R, Yudofsky S, et al: The effect of propranolol on uncontrolled rage outbursts in children and adolescents with organic brain dysfunction. *J Am Acad Child Psychiat* 21:129–135, 1982.
240. Wilson B, Moffat N: *Clinical Management of Memory Problems.* Frederick, MD, Aspen Publishers, 1984.
241. Winogron HW, Knights RM, Bawden HN: Neuropsychologic deficits following head injury in children. *J Clin Neuropsychol* 4:91–115, 1984.
242. Yager JY, Johnson B, Seshia SS: Coma scales in pediatric practice. *Am J Dis Child* 144:1088–1091, 1990.
243. Yamamoto, Bart RD: Transient blindness following mild head trauma. *Clin Pediatr* 27:479–483, 1988.
244. Ylvisaker M (ed): *Head Injury Rehabilitation, Children and Adolescents.* San Diego, College Hill Press, 1985.
245. Ylvisaker M, Weinstein M: Recovery of oral feeding after pediatric head injury. *J Head Trauma Rehabil* 4:51–63, 1989.
246. Zimmerman RA, Bilaniuk LT: Computed tomography in pediatric head trauma. *J Neuroradiol* 6:257–271, 1981.

12

Rehabilitation of the Child with Joint Disease

BARBARA M. KOCH

The most common form of joint disease in childhood is juvenile rheumatoid arthritis (JRA). Other conditions that produce arthritis and musculoskeletal complaints in childhood include dermatomyositis, scleroderma, ankylosing spondylitis, systemic lupus erythematosus, Kawasaki disease, infectious arthritis, and hemophiliac arthropathy. Each disease process will be defined and the nature of the expected disability discussed. Rehabilitation treatment techniques, including therapeutic exercise, splints, activities of daily living, and recreational activities will be reviewed.

Juvenile Rheumatoid Arthritis

The diagnosis of juvenile rheumatoid arthritis (JRA) requires 6 or more consecutive weeks of objective synovitis (57). JRA is characterized by chronic synovial inflammation of unknown cause and affects 60,000 to 200,000 children in the United States (47). Thus, it is a disease that produces a high incidence of childhood disability. The disease may present with typical systemic symptoms, arthralgia, rash, and fever. It is extremely important to exclude infections, neoplasms, orthopaedic conditions, and rheumatoid variants.

JRA appears to be a different disease than adult arthritis. The adult form usually has a relentless course with persistent deformities. Of those children with JRA, 75% have long periods of remission with ultimately no residual deformity (54). Several manifestations appear to accompany JRA more frequently than adult-onset arthritis. High fever and rheumatoid rash are prominent in children but present very rarely in adults. Iridocyclitis occurs in over 9% of the children and in less than 1% of the adults. Monoarticular manifestation is frequent in the pediatric age group but is rare in the adult population. Cervical apophysial disease is present in 25% of affected children and only in 10% of adults with arthritis. Leukocytosis, ranging from 15,000 to 18,000, is more common in the juvenile type than in the adult form.

On the other hand, subcutaneous nodules are frequent in adults but not in children.

It is important to realize that there is no laboratory test diagnostic for JRA. Rheumatoid factor (RF) is positive in 15% of the polyarticular population while antinuclear antibodies and HLA-B27 antigens may be present in children with pauciarticular disease. Other laboratory studies, such as the white blood cell count, erythrocyte sedimentation rate (ESR), and x-rays may be negative. Radiological studies are initially normal and not helpful in diagnosis but rather a means of determining late articular destruction. Although pediatric and adult rheumatoid arthritis are similar, differences include the role of the parents, growth and development, and prognosis (57).

CLASSIFICATION

Although JRA is described as a single disease, it is probably a group of diseases with distinct modes of onset and varied prognoses. Recognizing the different subtypes helps plan the most appropriate management for each child.

Systemic Onset Disease

Approximately 20% of children with JRA have systemic onset disease. Children with this type of disease present with fever of unknown origin, and generally appear toxic and listless. Diurnal temperature variations may be as much as 5°C, rising from the subnormal range to 41°C in the course of 1 day. An erythematous or maculopapular rash with central clearing may appear on the trunk, neck, or extremities (12). There may be significant lymphadenopathy, pericarditis, pneumonitis, hepatosplenomegaly, and enlarged mesenteric lymph nodes, which may produce severe abdominal pain suggestive of an acute abdomen (12). Much of this group has significant growth retardation (1) or delayed sexual maturation due to a chronic inflammatory state or long-term use of steroids. Elevation of ESR, white blood cell count, and a marked anemia may also be part of the systemic signs. At the onset, those may be only arthralgias and/or myalgias rather than true arthritis. Development of arthritis occurs within months to weeks after onset. Approximately 25% develop severe chronic arthritis which continues after systemic manifestations subside (29). The child often assumes a position of flexion and refuses to walk, even when frank arthritis is not evident. Involvement of the cervical spine is very common with systemic onset of the disease (54). The course may be recurrent episodes of systemic symptoms or development of polyarticular arthritis. Of those patients who have severe arthritis with progressive joint destruction, 25% show permanent joint deformity (54).

Polyarticular Disease

Of all children with JRA, 40% have polyarticular involvement with five or more joints affected. Children with polyarticular disease may have extra-articular symptoms, such as low-grade fever up to 39°C, slight organomegaly, mild anemia, malaise, and weight loss. Generally, there is symmetric involvement of the small joints of the hands and feet, as well as of the cervical spine, wrists, hips, and knees. The affected joints are warm with decreased range of motion (ROM) and swelling. Although joint pain may be absent, the child may wince on movement and may be reluctant to walk or play (12). Of this group, 85% are negative for RF and generally have less severe joint damage. However, the prognosis for these children is also related to age at the onset of symptoms. Girls under age 5 yr with negative RF have the most severe joint problems whereas those with RF negative polyarticular disease of later onset tend to have milder joint disease. The 15% who are rheumatoid factor positive with polyarticular disease are usually 8 yr or older at the onset of disease. These patients resemble adults with rheumatoid arthritis and have a greater likelihood of severe erosive disease and resultant disability (1). Within 4½ yr of onset, 50% of children in the polyarticular group have incurred considerable disability in a series observed by Schaller (53).

Pauciarticular Disease

The third group of patients are those with pauciarticular disease, which involves four or fewer joints within the first 6 months of the onset of the disease. Generally, the large joints are affected, including the knee, ankle, elbow, or wrist. Small joints of the hands or feet are rarely involved (53). Diagnosis may require synovial fluid analysis and synovial biopsy to rule out infection, malignancy, or foreign body as etiological factors (13).

In pauciarticular disease, there is a preponderance of females and 60% have a positive antinuclear antibody (ANA) test. The knee, ankle, or elbow are the most commonly affected joints and the joint disease is generally mild. However, asymmetrical growth of limbs and localized deformity are common in this group (1). Asymmetrical growth is secondary to increased vascular supply to the involved extremity. Of the children with pauciarticular type of disease, 10–50% will develop iridocyclitis, leading to permanent visual loss, including blindness in one or both eyes. Therefore, this group must have regular and frequent ophthalmological examinations.

The other subgroup of pauciarticular disease is seen primarily in boys over the age of 8 yr and is accompanied by the presence of HLA-B27 antigen and the absence of ANA or RF. The arthritis is asymmetric with primary involvement of the lower extremities. Sacroiliitis may be present or may develop later. Radiological evidence of sacroiliitis often appears years later. Although it may be years before the arthritis becomes manifest in the thoracic and lumbar spine, boys who are HLA-B27 positive are highly suspect for ankylosing spondylosis. If they develop sacroiliitis or arthritis of the thoracic or lumbar spine, they should be separated from the category of JRA and a different therapeutic approach taken (1).

There are also children with initial pauciarticular symptoms who do not conform to either of these subtypes; they slowly develop polyarticular manifestations. In this group, there is a prolonged course of chronic arthritis and morbidity that requires long-term monitoring and treatment.

EVALUATION

Evaluation of a child with JRA entails assessment of individual joints and overall functional status. Degree of fatigue and length of morning stiffness need to be determined (56).

Each joint should be examined for tenderness, heat, and erythema. Passive and active joint motion must be recorded and must include every component of the anatomic range. It is important not to neglect accurate assessment of seemingly less significant joint motion, for example, ankle eversion, inversion, or hip external and internal rotation since restriction in these movements may be the first sign of joint inflammation. Muscle strength examination and measurement of limb girth and leg length are essential for complete evaluation. One should observe posture in standing and sitting, record asymmetry of shoulders, hips, or any other abnormalities of body alignment. Gait evaluation includes a description of pathological features, lurching, shuffling, painful limp, and guarding or abnormal position of joints.

Several systematic methods of functional evaluation have been proposed. Pendleton and associates (46) formulated a numerical scale but the complex assessment and scoring system requires considerable time. The method is more appropriate as a research tool than for clinical evaluation. MacBain and Hill (32) devised a functional assessment that is more practical for clinical use. This method includes observations of strength, dexterity, and mobility. It measures grip strength and functional abilities in terms of timed performance on walking, running, stair climbing, donning and doffing socks, and a specially designed vest with ¾-inch buttons. An evaluation designed by Boone and coworkers (9) consists of gross and fine motor activities related to ambulation and self-care, which are graded for speed and quality. This method of assessment is applicable to children who are 5 yr or older.

Developmental expectations and the effect of maturation are two important considerations in selecting a method of functional assessment for children and in the interpretation of results. Some items, such as running or buttoning, may be difficult or inappropriate for 2- to 3-yr-old children. On the other hand, increased speed of performance is a natural consequence of maturation and does not necessarily reflect improvement of the underlying disease. However, regression in speed or endurance for an age-appropriate activity can be attributed to the disease process provided that the child fully cooperates.

A functional classification with rather broad but fairly standard catego-

Table 12.1.
Functional Classification of Arthritis

Class	Function
I	No functional handicap, the patient can perform usual activities
II	Discomfort and loss of motion in one or more joints but the patient can perform usual activities
III	Limitation of joint range of motion, the patient can perform only small portion of usual activities
IV	Bed to chair existence, little or no self-help skills

ries, which has gained universal acceptance for evaluating patients with arthritis, is shown in Table 12.1.

PRINCIPLES OF TREATMENT

The goals of rehabilitation as defined by Calabro (13) are "to halt the ravages of disease and to prevent as much crippling and disability as possible and to revert by constant vigilance serious complications with each mode of onset." One must keep in mind that it is easier to maintain function in the affected joints than to regain function after it has been lost. Therefore, it is imperative to preserve good range of articular motion and muscle strength so that when the disease process remits the child is not left with disabling deformities and permanent functional limitations.

Drugs

The indications, dosage, and side effects of various drugs used to control joint inflammation and systemic complications are summarized in Table 12.2 (49). Intra-articular injection of steroids is helpful to decrease pain and to improve exercise tolerance. Intra-articular corticosteroid injections may be indicated with disabling pain or flexion deformities of one or two joints.

Reye's syndrome occurs more frequently with chickenpox than with other viral infections. Long-term aspirin treatment for arthritis may increase the risk of Reye's syndrome. Management of chickenpox or of flu-like symptoms in children with JRA include temporarily discontinuing the aspirin. The current recommendations of the American Academy of Pediatrics are to consider children with JRA high risk for influenza; they should be immunized against this infection on an annual basis (16).

Rest

The use of bed rest and joint immobilization remains a matter of debate. A study of adults with rheumatoid arthritis showed no significant differences between patients who were active and those placed on bed rest for 10 weeks (38). Similarly, when the effect of joint immobilization by casting was compared with a regimen of bed rest and daily active exercises, improvement

Table 12.2.
Drug Therapy of Juvenile Arthritis

Drug	Dose	Recommended Usage	Side Effects
Aspirin	90–130 mg/ kg in 4 divided doses with meals and before bed	1st drug	Metabolic acidosis and hyperpyrexia Respiratory alkalosis Lethargy Tinnitus Vomiting Gastrointestinal pain, melena, and abdominal discomfort rare Liver dysfunction
Corticosteroids	0.5–1 mg/kg	Pericarditis Iridocyclitis Life-threatening febrile disease Disease unresponsive to ASA	Retards growth Cataracts Hypertension Diabetes Weight gain Osteoporosis and vertebral compression fracture Pseudotumor cerebri
IM Gold aurothiomalate (Myochrysine)	0.5–1 mg/kg weekly (to 50 mg)	Arthritis unresponsive to ASA (3 months to see effect)	Hematuria Proteinuria Bone marrow depression Rash Metallic taste Mouth ulcers
Oral Gold Auranofin	0.1 mg/kg/ day	Remains experimental in collaborative study	Diarrhea Rash Ulcers Less frequently anemia, hematuria, proteinuria
Hydroxychloroquine (Plaquenil)	5–7 mg/kg/ 1 ×/day	Arthritis unresponsive to ASA (3 months to see effect)	Loss of peripheral vision Bone marrow depression Ophthalmologic exam every 6 months
Tolmetin sodium (Tolectin)	20–30 mg/ kg (200 mg tabs) 3 or 4 divided doses	Alternative to ASA	Abdominal pain Increased SGOT Headache
Naproxen (Naprosyn)	10–15 mg/ kg day 2 divided doses	Alternative to ASA 2 daily doses Antipyretic and antiinflammatory	Gastric discomfort Hematuria Peptic ulcer
Ibuprofen (Motrin)	20–50 mg/ kg 4 divided doses	Alternative to ASA Antipyretic and antiinflammatory	Abdominal discomfort Hematuria Peptic ulcer

was noted in joint mobility and function in both groups of adults after four weeks of treatment (66). There are no comparable data available on children with rheumatoid arthritis.

In the case of acute symptoms, properly prescribed rest allows resolution of synovial inflammation and prevents additional damage to the articular surfaces. During this time, proper splinting and daily ROM exercises are necessary. If there is acute hip or knee involvement, skin traction to maintain good alignment is recommended (2). Bed rest must be used judiciously because it was shown that active or passive exercises without normal loading of the joints is insufficient for maintaining the integrity of articular cartilage (2). Prolonged inactivity should be avoided because it leads to muscle weakness of disuse at a daily rate of 5% strength loss (18), osteoporosis, and other potential complications.

Ideally, children should rest 10 minutes out of every hour. Because such a schedule is not practical, particularly for children in school, 8–10 hours of daily bed rest are recommended with 1 hour in the middle of the day (69). Alternating active periods with quiet play achieves a similar purpose. Children can generally pace their activities with restrictions placed only on those areas that produce overtiring and joint pain (54).

Localized joint immobilization requires special considerations in children. In our experience and that of others, stiffness develops quickly in JRA and loss of motion tends to be rapid and permanent after prolonged cast application. Therefore, cast immobilization is recommended as a method of treatment only for periods of less than 48 hours (14). There is a lack of controlled studies on prolonged joint immobilization in children and, therefore, minimal immobilization with daily ROM exercises is generally suggested (66).

Heat

For relief of pain and muscle spasm, heat application offers symptomatic relief. Heat increases the temperature of the connective tissue around the joint and, thus, enhances elasticity, allowing easier stretching of the joint (2). Moist heat is more effective than dry heating modalities (69) and is particularly useful prior to exercises. In most children, a 20-minute warm bath helps to overcome morning stiffness and is the most practical method for daily application at home. Toys placed in the tub and the relaxing effect of water will induce a youngster to move the affected limbs actively. Parents who plan to install a whirlpool in their bath should be informed that the agitation of the water does not provide additional therapeutic benefits over a warm bath. A formal exercise program in the Hubbard tank or a therapeutic pool is often advisable. Baldwin (5) compared the effects of a home exercise program with weekly pool therapy in two groups of children. Although there was no difference in respect to mobility, children who participated in supervised pool therapy sessions showed increased strength. This form of treatment was also preferred by both parents and children because it is pain-free, fun, and socially therapeutic. Young children who may be frightened in a large tank often find a low-boy type of device without agitation more comforting and acceptable. Water temperature must be carefully monitored in young children to avoid scalding. For total body immersion, the temperature should be limited to less than 38.9° for a period of 20–40 minutes (31). However, patients with systemic onset JRA may not be able to tolerate this degree of heat since total body immersion can lead to further elevation of the core temperature. Morning stiffness can also be minimized by having the child sleep in a sleeping bag or warm pajamas to retain the body's natural heat (10).

Moist hot packs are most applicable when one or two large joints are affected, whereas paraffin baths are useful for arthritis involving the small joints of hands and feet. Both types of heating modalities can be purchased for home use.

Application of deep heating modalities requires caution in growing children because of its potential effect on the epiphyseal plate. In experimental animals, ultrasound in very high intensities produced epiphyseal damage with growth arrest and short wave diathermy stimulated increased limb growth (28). Children cannot be expected to report the sensation of warmth accurately, which is necessary when using short wave diathermy. They usually do not sit still for precise local application. Since most patients have multiple joint inflammation, the use of short wave diathermy or ultrasound with topical effect is impractical in these cases. Deep heating is also considered contraindicated in rheumatoid arthritis (20) because the resulting local temperature elevation accelerates synovial collagenase activity, which may enhance enzymatic lysis and destruction of the articular cartilage.

Since cold can produce temporary analgesia and decrease muscle spasm, rubbing with ice blocks may be used before exercises (31). The principal contraindication to cold application is the arthritis variant associated with Raynaud's phenomenon.

Massage

Light superficial massage tends to alleviate painful muscle spasm. It is most often used for the hip, wrist, and finger joints but is not helpful in arthritis of the shoulder.

Principles of Exercises

Referring to the role of exercises in arthritis, Calabro (13) aptly said, "What you don't use you lose." In terms of specific goals, exercises are intended to maintain ROM strength, teach efficient use of muscles and joints, encourage functional activities and proper ambulation, and, after surgical procedures, restore strength and joint mobility.

A program to fulfill these expectations must consist of active, active assistive, and resistive ROM exercises, which should be performed at least twice daily. The rationale of active assisted motion is based on the elastic properties of connective tissue whereby prolonged moderate tension leads to elongation. Since forceful passive movements result in connective tissue tears and avulsion of articular cartilage, movements should be carried to the point of feeling stretch but not pain. Persistent or increased discomfort and pain for 10 to 15 minutes after exercises indicates that stretching was too excessive and that the force must be eased (69). Assisted movements are followed by a succession of active and resistive exercises to avoid loss of strength, particularly in conjunction with bed rest (41). Isometric contractions may have to be substituted for maintaining strength if resistive exercises are not tolerated because of joint pain. A single muscle contraction of 6 seconds performed daily in a position of two thirds maximal length was found to be sufficient for increasing strength in rheumatoid arthritis (33).

As in other childhood disabilities, exercises are best presented in the form of play selected to encourage the therapeutically desirable movements. Children with painful arthritis are often resistant and fearful of exercises. Initially, a great deal of effort may have to be spent on gaining their trust. One must establish credibility that severe pain will not be inflicted by the examiner if the child is truthful in reporting it. An important aspect of rehabilitation is education of the parents in a home program and appropriate activities.

Posture

Proper posture is of utmost concern in patients with JRA. A child with long-standing disease tends to stand with bent hips and knees, rounded shoulders, and head and neck in flexion (Fig. 12.1). Postural training consists of standing tall, shoulders retracted, chest expanded, abdomen pulled in, and the feet facing straight ahead. A child must be taught to control pelvic obliquity, resulting from partial weight-bearing on a painful joint; otherwise, a secondary scoliosis is likely to occur. In sitting, straight back posture is emphasized and feet should rest flat on the floor. Proper height of the chair and writing desk is important to encourage good posture. Sitting for long periods should be avoided because it will lead to joint stiffness and knee and hip flexion contractures. The children are instructed to stand up and walk around periodically when any activity, including school work, entails prolonged sitting. Sleeping in a correct posture is extremely important. The mattress should be firm with a bedboard underneath. A flat pillow, or none at all, is recommended to prevent shoulder protraction and flexion deformity of the cervical spine. Children with rheumatoid arthritis prefer side lying in a fetal position of flexion (Fig. 12.2). Sleeping in the prone or supine position will discourage this habit and prevent increasing flexion contractures. Sleeping in lower extremity extension splints often decreases morning stiffness allowing easier mobility in the morning.

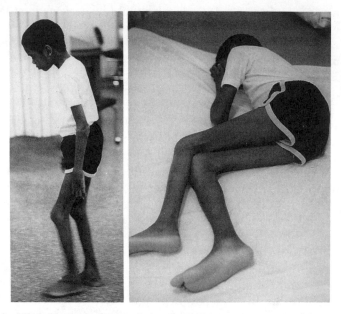

Figure 12.1. *Left,* Typical abnormal standing posture of juvenile rheumatoid arthritis patient with predominance of cervical spine flexion and protraction of shoulders.
Figure 12.2. *Right,* Patient in typical sleeping posture with hips and knees in flexion.

Ambulation

One can only give general outlines for the extent of walking. Any physical activity that involves walking should be modified or temporarily discontinued if it increases pain, swelling, or stiffness for 24 hours or more. Ambulation should be restricted in children with synovitis and flexion contracture of greater than 15° at the knee joint since malalignment will produce further articular damage. Therefore, partial weight-bearing is advisable. Children with severe arthritis and long-standing contractures may benefit from walking exercises in a therapeutic pool.

Ambulation training may be needed to emphasize correction of abnormal gait patterns, such as waddling, shuffling, stiff- or bent-knee walk, and, in arthritis of the ankle, lack of push-off. Reciprocal arm movements are stressed in arthritis of the upper limb, particularly when the elbow joint is affected, in order to avoid the habitual posture of resting the extremity against the pelvis or thigh.

Recreation

Well-selected sports and recreation are excellent exercises and offer the advantage of generally good compliance. Noncompetitive situations are preferable because the children are more likely to stop playing when discomfort appears. Trampoline, football, soccer, and other contact sports involving hard body impact must be avoided. Similarly, high joint stress, such as created by tennis or golf, is inadvisable. Nevertheless, the children are encouraged to participate in a variety of activities with adaptations if necessary. For example, volleyball, softball, and basketball are good activities to increase ROM, strength, and endurance; substitution of a beach ball or rubber ball will decrease potentially harmful joint impact. Ping-pong and badminton are nonstressful and fun. Baton twirling and playing yo-yo are appropriate for exercising the wrist and fingers. Among the arts and crafts, working with play-dough and clay, drawing, sewing, knitting, weaving, and model building represent some appropriate and enjoyable activities. Climbing and hanging on monkey bars are good for upper extremity stretching.

For preschool children, play cars, tractors, and other toys moved by pedals, or riding on a scooter will enhance hip and knee extension. Tricycle or bicycle seats should be elevated to provide maximal joint excursion.

Swimming is highly recommended for exercising all joints and is enjoyed by older children. Playing in a tub or wading pool is a substitute for preschoolers. Walking is a readily available exercise and stair climbing rather than riding the elevator may be encouraged in some cases.

Children with arthritis enjoy low impact aerobics. "People with Arthritis can Exercise", a 2-volume set of audio tapes, is available from the Arthritis Foundation. Studies of functional level and improvements in activities of daily living have been shown in rheumatoid patients who participate in endurance training (25).

Splints, Orthoses, and Shoe Modifications

Splints and braces must be light; they must be easy to apply and remove for the exercises that must be continued, even with localized joint rest. Dynamic hand splints with outriggers and other complicated features are generally not well tolerated by children. The compliance rate of any device is poor in children if they find that it disrupts their daily activities. With some exceptions, splints worn in the evening or night are more acceptable; however, they too must not immobilize so completely that the child cannot hold a doll or independently toilet during the night.

A detailed description of the different types of braces, splints, and shoe modifications and their indications are included in the section on treatment of specific joints.

Adaptive Devices and Techniques

The list of methods that can aid in performing daily activities and ambulation is virtually endless. Only a few samples are included here.

When there is limitation of shoulder or elbow motion, loosely fitted garments with front opening are recommended. Long-handled implements are helpful for combing or washing hard to reach body areas. Adapted utensils and implements with built-up handles may be necessary if there is loss of finger motion for making a fist or when grip strength is weakened.

Ambulation with crutches or other walking aids transfers part of the body weight to the arms, which may not be tolerable when upper extremity joints are affected. Arm platform attachments to crutches or a walkerette eliminate the pressure of weight-bearing from painful wrist and elbow joints. Of concern is that the patient who uses platform crutches for more than 3 months will lose elbow extension and the lost ROM is very difficult to regain.

Management of Specific Joints

Anticipating the problems that tend to occur in growing children who have inflammation of specific joints is the basis for planning an appropriate rehabilitation program.

Temporomandibular Joint. Although rarely involved in adults, this joint is commonly affected in children. The distance between the upper and lower teeth is measured to gauge the degree of movement limitation in these joints (Fig. 12.3). The children are encouraged to chew gum as an exercise to preserve maximal excursion of the jaw. Good oral hygiene, which is difficult to maintain with limited mouth opening, must be stressed. Micrognathia is not unusual and is attributed to the arthritic process or to secondary arrest of the mandibular epiphyses. Overcrowding of the teeth may necessitate orthodontic treatment.

Cervical Spine. Arthritis of the cervical spine affects the apophyseal joints with eventual fusion between C2 and C3 and, on occasion, other cervical vertebrae. ROM should be monitored serially. Although there is generally some loss of rotation and lateral flexion, the most severe limitation occurs in neck extension. Maximal attainable distance between the mandible and the manubrium sterni is an objective measurement of the range of extension. During the acute phase, the child should wear a cervical collar at

Figure 12.3. Significant involvement of temporomandibular joint with less than 1 cm between upper and lower teeth.

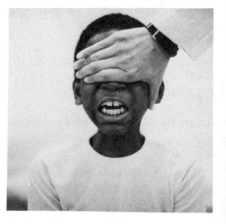

night and intermittently during the day to maintain the neck in extension, particularly while working at a desk to avoid a bent-over position (14). Unilateral arthritis of C2–C3 apophyseal joints leads to torticollis and requires a hard collar. Moist heat application followed by active neck extension, lateral flexion to touch ear to shoulder and turning the chin to the side, should be performed regularly.

Arthritis and anterior subluxation of the atlantoaxial joint due to erosion of the odontoid ligament may occur and result in spinal cord compression. If flexion-extension films of the spine demonstrate subluxation, the child must wear a hard cervical collar, especially while riding in a car or when sudden jolts to the neck are a possibility. Surgical stabilization has to be considered, particularly when subluxation is greater than 3 mm and neurological abnormalities are present.

Shoulder. In arthritis of the shoulder joint, the arm is held in adduction, internal rotation in front of the chest and resting on the abdomen. As the shoulder is elevated, a compensatory dorsal kyphosis develops. In addition to goniometric measurements of joint excursion, evaluation should also note the extent of complex movements used in functional activities; for example, hand to mouth, opposite shoulder, occiput, and back. Exercises should stress good postural alignment and prevention of joint deformity with emphasis on retraction and protraction. Loss of glenohumeral motion is not very disabling as long as the child can substitute with scapulothoracic motion. The ideal is to maintain 90° shoulder flexion, abduction, and extension as well as rotation for ADL (56). Appropriate positioning in bed and sitting is to rest the arm in abduction on a pillow or table top. Simon (58) feels that massage of the joint itself does not help; instead, he recommends relaxation exercises and massage of the trapezius to improve head and neck posture followed by isometric contractions of the deltoid, clavicular head of the pectoralis major, biceps, triceps, and internal rotators. In older children, traditional methods can be used for maintaining ROM progressing from Codman's exercises to finger climbing, shoulder wheel, and overhead pulleys (66). For the younger age group, ball games using a light inflatable ball or climbing on a slide or jungle gym are good activities. Volleyball will particularly encourage good joint excursion with overhead movements in forward flexion. Weaving is an excellent activity for children who enjoy crafts since it entails shoulder retraction and protraction, as well as forward flexion.

Elbow. Loss of extension and supination are the most common problems in the elbow and are extremely difficult to regain. A 30° elbow flexion contracture can be fairly well compensated in daily activities (66). However, flexion limited to less than 90° is a significant functional handicap and makes feeding difficult, particularly when the shoulder and wrist are also affected. In acute inflammation of the elbow joint, isometric exercises are used. The child lies supine with the elbow resting at the side and presses down on a towel roll placed under the wrist and hand for isometric exercises to the triceps. In the same position, with the hand tucked under the thigh or buttock, upward pressure will result in isometric biceps contraction. When the child has good ROM against gravity without significant pain, active assistive exercises are started, eventually progressing to movements against resistance. Rotating a ball or screw with gradually increasing resistance while holding the elbow at the side are practiced to maintain pronation and supination. Resistive exercise of the biceps and triceps are performed initially with a ½-lb wrist cuff weight using equal amount of weekly increments until a maintenance level of 2 to 3 lb is reached. Maximum resistance depends on the child's age, size, and the status of the elbow joint. For home use, socks filled with a measured weight of rice or beans are inexpensive substitutes (Fig. 12.4). All exercises should be performed twice daily and include 10 repetitions of each motion. Prolonged intermittent stretching of elbow flexion contractures can best be achieved by having the elbow supported on a pillow and a weighted cuff placed on the forearm for about 20 minutes. Air splints can be used with increasing gradients of pressure to increase extension at the elbow. The Dynasplint is now being fabricated in small enough sizes for children.

Wrist. Loss of motion at the wrist appears early; fibrosis and eventually, ankylosis are prone to develop. Granberry and Brewer (22) consider limitation of wrist extension a clinical barometer of the disease activity. Unlike adults, where ulnar wrist deviation is the standard deformity, in children, radial drift is equally common. Exercises recommended by Brewer and coworkers are shown in Figure 12.5 (22). The prayer position, in which both wrists are brought into maximal extension, is an excellent exercise for preventing wrist flexion deformity (Fig. 12.6). Craft play and recreation activities recommended for arthritis of the wrist have been mentioned earlier in this chapter. A dorsal cock-up splint supports the joint against gravity-induced flexion at night and provides pain relief during the day. Extension of 10° to 15° is usually well tolerated and correction for ulnar or radial devi-

Figure 12.4. Upper extremity strengthening at home using a sock filled with predetermined measure of rice.

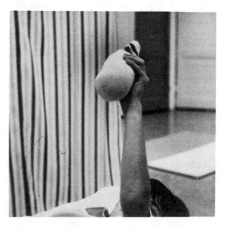

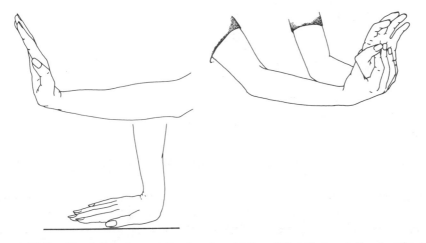

Figure 12.5. *Top left*, active wrist extension; *bottom left*, active assistive dorsiflexion using a table; and *right,* active assistive dorsiflexion using the other hand as the assist.

ation can be incorporated. If there is pain on using the wrist, or weakness of the wrist extensors, a working splint is desirable. A gauntlet splint fully supports the wrist allowing the child full, pain-free function (2) (Fig. 12.7). Rather than dorsal wrist splints, gauntlet splints hold the wrist in good alignment without interfering with work or play and compliance is generally good because of pain relief.

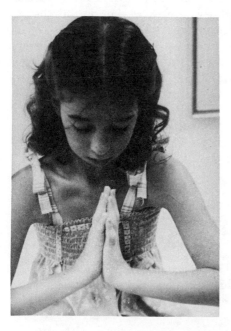

Figure 12.6. Prayer position for achieving maximal bilateral wrist extension.

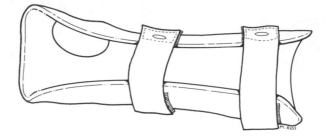

Figure 12.7. Gauntlet splint—supports the wrist allowing pain-free function.

Fingers. Involvement of the finger joints can be best assessed by measuring the circumference of each phalangeal articulation with a jeweler's ring. Extent of opening and closing should be measured as well as thumb abduction and opposition against the finger tips (46). Grip strength is recorded. Medial lateral drift of the index finger and wrist are interrelated and occur in the opposite direction. With ulnar deviation of the wrist, the second and third digits tend to have radial displacement and the reverse will develop when there is radial deviation at the wrist. These deformities are thought to represent compensatory realignment in order to maintain the index finger in line with the longitudinal and actual axis of rotation of the forearm. An individually designed program is needed in each case to prevent progression of the specific presenting deformities. There may be limitation of flexion or extension at the metacarpophalangeal articulation. Position of partial flexion protects these joints from subluxation and ulnar deviation. Strong interosseus muscles are particularly necessary to counteract the tendency to ulnar drift. Exercises to prevent progressive loss of motion (22) and to strengthen the finger extensors and interossei are extremely important. Squeezing a sponge for 6 seconds between the finger tips is one way to achieve this goal. On the other hand, making a fist or squeezing a ball in the whole hand will enhance imbalance between intrinsic and extrinsic muscles and hasten the deformity of ulnar deviation. Chaplin and his co-workers (15) found that, in young children, flexion contractures of the finger joints are most common. Swan neck and boutonniere deformities of the interphalangeal joints, characteristic of adult rheumatoid arthritis, are more likely to develop in older children and appear over the course of many years.

As we pointed out earlier, children do not accept elaborate splints. However, compliance is not a problem with the metal ring splint used for finger contractures because it looks like jewelry (Fig. 12.8). For swan neck deformity, the splint is applied so that it will allow flexion but limit extension of the proximal interphalangeal joint. In treating a boutonniere deformity, it is reversed to prevent excessive flexion. This splint can be used also to control hyperextension of the interphalangeal articulation of the thumb. The Bunnell knuckle bender splint assists with flexion of the metacarpophalangeal joints (23).

Hip. Loss of motion at the hip, more than at any other joint, leads to incapacity and the need for crutches and/or wheelchair. The most frequent complications are adduction and flexion deformities. Sometimes tightness of the iliotibial band develops. In the early phase of disease, the first radiological sign is narrowing of the articular space. Although ambulation is possible at this stage, pain and the resulting muscle spasm produce a habitual protective joint position, eventual soft tissue deformity, and progressive functional limitation. In generalized disease of the hip joint, adductor spasm and contracture can develop with gradual subluxation of the femoral head demonstrable on x-ray. A different problem arises in severe destructive arthritis, involving the synovia, bone, and cartilage, which allows medial displacement or central migration of the femoral head. This complication almost universally requires arthroplasty at maturity.

The primary concern of treatment is to prevent adduction, flexion deformities, and to increase the range and strength of hip abduction and extension. There is no adequate brace or splint for the hip and our approach is to use traction at night to avert deformities, and crutches during the day for joint protection. Furthermore, alignment in traction is recommended at 30° flexion, 15° abduction, and a position of external rotation. In this position, intra-articular pressure is lowest and, therefore, the threat of joint destruction is reduced. Prone lying, at least 1 hour in the daytime, should be strongly encouraged. Exercises in water are most valuable even while the arthritic process is active. Heat, massage, or intra articular cortisone injection prior to exercise may help decrease pain and enhance the child's tolerance of therapy. A beach ball is placed under the thigh and the patient is instructed to compress it by extending and abducting the hip in order to strengthen these muscles. Tricycling or bicycling with an elevated seat promotes maximal hip and knee extension. Hip flexion contracture may be initiated by a similar deformity at the knee and requires corrective measures at both joints. Destructive arthritis of the femoral neck and head leads to leg length discrepancy, which must be closely monitored and equalized with a shoe lift.

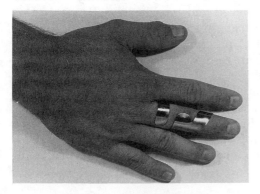

Figure 12.8. Metal ring splint for correction of swan neck or boutonniere deformity.

Knee. The characteristic posture is 30° flexion, which reduces intra-articular pressure and pain in the joint. In addition, genu valgum may develop as a result of iliotibial band contracture when there is concomitant arthritis of the hip. Surgical lengthening of the iliotibial band may be necessary and is usually adequate to correct valgus deformity of the knee. The patella may become adherent to the underlying femoral condyles with consequent limitation of active extension. Manipulation to restore patellar mobility will permit the quadriceps to extend the knee fully. In advanced articular disease, flattening and compression of the tibial plateau interferes with full range of both flexion and extension (63). In view of the potential deformities, examination of the knee joint must include serial measurements of flexion and extension as well as mediolateral angulation in valgus or varus attitude.

As the knee is a major weight-bearing joint, vigorous measures must be applied to avoid disuse weakness from the onset of the disease. In addition to the quadriceps and hamstrings, strengthening exercises should include other muscles of the lower limb. Similarly, in therapy for maintaining ROM, other joints of the leg have to be considered. Although movements are painful, isometric quadriceps exercises are indicated; a designated number of contractions must be performed supporting a tolerable amount of weight with the knee held in extension. Straight leg raising to 30° is sufficient to prevent atrophy of the quadriceps but does not increase its strength. Active and active-assistive exercises necessary to preserve joint mobility are started as soon as pain has subsided. The child performs knee flexion and extension in supine, sitting, and prone with assistance provided by the therapist to increase or complete the movements if active joint excursion is limited. It must be kept in mind that force applied to the distal part of the leg will lead to posterior displacement of the tibia on the femur due to tightness of the posterior joint capsule and anterior cruciate ligaments, which accompany knee flexion contractures. Therefore, any stretching force has to be applied just below the knee joint since this will allow the tibia to glide forward in a normal relationship to the femoral condyles (43). Active resistive exercises can be started when at least 90° knee motion, including all but the last 15° of extension, has been achieved and muscle strength within this range is good. In the young child, progressive resistive exercises begin with a 1-lb weight attached to the ankle. A program of 10 repetitions twice a day and weekly 1-lb weight increments are recommended. Maintenance therapy varies from 3 to 5 lb in young children to 15 to 20 lb in older adolescents. Evaluation of gait and posture should be provided particularly when there is knee flexion contracture with consequent leg length discrepancy, pelvic obliquity, and compensatory scoliosis. For this reason, postural exercises consisting of strengthening the trunk and hip extensors, as well as abdominal and scapular muscles should be incorporated in the program of all children with arthritis of the knee.

If a knee flexion contracture exists at the time of the evaluation, skin traction or serial splinting with plaster casts may be used. A cylinder plaster cast works to increase extension and is applied for 48 hours (2). It is then removed for 4 to 7 days of exercise using the cast in a bivalve form as a night splint. After several days of therapy, a new cylinder cast is applied for 48 hours and generally several more degrees of extension can be gained. This process may be repeated three or four times until the knee flexion contracture is less than 15°. The child can then use the cast in the position that has been achieved as a bivalved night splint. It is of importance that physical therapy continue to maintain an increasing ROM on a daily basis. A serious problem with correcting knee flexion contractures is producing a posterior tibial subluxation. To avoid this complication, Bianco and Peterson (7) use traction with additional perpendicular force applied to the proximal tibia. Subluxation is reduced if the tibia is brought forward and a gradual extension of the knee and hip is achieved. The extension desubluxation hinge (8) originally described for hemophiliac arthropathy tends to accomplish a similar purpose and may be used in a knee-ankle-foot orthosis (KAFO). Orthoses in rheumatoid arthritis should be easy to don and doff as the device will have to be removed to perform daily exercises.

Lower extremity orthotics are often designed to correct malalignment at the knee. KAFO can help control flexion contracture of valgus or varus at the knee (21). If the foot is kept in 5° of plantar flexion throughout the gait, dorsiflexion is blocked. A momentum of force is created that favors knee extension to help compensate for weak quadriceps. A solid ankle cushion heel (SACH) allows rapid compression of the heel and will also help increase knee extension (21).

Ankle. In arthritis of the ankle, loss of plantar flexion is accompanied by early restriction of eversion and inversion. Limited plantar flexion induces excessive knee flexion momentum immediately after heel strike. In addition, there is a lack of push off. Bed rest and wheelchair immobilization, on the other hand, can produce an equinus deformity. The shortened heel cord creates a stress on the tarsal joint and plantar fascia, which will encourage pronation of the foot. From late preschool age on, children can be taught to perform self-administered heel cord stretching exercises consisting of forward bending against a wall while keeping the foot flat on the ground and the knee straight to elongate both components of the triceps surae. Active exercises include dorsiflexion, plantar flexion, and circling the ankle. The children are encouraged to walk on heels and toes, which will maintain joint mobility and strength. Ankle pain on ambulation can be decreased by using an ankle cushion heel (SACH), which reduces the impact of heel strike and provides compensatory dorsiflexion and plantar flexion without actual joint motion. In some cases, the normally flexible tarsal joints become immobile. A deformity resembling cavovarus foot may develop and necessitates better corrective shoe inserts and eventual surgery.

Foot. Destruction and subluxation of the metatarsal heads, hammer toes, and hallux valgus (22) are the most common problems in the foot. Sweezey (64) feels that flexion and extension exercises of the interossei are helpful for hammer toes. Shoe inserts and modifications are very often used for arthritis affecting the foot. Ansell (2) suggests toe separators to hold the claw toes in extension. With severe pain at the ankle, one solution is an air splint that inhibits eversion and inversion while allowing dorsiflexion and plantar flexion. This reduces the pain significantly; however, children are rough on their orthotics and will often produce holes in the splint requiring replacement every few weeks. An alternative for some children with ankle pain is a leg-hind foot orthosis designed at the National Institutes of Health to reduce pain by supporting the subtalar and ankle joints (28). Again, motion is limited in eversion and inversion and free in dorsiflexion and plantar flexion. Many children in our clinic have been very satisfied with this orthosis, its limitation is difficulties to fit on days when there is a great deal of swelling of the ankle. Although several authors recommend orthopaedic shoes to maintain proper foot position, children with juvenile arthritis do not tolerate these shoes; they prefer soft shoes, such as Hush Puppies or sneakers in which the discomfort and impact of weight-bearing on walking is considerably reduced. Inserts to relieve weight-bearing over the painful metatarsal head or calcaneal area can be added to this type of footwear and are valuable for increasing the child's tolerance for walking (Fig. 12.9). In case of calcaneal spur, a ¼-inch sponge rubber bar placed 1 inch anterior to

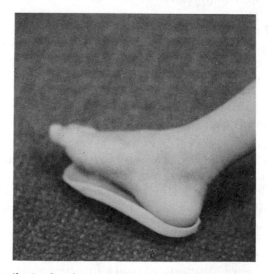

Figure 12.9. Plastizote shoe insert cushions the entire foot during weight-bearing and may be specifically designed to shift weight-bearing behind the metatarsophalangeal head.

the os calcis and extending fully under the longitudinal arch will transfer weight-bearing from the painful area. A bunion last shoe is often considered when hallux valgus begins to develop (63). Adolescents will often prefer surgery at this time to correct hallux valgus so they can wear more socially acceptable shoes.

Ankylosing Spondylitis

Ankylosing spondylitis is a chronic inflammatory disease that usually begins in the peripheral joints with no clinical or radiological involvement of the sacroiliac or spinal joints for years (57). The onset of ankylosing spondylitis in boys is often with asymmetric lower extremity arthritis. There may be a positive family history. Other diagnostic features include involvement of the first metatarsophalangeal head and an inflammatory enthesopathy that occurs at the infrapatellar ligament, Achilles tendon, and at the insertion of the plantar fascia (57). Subsequently, it extends to small posterior intervertebral or apophyseal articulations and the costovertebral joints. Ligamentous attachments surrounding these joints are characteristically involved. Among the extremity joints, hips and knees tend to be affected and there is ossification of the annulus fibrosis of the intervertebral discs (6).

DIAGNOSIS

After many years, clinical symptoms may consist of intermittent episodes of aching pain, back pain, and stiffness. Pain occurs most frequently in the morning. The children may complain of pain accentuated by intensive physical activity and relieved by mild exercise. Some patients have progressive stiffness and decreased ROM rather than significant pain. There may be associated iritis, aortic valvular insufficiency, temporomandibular arthritis, and erosion of the os calcis and pubic symphysis. Diagnosis is based on several clinical signs. Sacroiliac tenderness elicited either by direct palpation or positive Menell's sign, i.e., pain in the sacroiliac joint on hyperextension of the thigh is one symptom of ankylosing spondylitis (6). Chest expansion less than 3 cm measured at the level of the nipple is indicative of costovertebral involvement. Decreased mobility of the lumbar spine is suggested by inability of reaching the finger tips below the level of extended knees on forward bending. Another maneuver is the Schoeber test. A mark is made on the spine 10 cm above the level of the iliac crest when standing. Less than 5-cm increase of this distance on forward bending is an early sign of limited lumbar motion (14). Loss of cervical mobility is another but less common symptom in ankylosing spondylitis. Serial monitoring of these signs gives an indication of the course of the disease. Additional observations of value include measurements of height, time required for walking 50 feet and rising after lying supine for 10 minutes, duration of morning stiffness, onset of fatigue, and joint symptoms.

TREATMENT

The goals of treatment are to relieve pain and to prevent disabling deformities. Smythe (59) has aptly commented that it is the doctor's responsibility to control pain and the patient's job to keep moving.

Aspirin is the first line drug; however, tolmetin sodium and then indomethacin are often added or substituted relatively quickly in difficult cases (57). Steroids are recommended specifically for uveitis, vasculitis, and amyloid nephrosis. Because there is no specific treatment to influence the ankylosing arthritis, the most important aspect of management is education of the patient. Certain precautionary measures have to be observed throughout life; otherwise, the progressive disabling flexion deformity of the spine will be inevitable. From the time the first symptoms appear, the patient must develop the habit of sitting erect in a straight-backed chair, standing with extended spine; even squatting to pick up objects must be done with a straight back. Raising the height of the desk or lowering the chair will help maintain maximal elongation of the spine. The patient is advised to move about at regular intervals during the day because spondylitic joints rapidly become stiff with prolonged lack of mobility. Since morning stiffness is a particularly difficult problem in some patients, it was recommended that they should be awakened at 3 AM and walk around before going back to sleep. This measure should be explored as a means of decreasing morning stiffness. Night rest of 8 to 9 hours is advised using a firm mattress without pillows under the head or knees. In addition, there should be a midday rest period lying prone to decrease the tendency to flexion contractures. Patients with ankylosing spondylitis should exercise regularly in the morning following a hot shower, during the midday rest and periodically during the day to emphasize spine extenison and chest expansion. Figure 12.10 illustrates three simple exercises recommended to achieve these aims (11). Inflating a beach ball will also encourage maximal chest expansion (59). Stretching of the calf and hamstring muscles and exercises to maintain ROM in affected extremity joints should also be included. Recreational activities that entail similar movements are encouraged, specifically, archery, badminton, and tennis. As in other arthritides, swimming is an ideal sport because it promotes deep breathing, spinal extension, and full ROM of the extremities. Bowling, golf, and surf casting require spinal flexion and, therefore, are not advised (11). Wrestling, rugby, football, judo, and high diving are discouraged because these sports involve impact with potential damage to the spine.

Dermatomyositis

Dermatomyositis is an inflammatory disease of the muscles and skin associated with a characteristic rash. A diagnosis of juvenile dermatomyo-

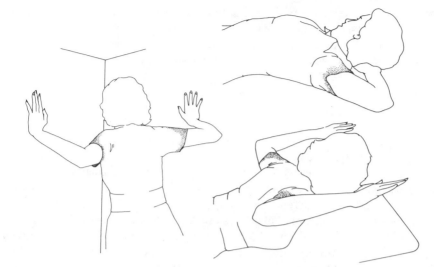

Figure 12.10. Chest expansion, spine extension in standing, supine, and prone positions.

sitis is made when, in addition to the rash, three of the following four criteria are documented: (*a*) increased muscle enzymes; (*b*) symmetric proximal muscle weakness; (*c*) vasculitis or chronic inflammation on muscle biopsy; (*d*) electromyography confirming inflammatory myopathy (2). It is characterized by pain, swelling, or atrophy of the affected muscles. Weakness tends to be generalized with some predilection for proximal musculature and particularly for neck flexors. Difficulties with stair climbing and dressing reflect the proximal distribution of weakness. Affected muscles are tender and may be stiff and brawny. Sullivan and associates (68) describe two cases of dermatomyositis in infancy with generalized weakness and floppiness. Involvement of the muscles of the palate and respiration may cause compromised breathing, asphyxia, aspiration, and pneumonia. There is a typical rash on the face and extensor surfaces of the limbs with brawny, nonpitting edema. Groton's sign, erythema, and hypertrophy or atrophy involve skin over the proximal interphalangeal joints (57). The skin is atrophic and scaly and the eyelids show a violet hue (54). Laboratory studies may show an elevated ESR. Elevation of SGOT, SGPT, LDH, CPK, and aldolase levels in the serum indicate muscle tissue breakdown. It was observed that a rise of these enzymes, particularly CPK, correlates with the activity of the disease. Serum muscle enzymes are important for diagnosis as well as for monitoring the effectiveness of therapy (14). Further observations are needed to determine the importance of strength measurements as a reflection of disease activity. EMG and muscle biopsy may confirm the presence of inflammatory myopathy. Other laboratory data that may be helpful include activated complement, increased levels of VIII:R Ag or fibrin peptide A, ANA, and 50% increase in HLA types B8 and DR3 (57).

Muscle weakness generally resolves after 6 to 8 weeks of treatment (14). Physical management in the acute period consists of ROM exercises and splints to prevent development of muscle contractures. Although there are no controlled studies as to when activation to increase strength and endurance can be started safely, there is general agreement that such exercises should not begin until there is clinical evidence of recovery (14). Precaution is recommended with resistive exercises in the early phases of healing as it is felt that strenuous muscle activity may damage the formation of new myofibrils (68). If rising serum enzyme levels indicate a relapse of the disease process, active and resistive exercise should be discontinued. In the chronic stage of dermatomyositis, one must emphasize prevention of deformities, maintenance of strength, pulmonary function, and achievement of highest possible level of independence in daily activities and ambulation. However, despite the most vigorous treatment, contractures can occur and may necessitate surgical correction (69).

The outcome of childhood dermatomyositis varies. The outcome is good in most cases although subcutaneous calcifications, scarring of skin, muscle atrophy, and mild contractures did occur in some children. Calcifications accumulate at pressure sites or points of previous trauma and are related to duration and severity of the disease (Figs. 12.11 and 12.12). In calcinosis universalis, there is a sheath-like deposit that can eventually erode the skin and may lead to ulceration. The treatment for these ulcers includes exercises and hydrotherapy, Furacin and scarlet red dressing, and occasional skin grafting.

Mortality in juvenile dermatomyositis has decreased from 20% to 7.2%, which may be related to steroid treatment or supportive care. Treatment is prednisone, 2 mg/kg, with slow tapering to 0.5 mg/kg once enzymes have returned to normal. With severe vasculitis, methylprednisolone may be necessary. In refractory cases, intravenous methotrexate may be used but additional research on the use of this drug is necessary (57). Serum enzymes may return to normal as soon as 2 weeks and muscle weakness resolves after 6 to 8 weeks of treatment (14).

Scleroderma

Scleroderma, meaning hard skin, is a chronic inflammatory process of the connective tissue, which primarily affects the skin. Scleroderma is rare in children. Only 1.5% of cases occur under 10 yr of age and 7% of the cases between 10 and 19 yr of age (57). The disease may also involve the gastrointestinal tract, heart, lungs, and kidney; hence, the designation of systemic sclerosis. Scleroderma is more frequently found in females than males.

Morphea is a localized form of scleroderma, which is more common in

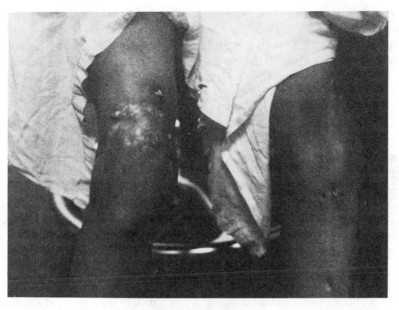

Figure 12.11. Calcification interferes with motion of the joint severely limiting flexion and extension of the knee.

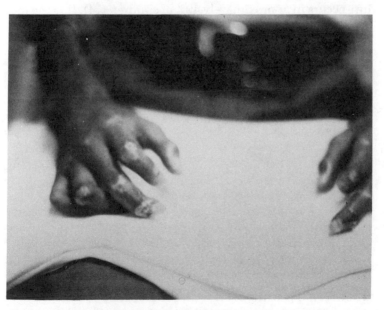

Figure 12.12. Sheath-like calcification occurs surrounding the joints inhibiting motion of the metacarpophalangeal and intercarpophalangeal joints.

children than in adults. The skin lesions are rarely severe except when they are located on the face. They may be patchy or linear in shape and extend into the subcutaneous fat tissue underlying muscle. Linear lesions may follow the course of peripheral nerves and can be associated with impaired bone growth, contractures, and progressive deformities (14). Synovitis may occur in joints adjacent and distal to a local skin lesion. Prognosis is good except for those children who develop systemic involvement (54).

Progressive systemic sclerosis affects both children and adults. The skin lesion is diffuse and involvement of multiple organs is usual in this form of disease. The skin becomes tough, shiny, and bound down to subcutaneous structures resulting in loss of normal skin folds and characteristic mask-like facies. Tightening of the facial skin produces microstomia, which makes eating and dental hygiene difficult (Fig. 12.13). The atrophic inelastic skin of the hands and fingers is particularly vulnerable to ulceration with secondary infection and autoamputation (Fig. 12.14). Raynaud's phenomenon may accompany systemic sclerosis and involves the tips of the fingers, nose, earlobes, and the toes. Polyarthritis affecting the elbow, wrist, and finger joints leads to flexion contractures. There may be myositis and, in long-standing disease, subcutaneous calcifications. X-ray studies frequently demonstrate decreased esophageal motility and small bowel involvement in up to 50% of patients (14).

Interstitial pulmonary fibrosis, nephritis, myocardial fibrosis, and gastrointestinal complaints are the most common systemic manifestations. Cardiac failure occurs in approximately 40% of children (14). It is the most com-

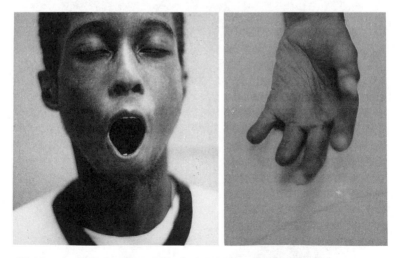

Figure 12.13. *Left,* Tightening of the facial skin producing microstomia.
Figure 12.14. *Right,* When the skin of the fingers and hands break down, a process of autoamputation may occur.

mon cause of demise in children and renal disease accounts for 10% of the deaths. Clinical evaluation entails recording ROM strength, posture, and gait. Length of both legs is measured. The skin must be carefully inspected particularly over the face, hands, and feet. Cutaneous ulcers, evidence of Raynaud's phenomenon, signs of synovitis, or tenosynovitis are noted.

The current drug regimen for patients with scleroderma includes the use of immunosuppressants, colchicine to inhibit the fibroproliferative process, and penicillamine to prevent the breakdown of collagen (14). Drugs to relieve vasoconstriction by sympathetic blockade can help alleviate the signs and symptoms of Raynaud's phenomenon and protect the fingers, toes, face, and ears from stress and cold. Severe ulceration of the digits can be treated with synthetic skin to promote healing (57). Goals of physical management range from treating the sclerodermatous skin lesions to alleviating the signs of Raynaud's phenomenon, arthritis, myositis, and the development of contractures. Bound fibrotic skin that adheres to cutaneous tissue will hamper the movement of underlying joints and lead to contractures. Friction massage with the application of mollifying creams, oils, or soaps relieves dryness of skin and helps mobilize adherent fibrotic tissues from the underlying joints and muscles (65). Stretching and massaging the tight perioral structures should be attempted to slow down progressive microstomia. Although local heat is used to relieve vasospasm produced by Raynaud's phenomenon, the application of these modalities requires caution (28). Warm water, paraffin baths, and, in older children, ultrasound are recommended for this purpose. Warm water soaks are also used for debridement of necrotic tissue from skin ulcers. Hyaluronidase may be added to the water and, thereafter, topical antibiotics should be applied to the ulcerated areas. Exposure to cold should be avoided. Local application of nitroglycerin paste with procaine jelly or dimethylsulfoxide has also been suggested for pain relief and improving circulation (69). Leg length discrepancy as a result of growth disturbance in linear scleroderma should be corrected by a shoe lift because it can lead to scoliosis in a growing child.

Systemic Lupus Erythematosus

Lupus erythematosus can affect any organ system; lung, heart, kidneys, gastrointestinal tract, and central nervous system are the most often involved. Other clinical signs are fever, malaise, arthritis, arthralgia, and a typical butterfly rash of the face with erythema of the malar areas and the bridge of the nose. Lupus nephritis is the most serious complication in children with systemic lupus erythematosus. Laboratory abnormalities include elevated immunoglobulins, positive test for ANA and lupus erythematosus preparation, and decreased complement. Involvement of the central nervous system including headache, schizophrenia, depression, hallucinations, and anxiety with or without pseudotumor cerebri is the second cause of morbidity and mortality (57). Drug treatment consists of high doses of daily prednisone with pulse methylprednisolone and cyclosporin experimentally. Arthritis occurs in 75% of children; however, the synovitis is usually not destructive or deforming. The use of ultraviolet and luminous heat is contraindicated because of extreme skin sensitivity to light. Exposure to cold should be avoided by patients who have signs of Raynaud's phenomenon (50). Participation in recreational activities is desirable with reasonable restrictions to avoid excessive fatigue and overexposure to sun.

Kawasaki Disease

Kawasaki disease is an acute febrile illness affecting predominantly infants and children less than 5 yr of age. The clinical course is well described as triphasic. The first phase is characterized by acute onset of fever followed in 1 to 3 days by conjunctival injection, erythema and fissuring of the lips, erythema of the oropharynx, swelling of the hands and feet, and erythematous rash, and lymphadenopathy. Desquamation of the skin of the fingers and toes begins under the nails and may involve the entire palm and sole. Children in this phase may also have aseptic meningitis, diarrhea, and hepatic dysfunction. The acute phase generally lasts 7 to 14 days. Rash, lymphadenopathy, and fever generally subside; however, anorexia and irritability persist with the next or subacute phase. During the convalescent phase, deep transverse grooves (Bow's lines) appear across each fingernail and toenail and grow out with the nail. If they are going to occur, arthritis, arthralgia, and myocardial dysfunction appear during this time between 10 and 15 days after the onset of fever. The convalescent phase lasts from this period until the sedimentation rate returns to normal, generally 6 to 8 weeks after the onset of the disease (36).

There is limited published information on the arthritis of Kawasaki disease. However, the Honolulu experience is that 30% of cases develop arthritis with an onset in the first 7 days of the disease. The arthritis is characterized by sudden onset of polyarticular symptoms with small and large joint involvement. Early arthritis is more frequent in those children who have severe multisystem disease especially those who develop coronary artery aneurysms. Joint fluid shows white blood counts with a mean of 135,000/ml and a predominance of polymorphonuclear cells. Two thirds of patients with arthritis have such symptoms affecting only a few joints in the subacute phase. Limping develops when lower extremity joints are involved. The joints are cool but quite swollen. Although no chronic arthritis has been observed, joint symptoms may persist as long as 120 days. While joint disease may appear in children already on high doses of salicylates, it generally responds to other nonsteroidal inflammatory agents, such as tolmetin sodium (26).

The etiology of this disease is not known. Acute symptoms are thought to be secondary to a microbial agent although the specific agent has not been identified. The subacute stage appears to be immunologically mediated with a rise and fall in all immunological classes (28).

Establishing the correct diagnosis and elimination of other treatable entities is the next step and includes supportive care, anti-inflammatory therapy, antiplatelet therapy, repeated evaluations to detect the complications of carditis, valvular dysfunction, arrhythmias, aneurysms, and arthritis. Long-term supervision will be necessary for children who develop aneurysms.

Drug treatment is initially 80 to 100 mg/kg/day of aspirin until fever is controlled. Thereafter, the dosage is reduced to less than 10 mg/day, which will help control platelet aggregation. This dose is designed to prevent coronary thrombosis and is given from 14 to 35 days when the risk of coronary artery disease is the greatest (36). As already stated, children who develop arthritis during this period respond best to tolmetin sodium.

BENIGN HYPERMOBILITY SYNDROME

In 1967, Kirk defined the hypermobility syndrome in a group of patients with hypermobility of joints and musculoskeletal complaints that, in the absence of demonstrable systemic rheumatological disease, were attributable to articular hypermobility (3). Gedalia also found a high frequency (66%) of hypermobility in juvenile episodic arthralgia seen at Texas Children's Hospital (19). The benign hypermobility syndrome has a marked female predominance. Symptoms first appear in children or young adults. Hyperextensible knees or elbows greater than 10° as well as hyperextensibility of the thumb and lumbar spine are characteristic. Without stability of normal ligaments, these hypermobile patients appear more vulnerable to the adverse effects of injury and overuse, sprains, traumatic synovitis, recurrent dislocations, tendonitis, and premature degenerative arthritis. An associated systemic connective tissue abnormality is possible but unlikely (48).

Acute Bacterial Arthritis

Acute septic arthritis occurs when pyogenic bacteria invade the synovial joint. Unless adequately treated, the infection will lead to joint destruction. Most commonly in childhood, septic arthritis is the result of a hematogenous spread of osteomyelitis at those joints where metaphysis is entirely intracapsular, mostly the hip and the elbow. Hematogenous dissemination to the joints from osteomyelitis is generally caused by Staphylococcus or, less commonly, Streptococcus, Pneumococcus, Haemophilus influenza, or Salmonella. Gonococcal arthritis evolves in the same manner in teenagers (27).

Septic arthritis is a serious infection because lysosomal enzymes of the polymorphonuclear cells and bacteria in the purulent exudate rapidly digest the articular cartilage. Granulation tissue that forms pannus over the articular cartilage blocks the nutritional supply of the joint. Since cartilage does not regenerate, the articular surface is permanently destroyed. As the joint capsule fills with purulent exudate and the fibrous capsule is stretched, pathological joint dislocation may develop. In an enclosed space, such as the hip joint, the increased articular pressure occludes the blood supply with resultant necrosis of the femoral head. Late sequelae of septic arthritis include degenerative joint disease and fibrous or bony ankylosis (51).

Infants usually present with irritability as the first sign. On examination, there is tenderness to joint motion. Fever and elevated white blood count may be minimal. Radiological examination during the first week may reveal only soft tissue swelling but, by the second week, there may be evidence of pathological dislocation. In the older child, there is obvious tenderness over a specific joint, restricted ROM, and muscle spasm. Fever and increased white blood cell count are present. Sedimentation rate is usually markedly elevated (51). The diagnosis is dependent on needle aspiration since early radiological studies may be nonspecific. A technetium 99M phosphate scan reflects an increased blood flow to the joint space and is helpful in detecting joint inflammation but it does not provide certain differentiation between inflammation and infectious arthritis. Gallium scans will identify the increased number of polymorphonuclear cells and infectious arthritis including septic arthritis (14). Neither of these diagnostic studies is currently accepted as a definitive diagnostic tool for septic arthritis.

Treatment of acute septic arthritis is a surgical emergency requiring immediate needle aspiration. This is followed by treatment with intravenous antibiotics. There is a controversy regarding other aspects of the treatment approach. Greene (24) states that aspiration and irrigation of the joint without surgical debridement is the appropriate treatment in every joint except the hip. The hip joint must always be surgically drained since this is far more effective than aspiration (51). The surgery consists of arthrotomy with aspiration of the joint and complete removal of the purulent exudate. After wound closure, continuous drainage, instillation of saline, antibiotics, and a detergent, such as Alevaire, are maintained (51). Intravenous antibiotic treatment for 5 to 14 days is followed by oral administration for a total of 4 weeks. The choice of antibiotics is based on the result of Gram's stain and culture. Cefuroxime is used for both Staphylococcus and *Haemophilus influenzae*. Institution of passive ROM exercises during this stage of antibiotic treatment is also controversial. Greene recommends joint immobilization for several days to allow decrease of the acute inflammation and to prevent pathological dislocation (24). For the hip joint, he uses split Russell traction. Other affected joints are splinted or casted. The length of immobilization varies. In some institutions, it may be only until the time the patient is free of pain, while in others it may be for 7 to 14 days of the intravenous antibiotic treatment or until the joint aspirate becomes sterile. On the other hand, opponents of immobilization recommend continued passive motion, suggesting that this treatment is not painful, that it prevents fibrosis, and that it assists in cartilage nutrition (40). Mooney, in a clinical study based on the experimental work of Salter (52), suggests that continued passive motion to a septic joint is far better than rest and immobilization. Indeed, in this study, passive motion appears to improve cartilage repair (40). However, this treatment has not been universally accepted. It depends on the treatment practice of the orthopaedic surgeon or the infectious disease specialist managing the case whether immobilization or active assistive ROM is selected. When exercises are allowed, the child should have a program of both ROM and strengthening to restore joint mobility, periarticular tissue flexibility, and stability through increasing muscle strength. Because the hip joint in particular may show late changes, follow-up radiological studies of the involved and uninvolved sides 6 to 12 months after the infection is indicated. If significant damage has occurred with pain and loss of function, reconstructive surgery is often necessary (55).

INFECTIOUS ARTHRITIDES FROM OTHER CAUSES

Viral arthritis is more common in adults than in children. Arthralgia is more common than frank arthritis. It is usually migratory and 1 to 2 weeks in duration. Symptoms generally disappear after residual joint disease. Viruses may be isolated from joints or only virus-containing immune complexes.

The most common virus associated with arthritis is rubella-associated arthropathy. It is also known that musculoskeletal symptoms after rubella vaccine are common in young women but unusual in preadolescent females and males after natural infection. Arthralgia usually begins within 17 days of the rash or 10 to 28 days after immunization. There is involvement of fingers and knees. Symptoms usually disappear in 3 to 4 weeks but occasionally persist for months or years. Hepatitis viral arthritis is rare in children under the age of 14 yr. Usually, dermatitis followed by symmetric arthritis of the interphalangeal joints and, less frequently, knee and ankle involvement occurs. Joint symptoms last up to 4 weeks and respond to nonsteroidal anti-inflammatory agents.

Epstein-Barr virus, cytomegalic virus, and varicella zoster are also known to be associated with arthritis but are all quite rare. Rarely, paramyxovirus, i.e., mumps, causes arthritis but there is no association with the mumps vaccine. Transient synovitis, presumably viral in origin, occurs predominantly in males 3 to 10 yr of age with onset in the hip, thigh, and knee and lasts approximately 6 days. Physical examination reveals loss of internal rotation and abduction. The sedimentation rate and white blood count are normal. X-rays may show widening of the joint space. Diagnostic studies may include hip aspiration to rule out a septic joint. Treatment includes analgesics, nonsteroidal anti-inflammatory agents, bed rest, and skin traction. Long-term sequelae have included Legg-Calve-Perthes disease in approximately 1.5% of patients.

Fungal and tuberculosis infections are rare in pediatrics. However, they are important because they are treatable. Candida septic arthritis, often with osteomyelitis, occurs in the newborn, immunocompromised individuals, and infected prosthetic joints. Fungal infections (14) are treated with amphotericin B alone or in conjunction with other antifungal agents. Tuberculous joint involvement may develop from osteomyelitis or hematogenous spread. Of all cases, 50% affect the spine. Other joints involved are those of the lower extremities. The diagnosis is made by histological examination and culture. Recommendation is initial treatment with Isoniazid (5 mg/kg up to 300 mg orally daily), Rifampin (10 mg/kg up to 600 mg orally), and Pyrzinamide (15 to 30 mg/kg up to 2 g daily). The treatment of these drugs is a minimum of 9 months with clinical determinations of cure (37).

Lyme Disease

Lyme disease is a complex multisystem disease via the tick-bone spirochete, Borrelia burgdorferi. The tick-borne vector responsible for the disease is dependent on the geographic location of the disease. However, the disease is widespread in the northeast USA, from Massachusetts to Maryland, in the Midwest in Wisconsin and Minnesota, on the West Coast in California and Oregon as well as throughout Europe from France to Scandinavia and Russia. Clinical features include erythema chronicum migrans (ECM), a red macule or papule that occurs at the site of the tick bite 3 to 32 days later and expands to form a large annular lesion with a bright outer border and a central clearing (60). The skin lesion may be accompanied by fever, minor systemic symptoms, and/or regional lymphadenopathy. The laboratory test for Borrelia burgdorferi antigen is often negative at this time (60).

In stage 2, there is early disseminated infection with Borrelia burgdorferi cultivated from blood and multiple organs. There may be additional dermatological reactions, including a secondary annular skin lesion, malar rash, diffuse erythema, or urticaria. Skin involvement may be accompanied by headache, mild stiff neck, fever, chills, myalgias, arthralgias, profound malaise, and fatigue. Less commonly, there may be general lymphadenopathy, splenomegaly, sore throat, hepatitis, testicular swelling, conjunctivitis, uveitis, or panophthalmitis.

Neurological symptoms, such as meningeal irritation, may occur at the time of ECM. Of these patients, 15% develop frank neurological abnormalities, such as meningitis, encephalitis, cranial neuritis (including bilateral facial palsy and optic atrophy), motor and sensory neuropathy, plexitis, mononeuritis multiplex, chorea, or myelitis (45). The cerebrospinal fluid (CSF) generally shows a lymphocytic pleocytosis. Borrelia burgdorferi may also produce a chronic infection of the central nervous system with organic mental symptoms or signs resembling multiple sclerosis (44).

Cardiac involvement may occur in about 8% of patients. The most common abnormality is varying degrees of atrioventricular block. Other patients have more diffuse cardiac pathology including myopericarditis, left ventricular dysfunction, cardiomegaly, or pancarditis (61). Usually, cardiac involvement is brief, lasting 3 days to 6 weeks, but it may recur (14).

At the average, 6 months after the onset of disease (2 weeks to 2 yr) following intermittent episodes of arthralgia or musculoskeletal pain, 60% of the patients have brief attacks of asymmetric oligoarthritis, especially of the knee (63). The third stage of the Lyme disease or persistent infection may include episodes of arthritis in the second or third year of the disease with arthritis lasting months rather than weeks. Typically, only a few joints are affected; again, primarily the knee. Occasionally, Baker's cysts may develop. Joint involvement includes the temporomandibular joint, shoulder, elbow, wrist, hip, knee, ankle, fingers, and toes. Episodes of arthritis are often separated by months or even years of complete remission. However, some patients develop periarticular symptoms, arthralgia, or periods of fatigue between attacks of overt arthritis. At the severe end of the spectrum, chronic synovitis occurs after earlier arthralgia or intermittent arthritis in approximately 11% of patients, erosion of cartilage and bone in approximately 4% of patients (61), and permanent joint disability in approximately 2% (63).

Acrodermatitis is another late stage manifestation of Lyme disease characterized years after the onset by a red, violaceous skin lesion, sometimes becoming sclerotic or atrophic (4). Below the skin lesion, subluxation of the small joints of the hands may occur. Periostitis, erosion of cartilage and bone might appear.

The pathophysiology of Lyme disease is based on immunological theory. One theory is that the immune complex consisting of antigens from the spirochete and complement from the human host accumulate in the joint. This complex attacks neutrophils with release of enzymes, which then destroy the joint. The second immunological theory is that the Borrelia spirochete releases interleukin 1, which stimulates collagenase and prostaglandin, both of which degrade collagen and result in erosion of cartilage, clinical symptoms, and pain of arthritis (42).

There have been reports of 19 women with Lyme disease, five of whom had infants with problems of syndactyly, cortical blindness, prematurity, rash, and even fetal death (35).

For pediatric treatment, phenoxy penicillin is effective in doses of 50 mg/kg/day (up to 2 g day for 10 to 20 days). For children allergic to penicillin, erythromycin can be given. Later in the illness, parenteral antibiotics are usually necessary. For established arthritis, 2.4 million units per week for three weeks or intravenous penicillin 20 million units per day in divided doses seem to be curative in 50% of cases (62). Patients with chronic arthritis have been treated conservatively with nonsteroidal anti-inflammatory agents, partial weight-bearing, and intra-articular steroids (63). Strenuous activity may prolong active disease. Synovectomy has been a successful form of treatment in a small number of patients with the chronic form of arthritis (34).

Hemophiliac Arthropathy

PATHOPHYSIOLOGY

Hemophilia is a sex-linked hereditary bleeding diathesis caused by defective plasma coagulation factors. The classical hemophilia A is a deficiency of Factor VIII. In hemophilia B, or Christmas disease, Factor IX is deficient. Depending on the level of circulating coagulation factor, hemophilia is classified as mild, moderate, or severe. In children with severe hemophilia, the plasma coagulation factor is less than 1% and spontaneous articular bleeding may occur without history of trauma. In moderate and mild disease, hemarthrosis is usually precipitated by an injury, which is sometimes relatively slight. In cases of moderate deficiency, plasma coagulation factor ranges from 1% to 5% whereas, in mild hemophilia, it is above 5%.

There are three stages in the development of hemarthrosis. In the acute phase, the joint is hot, tender, and distended as a result of fresh intra-articular bleeding. Today 10% to 15% of adolescents and 75% of adults with hemophilia have chronic arthropathy. In the past, all patients with severe disease developed the arthropathy by the age of 10 yr. With moderate disease, arthropathy developed by adulthood. This should not be true of patients who are treated at the first signs of tingling rather than after 4 to 6 hours of bleeding (17) when accumulation of blood in the joint space, consequent pain, muscle spasms, and guarding positions that relieve intra-articular pressure are already present.

Current medical treatment is replacement of the defective coagulation factor. Fresh frozen plasma contains all clotting factors but its use is limited by physiological tolerance of plasma volume increase. This limitation allows safe treatment with only 10 to 15 ml/kg, which is expected to result in a 10% to 20% rise in factor VIII activity. However, to control an acute hemarthrosis, a plasma factor level of 40% to 50% is needed for hemostasis and to provide coverage for at least 24 hours. Therapy can be repeated in 48 hours if necessary. Cryoprecipitate in fresh frozen plasma recovers 30% to 50% of Factor VIII and fibrinogen. One advantage of this treatment is decreased risk of a blood-borne virus infection. Lyophilized concentrate made from pooled plasma is purified after cryoprecipitation by a variety of methods and is generally highly acceptable. The disadvantage of plasma pooling is that some concentrates may contain as many as 20,000 donors, which increases the possibility of infection. Between 1977 and 1984, 90% of severe hemophiliacs were exposed to human immunodeficiency virus (HIV) (17).

If treatment is delayed, inadequate, or ineffective due to the presence of plasma inhibitors or antibodies to the replacement factor, the hemarthrosis may progress to a subacute stage. The synovial membrane becomes thickened, vascularized with propensity for subsequent bleeding. Once this process is set in motion, the patient will have repeated hemorrhages in the same joint and chronic hemarthrosis develops with intra-articular fibrosis, cartilage destruction, and severe movement limitation. Intra-articular bleeding tends to occur in the knee, elbow, ankle, shoulder, hip, and wrist joints in this order of frequency. On occasion, small articulations of the hand may be affected. Weight bearing joints and those without soft tissue protection are most vulnerable.

EVALUATION

Examination of children with hemarthrosis should include measurement of articular motion in all large joints as well as small articulations with a history of bleeding. Gait and posture must be observed. Leg length and extremity girth are recorded, particularly in the thigh and calf where muscle atrophy is most common and has significant functional implications. It is important to review the status of replacement therapy, compliance, use of assistive devices, general functional level, and recreational activities of the child.

JOINT MANAGEMENT

Prevention of joint deformities and preservation of muscle strength are two equally important aims of rehabilitation in hemophiliac arthritis. In the lower extremities, especially abnormal joint alignment will enhance the stress of weight-bearing, thereby creating an increased risk of subsequent trauma and intra-articular hemorrhage. Furthermore, joints are more prone to injury when they are deprived of normal shock-absorbing protection provided by supportive muscles (8).

Acute intra-articular bleeding requires clotting factor replacement therapy, joint immobilization for 48 hours that, in the case of a lower extremity joint, also means nonweight-bearing and a graduated regimen of exercises thereafter. Regardless whether the hemarthrosis is acute, subacute, or chronic, therapeutic exercises must follow a course of slowly progressive intensity, which is determined by subjective symptoms and clinical findings. Initially, the child is taught isometric exercises to muscles surrounding the affected joint. In 2 to 3 days, active and assistive movements can be started proceeding from gravity eliminated to antigravity positions. After the pain has subsided and the child is able to perform active motion against gravity without any difficulty, a program of progressive resistive exercise can be instituted. It is essential to avoid the use of excessive resistance that could inflict additional joint damage and bleeding. Therefore, movements must be performed in a slow, steady fashion and the amount of resistance should not exceed ½ to 1 lb at first with similar increments added at weekly intervals unless exacerbation of symptoms appears. Passive ROM exercises should not be used in hemophiliac arthritis since they cause minor trauma with bleeding. Local application of cold or ice compresses can be helpful to alleviate pain in the acute stage. Heat must be avoided because it tends to increase bleeding tendency.

Splints and Orthoses

Splints are used for joint immobilization during the acute phase and the most frequent indication is bleeding in the knee joint. In chronic hemarthrosis, splinting at night is suggested to avoid recurrent bleeding. A traditional KAFO may be recommended to support the knee on ambulation and to provide slow maintained stretching of flexion contractures (39). A Dynasplint can be used on the elbow or knee to gain progressive extension. It must be stressed that orthotic support of the knee is not a substitute for stability provided by effective muscle action. In fact, once muscle strength is restored, recurrent episodes of hemarthrosis generally decrease.

Temporary splinting may be needed to immobilize a painful ankle with acute hemarthrosis. Air splints to prevent inversion and eversion of the ankle may be useful in the active child with hemophilia who has chronic bleeding into one or both ankles. The practical difficulty with air splints is their low durability and need for frequent replacement.

MANAGEMENT OF SPECIFIC JOINTS

Knee

This joint is the most common site of hemarthrosis. Acute bleeding requires immobilization during the first 48 hours. A light knee immobilizer splint is suitable for this purpose and should be kept on hand in cases with recurrent bleeding episodes (Fig. 12.15). The child is not allowed to bear weight on the affected extremity and must use crutches for walking. If the elbow joint is also involved, the crutches are modified with a platform attachment for the arm. During the period of immobilization, the child should perform isometric exercises of the muscles surrounding the knee in order to alleviate disuse weakness. For maintaining strength and ROM at the unaffected lower extremity joints, active exercises to the hip and ankle are advised. After 48 hours, active motion of the knee can be started progressing to extension against gravity. When active movements are at least partially regained and the knee is free of pain, the immobilizer splint may be removed. Full weight-bearing is allowed after the pain has subsided and limitation of active knee extension is not more than 15°. Active resistive exercises using progressive weight increments as outlined earlier can begin when 90° knee motion is restored. Depending on the child's age, 3 to 5 lb of resistance for 10 repetitions twice daily is used for a maintenance program.

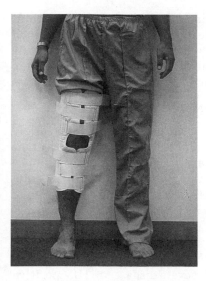

Figure 12.15. Commercially available knee immobilizer with Velcro closures for the first 48 hours after a bleeding episode.

If another episode of acute hemarthrosis develops, resistive exercises must be discontinued and the sequential program should be started again beginning with isometric contractions.

Chronic hemophiliac arthropathy of the knee affects the mobility of the ipsilateral hip and ankle. Furthermore, deformity of one knee places excessive stress on the contralateral lower extremity and leads to postural malalignment with pelvic obliquity and resultant scoliosis. Gait training and postural exercises must be instituted to alleviate these consequences.

Elbow

The second most common site of hemarthrosis is the elbow. As in the case of other joints, an acute episode of bleeding is treated with immobilization and isometric exercises of the musculature around the elbow in the manner described. Active exercises of the shoulder and wrist are used to ensure that no loss of movement occurs at these joints during the period of immobilization. After the acute episode, the program proceeds from active exercises for restoring ROM to progressive resistive exercises for increasing strength. For a chronic maintenance program in children, 2 to 3 lb of resistance in the form of a weighted wrist cuff is adequate. All exercises must include elbow flexion, extension, supination, and pronation. Because it is particularly difficult to regain extension and supination, these movements should be stressed as soon as the intra-articular bleeding has ceased.

Ankle

Hemarthrosis of this joint usually leads to limitation of dorsiflexion, eversion, and inversion. Use of an air splint for a period of months allows resolution of chronic synovitis. At the same time, the child needs to perform active assistive ROM to maintain full ankle motion. A good exercise, which includes every possible motion, is to make circular movements with the ankle. The children are taught to make a daily habit of toe and heel walking after the acute stage of bleeding has subsided.

RECREATION

Children with hemophilia are encouraged to participate in recreation. However, they must learn to observe certain precautions to live with their disease, to gauge the relative safety of different activities, and to avoid those that are potentially injurious. It is important to plan with each child a suitable activity program, considering individual preferences and the severity of disease. For proper guidance, one must know whether the child receives regular replacement at home or in a hospital and whether treatment is easily available. Patients with plasma inhibitors or antibodies are more difficult to treat and recreational activities should be chosen with a more conservative approach. Many of the adolescents with severe disease are HIV positive and concern of morbidity and mortality from this complication may supersede other treatment complications.

Competitive sports and those that involve high impact and body contact are generally contraindicated. Swimming is an excellent activity for all children with hemophilia and, as an exception, it is a sport that may be allowed on a competitive basis. However, diving and playing in the shallow pool should be avoided because of the potential risk of injury. Walking, hiking, jogging, badminton, and jumping rope may be appropriate in individual cases. Some children may prefer golf or tennis but these sports are inadvisable when there is chronic or recurrent hemarthrosis of the upper extremity joints because of the strong forces produced, in particular, at the elbow.

For very young children, low carts propelled with the arms or legs present a good opportunity to be active. Tricycling on an elevated seat promotes hip and knee extension. The popular "Big Wheel" tends to be unstable at high speeds and should be used with caution. Bicycling is a good sport provided the child is mature enough to be concerned about personal safety and is reliable in observing precautionary rules. Softball, soccer, and basketball may be considered in some cases but only on a noncompetitive basis because, in the excitement of competition, children are prone to ignore pain and injury. Wrestling, boxing, and downhill skiing are strongly discouraged in all instances.

REFERENCES

1. Ansell BM: Juvenile arthritis. *The Practitioner* 230:343–350, 1986.
2. Ansell BM: Pediatric rehabilitative rheumatology. In *Rheumatic Disorders in Childhood.* Boston, Butterworth, 1980.
3. Arroyo IL, Brewer EJ, Giannini EH: Arthritis/arthralgia and hypermobility in school children. *J Rheumatol* 15:978–980, 1988.

4. Asbrink E, Brehmer-Anderson E, Houmark A: Acrodermatitis chronica atrophicans—a spirochetosis: Clinical and pathological picture based on 32 patients; course and relationship to erythema chronicum migrans. Afzelius. *Am J Dermatopathol* 8:209, 1986.
5. Baldwin J: Pool therapy compared with individual home exercise therapy for juvenile rheumatoid arthritis. *Physiotherapy* 58:230, 1972.
6. Ball GV: Ankylosing spondylitis. In McCarty DJ (ed) *Arthritis and Allied Conditions*. Philadelphia, Lea & Febiger, 1989.
7. Bianco AJ, Peterson HA: Juvenile rheumatoid arthritis. *Orthop Clin North Am* 2:745, 1971.
8. Boone DC: Common musculoskeletal problems and their management. In Boone DC (ed): *Comprehensive Management of Hemophilia*. Philadelphia, FA Davis Co, 1976.
9. Boone JE, Baldwin J, Levine C: Juvenile rheumatoid arthritis. *Pediatr Clin North Am* 21:885, 1974.
10. Brewer EJ: Reduction of morning stiffness and/or pain using a sleeping bag. *Pediatrics* 56:621, 1975.
11. Calabro J: Early diagnosis and management of ankylosing spondylitis. *Med Times* 105:80, 1977.
12. Calabro JJ: Juvenile rheumatoid arthritis. In McCarty DJ (ed): *Arthritis and Allied Conditions*. Philadelphia, Lea & Febiger, 1989.
13. Calabro JJ: Management of juvenile rheumatoid arthritis. *J Pediatr* 77:353, 1970.
14. Cassidy JT, Petty RE: *Textbook of Pediatric Rheumatology*. New York, Churchill Livingstone, Inc. 1990.
15. Chaplin D, Pulkki T, Soarimaa A, Vainto K: Wrist and finger deformities in juvenile rheumatoid arthritis. *Acta Rheumatol Scand* 15:206, 1969.
16. Committee on Infectious Disease. American Academy of Pediatrics. Elk Grove Village, IL 1988.
17. Corrigan JJ: Hemostasis: General considerations. In Miller DR, Baehner RL (eds): *Blood: Diseases of Infancy and Childhood*. St. Louis, CV Mosby Co, 767–777, 1984.
18. Gault SJ, Spyker JM: Beneficial effect of immobilization of joints in rheumatoid and related arthritides: A splint study using sequential analysis. *Arthritis Rheum* 12:34, 1969.
19. Gedalia A, Person DA, Brewer EJ, Giannini EH: Hypermobility of the joints in juvenile episodic arthritis/arthralgia. *J Pediatr* 107:873–876, 1986.
20. Gerber LH: Principles and their application in the rehabilitation of patients with rheumatic disease. In Kelly WN, Harris ED, Ruddy S, Sledge CB (eds): *Textbook of Rheumatology*. Philadelphia, WB Saunders, Vol II, 1981.
21. Gerber LH: Rehabilitative therapies for patients with rheumatic disease. In Schumacher HR (ed): *Primer on Rheumatic Diseases*. Atlanta, Arthritis Foundation, 1988.
22. Granberry WM, Brewer EJ: The combined pediatric approach to management of juvenile rheumatoid arthritis. *Orthop Clin North Am* 9:481, 1978.
23. Granberry WM, Magnum GL: The hand in the child with juvenile arthritis. *J Hand Surg* 5:105, 1980.
24. Greene NE, Edwards K: Bone and joint infections in children. *Orthop Clin North Am* Oct. 18(4):555, 1987.
25. Hicks JE: Exercise for patients with inflammatory arthritis. *J Musculoskel Med* 6(10):40, 1989.
26. Hicks RQ, Melish ME: Kawasaki syndrome. *Pediatr Clin North Am* 33(5):1151, 1986.
27. Ho S: Bacterial Arthritis. In McCarty DJ (ed): *Arthritis and Allied Conditions*. Philadelphia, Lea & Febiger, 1989.
28. Hunt GC, Fromherz WA, Gerber LH, Hurwitz SR: Hindfoot pain treated by a leg-hindfoot orthosis. A case report. *Physical Therapy* 67:1384, 1987.
29. Jacobs JC: Pediatric Rheumatology for the Practitioner. New York, Springer Verlag 1–556, 1982.
30. Lehman J, De Lateur BJ: Therapeutic heat. In Lehman JF (ed): *Therapeutic Heat and Cold,* ed 3. Baltimore, Williams & Wilkins, 1982.

31. Lehman JF, de Lateur B: Diathermy and Superficial Heat, Laser and Cold Therapy. In Krusen's Handbook of Physical Medicine and Rehabilitation. Philadelphia, WB Saunders, 1990.
32. MacBain KP, Hill RH: A functional assessment of juvenile rheumatoid arthritis. *Am J Occup Ther* 27:326, 1973.
33. Macover S, Satsky AJ: Effective isometric exercise on the quadriceps muscle. Patient with rheumatoid arthritis. *Arch Phys Med Rehabil* 47:737, 1966.
34. McLaughlin TP, Zemel L, Fisher RL, Gossling HR: Chronic arthritis of the knee in Lyme disease. *J Bone Joint Surg* 68-A(7):1057, 1986.
35. Marbowitz LE, Steere AC, Benach J: Lyme disease in pregnancy. *JAMA* 256:3394, 1986.
36. Melish ME: Kawasaki syndrome. (The mucocutaneous lymph node syndrome). *Ann Rev Med* 33:569, 1982.
37. Messher RP: Arthritis due to Mycobacteria, Funghi and Parasites. In McCarty DJ (ed): *Arthritis and Allied Conditions.* Philadelphia, Lea & Febiger, 1989.
38. Mills JA, Pinals RS, Ropes MW, Short CL, Sutcliff J: Value of bed rest in patients with rheumatoid arthritis. *N Engl J Med* 284:453, 1971.
39. Molnar G: Orthotic management in children. In Redford JB (ed): *Orthotics Etcetera.* Baltimore, Williams & Wilkins, 1986.
40. Mooney V, Stills M: Continuous passive motion with joint fractures and infections. *Orthop Clin North Am* 18(1):1, 1987.
41. Muller EA: Influence of training and inactivity on muscle strength. *Arch Phys Med Rehabil* 55:449, 1970.
42. Myerhoff J: Lyme disease. *Am J Med* 75:663, 1983.
43. Ozel AT, Kottke FJ: Rheumatoid arthritis in children. *Minn Med* 60:637, 1977.
44. Pachner AR, Steere AC: Tertiary Lyme disease—central nervous system manifestations of long standing infections of borrelia burgdorferi. *Zki Bakt Hyg* 263:301, 1986.
45. Pachner AR, Steere AC: The triad of neurologic manifestations of Lyme disease: Meningitis, cranial neuritis and radiculoneuritis. *Neurology* 35:47, 1985.
46. Pendelton TR, Coleman MR, Grossman, BJ: Numerical scale for evaluation of patient with inflammatory joint disease. *Phys Ther* 53:373, 1973.
47. Petty RE: Epidemiology and genetics of the rheumatic disease of childhood. In Cassidy JJ (ed): *Textbook of Pediatric Rheumatology.* New York, John Wiley & Sons, 15, 1982.
48. Pinals RS: Traumatic Arthritis and Allied Condition. In McCarty DJ (ed): *Arthritis and Allied Conditions.* Philadelphia, Lea & Febiger, 1989.
49. Rosenberg AM: Advanced drug therapy for juvenile rheumatoid arthritis. *J Pediatr* 114(2):171, 1989.
50. Rothfield NF: Systemic lupus erythematosus: Clinical aspects and treatment. In McCarty, DJ (ed): *Arthritis and Allied Conditions.* Philadelpia, Lea & Febiger, 1989.
51. Salter RB: *Textbook of Disorders and Injuries of Musculosketal System.* Baltimore, Williams & Wilkins, 1970.
52. Salter RB, Kelley FW: The protective effect of continuous passive motion on living articular cartilage in acute septic arthritis. *Clin Orthop Rel Res* 159:223, 1981.
53. Schaller JG: Treatment of juvenile rheumatoid arthritis. In McCarty DJ (ed): *Arthritis and Allied Conditions.* Philadelphia, Lea & Febiger, 1989.
54. Schaller JG, Wedgewood RJ: Rheumatic Disease of Childhood. In Behrman RE, Vaughn VC (eds): *Nelson's Textbook of Pediatrics.* Philadelphia, WB Saunders, 1987.
55. Schmid FR: Routine drug treatment of septic arthritis. *Clin Rheumatic Dis* 10(2):293, 1984.
56. Seull SA, Dow MD, Athreyea BH: Physical and occupational therapy for children with rheumatologic disease. *Pediatr Clin North Am* 35(5):1073, 1988.
57. Singsen BH: Pediatric rheumatic diseases. Non-articular rheumatism, JRA, juvenile spondyloarthropathies. *Primer on the Rheumatic Disease.* Atlanta, Arthritis Foundation, 160, 1988.

58. Simon L: Rehabilitation of rheumatoid shoulder. *Rheumatol Rehabil (Suppl)* 18:81, 1979.
59. Smythe H: Therapy of the spondyloarthropathies. *Clin Orthop* 143:84, 1979.
60. Steere AC: Lyme disease. *N Engl J Med* 321(9):586, 1989.
61. Steere AC, Batsford WP, Weinberg M: Lyme carditis: cardiac abnormalities of Lyme disease. *Ann Intern Med* 93:8, 1980.
62. Steere AC, Greene J, Schoen RT: Successful parenteral penicillin therapy of established septic arthritis. *N Engl J Med* 312:869, 1985.
63. Steere AC, Schoen RT, Taylor E: The clinical evaluation of Lyme arthritis. *Ann Intern Med* 107:725, 1987.
64. Sweezey RL: Approaches to deformities in rheumatoid arthritis. *Postgrad Med J* 45:146, 1969.
65. Sweezey RL: Essentials of management and rehabilitation in arthritis. *Semin Arthritis Rheum* 3:349, 1974.
66. Sweezey RL: Rehabilitation in Arthritis and Allied Conditions. In Kottke FJ, Lehman JF (eds): *Krusen's Handbook of Physical Medicine and Rehabilitation.* Philadelphia, WB Saunders, 1990.
67. Sweezey RL: Rehabilitation Medicine and Arthritis. In McCarty DJ (ed): *Arthritis and Allied Conditions.* Philadelphia, Lea & Febiger, 1989.
68. Sullivan DB, Cassidy JT, Petty RE, Burt A: Prognosis in childhood dermatomyositis. *J Pediatr* 80:555, 1972.
69. Szer IS: Systemic lupus erythematosus, dermatomyositis, scleroderma & vasculitis in childhood. In Kelly WN, Harris S, Ruddy C, Sledge B (eds): *Textbook of Rheumatology.* Philadelpia, WB Saudners, 1989.
70. Vance PW: Chronic state treatment of dermatomyositis. *Arthritis Rheum* 20:342, 1971.

13

Spinal Cord Injury

JAMES BOYD AND JANE C. S. PERRIN

For the child and adolescent, the profound multisystemic effect of a spinal cord injury is compounded by impairment of growth, development, and personality adjustment. Although physiological consequences are similar in children and adults, the differences are most striking in the young patient. Adolescents are more like adults except for a greater tendency to develop scoliosis and more pronounced psychological reactions. Rehabilitation is a long process involving child, immediate family, hospital-based health team, school, and community agencies. The discussion in this chapter is often focused on body parts but the implication is to appreciate and treat the needs of the whole child.

Epidemiology

Pediatric spinal cord injury is defined as an acute traumatic lesion of the cord and roots resulting in motor and sensory deficit or both from newborn to adolescent age group. Of the estimated 11,000 new cases of spinal cord injury in the United States each year, nearly 10% occur in children of 1 to 15 yr of age (65).

Motor vehicle accidents cause 50% to 65% of injuries, followed by trauma from sporting accidents, falls and gunshot wounds, and occasional birth trauma. In Kewalramani's study of pediatric spinal cord injuries (64), mortality rate from all causes was 59% and from motor vehicle accidents 84%. The mortality rate for patients reaching a hospital is 4.2% in the 0- to 19-yr age group (5).

Pathophysiology

Although spinal fractures are the rule in adults, up to half the children under 10 yr of age suffer traction, contusion, or ischemic injury of the spinal cord without radiologic evidence of fracture or dislocation (12, 65, 95, 101, 121). For this reason, the pediatric trauma victim must be examined carefully for clinical evidence of cord injury. This is particularly difficult in the presence of head injury (113). A further problem is a 2- to 4-day delay in the appearance of neurological findings that has been described in children after traumatic infarction of the spinal cord (13). Anatomic variation and osseous immaturity of the young child can masquerade as a fracture or subluxation injury (35, 114). Magnetic resonance imaging (MRI) is useful in identifying the site and extent of the cord injury, particularly when skeletal findings are absent (4). Minor contusion can increase permeability of intramedullary microvasculature producing edema, microhemorrhage, decreased perfusion, and secondary elevation of lysosomal enzymes (129). After experimental spinal cord trauma, hemorrhage appears in the central gray matter by 30 minutes and, within 24 hours, gray and white matter is necrotic (123). The injury zone can extend over time in a transverse, caudal, or rostral direction (17). A syrinx may develop immediately or many years after injury, creating additional neurological deficit (25, 40). If an MRI is obtained soon after the injury, subsequent films can verify the development of a new lesion or its progression (Fig. 13.1).

Damage to the major spinal cord vessels, such as the anterior, posterior,

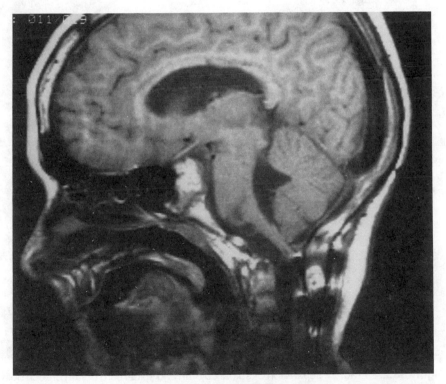

Figure 13.1. Cystic lesion of the brainstem and cervical cord in a child with complete C1 quadriplegia and multiple cranial nerve deficits affecting ocular movements, swallowing, and speech.

or Adamkiewicz artery, can result in extensive infarction. Cross-clamping of the aorta can cause spinal cord injury (102). Decreased distal aortic pressure below 60 mm Hg is correlated with a loss of somatosensory-evoked potentials and subsequent paraplegia (69). Recent studies correlated the risk of injury with pressure of the cerebral spinal fluid (CSF) in the lumbar canal and have suggested prevention by removing CSF prior to clamping (2, 85). Monitoring somatosensory-evoked potentials is recommended.

Although rare, spinal cord injury does occur at birth in association with breech delivery. A particular snapping noise has been described during breech delivery that is associated with quadriplegia and seen in the absence of radiologic evidence of injury (10, 67). Leventhal (73) demonstrated with neonatal autopsy specimens that the spinal column could be stretched 2 inches without disruption but the spinal cord only ¼ inch before tearing (Fig. 13.2). Neonatal traction injury with vascular compromise and hemorrhage

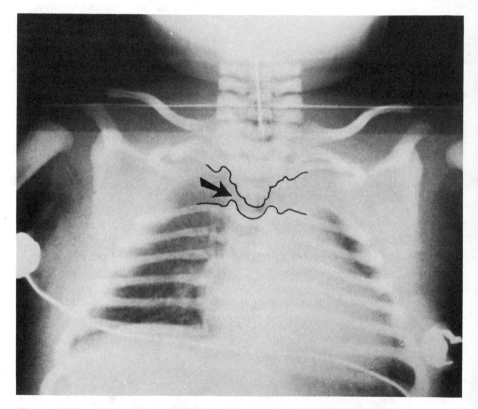

Figure 13.2. Fracture separation of spinal column and spinal cord during breech delivery. Neonatal chest radiograph courtesy of Dean Ross, MD, Department of Physical Medicine and Rehabilitation, University of Michigan, Ann Arbor, MI.

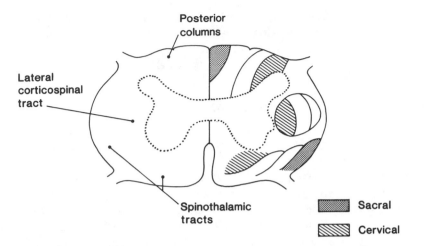

Figure 13.3. Cross-section cervical spinal cord illustrating central location of cervical tracts and peripheral sacral tracts ascending and descending. Modified from Chusid (14).

is likely to cause extensive damage along the spinal cord axis and the child generally does not regain reflex innervation.

Patients with incomplete motor or sensory loss have a better prognosis for neurological recovery. Evidence of motor function should be sought below the level of the lesion and carefully differentiated from spinal cord reflex activity, such as the triple flexion or withdrawal reflex. In the young child, testing of sensory modalities may be limited to pain sensation but careful examination is warranted. In older children, position sense can be tested and may reveal sparing of the posterior columns. Preservation of sacral sensation is the major early indicator of an incomplete lesion, such as occurs with central cord injury, anterior spinal artery infarction, and cord contusions. Peripheral anatomic location of sacral and lumbar sensory and motor fibers accounts for the sacral sparing in partial cord injuries as illustrated in Figure 13.3. The Brown-Sequard syndrome is characterized by preserved motor function and absent pain sensation on one side, with loss of motor function and spared pain sensation on the other side.

In a follow-up of neurological evolution of 300 patients examined with 24 hours of spinal cord injury, Philippi and associates (100) found that spinal cord concussion (spinal shock) may mask motor and sensory levels up to 48 hours. A lesion can be considered complete when anal reflexes return in the absence of sensation or movement below the dermatome/myotome level of the injury. Children with incomplete lesions recover function most rapidly in the first 2 months but may continue to improve up to 1 yr.

Somatosensory-evoked potentials (SSEP) are useful if severity of the lesion is in doubt. Rowed and co-workers (109) demonstrated altered but elicitable response during the first week in patients with incomplete lesions. Recovery of physiological responses preceded clinical improvement. SSEP are absent to peripheral nerve stimulation below the level of the injury in patients with complete lesions.

Treatment of Acute Stage

Because the majority of spinal cord injuries arrive in the emergency room as definite or possible incomplete lesions, early aggressive treatment is indicated. In a review of acute management, Green and associates (47) attribute reduction of sequelae to proper emergency care, attention to respiratory and cardiovascular stabilization, immobilization of the patient on a spine board, efficient transportation, and team management in the emergency roor

Clinical and radiological examinations for concurrent injuries are andatory. Central and peripheral intravenous lines are placed to maintain dequate tissue perfusion and corticosteroids are given. Bracken and associ ites (6) demonstrate that the administration of a high dose of methylprednisolone given over 23 hours and beginning within 8 hours of injury are beneficial to patients with both incomplete and complete injury. A variety of other treatments for reversal of paralysis have been tried with uncertain results. These include regional hypothermia, dimethylsulfoxide, hyperbaric oxygen, α-adrenergic blockers such as phenoxybenzamine, antifibrinolytic therapy with ϵ-aminocaproic acid, pyrogenic polysaccharides, and nerve growth factor.

Animal experiments suggest that combination of nimodipine with dextran 40, commencing 1 hour after compression clip injury, improves spinal cord blood flow, motor-evoked potentials and somatosensory-evoked potentials (32). Direct-current stimulation with electrodes placed against the dura in rats provides significant improvement in motor performance, amplitude of motor-evoked potentials, and axon cell counts in the motor cortex and brain stem nuclei (33).

In childhood, spinal fractures with neurological deficit occur at all levels but are most commonly cervical. These include fractures with and without dislocation, which are unstable if the ligaments and discs rupture (54). In children under 8 yr of age, the cord injury is primarily in the upper cervical region (52, 110). Thoracic fractures are inherently more stable but may also require stabilization of realignment. Denis (23) has proposed the "three column spine" in order to analyze more accurately the stability of various injuries. Availability of CT and MRI scans have improved the accuracy of the classification of skeletal injury.

After the acute medical problems have been controlled, definitive treatment of the spinal injury may require closed or open reduction for decompression of neurological structures and/or for restoring vertebral alignment and stability to permit early mobilization. If impingment of cord or roots is suspected, metrizamide myelography, computed tomography (CT), and/or MRI may be useful. Wilmot and Hall (124) report their surgical indications in adults and compare the surgical approach to conservative management. The halo cervical device provides the most effective immobilization and may be used as the primary method of closed reduction and fixation. The halo also permits open reduction while providing stability.

In general, surgical techniques consist of reduction followed by posterior fusion for subluxation or dislocations, whereas the anterior approach may be necessary for compression fractures (57, 61). Fusion and stability are enhanced with the use of wiring, spinal plates, distraction rods, and/or external orthoses. Farcy and Weidenbaum (30) report that the Cotrel-Dubousset instrumentation offers three-dimensional restoration of spinal injuries with greater stability in torsion and axial loading. Surgical complications are infrequent. Patients who are expected to cooperate can be safely managed without restrictive body jacket, allowing advanced self-care training within 2 to 3 weeks after the procedure (84).

Early management is best done in a pediatric intensive care unit. Cardiopulmonary support is particularly important in cervical cord injuries and may be necessary at least temporarily in high thoracic cord injuries. Atelectasis and pneumonia are frequent complications in cervical and thoracic injuries (37, 86, 107). Optimal nutrition (Table 1.1) and pressure relief of vulnerable skin areas are special concerns. The use of a kinetic bed that remains in motion throughout the day enhances skin pressure relief, venous return, and postural drainage while immobilizing the unstable spinal column. Psychological support for the patient and family should begin at this time. The child without complications who has been stabilized for early mobilization can progress to a rehabilitation unit in 2 to 3 weeks after the injury.

Rehabilitation Management of the Flaccid Phase

There are many differences in the management of the child with spinal cord injury in the flaccid phase compared to the spastic stage. The flaccid phase may last a few days or months and occasionally is permanent.

RESPIRATORY SUPPORT

Children with quadriplegia at the C3 level or above have insufficient diaphragmatic innervation to maintain functional respiration and need tracheostomy with mechanical ventilation. Quadriplegia at the C4 segment requires ventilation until respiratory musculature can be strengthened. Even quadriplegia at lower cervical or thoracic levels can cause insidious respiratory distress necessitating short-term intubation and artificial ventilation due to the absence of intercostal muscle function.

Exercises should be instituted at the earliest possible time in order to utilize and strengthen neck and shoulder muscles, which play an accessory role to expand the rib cage (43, 48). Strengthening of the clavicular portion of the pectoralis muscle to increase the force of expiration is recommended by De Troyer and associates (21). Since diaphragmatic muscles develop disuse atrophy after mechanical ventilation for a long period, these muscles also need strengthening. Children generally require additional exercises to identify and coordinate diaphragmatic movement. Independent breathing has to be increased gradually and performed several times during the day to avoid exhaustion of the available musculature, which may demoralize the child and staff. Preceding the sessions with postural drainage and shallow tracheal suctioning will reduce airway resistance. Suctioning beyond the opening of the tracheostomy tube is irritating to the tracheal mucosa and should be minimized. β-Adrenergic aerosol acts directly on the mucociliary system to accelerate clearance of tracheal secretions (39, 70) and reduces bronchospasm by smooth muscle relaxation. Adapted cough techniques should be taught to both the child and family (8). In the upright position, an abdominal binder improves mechanical function of the diaphragm (46).

Monitoring with a pulse oximeter is useful to reassure the child that oxygenation is adequate. Formal pulmonary function testing including arterial blood gas determination, measurement of maximal inspiratory and expiratory pressures, responses to hypoxia and hypercarbia, and spirometry should be performed at regular intervals. Braun and colleagues (7) report that unilateral diaphragmatic dysfunction tends to create oxygen desaturation during sleep.

Respiratory obstruction by airway secretions, granulation tissue, plugged tracheostomy tube, and intercurrent infection, such as tracheitis or pneumonia, will require careful vigilance and modification of ventilatory assistance.

CARDIOVASCULAR CARE

During the flaccid phase of quadriplegia, there is lower diastolic blood pressure, feeble spinal sympathetic cardiovascular reflexes, and decreased plasma epinephrine and norepinephrine (80). Winslow and colleagues (125) demonstrated that tracheal suctioning and/or prone positioning precipitated the most episodes of bradycardia and asystole in children with quadriplegia. Vagolytic agents rapidly reversed these episodes.

Orthostatic hypotension is controlled with elastic stockings, abdominal compression, and air splints. Graduated upright positioning on a tilt table while monitoring pulse and blood pressure allows for readjustment over a period of time. Helpful medications are salt tablets and ephedrine or pseudoephedrine before getting out of bed.

The risk of deep vein thrombosis and pulmonary embolism is extremely low in children prior to puberty (50, 103). Complications from preventive treatment probably outweigh benefits for the young patient. However, prophylaxis with low-dose heparin is recommended for the postpubertal adolescent who resembles the adult more than the child in this respect. The regimen starts 12 hours after the injury with 150 units/kg/12 hours subcutaneously not to exceed 5000 units per single dose. If lower extremity swelling occurs and deep venous thrombosis is documented, heparin doses must be increased and monitored by partial thromboplastin time. Heparinized patients should not receive aspirin because platelets are the only blood components providing hemostasis (97).

GASTROINTESTINAL COMPLICATIONS

Adynamic ileus may occasionally persist for several days or weeks. Prolonged ileus has been treated successfully with metoclopramide (89).

Upper intestinal bleeding may occur in the early weeks after a cord injury. In studies of mixed age groups. the youngest patients being 12 yr old, the risk varied from 4% (63) to 20% (27), and increased with full heparinization but not with low-dose heparin or steroids. Duodenal and gastric ulcers are common bleeding sites in children. Fiberoptic endoscopy is the most reliable method of finding the source of bleeding. Cimetidine can be given in doses of 10 to 20 mg/kg/24 hours to reduce gastric acidity. In persistent flaccid phase, the anal sphincter remains patulous. These cases arc best managed by a constipating diet low in fiber and spice. Bowel evacuation by Valsalva maneuver and/or digital disimpaction are the usual methods but fecal soiling may continue. Medications, such as kaopectate and probanthine, may be useful to maintain firm consistency of stools and to decrease peristalsis.

URINARY SYSTEM

In the early weeks after spinal cord injury, the bladder remains asensory, atonic, and flaccid. Unless it is artificially drained, distension occurs. Cumulative experience leaves no doubt that intermittent catheterization is the technique of choice (9, 115) replacing indwelling catheters after initial hydration is completed. Percutaneous suprapubic catheter placement is reported to be a safe and effective alternative to intermittent catheterization for early management of the bladder in adolescents and adults (93). This study extended for only 35 days and does not imply that long-term use is without risk.

SYMPTOMATIC HYPERCALCEMIA

Beware the pubertal child with increasing irritability and anorexia (82). Hypercalcemia may reach alarming pathological levels of 13 to 14 g/ml at 6 to 12 weeks after the injury. Symptoms are anorexia, nausea and vomiting, constipation, polyuria, and polydypsia and/or emotional lability. Dehydration makes renal excretion even more difficult. Parathyroid hormone and alkaline phosphatase levels are normal. Inability to concentrate urine, nephrocalcinosis, renal stones, and hypertension are significant but reversible complications.

Standing and mobilization alone are inadequate to control hypercalcemia. The usefulness of electrical stimulation of paralyzed muscles is undocumented. Elimination of vitamin D intake, low calcium diet down to 200 mg/day, intravenous saline infusion, and furosemide may result in temporary control only. Other treatments with serious potential side effects are mithromycin, a cytotoxic platelet inhibitor, and high doses of corticosteroids. Calcitonin, a direct inhibitor of bone resorption with low toxicity, is a definitive treatment of choice for short-term therapy (1).

There is no established relation between hypercalcemia and heterotopic ossification, or of the decreased growth rate of the lower extremities that occurs in injured children. Duval-Beaupere et al. (24) discuss possible causative factors related to growth problems in the trunk and lower extremities after spinal cord injury.

Rehabilitation Management of the Spastic Phase

The onset of spasticity heralds important new problems and warrants a different management strategy.

HYPERACTIVE REFLEXES

Exaggerated stretch reflexes activated by the muscle spindle and nociceptive reflexes precipitated by cutaneous stimuli contribute to hyperreflexia, hypertonicity, and muscle spasm. From a clinical viewpoint, these symptoms interfere with transfer, ambulation, and bed mobility. Proper positioning to prevent hip, knee, and plantarflexion contractures, slow sustained stretching sometimes preceded by icing, and the use of splints to resist spastic posturing are therapeutic measures.

Diazepam and baclofen are useful medications to achieve skeletal muscle relaxation (60, 130). Intramuscular phenol neurolysis guided by nerve stimulation or selected peripheral nerve blocks may reduce spasticity for several weeks or months. Residual low-level spasticity is desirable for maintaining muscle tone and to assist transfer. Fixed contractures require surgical intervention including tendon releases and transfers.

AUTONOMIC DYSREFLEXIA

Autonomic dysreflexia is paroxysmal dramatic hyperactivity of the uninhibited sympathetic and parasympathetic nervous system in patients with lesions proximal to T6, above the major sympathetic splanchnic outflow. Triggers are bladder overdistension, fecal impaction, skin breakdown, fractures, and other noxious stimuli below the level of the lesion. High intravesical pressures associated with detrusor-sphincter dyssynergy can trigger dysreflexia even at normal bladder volumes.

Common symptoms are sweating, flushing, and pounding headache. Hypertension, bradycardia, and pilo-erection are clinical signs (62). However, some patients with high cervical injury do not have bradycardia. Death and cerebral vascular accident can result in extreme cases. A high index of suspicion must be maintained by those caring for persons with quadriplegia. Good care is preventive; it includes family education and informing consulting specialists of possible risks prior to surgical procedures, particularly intravesical manipulation (28). Management of an acute episode includes locating and eliminating the stimulus, stopping any procedure in progress, moving to a sitting position to take advantage of orthostatic hypotension, emptying the bladder and rectum, normalizing body temperature, and continuing to monitor vital signs. The use of anesthetic gel or ointment is recommended when examining and disimpacting the rectum so that afferent stimulus is reduced.

For emergency treatment of hypertension, effective drugs are sublingual nifedipine, 0.24 mg/kg (29, 112), or hydralazine in 5- to 10-mg doses intramuscularly or intravenously. Oral drugs used to prevent recurrent episodes are phenoxybenzamine, an adrenergic blocker, and guanethidine. Sweating can be controlled by anticholinergics, such as propantheline or glycopyrrolate. The latter has minimal adverse effect on bladder emptying. Prior to radiological or surgical bladder procedure in the susceptible individual oral administration of mecamylamine is recommended and is more effective than instillation of topical anesthesia (28).

RESPIRATORY CARE

With enhanced muscle tone, the chest wall is subject to increased stability allowing a more effective diaphragmatic ventilation. However, spasticity of the abdominal muscles may reduce tidal volume and lead to progressive respiratory difficulty (49). Continued efforts to improve diaphragmatic strength and the effectiveness of accessory muscles is important to maintain independence from mechanical ventilation even if this is only for short periods during the day. When daytime ventilator dependency cannot be avoided, the use of a portable wheelchair-mounted unit greatly facilitates social interactions, community mobility, and attendance at school.

Phrenic nerve stimulation is another alternative (11, 94, 111). Prerequisites are intact phrenic nerve and diaphragmatic function as demonstrated by phrenic nerve conduction studies (74). Electrodes are placed around the phrenic nerve in the neck or, if necessary, in the thorax. The procedure is technically more difficult in children under 6 yr of age (111). Disuse atrophy of the diaphragm requires gradually increased pacing to avoid muscle fatigue (44, 111).

GASTRIC EMPTYING

Injuries above the sympathetic outflow may cause delayed gastric emptying (31) and lead to reflux, esophagitis, and aspiration.

BOWEL REGULATION

Poor colonic compliance is probably related to hyperreflexia (45). The anal sphincter becomes overactive and constipation with subsequent megacolon may develop. The most reliable method of control is maintenance of a soft bulky stool with high fiber content, digital stimulation, and/or bisacodyl suppository used on a regular schedule for daily or every other day toileting. The gastrocolic reflex should be utilized to aid in colonic evacuation by performing the digital stimulation 20 to 30 minutes after a meal. Oral stool softeners such as docusate sodium and mild laxatives, for example, senna preparations, can be useful adjuncts.

URINARY TRACT

When bladder reflex activity returns, detrusor-sphincter dyssynergy may interfere with effective emptying. Abnormally high intravesical pressures are likely to damage the upper urinary tracts. Urodynamic evaluation provides the most accurate assessment of detrusor-sphincter function, storage capacity, leakage pressure, and the effectiveness of emptying techniques such as bladder tapping (127, 128). Perkash and Friedland (98) report hyperreflexia caused by the catheter used during urodynamic study, suggesting the addition of sonography as a clarification. Renal ultrasound is a safe, reliable technique that should be performed on an annual basis to monitor the function of the upper urinary tracts.

The goals of bladder management are prevention of hydronephrosis and deterioration of renal function as well as avoidance of urinary infection by emptying the bladder completely at regular intervals and urinary continence.

Intermittent clean catheterization is the preferred method of bladder emptying (9, 115) and is effective in preventing hydronephrosis (58). An additional benefit is that complete bladder emptying also reduces bacterial growth (20, 72). Fluid intake should be maintained at a level that creates an adequate flushing action of the urinary system. The timing of catheterization should be at least four times a day to avoid stretching the bladder beyond the normal maximal volume. Standards for bladder capacity and average daily urine output are shown in Table 1.1.

Bladder tapping to promote micturition may be successful in selected cases (127). Transurethral electrostimulation to improve micturition (77) and botulinum toxin to decrease bladder dyssynergia (26), tried in adults, has not been used in children. Pharmacological manipulation is based on the pattern of detrusor and sphincter function: incontinence secondary to sphincter weakness as opposed to sphincter-detrusor dyssynergy with overflow incontinence. An outline of selection and indication for various drugs is shown in Table 13.1. Oxybutynin inhibits detrusor activity, reduces the risk of reflux, and improves bladder storage capacity.

Table 13.1.
Classification and Drug Therapy of Neurogenic Bladder Dysfunction [a]

Detrusor areflexia	Bethanecol (Urecholine):
	Parasympathetic stimulator (cholinergic)
	Contraindicated in asthmatics
Bladder neck (smooth muscle)	Ephedrine
hypotonic dyssynergy	Pseudoephedrine (Sudafed)
	Imipramine (Tofranil):
	α-and β-adrenergic sympathetic stimulators
Nonrelaxing bladder neck	Phenoxybenzamine (Di-Benzyline):
(smooth muscle)	α-adrenergic blockers
Nonrelaxing external sphincter	Diazepam (Valium): brain and spinal cord
(striated muscle)	Polysynaptic reflex inhibition
	Baclofen (Lioresal): spinal cord monosynaptic reflex inhibition
	Dantrolene sodium (Dantrium): muscle excitation—
	contraction coupling inhibition
	Dantrolene is contraindicated in marginal pulmonary function
Detrusor hyperreflexia	Propantheline (Probanthine)
	Oxybutynin (Ditropan):
	Parasympathetic inhibitors (anticholinergics)

[a] Adapted from Halstead and Claus-Walker (51) and Hachen (50).

Antimicrobial prophylaxis is safe and may further reduce the incidence of clinical infection (68, 83, 87). Symptomatic urinary infection should be treated with antimicrobial agents and mechanical flushing by increased fluid intake. Children with spinal cord injury rarely experience dysuria but frequently note that they cannot stay dry when infection is present. In addition, they may have systemic symptoms including fever, malaise, and anorexia. Kass et al. (59) describe persistent and asymptomatic bacterial colonization of the bladder in 56% of children with neurogenic bladder and demonstrate that this is innocuous. Treatment with antimicrobials is unnecessary. However, prophylactic antibiotics should be considered for protection of the upper urinary system in the presence of vesicoureteral reflux.

Artificial sphincter implantation is an option, particularly for the adolescent patient with severe sphincter weakness (75). Bladder augmentation has improved bladder storage capacity in selected patients including children (22, 66). In rare cases, vesicostomy may be necessary but colonic urinary diversion has been abandoned for late complications.

Urolithiasis is as high as 20% in spinal cord injured children, with propensity for nephrolithiasis in those with hypercalcemia, and for vesicolithiasis in those with chronic urinary tract infections, especially proteus.

CHRONIC PAIN

Pain is a common complaint in cauda equina injury. Central pain reported as dysesthesias and paresthesias is almost universal in adolescents with spinal cord injury compared to younger children who seldom complain.

In recognition of physiological and psychological components of pain, therapy consists of controlling both generation and interpretation of pain. Newberger and Sallan (92) emphasize analgesic regimes in adequate dosage and regular scheduling to avoid reinforcing pain behavior. Oral analgesics including aspirin, acetaminophen, and other nonsteroidal anti-inflammatory drugs (NSAIDS) are offered in this manner early in the course of central pain. Long-term use of narcotic analgesics must be avoided. Amitriptyline at bedtime is often useful. Heat and relaxation provided by hydrotherapy, passive range of motion, and weight-bearing on the lower extremities may also help. Behavior modification with parents entering the contract to alter pain behavior is a worthwhile technique (120).

DECUBITI

Skin lesions tend to occur on the legs and buttocks from careless transfer techniques and prolonged pressure. In bed, the bony prominences are the most likely locations. Prone positioning on pillows or using a waterbed are simple preventive modifications at home. All children who use a wheelchair should undergo training with biofeedback or a timer to develop the habit of shifting weight or buttock pushup from the chair every 15 minutes. Electric sensors can be implanted in the seat to signal the advent of intolerable pressure level. Wheelchair cushions should maintain subischial pressures below 40 mm Hg. Available cushions include foam blocks with sacral/ischial relief, gel material, or air cells. If full-thickness skin breakdown presents, substitution of prone cart or prone scooter offers complete relief of weight-bearing. A high-protein intake with vitamin and zinc supplement, correction of anemia, and treatment of spasticity and contractures are additional measures.

There are numerous routines for debridement and promotion of granulation of full-thickness undermined decubiti. The wet-to-dry technique using an antiseptic solution of equal parts normal saline, 2% hydrogen peroxide, and ¼% acetic acid is effective and low in cost. Gauze saturated with the solution is well packed into the wound recesses and allowed to dry over 6 to 8 hours, then removed and repacked. Necrotic tissue adheres to the extracted gauze but sharp debridement may be required as well. Complementing this regimen is daily hydrotherapy in saline detergent solution and ultraviolet cold quartz radiation.

Although complicated decubiti are uncommon in childhood, in deep lesions, additional complications may occur such as hidden abscess, osteomyelitis, or myositis ossificans. A radionucleotide scan can only rule out osteomyelitis (118) while a CT scan can identify each of these problems (36).

A reasonably nourished physically stable child with a large clean granulating wound is ready for surgical closure. Primary plastic procedures include skin grafts and skin flaps with or without muscle interposition. A sensate flap may be possible in some cases (16). Postoperative care includes gradually increasing periods of weight-bearing after the initial healing occurs and avoidance of wound contamination.

MUSCULOSKELETAL PROBLEMS

The effect of growth creates special complications for children, particularly of the hips and spine.

All children and adolescents who sustain cervical or high thoracic spinal cord injury are at risk for spinal curvature. Those injured by age 10 yr have the highest incidence (71, 81). Thoracolumbar scoliosis and lumbar kyphosis are the commonest deformities. A thoracolumbosacral orthosis (TLSO) is a temporizing measure allowing children to achieve skeletal maturity before surgical instrumentation but curves with apex above the midthoracic level are inadequately held. Spinal deformities are monitored by posteroanterior and lateral sitting x-rays, using discretion in order to minimize radiation dose. Spine fusion is indicated for progressive curves greater than 40°. Children with low thoracic injury level require a TLSO throughout the growing years and often avoid surgical intervention.

Hip dislocation and dysplasia are common sequelae in young children. Paralytic or spastic muscle creates abnormal forces around the hip joint, which prevents normal formation of the acetabulum and promotes dislocation. Unilateral dislocation creates pelvic obliquity, which aggravates scoliosis.

HETEROTOPIC OSSIFICATION

Heterotopic bone formation can develop after spinal cord injury. Often manifested bilaterally, propensity is for hip, knee, elbow, and shoulder, in that order. Ankylosis in hip extension can make sitting impossible. Reports of 20% prevalence in mixed age groups with spinal cord injuries compare with a much lower incidence of 10% among children under 16 yr of age (41).

Symptoms and signs usually appear between 2 and 6 months after injury as pain, swelling, and restricted motion. Serum alkaline phosphatase is elevated. Bone scan is positive before radiological visualization and remains positive during acute accelerated and chronic decelerating phases of activity but returns to normal when ossification is mature with distinct margins and trabeculation on x-ray (119).

Operative resection is contraindicated until the lesion is mature and is necessary only for severe dysfunctional ankylosis. Some pediatric cases show partial or complete resolution over time (41). Preventive measures—including decubitus and infection control, regular range of motion, which is continued through the stage of ossification—are helpful but incompletely successful. Disodium etidronate (Didronel), which blocks formation of crystalline hydroxyapatite, has been prophylactic (116). Didronel should be used cautiously in children because of concern about the interference with bone metabolism in the growing skeleton. Aspirin may be a useful medication to prevent recurrence after surgical excision (90).

SEX EDUCATION AND COUNSELING

Adolescents in the under 16-yr age group range from having considerable to no experience with sexual intercourse, but all are curious about it. Sophistication in sexual anatomy, physiology, and psychology depends on family, school, and social background ("street versus protected") and needs assessment before sexual counseling. Although the mature adolescent will give high priority to sexual function, primary interest in the young child is mobility.

Comarr and Vigue (19) have developed guidelines for assessment and sexual counseling for individuals aged 13 yr and older. Neurological examination to determine sensation of scrotum, penis or clitoris, perianal area, and volitional control of external sphincter separates complete from incomplete lesions. Six months to a year are required to determine return of erection (psychogenic, spontaneous, or by external stimulation), ejaculation, and orgasm. Early pessimism is unwarranted.

Vibratory stimulation of the penis can accomplish erection and ejaculation (3, 117). The spermatozoa count is adequate but motility is impaired. Perkash and associates (99) describe effective rectal probe electroejaculation in patients with upper motor neuron, conus, and cauda equina lesions.

Personal counseling of the adolescent by the physician and/or psychologist determines and enhances the knowledge of the patient in areas of anatomy and sexuality. Explicit anatomic illustrations are useful. Basic elements of social life, body image, and self acceptance are dealt with before such details as position and intercourse.

The preadolescent and younger child is given opportunity to ask questions generated by illustrative material and discussion.

Psychoemotional Reactions

A child with acquired paralysis undergoes a devastating experience: loss of body sensation that may feel like the head is free floating, loss of control over the body and environment, separation from family, and placement in a hostile world of strange machines, multiple changing caretakers who mutilate him with needles and tubes.

Greatest support for the younger child comes from the parent rooming in or maintaining a very close vigil. The rehabilitation team—physicians, nurses, and therapists—do the greatest service by treating the child consistently and patiently. A sympathetic attitude must be maintained toward the parents who may be overly anxious or accusative and hostile.

Preparation for new procedures, honesty and trustworthiness in communications with the child ("tell me when this stretching hurts and we won't stretch any further today"), and consistency in setting limits are imperative for the child's coping with further rehabilitation and a new kind of life. In the rehabilitation unit, there should be a playroom retreat where white coats and procedures are forbidden.

Children with personalities centered around physical and sport activities face the most difficulty with adjustment and sublimation. Preceding personality problems, such as phobias, hyperactivity, shyness, and withdrawal will be exaggerated by the injury and the child is apt to interpret the injury as punishment.

Compounding the injury are increased dependency, pain, medications, and absence from school and peer group. The parents experience loss of the child they knew, radical changes in family life and financial costs, and suffer through the throes of denial, guilt, depression, resentment, and anger.

Management starts with simple and repeated explanation of diagnosis and prognosis. If the lesion is complete, implications should not be presented in one sitting. Periodic review with parents elicits their understanding of what they have been told of the illness and the management. Physicians must accept projected hostility as nonpersonal and allow parents to vent emotions. Recognizing that family crisis needs resolution before it becomes chronic or causes the family to disintegrate, the social worker intervenes to catalyze the working through of grief by guiding family members to open discussion of feelings. The social worker also helps with family referral to resources such as State Crippled Children and Supplemental Income (SSI) programs.

Injury in early adolescence, i.e., from 12 to 15 yr, is an especially devastating blow to the usual adolescent megalomania and narcissism and results in humiliation and panic, giving way to anger (42). Adolescent tasks, which include adjustment to adult body image, sexuality, self-determination, and independent living, are now more complicated.

Immediate arrangements include access to the call button, input from staff and family, radio, and TV. Short-term low-dose tranquilizer or antidepressant medication may be justified in extreme circumstances. For prolonged or severe anger, temper tantrums, or depression, psychiatric counseling and behavior modification programs are warranted. The latter is based on a staff-patient protocol placing the patient in control, with baseline privileges expanded for positive behavior and restricted for negative behavior (126). Full adjustment to disability may take years. Contact with other spinal cord injured children and adults who have made successful adaptation provides a positive role model. Long-term support is aimed at avoiding social isolation.

Functional Rehabilitation

At the transfer to a rehabilitation unit, functional goals and a problem list are established on the basis of the spared motor and sensory function, spasticity, urinary status, behavior, and other consequences of the injury, as out-

Table 13.2.
Rehabilitation Goals

Education of the child and family in spinal cord function and lesion
Training in appropriate locomotion
Training in self-care and daily activities
Prevention of deformities, decubiti, and renal complications
Bowel and bladder regulation
Control of vasomotor dysfunction (autonomic hyperreflexia, orthostatic hypotension)
Maintenance of nutrition without obesity
Control of pain
Sex education
Communication
Emotional and social adjustment
Introduction to recreation and wheelchair sports
Information on financial assistance and community agencies
Return to home and appropriate school

lined in Table 13.2. Although neurological level is a significant prognosticator of anticipated phsyical function (Table 13.3), attainment of maximal expectations depends on the child's motivation, emotional health, and intelligence; on the support and adjustment of the family; on intercurrent medical complications and skills of the management team.

In conjunction with the family, the team must set realistic goals for physical independence. Education of the child and members of the support team is an important aspect of the rehabilitation process. Progress in adjusting to a permanent disability is fostered by the achievement of new adaptive skills and success is the best reward for maintaining motivation and to avert depression arising from a feeling of helplessness.

NURSING CARE

Next to parents, pediatric nurses spend the most time with the child. The nurses provide a structured environment with limit-setting and behavior management which, as a minimum, provides predictable rewards for appropriate behavior and appropriate restriction of privileges as a consequence to negative behavior. At the same time, they are the advocates for the child and parents. Reassurance regarding the therapeutic and medical management as well as reinforcement of the formal therapeutic activity is essential.

Specialized nursing care includes operation of the respiratory equipment and management of secretions. With the assistance of respiratory therapists, postural drainage, gentle percussion, and aerosol treatments are applied to mobilize sputum and prevent atelectasis and pneumonia. Daily inspection of the skin, turning and alternate positioning for pressure relief at least every 2 hours, cleansing, lubricating, and instructing the child and family of the potential hazards of heat and careless transfers are necessary to prevent skin breakdown.

If the patient is in a halo or other traction device, the screw sites must be

Table 13.3.
Functional Levels of Injury[a]

Level	Spared	Independence	Equipment and Abilities
C3	Head rotation	No	Requires respirator or electrophrenic implant
C4	Neck stability, diaphragm (respiratory insufficiency)	No	Electric wheelchair propulsion, puff control, powered environmental control
C5	Elbow flexion, supination	Variable	Electric wheelchair or rim projections, assisted sliding board transfer, pressure relief; powered wrist-hand orthosis
C6	Wrist extension, elbow pronation, fair shoulder stability	Independent: in feeding, grooming, dressing, upper extremity; may be independent in wheelchair	Wrist-driven flexor hinge orthosis prehension; wheelchair hand rim projections, relief skin pressure; drive with cuff, hand controls, lift for transfer; may do self-catheterization
C7	Finger, elbow extension, weak finger flexion	Independent in wheelchair	Self-catheterization, bed/car transfer, electric typewriter; drive with hand control; travel on plane
C8-T1	Hand intrinsics	Independent in wheelchair	Standard wheelchair rims, write, touchtype, drive with hand control
T2-T12	Trunk stability	Independent in wheelchair	Bath transfer, wheelchair to 6-inch curbs and into car, drive with hand control
L1-L3	Hip flexion, knee extension weak	Household ambulation with KAFO[b], crutches	Bladder management program remains necessary
L4	Knee extension	Community ambulation, usually with crutches	Bladder management program remains necessary
L5-S2	Hip abduction, extension; foot dorsiflexion strong, plantar flexion	Ambulation with AFO[c] or none, possibly canes	Bladder management program remains necessary, bus travel

[a]Capabilities of patients vary, depending on level of lesion, general health, motivation, and training.
[b]KAFO, knee-ankle-foot orthosis.
[c]AFO, ankle-foot orthosis.

maintained scrupulously and transfer techniques taught carefully to avoid dislodging the apparatus.

Care of the urinary system entails maintaining intake and output record; performing and teaching intermittent catheterization; and monitoring maximal and residual bladder volumes, urinary leakage, infection, and stone formation. Bowel emptying should be recorded and a program of regularity established using digital stimulation with the assistance of stimulant suppository when necessary. Digital disimpaction and other supplemental methods of bowel emptying should also be taught.

Bedside range of motion exercises supplement the formal therapy sessions to prevent contractures.

THERAPEUTIC EXERCISES

Early management requires passive range of motion exercises with sustained, slow, gentle stretching to the paralyzed extremities applied twice daily. Active strengthening exercises are given to the nonparalyzed muscle groups, especially shoulder depressors, latissimus dorsi, and triceps for wheelchair pushup to relieve skin pressure. Exercises in hydrotherapy are a useful adjunct to support weak movement, to increase sensory awareness, and to debride decubiti. Sitting and elevation to vertical position on the tilt table are achieved gradually. Training in bed mobility is followed by mat activities for balance as preparation for transfer training. For children, exercises incorporated into games and other enjoyable activities are more successful than repetitive movements. A reward system for improved performance is generally helpful.

In the training of children who require a wheelchair for mobility, the rules of safety must be emphasized. Propelling, turning, maneuvering, and transfer are taught in various situations, including negotiating curbs, "wheelies," outdoor mobility, and wheelchair sports. Regular pushups and weight shifting must become ingrained habits from the beginning.

Even the child with high quadriplegia will want to stand and walk. However, the energy requirement for paraplegic ambulation is four to six times normal (38). Standing in parallel bars is initiated with posterior splints or pneumatic orthoses to learn hand and shoulder control, weight shifting, progressing to a "drag-to" or "swing-to" gait with walker or crutches.

In quadriplegia, full range of scapulothoracic and glenohumeral joint motion, web space of the hands, and wrist extension is critical for maintenance of functional positioning, including tenodesis of the finger flexors. Strengthening of cervical and other functioning muscles, breathing exercises, and wheelchair propulsion by use of traction knobs or a joy stick constitute a progressive program. Specialized electronic wheelchair controls are required for patients lacking hand and shoulder function. Group activities and quite vigorous exercises on the mat or large balls may be enjoyed by the previously physically active quadriplegic child.

FUNCTIONAL ELECTRICAL STIMULATION

For highly motivated patients, computer-coordinated electrical stimulation of lower extremity muscle groups provides aerobic conditioning, which can improve cardiopulmonary conditioning and increase strength, endurance, and bulk of stimulated muscles without ill effect (104, 105).

Marsolais and Kobetic (79) report walking distances from 50 to 330 meters at a speed of 1.5 meters per second with the use of computer-activated percutaneously implanted muscle electrodes in patients with paraplegia proximal to the T10 level. Breathlessness and knee extensor fatigue are described as the limiting factors. The metabolic energy cost ranged from two to three times normal (78). Electrode failure, burns, infection, and fractures are reported complications (78). Hirokawa and colleagues (53) report advantages of a reciprocating gait orthosis powered by functional electrical stimulation of the thigh muscles in six adults with paraplegia.

Peckham and associates (96) employed electrical stimulation of upper extremity muscles to provide improved grasp, control, and release of objects encountered in daily living as an alternative to standard upper extremity orthoses.

HAND FUNCTION AND ADAPTIVE SKILLS

Activities and games that the child wishes to try and enjoys play a supporting role through the stages of denial, depression, and acting out.

Functional assessment of the upper extremities consists of an evaluation for active muscle function, sensation, joint motion, speed, and skill of manipulating games and implements. The therapy program utilizes activities appropriate for age and adaptive development to increase range, strength, coordination of upper extremities, and independence in self-care. Progress in daily activities should be evaluated and demonstrated for parents so that the child is allowed and encouraged to do as much as possible without help. Encouragement toward stepwise progress may be enhanced with a reward chart, privileged use of electronic games, or other rewards. As soon as possible, the child is allowed to have a therapeutic pass to practice skills at home. A follow-up report of successes and problems are required from the child and parent. Home visit to recommend structural modifications and equipment is done prior to discharge.

In spinal cord injury affecting the upper extremities, surgical transfer of preserved muscles is helpful for improving hand function. In C5 quadriplegia, the brachialis graded as having at least good strength can be transplanted into the extensor carpi radialis brevis and will function as a wrist extensor, but residual elbow flexion will be weakened. Flexor pollicis longus tenodesis creates a key pinch function in C6 lesion (18). Transfer of the posterior deltoid provides substitution for triceps function. Surgical procedures are deferred usually until 1 year after the injury. Because transferred muscles are expected to lose about one grade of strength, re-education and strengthening of the rerouted muscle is needed.

ASSISTIVE DEVICES

Young children need to be as free as possible from orthoses and cumbersome equipment, as well as to become dexterous with what is truly useful.

Thermoplastic splints can be fabricated for preventive purposes to maintain the ankle at 90° and to hold the wrist in extension and the hand in position of function for preserving the integrity of intrinsic muscles.

Wheelchair prescription is a joint decision by the team and family. General considerations and accessories for a pediatric wheelchair are discussed in Chapter 8. A solid seat base with cushion is important in the young child to maintain hip alignment. If possible, costly electric wheelchair models should be tried before ordering them. Prone scooters and arm-propelled carts, caster carts, and motor caster carts are devices that provide pleasure as well as mobility (Fig. 13.4).

For the paraplegic ambulator, lower extremity orthoses are designed for limb support and spasticity control (106). Facility of donning and doffing is an important consideration. Metal uprights allow for growth but plastic orthoses offer the advantage of being light in weight. Craig Scott orthoses meet the above criteria for the strong paraplegic. The reciprocal gait orthosis provides coordinated hip flexion and extension operated by hip flexors. Some children use trunk movement when hip flexors are weak or absent.

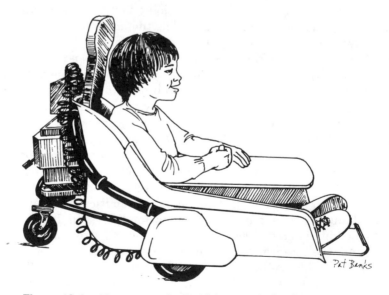

Figure 13.4. Young paraplegic driving a motorized caster cart.

Children who lack hip flexors or have hip flexion contractures frequently revert to a swing-type gait. The hip guidance orthosis is another alternative for the child with thoracic or high lumbar lesion (91, 108). For the less agile child with high paraplegia, the parapodium or ORLAU swivel walker (76) is useful for household or exercise ambulation and allows standing with hands free for functional use. Regardless of brace type, the most reliable indicator of ambulatory speed and energy cost in the motivated patient is the strength of the hip and knee muscles (122). Without strong knee extensors, ambulation is generally of the exercise level, regardless of the orthosis employed.

Because of time required for donning and the energy cost of walking, rejection rate is high among teenagers and young adults (15). Nevertheless, the opportunity for standing upright and experiencing the ambulation should be offered. Young children are more interested and able to ambulate despite extensive paralysis. In wheelchair-bound quadriplegics, plastic, solid ankle-foot orthoses prevent equinus contractures.

Virtually all children with high spinal injuries before puberty are at risk for scoliosis (71). Early scoliosis measuring less than 20° warrants placement of the seated quadriplegic child in a plastic or plastic mesh spinal orthosis and a separate or attached molded seat insert to prevent pelvic obliquity.

For most children, the simpler the devices, the more likely the acceptance and long-term use. Adapted eating utensils with hand cuff, straw adapters, writing, typing, personal hygiene aids, and clothing modifications are used for paraplegics with lesions as high as C6 (105). For the accepting and motivated adolescent with C6 quadriplegia and preservation of radial wrist extension against gravity, training is offered with a tenodesis splint. The principle of wrist-driven finger flexor hinge orthosis or ratchet splint is to activate a three-jaw chuck thumb-finger prehension by active wrist extension. These dynamic splints enable their users to manipulate objects, dial a telephone, and handle tools independently (88). However, by allowing mild flexion contractures to develop at the metacarpophalangeal (MP) and proximal interphalangeal (PIP) joints and strengthening wrist extensors, the person can perform the same tasks without prehension orthosis. To achieve a similar tenodesis effect in the absence of wrist extension in C5 lesions, an externally powered orthosis may be considered with the addition of the balanced forearm orthosis for C4 level (106) (Fig. 8.5).

Static splints for night-time positioning and clip-on equipment are the short and long opponens type in the presence or absence of wrist extensors, respectively.

The high quadriplegic child benefits from an electric wheelchair equipped with portable ventilator. The control lever must be adjusted for manipulation by the weaker hand, chin, or puff and sip. Adaptable head- or mouthpiece may be used to operate television, typewriter, and other household appliances. Personal computers with keyboards suitable for mouth stick operation and a variety of electronic environmental control systems are available (106).

SOCIAL REINTEGRATION

The older child's and adolescent's job and friendships are based in school and absence interferes with both. Hospital tutoring is an integral part of rehabilitation as soon as the child feels well enough to concentrate on mental tasks. Discharge planning includes a schedule for return to school; home tutoring is not a viable substitute. For a child with paraplegia who is independent from wheelchair and self-sufficient in bladder care, return to the previous regular classroom and friends is recommended. Architectural barriers have to be overcome and transportation provided. Advantages of academic and social reintegration outweigh special placement for the sake of therapies. The elementary or middle school-aged child with quadriplegia who is dependent in toileting and self-care needs special services mandated by public law. Mainstreaming with the availability of an aide is preferred to placement in a handicapped classroom. The high schooler with quadriplegia who has a helping family, friends, electric wheelchair, and tape recorder is supported in a trial return to the previous school. Special arrangements must be made for privacy and assistance in toileting, and allow time-out periods for lying down. Returning to school on a part time basis is recommended before full commitment. When age 16 yr is reached, specialized driver training should be provided through the school.

Depending on personal adjustment, competitiveness, and comfort, the adolescent benefits both from groups of able-bodied teenagers with similar interests, for example, chess and computer use, and from participation in groups of disabled persons with similar abilities for wheelchair sports.

Exploration of recreational possibilities, organized sports, accessible parks and camping areas, and travel is facilitated through community agencies and national organizations, such as the National Spinal Cord Injury Foundation. A guide for the handicapped teenager (34) includes comprehensive listing of travel agencies, sport associations, civil rights organizations, technological aids, and other useful information. Travel safety devices for children in wheelchairs are discussed in Chapter 8.

Long-term Follow-up

Children with spinal cord injury are at risk for deterioration of urinary, musculoskeletal, and other systems during the years of growth. Long-term care is essential to prevent complications and to provide support for functional adjustment at home and school. The early weeks after discharge are the most difficult while the family and the child develop new lives together. Home visits combined with outpatient therapy and office follow-up should be supplemented by conferences and telephone contacts with the family and the school.

Regional Centers, Research, and Prevention

The Regional Service Administration of the Department of Health and Human Services funds regional Spinal Cord Injury Centers across the United States. Information pooled from the centers is collected at the National Spinal Cord Injury Center in Phoenix and provides cumulative data on health care delivery, cost, and significant events to persons with spinal cord injury and their families.

The majority of severe or fatal neck injuries are suffered in motor vehicle accidents. Approximately 6000 car passengers per year die of a broken neck and 500 others become quadriplegic. In a population of 62,000 occupants of cars in serious accidents, almost all severe and fatal neck injuries are sustained by persons not using proper seat belts or infant carriers (55). Any child restraint system reduces fatalities as much as 90% (56). In 1977, over 2400 motor vehicle occupants age 15 yr or younger died in traffic crashes. Legislation for compulsory wearing of seat belts decreases fatalities and injuries (Chapter 8).

Health professionals are in a position to support mandatory seat restraint legislation and to educate families on the use of infant carriers and child restraints from the day the newborn is driven home from the hospital. Rehabilitation professionals have the additional special concern for safe transport of already handicapped children in automobiles and school buses (Chapter 8).

High-risk sport and recreational activities deserve further preventive measures. Diving into rivers, use of all-terrain vehicles without proper instruction or safety gear, and unsafe football tackles (spearing) continue to cause quadriplegia despite medical and public awareness.

REFERENCES

1. Austin LA, Heath H: Calcitonin. *N Engl J Med* 304:269–278, 1981.
2. Berendes JN, Bredee JJ, Schipperheyn JJ, Mashhour YAS: Mechanisms of spinal cord injury after cross-clamping of the descending aorta. *Circulation* 66:I-112–I-116, 1982.
3. Beretta G, Chelo E, Zanollo A: Reproductive aspects in spinal cord injured males. *Paraplegia* 27:113–118, 1989.
4. Bondurant FJ, Cotler HB, Kulkarni MV, McArdle CB, et al: Acute spinal cord injury. A study using physical examination and magnetic resonance imaging. *Spine* 15:161–168, 1990.
5. Bracken MB, Freeman DH, Hellenbrand K: Incidence of acute traumatic hospitalized spinal cord injury in the United States, 1970–1977. *J Epidemiol* 113:615–622, 1981.
6. Bracken MB, Shepard MJ, Collins WF, Holford TR, et al: A randomized controlled trial of methylprenisolone or naloxone in the treatment of acute spinal cord injury. *N Engl J Med* 322:1405–1411, 1990.

7. Braun SR, Giovannoni R, Levin AB, Harvey RF: Oxygen saturation during sleep in patients with spinal cord injury. *Am J Phys Med* 61:302–309, 1982.
8. Braun SR, Giovannoni R, O'Conner M: Improving cough in patients with spinal cord injury. *Am J Phys Med* 63:1–10, 1984.
9. Brock WA, So EP, Harbach LB, Kaplan GW: Intermittent catheterization in the management of neurogenic vesical dysfunction in children. *J Urol* 125:391–399, 1981.
10. Byers RK: Spinal-cord injuries during birth. *Dev Med Child Neurol* 17:140–146, 1975.
11. Cahill JL, Okamoto GA, Higgins T, Davis A: Experiences with phrenic nerve pacing in children. *J Pediatr Surg* 18:851–854, 1983.
12. Chen LS, Blaw M: Acute central cervical cord syndrome caused by minor trauma. *J Pediatr* 108:96–97, 1986.
13. Choi J, Hoffman HJ, Hendrick EB, Humphreys RP, et al: Traumatic infarction of the spinal cord in children. *J Neurosurg* 65:608–610, 1986.
14. Chusid JG: *Correlative Neuroanatomy & Functional Neurology.* East Norwalk, CT, Appleton-Century-Crofts, CT, 1985.
15. Coghlan TK, Robinson CE, Newmarch B, Jackson G: Lower extremity bracing in paraplegia—a followup study. *Paraplegia* 18:25–32, 1980.
16. Coleman JJ, Jurkiewicz MJ: Methods of providing sensation to anesthetic areas. *Ann Plast Surg* 12:177–186, 1984.
17. Collins WF: A review and update of experimental and clinical studies of spinal cord injury. *Paraplegia* 21:204–219, 1983.
18. Colyer RA, Kappleman B: Flexor pollicis longus tenodesis in tetraplegia at the sixth cervical level. *J Bone Joint Surg* 63A:376–379, 1981.
19. Comarr AE, Vigue M: Sexual counseling among male and female patients with spinal cord and/or cauda equina injury. *Am J Phys Med* 57:107–122; 215–227, 1978.
20. Cox CE, Hinman F: Experiments with induced bacteriuria, vessical emptying and bacterial growth on the mechanism of bladder emptying. *J Urol* 86:739, 1961.
21. De Troyer A, Esteene M, Heilporn A: Mechanism of active expiration in tetraplegic patients. *N Engl J Med* 314:740–741, 1986.
22. Decter RM, Bauer SB, Mandell J, Colodny AH, et al: Small bowel augmentation in children with neurogenic bladder: An initial report of urodynamic findings. *J Urol* 138:1014–1016, 1987.
23. Denis F: The three column spine and its significance in the classification of acute thoracolumbar spinal injuries. *Spine* 8:817, 1983.
24. Duval-Beaupere G, Lougovoy J, Trochellier L, Lacert P: Trunk and leg growth in children with paraplegia caused by spinal cord injury. *Paraplegia* 21:339–350, 1983.
25. Dworkin GE, Stas WE: Posttraumatic syringomyelia. *Arch Phys Med Rehabil* 66:329–331, 1985.
26. Dykstra DD, Sidi AA, Scott AB, Pagel JM, et al: Effects of botulinum A toxin on detrusor sphincter dyssynergia in spinal cord injury patients. *J Urol* 139:919–922, 1988.
27. Epstein N, Hood DC, Ransohoff J: Gastrointestinal bleeding in patients with spinal cord trauma. *J Neurosurg* 54:16–20, 1980.
28. Erickson RP: Autonomic hyperreflexia: Pathophysiology and medical management. *Arch Phys Med Rehabil* 61:431–440, 1980.
29. Evans JKH, Shaw NJ, Brocklebank JT: Sublingual nifedipine in acute severe hypertension. *Arch Dis Child* 63:975–977, 1988.
30. Farcy JP, Weidenbaum M: A preliminary review of the use of Cotrel-Dubousset instrumentation for spinal injuries. *Bull Hosp Joint Dis Orth Inst* 48:44–51, 1988.
31. Fealey RD, Szurszewski JH, Merritt JL, DiMagno EP: Effect of traumatic spinal cord transection on human upper gastrointestinal motility and gastric emptying. *Gastroenterology* 87:69–75, 1984.

32. Fehlings MG, Tator CH, Linden RD: The effect of direct-current field on recovery from experimental spinal cord injury. *J Neurosurg* 68:781–792, 1988.
33. Fehlings MG, Tator CH, Linden RD: The effect of nimodipine and dextran on axonal function and blood flow following experimental spinal cord injury. *Neurosurgery* 71:403–416, 1989.
34. Feingold S, Miller H: Your Future: *A Guide for The Handicapped Teenager.* New York, Richard Rosen Press Inc, 1981.
35. Feshmire FM, Luten RC: The pediatric cervical spine: Developmental anatomy and clinical aspects. *J Emerg Med* 7:133–142, 1989.
36. Firooznia H, Rafii M, Golimbu C, Lam S, et al: Computed tomography of pressure sores, pelvic abscess, and osteomyelitis in patients with spinal cord injury. *Arch Phys Med Rehabil* 63:545–548, 1982.
37. Fishburn MJ, Marino RJ, Ditunno JF: Atelectasis and pneumonia in acute spinal cord injury. *Arch Phys Med Rehabil* 71:197–200, 1990.
38. Fisher SV, Gullickson G: Energy cost of ambulation in health and disability: A literature review. *Arch Phys Med Rehabil* 59:124–133, 1978.
39. Foster WM, Langenback EG, Bergofsky EH: Respiratory drugs influence lung mucociliary clearance in central and peripheral ciliated airways. *Chest* 80:877–880, 1981.
40. Gabriel KR, Crawford AH: Identification of acute posttraumatic spinal cord cyst by magnetic resonance imaging: A case report and review of the literature. *J Pediatr Orthop* 8:710–714, 1988.
41. Garland DE, Shimoyama ST, Lugo C, Barras D, et al: Spinal cord insults and heterotopic ossification in the pediatric population. *Clin Orthop Rel Res* 245:303–310, 1989.
42. Geller B, Greydanus DE: Psychological management of acute paraplegia in adolescence. *Pediatrics* 63:562–564, 1979.
43. Gilgoff IS, Barras DM, Jones MS, Adkins HV: Neck breathing: A form of voluntary respiration for the spine-injured ventilator-dependent quadriplegic child. *Pediatrics* 82:741–745, 1988.
44. Glenn WW, Hogan JF, Loke JS, Ciesielski TE, et al: Ventilatory support by pacing of the conditioned diaphragm in quadriplegia. *N Engl J Med* 310:1150–1155, 1984.
45. Glick ME, Meshkinpour H, Haldeman S, Hoehler F, et al: Colonic dysfunction in patients with thoracic spinal cord injury. *Gastroenterology* 86:287–294, 1984.
46. Goldman JM, Williams SJ, Silver JR, Denison DM: Effect of abdominal binders on breathing in tetraplegic patients. *Thorax* 41:940–945, 1986.
47. Green BA, Callahan RA, Klose J, De La Torre J: Acute spinal injury: Current concepts. *Clin Orthop* 154:125–135, 1981.
48. Gross D, Ladd HW, Riley EJ, Macklem PT, et al: The effect of training on strength and endurance of the diaphragm in quadriplegia. *Am J Phys Med* 68:27–35, 1980.
49. Haas F, Axen K, Pineda H, Gandino D: Temporal pulmonary function changes in cervical cord injury. *Arch Phys Med Rehabil* 66:139–143, 1985.
50. Hachen HJ: Spinal cord injury in children and adolescents: Diagnostic pitfalls and therapeutic considerations in the acute stage. *Paraplegia* 15:55–64, 1977–78.
51. Halstead LS, Claus-Walker J: *Neuroactive Drugs of Choice in Spinal Cord Injury.* Houston, Institute Rehabilitation Research, 1980.
52. Hill SA, Miller CA, Kosnik J, Hunt WE: Pediatric neck injuries: A clinical study. *J Neurosurg* 60:700–706, 1984.
53. Hirokawa S, Grimm M, Solomonow M, Baratta RV: Energy consumption in paraplegic ambulation using the reciprocating gait orthosis and electric stimulation of the thigh muscles. *Arch Phys Med Rehabil* 71:687–694, 1990.
54. Holdsworth F: Fractures, dislocations and fracture-dislocations of the spine. *J Bone Joint Surg* 52A:1534, 1970.

55. Huelke DF, O'Day J, Mendelsohn RTA: Cervical injuries suffered in automobile crashes. *J Neurosurg* 54:316–322, 1981.
56. Huelke DF, Weber KB: Children in crashes: How serious a problem? *Univ Mich Ctr J* 46:38–39, 1980.
57. Jacobs RR, Asher MA, Snider RK: Dorso-lumbar spinal fractures: Recumbent vs. Operative treatment. *Paraplegia* 18:358–376, 1980.
58. Kass EJ, Koff SA, Diokno AC: Fate of vesicoureteral reflux in children with neurogenic bladders managed by intermittent catheterization. *J Urol* 125:63–64, 1981.
59. Kass EJ, Koff SA, Diokno AC, Lapides J: The significance of bacilluria in children on long-term intermittent catheterization. *J Urol* 126:223–225, 1981.
60. Katz RT: Management of Spasticity. *Am J Phys Med* 67:108–116, 1988.
61. Kelly EG: Orthopedic management of the patient with spinal injury. *Curr Probl Surg* 17:205–215, 1980.
62. Kewalramani LS: Autonomic dysreflexia in traumatic myelopathy. *Am J Phys Med* 59:1–21, 1980.
63. Kewalramani LS: Neurogenic gastroduodenal ulceration and bleeding associated with spinal cord injuries. *J Trauma* 19:259–265, 1979.
64. Kewalramani LS, Kraus JF, Sterling HM: Acute spinal-cord lesions in a pediatric population: epidemiological and clinical features. *Paraplegia* 18:206–218, 1980.
65. Kewalramani LS, Tori JA: Spinal cord trauma in children. *Spine* 5:11–18, 1980.
66. King LR, Webster GD, Bertram RA: Experiences with reconstruction in children. *J Urol* 138:1002–1006, 1987.
67. Koch BM, Eng GM, Neonatal spinal cord injury. *Arch Phys Med Rehabil* 60:378–380, 1980.
68. Krebs M, Halvorsen RB, Fishman IJ, Santos-Mendoza N: Prevention of urinary tract infection during intermittent catheterization. *J Urol* 131:82–85, 1984.
69. Krieger KH, Spencer FC: Is paraplegia after repair of coarctation of the aorta due principally to distal hypotension during aortic cross-clamping. *Surgery* 97:2–7, 1985.
70. LaFortuna CL, Fazio F: Acute effect of inhaled salbutamol on mucociliary clearance in health and chronic bronchitis. *Respiration* 45:111–123, 1984.
71. Lancourt JE, Dickson JHM, Carter RE: Paralytic spinal deformity following traumatic spinal-cord injury in children and adolescents. *J Bone Joint Surg* 63A:47–53, 1981.
72. Lapides J, Diokno AC, Silber SJ, Lowe BS: Clean intermittent self-catheterization in the treatment of urinary tract disease. *J Urol* 107:458, 1972.
73. Leventhal HR: Birth injuries of the spinal cord. *J Pediatr* 56:447, 1960.
74. Lieberman JS, Corkill G, Nayak NN, French BN, Taylor RG: Serial phrenic nerve conduction studies in candidates for diaphragmatic pacing. *Arch Phys Med Rehabil* 61:528–531, 1980.
75. Light JK, Scott FB: Use of the artificial urinary sphincter in spinal cord injury patients. *J Urol* 130:1127–1129, 1983.
76. Lough LK, Nielsen DH: Ambulation of children with myelomeningocele: parapodium versus parapodium with Orlau swivel modification. *Dev Med Child Neurol* 28:489–497, 1986.
77. Madersbacher H, Pauer W, Reiner E: Rehabilitation of micturition by transurethral electrostimulation of the bladder in patients with incomplete spinal cord lesions. *Paraplegia* 20:191–195, 1982.
78. Marsolais EB, Kobetic R: Development of a practical electrical stimulation system for restoring gait in the paralyzed patient. *Clin Orthop Relat Res* 233:64–74, 1988.
79. Marsolais EB, Kobetic R: Functional electrical stimulation for walking in paraplegia. *J Bone Joint Surg* 69A:728–733, 1987.
80. Mathias JC, Christensen NJ, Frankel HL, Spalding JMK: Cardiovascular control in recently injured tetraplegics in spinal shock. *Q J Med* (N Series XLVIII) 190:273–287, 1979.

81. Mayfield JK, Erkkila JC, Winter RB: Spine deformity subsequent to acquired childhood spinal cord injury. *J Bone Joint Surg* 63A:1401-1411, 1981.

82. Maynard FM: Immobilization hypercalcemia following spinal cord injury. *Arch Phys Med Rehabil* 67:41-44, 1986.

83. Maynard FM, Diokno A: Urinary infection and complications during clean intermittent catheterization following spinal cord injury. *J Urol* 132:943-946, 1984.

84. McBride GG: Cotrel-Dubousset rods in spinal fractures. *Paraplegia* 27:440-449, 1989.

85. McCullough JL, Hollier LH, Nugent M: Paraplegia after thoracic aortic occlusion: Influence of cerebrospinal fluid drainage. *J Vasc Surg* 7:153-160, 1988.

86. McMichan JC, Michel L, Westbrook PR: Pulmonary dysfunction following traumatic quadriplegia. *JAMA* 243:528-531, 1980.

87. Merritt JL, Erickson RP, Opitz JL: Bacilluria during follow-up of patients with spinal cord injuries: II. Efficacy of antimicrobial suppressants. *Arch Phys Med Rehabil* 63:413-415, 1982.

88. Meyer CMH, Shrosbee RD, Abrahams DL: A method of rehabilitating the C6 tetraplegic hand. *Paraplegia* 17:170-175, 1979-80.

89. Miller F, Fenze TC: Prolonged ileus with acute spinal cord injury responding to metoclopramide. *Paraplegia* 19:43-48, 1981.

90. Mital MA, Garber JE, Stinson JT: Ectopic bone formation in children with head injuries: Its management. *J Pediatr Orthop* 7:83-90, 1987.

91. Nene AV, Patrick JH: Energy cost of paraplegic locomotion with the Orlau Parawalker. *Paraplegia* 27:5-18, 1989.

92. Newberger PE, Sallan SE: Chronic pain: Principles of management. *J Pediatr* 98:180-184, 1981.

93. Noll F, Russe O, Kling E, Botel U, et al: Intermittent catheterization versus percutaneous suprapubic cystostomy in the early management of traumatic spinal cord lesions. *Paraplegia* 26:4-9, 1988.

94. Oakes DD, Wilmot CB, Halverson D, Hamilton RD: Neurogenic respiratory failure: A 5-year experience using implantable phrenic nerve stimulators. *Ann Thorac Surg* 30:118-121, 1980.

95. Pang D, Wilberger JE: Spinal cord injury without radiographic abnormalities in children. *J Neurosurg* 57:114-129, 1982.

96. Peckham PH, Keith MW, Freehafer AA: Restoration of function by electrical stimulation in the upper extremity of the quadriplegic patient. *J Bone Joint Surg* 70A:144-148, 1988.

97. Perkash A: Experience with the management of deep vein thrombosis in patients with spinal cord injury. *Paraplegia* 18:2-14, 1980.

98. Perkash I, Friedland GW: Catheter induced hyperreflexia in spinal cord injury patients: Diagnosis by sonographic voiding cystourethrography. *Radiology* 159:453-455, 1986.

99. Perkash I, Martin DE, Warner H, Speck V: Electroejaculation of spinal cord injury patients: Simplified new equipment and technique. *J Urol* 143:305-307, 1990.

100. Philippi R, Kuhn W, Zach GA, Jacob-Chia D, Dollfus P: Survey of the neurological evaluation of 300 spinal cord injuries seen within 24 hours after injury. *Paraplegia* 18:337-346, 1980.

101. Pollack IF, Pang D, Sclabassi R: Recurrent spinal cord injury without radiographic abnormalities in children. *J Neurosurg* 69:177-182, 1988.

102. Puntis JW, Green SH: Ischaemic spinal cord injury after cardiac surgery. *Arch Dis Child* 60:517-520, 1985.

103. Radecki RT: Deep vein thrombosis in the pediatric disabled patient. *Arch Phys Med Rehabil* 69:743-744, 1988.

104. Ragnarsson KT: Physiologic effects of functional electrical stimulation-induced exercise in spinal cord injured patients. *Clin Orthop Relat Res* 233:53-63, 1988.

105. Ragnarsson KT, Pollack S, O'Daniel W, Edgar R, et al: Clinical evaluation of computer-

ized functional electrical stimulation after spinal cord injury: A multicenter pilot study. *Arch Phys Med Rehabil* 69:672–677, 1988.

106. Redford J (ed): *Orthotics Etcetera*. Baltimore, Williams & Wilkins, 1986.
107. Reines HD, Harris RC: Pulmonary complications of acute spinal cord injuries. Neurosurgery 21:193–196, 1987.
108. Rose GK, Stallard J, Sankarankutty M: Clinical evaluation of spina bifida patients using hip guidance orthosis. *Dev Med Child Neurol* 23:30, 1981.
109. Rowed DW, McLean JAG, Tator CH: Somatosensory evoked potentials in acute spinal cord injury. Prognostic value. *Surg Neurol* 9:203–210, 1978.
110. Ruge JR, Sinson GP, McLone DG, Cerullo LJ: Pediatric spinal injury: The very young. *J Neurosurg* 68:25–30, 1988.
111. Sharkey PC, Halter JA, Nakajima K: Electrophrenic respiration in patients with high quadriplegia. *Neurosurgery* 24:529–535, 1989.
112. Siegler RL, Brewer ED: Effect of sublingual or oral nifedipine in the treatment of hypertension. *J Pediatr* 112:811–813, 1988.
113. Sneed RC, Stover SL: Undiagnosed spinal cord injuries in brain injured children. *Am J Dis Child* 142:965–967, 1988.
114. Stauffer ES, Mazur JM: Cervical spine injuries in children. *Pediatr Ann* 11:502–511, 1982.
115. Stover SL, Lloyd K, Waites KB, Jackson AB: Urinary tract infection in spinal cord injury. *Arch Phys Med Rehabil* 70:47–54, 1989.
116. Stover SL, Niemann KM, Miller JM: Disodium etidronate in the prevention of post operative occurrence of heterotopic ossification in spinal cord injury patients. *J Bone Joint Surg* 58A:683–688, 1976.
117. Szasz G, Carpenter C: Clinical observations in vibratory stimulation of the penis of men with spinal cord injury. *Arch Sexual Behav* 18:461–474, 1989.
118. Thornhill-Joynes M, Gonzalse F, Stewart C, Kanel GC, et al: Osteomyelitis associated with pressure ulcers. *Arch Phys Med Rehabil* 67:314–318, 1986.
119. Tibone J, Sakimura I, Nickel VL, Hsu JD: Heterotopic ossification around the hip joint in spinal cord injured patients. *J Bone Joint Surg* 60A:769–775, 1978.
120. Varni JW, Bessman CA, Russo DC, Cataldo MF: Behavioral management of chronic pain in children: Case study. *Arch Phys Med Rehabil* 61:375–379, 1980.
121. Walsh JW, Stevens DB, Young AB: Traumatic paraplegia in children without contiguous spinal fracture or dislocation. *Neurosurgery* 12:439–445, 1983.
122. Waters RL, Yakura JS, Adkins R, Barnes G: Determinants of gait performance following spinal cord injury. *Arch Phys Med Rehabil* 70:811–818, 1989.
123. White JR: Pathology of spinal cord injury in experimental lesions. *Clin Orthop* 112:16, 1975.
124. Wilmot CB, Hall KM: Evaluation of the acute management of tetraplegia: Conservative versus surgical treatment. *Paraplegia* 24:148–153, 1986.
125. Winslow EB, Lesch M, Talano JV, Meyer PR: Spinal cord injuries associated with cardiopulmonary complications. *Spine* 11:809–812, 1986.
126. Woolston FL, Schowatler JE: Behavior modification protocol on a pediatric adolescent unit. *Pediatrics* 66:355–358, 1980.
127. Wyndaele JJ: A critical review of urodynamic investigations in spinal cord injury patients. *Paraplegia* 22:138–144, 1984.
128. Wyndaele JJ: Urethral sphincter dyssynergia in spinal cord injury patients. *Paraplegia* 25:10–15, 1987.
129. Yashon D: Pathogenesis of spinal cord injury. *Orthop Clin North Am* 9:247–261, 1978.
130. Young PR, Delwaide PJ: Spasticity. *N Engl J Med* 304:28–33(part one), 304:96–99(part two), 1981.

14

Rehabilitation of Children with Neuromuscular Diseases

GLORIA D. ENG

Neuromuscular diseases in children encompass a broad spectrum of complex disorders that are sometimes difficult to diagnose. Their patterns of genetic transmission are frequently obscure and the cause is mostly unknown. Although with histological and electronmicroscopic techniques their structural patterns are becoming more apparent, the natural pathophysiology and ultimate prognosis is not always well defined. Yet, it remains for us to attempt diagnostic differentiation in order to develop a realistic approach to management.

Definition

Neuromuscular diseases affect some part of the motor unit, namely, the anterior horn cell, spinal roots, peripheral nerves, neuromuscular junction, or the muscle fibers themselves. The cardinal manifestation of these disorders is *weakness,* presenting as hypotonia in infants and young children.

General Considerations

HISTORY

The importance of gestational and delivery history in an infant suspected of having neuromuscular disease cannot be underestimated. Paucity of fetal movements may suggest intrauterine weakness. Intermittent bleeding throughout the course of gestation may indicate nature's attempt to abort the infant spontaneously. A protracted labor may be due to uterine incompetence or a hypotonic infant. The neonatal course is often significant for feeding difficulties, choking spells, respiratory problems, apnea, general lethargy, and limpness.

In taking the history, it is imporant to determine the time of onset of weakness; whether the symptoms are static, fluctuating, or progressive; whether the child complains of cramps, paresthesias, or passes dark urine especially after strenuous exercise; and, whether significant preceding events such as an upper respiratory infection or exposure to insect bites or toxins occurred. A history of delayed milestones or a peculiar way of standing or walking are suspicious signs of weakness. For additional details of history-taking, the reader is referred to Chapter 1.

The family history of hereditary disorders is of utmost importance. Since many neuromuscular disorders are genetically transmitted, it may be the key to the diagnosis. In some autosomal-dominant inherited disorders, it is not unusual for a parent to be afflicted without realizing it. In autosomal-recessive conditions, the parents need not be affected but there may be siblings or members of the extended family who have the disease. Consanguinity of the parents will increase the chances of a combination of recessive genes. In X-linked afflictions, the mother's lineage must be traced with particular reference to male relatives to establish the possibility of carrier state.

CLINICAL EXAMINATION

Since conduct of physical examination is discussed in Chapter 1, only some leading signs of neuromuscular disease will be mentioned here.

An infant with generalized weakness will show paucity of movements with inability to kick and reach. In supine position, the arms assume a characteristic "jug handle" position and the legs the frog position. There may be paradoxical breathing, a weak cry, and a long, expressionless face. The infant is floppy, the physiological infantile reflexes are weak or absent. Lack of head and trunk control is readily evident from the collapsed kyphotic posture in supported sitting.

The child with proximal weakness will slide through the examiner's hands when held under the axillae and may be unable to wheelbarrow walk on extended arms because of decreased strength of the shoulder girdle. Struggling to rise from the floor, strenuously clutching the rails to ascend or descend stairs indicates weakness of the pelvic girdle. Inability to toe or heel walk suggests distal extremity weakness.

Localized or diffuse wasting, muscle hypertrophy, unusual texture of palpated muscle, fasciculations of the tongue, and/or tremor of the hands should be noted. Postural aberrations, such as scapular winging; increased lordosis; pelvic obliquity or kyphoscoliosis; cavus or valgus feet; presence or absence of deep tendon reflexes are recorded.

Throughout the evaluation, it is important to observe the parents. Not uncommonly, a nasal quality of voice, facial features with thinning of the temporalis and masseter muscles, transverse smile, thin arms and legs, or balding could suggest the possibility of myotonic dystrophy. Weak, thin facial muscles, sloping shoulders and scapular winging arouse the suspicion of facioscapulohumeral dystrophy. A parent who has pes cavus or equino-varus may have a neuropathic disorder with transmission to the offspring without recognizing the problem.

LABORATORY STUDIES

Careful history and physical examination enable the examiner to formulate a systematic categorization of possible anatomic and clinical differential entities. The presumptive diagnosis needs to be confirmed by appropriate laboratory studies.

Serum Enzymes

Elevated levels of creatine kinase, aldolase, and transaminase in the serum reflect breakdown of muscle tissue. These values may be slightly elevated in neurogenic disease and show a mild to marked rise in some myopathies and dystrophies. In normal infants, creatine kinase may be considerably elevated during the first 24 hours of life tapering to a normal level by 5 days of age; however, it may remain high throughout the first year of life.

In the metabolic myopathies, specific biochemical tests may be necessary, i.e., lactate and pyruvate levels during the ischemic exercise test in myophosphorylase deficiency, or carnitine and carnitine palmityl transferase levels in serum and muscle in some of the lipid myopathies. Fasting may be a provocative test in carnitine palmityl transferase deficiency.

Electrodiagnosis

Electrodiagnostic studies are a natural extension of assessment in suspected neuromuscular disorders and are reasonably well tolerated by infants and young children. The interpretation of electromyography, nerve conduction velocity, and neuromuscular transmission studies is based on a knowledge of the normal maturation of the peripheral nervous system. Nerve conduction velocity in term babies is approximately one-half of that in adults and reaches mature values by 3 to 5 yr of age. Similarly, neuromuscular transmission improves with maturation. Electromyography is easily performed in a weak infant or child although the findings may prove to be nonspecific and difficult to interpret. The duration of voluntary motor unit potentials is normally shorter in infants but the amplitude remains much as adult measurements. It is frequently difficult to induce an infant to respond with a maximal volitional contraction in order to assess recruitment patterns. Fibrillation-like potentials seen in premature and young infants do not necessarily indicate denervation. Endplate potentials, which are profuse and easily found, may lead to misinterpretation. Positive iterative discharges, as seen in adults with myotonic dystrophy, are frequently abbreviated in infants. For further discussion of electrodiagnosis, the reader should consult Chapter 6.

Muscle Biopsy

Meticulous handling of biopsy material is emphasized, especially when the possibility of an obscure myopathy exists (27, 44). Selection of a biopsy site should reflect active tissue pathology; severely atrophic or fibrotic muscles usually represent a burned-out disease process and yield inadequate material for histological studies. A muscle that has been recently studied electromyographically or received intramuscular injections should not be the site of biopsy. Hackmatt and Dubowitz advocate the use of ultrasound to locate appropriate muscle for biopsy. (56).

DIFFERENTIAL DIAGNOSIS

It is sometimes difficult to discriminate between cerebral dysfunction and a neuromuscular disorder in an infant presenting with hypotonia. Presence of deep tendon reflexes, imposable or persistent infantile reflexes, and tone alterations in response to position change suggest cerebral damage. Mental retardation with or without a known genetic marker may likewise present with hypotonicity and delayed motor development. The stigmatizing features are evident at first glance in genetic entities, such as Down's syndrome. In all forms of mental retardation, there is a global developmental delay affecting personal, social, and language skills. With a few possible exceptions, in neuromuscular disorders these areas of function are generally not impaired.

Another unusual cause for hypotonia to be considered is the Prader-Willi syndrome (10). Most of these children are hypotonic, short in stature; they have mental retardation, obesity, and, in the male, undescended testes. Although motor development is usually delayed, there is no muscle disease. These children may develop diabetes of the adult type in adolescence.

A differential diagnostic possibility, important because of its good prognosis, is benign congenital hypotonia (10). It affects primarily gross motor development without delay in cognitive skills and fine hand function. Deep tendon reflexes, serum enzymes, and electrodiagnostic and biopsy studies remain normal.

In a survey of hypotonia, the infant who suffers a traction injury of the spinal cord should not be forgotten. Infantile poliomyelitis, although rare, must be kept in mind especially in this day of haphazard immunizations. Connective tissue disorders, such as Ehlers-Danlos syndrome, may present as floppiness without muscle weakness. Many of these disorders are dominantly inherited with a history of double jointedness in one of the parents.

Although not hypotonic, infants with arthrogryposis multiplex congenita may have a "burned out" intrauterine neuromuscular disorder of neuropathic or myopathic origin and deserve careful evaluation (3).

Table 14.1.
Differential Diagnosis of Neuromuscular Disorders in Childhood

Brain	Cerebral palsy, dysgenetic brain, infection, degenerative CNS lesions
Spinal cord	SMA
	Infantile poliomyelitis
	Spinal cord traction injury
	Tumor or malformation
Roots and nerves	Infectious polyneuropathy
	Hereditary polyneuropathy
	Toxic polyneuropathy
	Traumatic neuritis, etc.
Neuromuscular junction	Myasthenia gravis
	Tick paralysis
	Toxic paralysis—antibiotics
	Insecticides, crop sprays
	Botulism
Muscle disease dystrophy	Duchenne muscular dystrophy
	Facioscapulohumeral dystrophy
	Becker dystrophy
	Scapuloperoneal dystrophy
	Emery-Dreifus disease
	Oculopharyngeal dystrophy
	Myotonic dystrophy
Congenital myopathies	Type I hypotrophy
	Mitochondrial
	Nemaline
	Central core
	Fiber-type disproportion
	Finger-print myopathy, etc.
Metabolic myopathies	Glycogenosis
	Endocrine
	Lipid

Diagnosis and Management of Specific Disorders

A practical approach to the diagnosis of neuromuscular disorders is by anatomic categorization. After excluding cerebral damage and other previously mentioned conditions as possible causes of hypotonia, the focus should shift to the anterior horn cells, dorsal and ventral roots, peripheral nerves, neuromuscular junction and, finally, to the muscles (Table 14.1).

SPINAL MUSCULAR ATROPHIES

The most common neuromuscular disorder affecting infants and children is spinal muscular atrophy (SMA). Its incidence has been estimated at 1 in 15,000 to 25,000 live births.

Classification

Much confusion exists in the classification of SMAs. Some feel that Werdnig-Hoffman disease, the infantile form or type I SMA, is a distinct and sep-

Table 14.2.
Classification of the Spinal Muscular Atrophies[a]

Class	Synonyms	Clinical Features	Genetics
SMA type I	Werdnig-Hoffman disease	⅓ show prenatal onset 95% show clinical signs by 3 months Median age of death, 7 months	Autosomal recessive
SMA type II	Arrested Werdnig-Hoffman disease Chronic generalized SMA	Clinical signs under 3 yr of age, variable severity Median age of death exceeds 10 yr	Autosomal recessive
SMA type III	Kugelberg-Welander syndrome	Clinical signs 3–15 yr Milder course	Occasional autosomal dominant
Distal SMA	Progressive SMA	Onset at birth or infancy Frequently confused with Charcot-Marie-Tooth Slow progression; normal life span	Autosomal recessive, occasional autosomal dominant
Scapuloperoneal atrophy		Onset in late childhood, early teens Progress slow from scapuloperoneal to generalized weakness in adult life	Autosomal dominant or recessive
SMA with cerebral dysfunction	Neuraxonal dystrophy variants	Onset in childhood, slowly progressive, associated with mental retardation	Probably rare, recessive

[a]From Pearn J: Classification of spinal muscular atrophies. *Lancet* 1:919–922, 1980.

arate entity because the course of this disorder is so ominous and different from the other forms of the disease. However, many authors (37, 54, 81, 85) believe that these disorders are a spectrum of one common pathological entity. A chronic form of infantile SMA is type II, which has a more insidious onset. The juvenile type III or Kugelberg-Welander disease (8, 61, 68) affects children between 5 and 15 yr of age and is slowly progressive. Another chronic form is the distal SMA (59), which accounts for 10% of all cases described in northeastern England but is only seen occasionally in this country. Table 14.2 shows a summary of the different clinical types.

Inheritance

The infantile form, or Werdnig-Hoffman disease, is generally believed to be transmitted by autosomal recessive genes. According to Pearn and associates (81), a single autosomal recessive gene is responsible for 90% of subacute and chronic cases of childhood. Gomez (54) feels that the juvenile onset type is due to one or more autosomal recessive genes and that the dominant trait is rare. Two separate autosomal recessive genes and perhaps one dominant gene have been incriminated in the transmission of distal SMA (59, 61). The late sporadic onset variety may represent a new dominant mutation. A recent molecular genetic research technique known as linkage analysis shows the defect to be on chromosome five.

Pathology

The underlying pathology is degeneration of the anterior horn cells in the spinal cord and the neurocytes in the motor nuclei of some cranial nerves. Active axonal degeneration has been described in both anterior and posterior spinal roots. Perhaps it is for this reason that, in 30% of SMAs, nerve conduction velocity is prolonged. These findings are more significant in type IA of the disease (62). It is interesting to note that, on autopsies of children with Werdnig-Hoffman disease, a small thymus has been found. In some, a decreased cellular immunity has been demonstrated, which may account for the children's susceptibility to respiratory infections and their frequent stormy terminal course.

Laboratory Studies

The serum level of muscle enzymes is usually normal with the exception of creatine kinase. This enzyme may be slightly elevated in young infants and in type III spinal muscular atrophy where increased serum values can be found in 50% of cases.

Electromyographic assessment of patients with Werdnig-Hoffman disease shows nonspecific findings with diminution of recruitment pattern and some fibrillations. Regular motor unit activity occurring at a frequency of 5 to 15/sec (myokymic discharges) in relaxed muscles has been described. In the more chronic forms of SMA, one begins to see high-amplitude, long-duration potentials, and an increasing number of long-duration polyphasic potential (62) (see Chapter 6).

Histochemical examination of muscle biopsy specimen in the infantile form may show abundance of round atrophic fibers with compensatory hypertrophy, usually consisting of type I muscle fibers. Serial biopsies are sometimes necessary because persistent fetal muscle characteristics may make it difficult to arrive at a definitive diagnosis in early infancy. The importance of a correct diagnosis is evident for prognostic implications and genetic counseling. In the more chronic forms of SMA, one begins to see type grouping with atrophy of small and large fibers as well as some markedly hypertrophied fibers. It is not unusual in these forms of the disease, especially Kugelberg-Welander type, to encounter myopathic fiber changes and proliferation of the endomysium. Hausmanowa-Petrusewicz and associates (61) postulate that a fetal defect is responsible for the pathological features in this form of the disease but feel that these changes probably occur later in fetal life than those seen in Werdnig-Hoffman disease.

Clinical Course

Early demise is the outcome in Werdnig-Hoffman disease. Some babies are limp at birth whereas others may appear fairly normal at first and become suddenly weak. Feeble cry, sucking, and swallowing difficulties in contrast to their alert faces are characteristic of these infants. Although in some cases there may be greater proximal involvement, most infants have diffuse weakness with the exception of occasional finger and toe movements. They lie virtually immobile in the position described earlier. Breathing is paradoxical and there is areflexia. Some cases demonstrate fibrillations of the tongue and eyelids, but fasciculations are not discernible in the skeletal muscles.

In the clinical type II of the disease, there is a more chronic course. Pearn and associates (82) reviewing 141 cases of SMA, reported on the findings of those who survived beyond 18 months. In some cases, symptoms were present at birth. Ninety-five percent were diagnosed at least by 3 yr although, in a few children, the disease was not identified until 8 yr. Boys were more severely affected than girls. Despite early onset, some children with the chronic form are able to attain motor milestones (Fig. 14.1). One third can roll over and some may be able to maintain a precarious sitting position balancing their head and trunk mechanically with very little muscle control. In

Figure 14.1. Two sisters with spinal muscular atrophy type II. Both are ambulatory, have pes planus, and fine tremor of the hands.

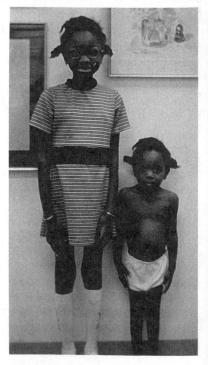

the same series, 50% of children never walked and 37% could walk with braces and crutches at some stage, but none of them could run after 12 yr. Calf hypertrophy has been described in boys with this type of spinal muscular atrophy. We have noted fasciculation and wasting of the tongue in one half of the children and more weakness of the proximal muscles compared to the distal ones, as well as tremor in the hands and forearms of some children (37).

Merlini and associates (73) reviewed the course of 113 patients with SMA between 1974 and 1987. Twenty-one had severe SMA with the average age of demise at 6 months. Fifty-two had the intermediate type. Of these, six died between 5 and 12 yr of age. Forty patients had the mild form of SMA, ranging in age from 3 to 47 yr, and all were alive at the time of report. However, almost one half of the patients with mild SMA lost the ability to walk. All nonambulatory patients developed scoliosis of the paralytic type leading to kyphosis and pelvic obliquity, representing the single most demanding therapeutic challenge in their care. Total contact plastic thoracolumbosacral orthoses did not slow the progression of spinal deformities although the braces allowed weaker patients to sit upright. Spinal instrumentation and stabilization procedures resulted in stable corrections with improvement in cosmesis and function. The authors recommend surgical consideration in anticipatory management of all SMA II and some SMA III patients.

The later onset type III Kugelberg-Welander disease (68) is slowly progressive although occasional sudden exacerbations may occur. The distribution of muscle weakness is proximal and the pelvic girdle is usually more affected than the shoulder girdle. Pseudohypertrophy of the calves has been described in 20% of cases. Facial weakness is rare but may appear in the course of the disease. Fasciculations can be observed in approximately 50% of cases. Most patients need a wheelchair by their middle 30s. Type III SMA may be mistakenly diagnosed as Becker muscular dystrophy or limb-girdle dystrophy because of the slowly progressive course, enlarged calves, and pattern of muscle weakness.

Distal SMA is slowly progressive and does not shorten life span (59, 82) but the disorder must be differentiated from other hereditary polyneuropathies because of the common manifestation of pes cavus or equinovarus deformities.

Management

Rehabilitation of a child with SMA is based on a premise that despite the relative briefness of life in some cases, it must approximate normal as much as possible and be free of severe discomfort. The parents are encouraged to develop a level of comfort in nurturing, feeding, and providing mobility to an otherwise immobile child (6, 34–37).

Feeding. The use of proper nipples such as a premature baby nipple with a large opening; thickening of the formula; proper jaw control and support of the buccinators with the baby in semireclined position; frequent small feedings to prevent fatigue; and supplemental feedings with nasogastric tube drip rather than bolus, which may encroach on diaphragmatic excursion, are recommended. Problems with constipation are necessarily addressed as impaction can also interfere with respiratory effort.

Respiratory Care. Suctioning with small bulb syringes can clear the airway prior to feeding. Catheter suctioning using a portable apparatus is sometimes indicated. Postural drainage is useful if there are increased secretions. The young child may have to be helped to cough effectively by applying gentle pressure on the abdomen. In the event of respiratory infection, vigorous specific antimicrobial treatment and oxygen can alleviate the child's distress. If respiratory failure supervenes, intubation and respiratory support remain a case by case decision.

Mobility. The infant with Werdnig-Hoffman disease who is limp and immobile should be positioned in appropriate seating supported by extra foam wedges to allow his or her hands to come together in midline. The infant can be placed in supine or side-lying position on a wedge so his or her head is elevated; or the child can be gently rocked in a hammock. The child should be given lightweight toys of different textures to feel, transfer, and explore orally. Most infants with SMA I do not tolerate prone-lying. Gentle exercise of the extremities and maintaining good spinal alignment not only provide mobility but ensure comfort.

For the older child, positioning and daily passive range of motion exercises must be instituted to prevent joint and soft tissue contractures. In the less severe forms of the disease and when the child is old enough, selected play and other daily activities can serve as active exercises. Physical therapy cannot alter the course of the disease. Reservations about vigorous overload exercises are similar to those described in muscular dystrophy. Although reduced activity level could theoretically create additional disuse weakness, these youngsters are generally bright and well motivated to maintain all functional activities as long as they can.

For the children who have delayed and restricted development affecting only the area of physical function, assistive devices are important to provide substitutive means of gross and fine motor activities. Custom seating may be necessary for the more severe group of SMA II (intermediate) for head and trunk control. For those who have head control, with or without the ability to sit, the use of standing frames or a parapodium allows erect posture, normal joint alignment, and facilitates socialization. Crawling devices, adapted walkerettes, and scooters can be managed by some of the children. For the 3-yr-old intelligent child who will never walk and who has weak upper extremities, a motorized wheelchair should be considered.

Braces. Children with SMA II (intermediate) may be able to stand and to walk with lightweight braces such as polypropylene ankle-foot orthoses

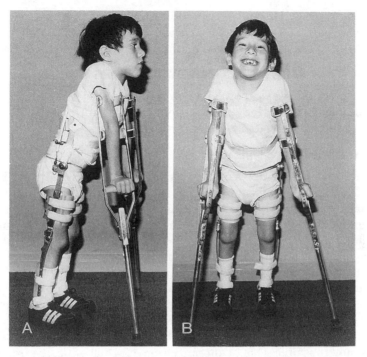

Figure 14.2. Boy with spinal muscular atrophy type II walking with reciprocal brace, front view (*A*) and back view (*B*).

(AFOs). Ischial weight-bearing knee-ankle-foot orthosis (KAFO) is sometimes appropriate for flaccid paralysis of the legs. According to Granata and associates (55), fitting the child with these braces is best done under 2 yr of age, to permit standing, to prevent contractures and scoliosis, and to provide functional and psychological benefits. The reciprocating orthosis may also assist in ambulation while it prevents contractures. This device can be used effectively until ages 10 to 12 yr (Fig. 14.2). The longer a child maintains erect stance, the longer will his or her need for wheelchair mobility be delayed. Secondary complications of kyphoscoliosis and associated restrictive lung disease will be delayed as well.

As the children grow, their muscle strength may become inadequate to support the growing limbs and trunk even though there is no overt progression of the disease. Shoulder girdle and hand weakness can interfere with the use of crutches. For the same reason, transfer activities are particularly laborious in wheelchair-bound children with shoulder depressor weakness and precarious trunk balance.

Because these children are usually of normal intelligence, scholastic pursuits are especially important. Electronic aids and environmental controls enable the severely affected bright youngster to function independently in school, college, and to prepare for a career. Supportive emotional counseling of the children and their parents should be a continuing intervention.

MUSCULAR DYSTROPHIES

The etiology of these genetically determined diseases remains unknown. A reasonable classification of various entities was outlined by Walton and Gardner-Medwin (100) and is shown in Table 14.3.

Duchenne Muscular Dystrophy

This disease affects males and is transmitted by X-linked mode of inheritance. Therefore, it is of utmost importance in genetic counseling to identify potential carriers. In addition to the child's mother, his sisters and maternal aunts are at risk. Previously, one of the most reliable tests was the measurement of serum creatine kinase levels. Three random samples were examined and vigorous exercise was to be avoided for 48 hours prior to obtaining the blood. Results have not always been definitive and, because mutations are rare, mothers of affected sons have been presumed genetic carriers. Recent extraordinary advances using molecular genetic techniques have located the gene for Duchenne and Becker dystrophy on the short arm of the X-chromosome at position Xp21 (75, 94). In utero diagnosis of the disease is now possible (17). Differentiation of Duchenne dystrophy from Becker type is by qualitative difference of the protein moiety called dystrophin. In Duchenne dystrophy, there is almost no dystrophin present, whereas in Becker dystrophy, the protein is present but usually of abnormal weight (63, 64). Myoblast transfer is currently an experimental procedure that results in fusion of donor myoblasts with the dystrophic reception fibers as indicated by the presence of dystrophin in the receptor cells. It is not clear whether the strength of the receptor muscle improves (66, 69).

Laboratory examinations to establish the diagnosis of Duchenne muscular dystrophy include serum creatine kinase, electromyography, and muscle biopsy. Serum enzyme level is extremely high, often elevated by 10 to 20

Table 14.3.
Classification of Muscular Dystrophies

A. X-linked muscular dystrophy
   Duchenne—severe
   Becker—benign
B. Autosomal recessive muscular dystrophy
   Limb girdle
   Congenital muscular dystrophy
C. Facioscapulohumeral muscular dystrophy
   Distal muscular dystrophy
   Ocular muscular dystrophy
   Oculopharyngeal dystrophy

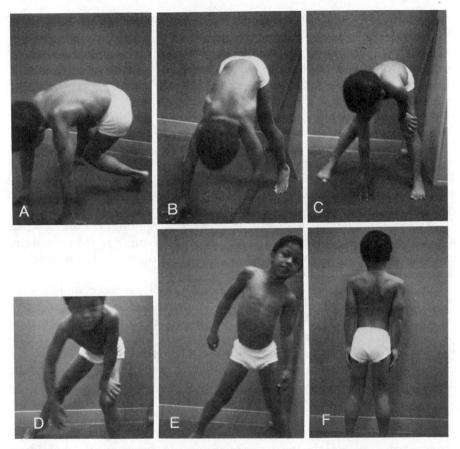

Figure 14.3. Duchenne's muscular dystrophy patient has difficulty rising from the floor; *A–D;* typical Gower sign; *E,* waddling gait; *F,* pseudohypertrophy of the calves.

times above normal in young infants who later develop overt clinical symptoms (10). As the disease progresses, the serum enzyme values drop but never return to normal. Electromyograms show small, low-amplitude, short-duration motor unit action potentials with increased recruitment pattern on effort. An increased number of polyphasic potentials and occasional fibrillations are present. Muscle biopsy demonstrates focal necrosis and hyalinization of muscle fibers. As the disease progresses, there is increasing fatty infiltration and endomyseal proliferation.

The characteristic history involves a young boy who may have been a late walker but showed no overt symptoms until 3 to 6 yr of age. He begins to fall frequently, has difficulty climbing stairs, and rising from the floor. His gait is waddling with increased lordosis and toe walking (Fig. 14.3). There is usually minimal progression until 7 yr when a precipitous decline sets in. Most children are in wheelchairs between 9 and 12 yr of age. In the past, many did not survive the second decade.

Muscle weakness and contractures account for the abnormalities and deterioration of gait. Hip flexor, tensor fascia latae, and triceps surae contractures limit ambulation. There is hip extensor weakness with exaggerated lumbar lordosis, which increases in the course of the disease. The knees are locked in genu recurvatum to prevent collapse of that joint. As the triceps surae becomes shorter and the quadriceps becomes weaker, the knee can no longer maintain extension. The child begins to fall more often and he assumes a wide-based gait for balance. Soon he is unable to climb stairs and, usually within 6 to 12 months he cannot walk independently. Hip, knee, and elbow flexion contractures as well as equinovarus foot deformities appear rapidly and a progressive scoliosis develops in the wheelchair-bound child. Obesity is a frequent problem at this stage although muscle bulk becomes lost as the disease progresses. In late stage of Duchenne dystrophy, muscles of the face may be involved, the head begins to loll against the back of the chair as neck weakness develops (10).

Cardiomyopathy of Duchenne muscular dystrophy is detectable by serial ECGs that frequently show tall R waves or increased R/S ratios in the precordial leads; decreased left ventricular ejection fraction on echocardiography; arrhythmias and ventricular ectopy (25, 83). Yotsukura and associates (102) noted that even in the terminal stage of Duchenne dystrophy, left ventricular function may not be markedly involved, and that respiratory failure with associated precapillary pulmonary hypertension and right ventricular failure ultimately leads to death.

Cardiac abnormalities are further complicated by restrictive pulmonary disease. Vignos (97) studied the correlations among physical abilities, pulmonary function, and the incidence of respiratory infections in 38 children. Based on physical function, he divided the group into nine classes (Table 14.4). The total lung volume remained nearly normal until class V and progressively declined beyond this functional level. In the absence of infection, the patients were usually able to maintain blood gas homeostasis. Pulmonary pathology was of the restrictive type and correlated with the loss in muscle power. Diaphragmatic action was well preserved even in advanced disease.

Scoliosis associated with Duchenne muscular dystrophy further compromises respiratory function. In a review of 105 patients by Cambridge and Drennan (13), scoliosis developed in 95% of the patients after loss of ambulation. Miller and associates (74) found decline of forced vital capacity (FVC) most rapid at the adolescent growth spurt. Rideau and co-workers (84) could predict longevity of the patients based on reduction of FVC at age 10 to 12 yr, relating the decline directly to the severity of the scoliosis. There is general agreement (13, 16, 78, 91, 92, 95) that the use of a spinal orthosis

Table 14.4.
Functional States of Duchenne Muscular Dystrophy[a]

    I. Walks and climbs stairs without assistance
   II. Walks and climbs stairs with the aid of railings
  III. Walks and climbs stairs slowly with the aid of railings (greater than 25 sec for eight standard steps)
  IV. Walks unassisted and rises from chair, but cannot climb stairs
   V. Walks unassisted but cannot rise from chair or climb stairs
  VI. Walks only with assistance or walks independently with long-leg braces
 VII. Walks in long-leg braces but requires assistance for balance
VIII. Stands in long-leg braces, but unable to walk, even with assistance
  IX. In a wheelchair or bed

---

[a]From Vignos PJ Jr: Respiratory function and pulmonary infection in Duchenne muscular dystrophy. *Isr J Med Sci* 13:207–214, 1977.

does not control curve progression and surgical stabilization should be considered when the curve progresses beyond 35°. Smith and associates (92) noted in a review of 51 boys that early maintenance of the lumbar spine in extension rarely prevented the development of a severe curve. Sitting became difficult and painful with skin breakdown in many cases. They urge spinal surgery when ambulation is no longer possible.

Experience has increased in the management of end-stage respiratory failure in Duchenne muscular dystrophy (2, 20). Mouth intermittent positive pressure ventilation in combination with other techniques of ventilatory assistance has increased longevity while allowing for optimal function (1). The psychosocial aspects that surround the use of ventilators as well as the demand on health-care providers and families remain controversial issues (7, 74, 93).

As patients with Duchenne muscular dystrophy live longer, symptoms referable to smooth muscle dysfunction become apparent. This includes intestinal pseudo-obstruction and gastric hypomotility with gaseous eructation and pain (5, 71). Urinary retention can also be a problem.

A number of studies indicate low cognitive function among children with Duchenne dystrophy (70, 101). Karagan and associates (65) demonstrated more significant differences in verbal IQ than on performance tests, with low scores on subtests requiring memory for patterns, numbers, and verbal labeling. Brooke (10, pp. 117–190) observed a mean IQ score of 85. The retardation is not progressive and may precede the onset of muscle weakness.

Becker Muscular Dystrophy

This form is similar to Duchenne dystrophy in terms of distribution of weakness but has a later onset and a more benign course (9, 10). It is also an X-linked inherited disorder with gene localization (67). Intellectual impairment is not a prominent feature of Becker dystrophy.

Limb-Girdle Dystrophy

This type of dystrophy presents primarily with proximal weakness and greater involvement of the pelvic girdle than the shoulder musculature (100). The rapidly progressive form may resemble Duchenne dystrophy but cases with more benign course and mild weakness may be difficult to differentiate from Becker dystrophy or type III SMA. Prognostication is also difficult in individual cases because of the variable course and severity. The disorder affects both sexes and is transmitted by autosomal recessive inheritance.

Congenital Muscular Dystrophy

This condition appears as marked hypotonia at birth and affects muscles of the limbs and face (72). Contractures are frequent and tend to be progressive, although muscle weakness may remain static for years.

Cardiomyopathy and mental retardation are generally not associated with this disease. However, Fukuyama and associates (52, 79) described congenital muscular dystrophy with severe mental retardation and seizures.

Facioscapulohumeral Dystrophy

Face, neck, and shoulder girdle muscles are primarily affected (10, pp. 117–190). Symptoms usually appear between the end of the first decade and adolescence. Both sexes are affected and inheritance is generally by dominant genetic transmission. A fetal form of the disease with rapid progression and demise in adolescence has been recognized (10, pp. 117–190). Cochlear dysfunction is a specific and frequent phenomenon resulting in high-frequency hearing loss in these children (99).

Oculopharyngeal Dystrophies or Myopathies

These relatively rare disorders present with ptosis, ophthalmoplegia, and limb-girdle weakness (10, pp. 117–190). When carefully assessed, some children have congenital myopathy of the mitochondrial or myotubular variety. In others, muscle biopsy shows ragged red fibers characteristic of the oculocranial somatic syndrome. These conditions are usually transmitted by autosomal dominant inheritance and their course may be a gradual improvement with time.

Management

At the present time, there is no treatment for muscular dystrophies except for preventive and functional management of the presenting disability and medical treatment of cardiopulmonary complications. A variety of drugs to include calcium channel blockers, the amino acids leucine and penicillamine, have been tried without changing the progressive course in Duchenne muscular dystrophy (77). Brooke and associates (11), in a collaborative study of Duchenne muscular dystrophy boys, used high doses of prednisone for 6 months. With this treatment, a 50% slowing of progression rate was demonstrated but development of contractures continued. Their study was based on the work of DeSilva and associates (22) who found that ambulation was prolonged by approximately 2 yr in the prednisone-treated group. Further studies are contemplated to evaluate optimal treatment schedules and deal with the side effects of steroid therapy.

Supportive management programs have been detailed in several excellent reviews (15, 48–51). Specific objectives include a reasonable life-style, encouraging self-help skills and ambulation, anticipating treatment of complications, providing recreational and vocational programs adapted to the boy's capabilities, and counseling of siblings, parents, and the boy himself throughout his life.

Specific management strategies relate to the stages of the disease. As stated, until 7 yr, most children with muscular dystrophy do not require intensive treatment. The patient and parents should be instructed in range of motion exercises emphasizing stretching the tensor fascia latae, iliopsoas, hamstrings, tendo Achilles, and elbow and finger flexors. Correct posture and alignment both in standing and sitting is critical. Exercise in the "submaximal" or "underload" zone does not appear to be deleterious in early phases of the disorder (51). Supervised swimming affords mobility, maintains joint range of motion, good respiratory exchange, general conditioning, and can be continued even when the child is no longer walking. As the child becomes weaker and has difficulty going up and down stairs, or even walking, contractures develop more rapidly because of compensatory postural adjustments. Flexion contractures can be stretched by placing the child in prone position several times a day. The use of orthotic devices has to be individualized. Night splints and some of the lighter-weight polypropylene KAFOs with ischial seating may be tried. Achilles tendon release and plantar fasciotomy may be helpful when severe toe walking interferes with balance. The knee extensors must be at least fair in grade for walking to be prolonged for several months or years after the orthopaedic procedure. Polypropylene AFOs may be used in an effort to maintain the feet in plantigrade position. The reciprocal walking brace permits forward propulsion in a few selected patients.

Because of the increased effort for walking, persistence in this endeavor is not always practical. It is advisable to prepare the child and his parents for wheelchair existence at least 6 months to 1 year ahead of time. Most children with Duchenne muscular dystrophy need a wheelchair between 9 and 13 yr of age. Some children prefer and are capable of using other mobility devices, such as the Amigo or Pony motorized chairs. These vehicles can be extremely enjoyable and allow the child freedom in movement that he may never have experienced before. Finally, when he needs a wheelchair, it can be a "passport" to more, rather than less, social and educational activity.

Careful selection of a wheelchair for the patient with muscular dystrophy is of extreme importance. The seat and back should be firm. The side arms should be removable so that the child does not lean to one side or the other. It is sometimes necessary to provide a neck collar or extension of the back of the seat to support the head. Foot rests should hold the feet in plantigrade with straps to prevent the progression of equinovarus deformity (Fig. 14.4). An occasional child will eliminate the foot rests in order to assist in propelling the chair with his feet. He should be encouraged to use a chair that he wheels himself in order to maintain upper extremity strength. A motorized chair becomes necessary for the child who is essentially quadriparetic. A contour-U insert or other customized molded seat in a powered base wheelchair may be an option.

Other adaptive devices useful in dystrophy patients include overhanging slings to assist shoulder abduction and balanced forearm orthoses to help with hand function. However, adolescent patients usually discard most devices prescribed for them. In their desire to appear as normal as other children, they become clever in adaptive maneuvers for self-care.

As the boy becomes weaker and the hip and knee flexion contractures progress inexorably, it may be difficult to attain comfortable sleeping postures. The use of a hospital bed with electric controls and side rails may allow the child to shift his position independently. Raised stools, chairs, lap boards, tables, raised toilet seats with side rails, accessible shower stalls with grab bars, and a shower head adjusted at chest level are modifications that can facilitate care.

Housing for the patient with dystrophy must be wheelchair accessible with necessary adaptations to allow for privacy and independence. Vans with lifts facilitate transportation of a wheelchair-bound child.

Deterioration of pulmonary function parallels the increasing scoliosis in Duchenne dystrophy. As in patients with SMA, a Jewett hyperextension brace or other types of total contact orthosis do not prevent progression of the curve (16). Some authors (84, 91, 92, 95) recommend spinal fixation for curves exceeding 35° and the vital capacity less than 40% of predicted normal value.

Obesity is a problem in the patient with Duchenne dystrophy when immobility sets in. Proper dietary management should be introduced early and regularly monitored. During the late stages of the disease, severe weight loss and inanition occur as muscle mass disappears and self-feeding may no longer be possible.

The management of end-stage respiratory failure in Duchenne muscular dystrophy has extended the lives of many young men and has allowed optimal function, pursuance of educational goals, and even the option of living at home (2). The decision of prolonging life by means of ventilator support is controversial and a choice to be made on an individual basis (74).

The psychosocial aspects of this disease remain a long-term challenge (7, 33, 48). As it is a disorder with a slow and arduous course, it has all the con-

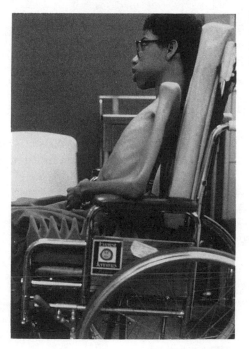

Figure 14.4. Duchenne's muscular dystrophy. Note marked muscle wasting, lordotic posture in advanced wheelchair stage.

comitant strains of an illness with considerable psychological stress and prolonged grieving. The initial guilt in the mother may cause marital conflicts; the father's expectation of his son is destroyed. There are many practical problems including the physical hardship of lifting, the need for continuing medical attention, potential financial burdens, and restriction in freedom of activity for both child and family. The coping mechanisms range from initial denial hoping that the disease really does not exist to overprotection, which leads to isolation of the child. Lack of discipline, which makes a child tyrannical, and problems with sibling stress ensue. As he grows to an adolescent, the child himself becomes frustrated over the lack of sexual expression, increasing immobility, fear of impending death, the realization that he is not attractive and that he is a burden to his friends or family.

Group psychotherapy and individual sessions have been helpful to both the child and parents and should be initiated early and continued even after the child's death.

The same principles of management apply to the less severe dystrophic disorders with modifications determined by the presenting problems.

MYOTONIC DISORDERS

Myotonic Dystrophy

There is a fetal form of myotonic dystrophy that deserves special emphasis (60). The gestational history may include polyhydramnios because of inability of the fetus to swallow amniotic fluid. The mother might feel diminished fetal movements. There may be increased fetal wastage. At birth, the newborn infant is frequently floppy with low Apgar scores, is unable to close the eyes fully, exhibiting a loose slack facies, a tented mouth (Fig. 14.5). On further examination, elevation of the diaphragm might be noted. Cryptorchidism, talipes equinovarus as well as lower extremity hirsutism have been described. The baby is liable to have feeding difficulties, sleep apnea, and respiratory failure. It is not uncommon in the neonatal type to find mental retardation that is more severe than in Duchenne muscular dystrophy. In our experience, these children remain floppy for the first few years of life and gradually show slow motor gains. Some of them walk by 3 yr of age, others not until 5 or 6 yr of age.

The creatine phosphokinase is normal to slightly elevated. Electromyographic examination in infants may be nonspecific. In the fetal form, the biopsy may be entirely normal or there may be a few angulated fibers and some type I hypotrophy. It is frequenty advisable to wait several months until an infant is older to obtain a muscle biopsy. Sarnst and co-workers (86) described severely affected neonates with congenital cataracts and ECG changes. Conduction blocks are common even in the fetal form of the disorder. The mother is the affected parent in 94% of the cases.

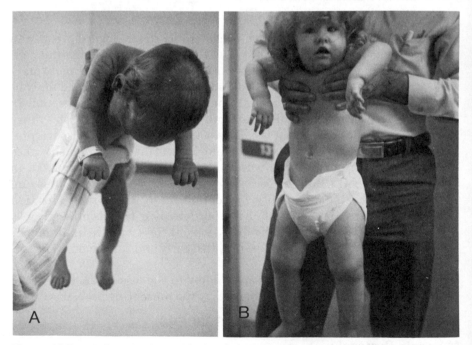

Figure 14.5. *A,* floppy infant with myotonic dystrophy. *B,* slack facies, tented mouth, shoulder-girdle weakness.

In the childhood form of myotonic dystrophy, the youngster may be symptom free, except for a myopathic facies. Some cases appear with subluxed or dislocated hips, as well as club feet; dysphagia, urinary tract, and uterine involvement. Malabsorption has been noted in some affected individuals secondary to smooth muscle dysfunction.

Central nervous system abnormalities including hydrocephalus, EEG abnormalities with overt seizures, and myocardial conduction blocks manifested by arrhythmias have been found in some patients. It has been described that certain cases of myotonic dystrophy are at risk during anesthesia, developing episodes of cardiac arrhythmias, and/or malignant hyperthermia.

In the work-up of the children, the diagnosis is frequently made in one or the other parent because overt myotonia may not become evident until age 4 or 5 yr. Sometimes it is difficult to identify the carrier parent because some of the clinical manifestations may not be obvious until old age. Evaluation for cataracts, deafness, and ECG abnormalities must be pursued.

Myotonia Congenita

Differentiated from myotonic dystrophy is a disorder known as myotonia congenita (Thomsen disease) (10, pp. 197–205). This is usually an autosomal dominant disorder, although occasionally a recessive form may be encountered. Patients affected with this disease are usually stiff after prolonged rest and inactivity. The myotonia is aggravated by cold, fatigue, and sometimes the muscles are so hypertrophied that these children appear as infantile Hercules. There is no weakness associated with this disorder. Biopsy is normal.

Paramyotonia Congenita (Eulenburg Disease)

Paramyotonia congenita is a disorder that includes myotonia, hypertrophy of muscles, and stiffness that can be followed by transitory weakness (43). It may be confused with the so-called hyperkalemic paralysis (Gamstorp disease), which may have long periods of paralysis.

Management

The approach to the infant with myotonic dystrophy includes cardiorespiratory monitoring and careful feeding with occasional need for a gastrostomy. Talipes equinovarus deformities require serial casting and corrective splinting. The infant must be carried in a seating arrangement that maintains good support and alignment. The parents are taught range of motion exercises to prevent joint contractures. Postural drainage techniques may be necessary in the event of pulmonary infections. Exercises are added to facilitate head and trunk control and increased mobility. As the child assumes upright stance, the use of supportive lightweight braces and spinal orthoses to prevent rapid progression of scoliosis may be necessary. Most of

Table 14.5.
Congenital Myopathies

	Onset	Course	Inheritance	DTR
Central core disease	Birth to infancy	Mild to moderate Disability—progressive Adult life Slow development	Autosomal dominant	Normal or decreased
Nemaline rod myopathy	Early infancy	Slow development Variable Occasionally severe	Autosomal dominant	Decreased to absent
Finger-print body myopathy	Infancy	Unknown Probably adult life	Autosomal recessive	Decreased to absent
Multicore disease	Infancy to childhood	Probably adult life	Autosomal recessive	Decreased
Myotubular or central nuclear myopathy	Early infancy to childhood	Variable Benign to progressive	X-linked Autosomal recessive or dominant	Decreased to absent
Mitochondrial myopathy megaconial	Late infancy to childhood	Slow progression	Autosomal recessive	Decreased to absent
Mitochondrial myopathy pleoconial	Early infancy	Variable Slow progression	Autosomal recessive	Decreased to absent

the children will walk but sometimes not until 5 yr of age. A well-structured, individualized educational plan must be specially designed if mental retardation is present. Self-help skills are fostered. The cardiac and neurological complications may require extensive consultation with the appropriate specialists.

In the patient with myotonia congenita, the treatment is medical. Administration of quinine, procainamide, phenytoin, and corticosteroids has had varied success (10, pp. 197–205). Because a child with this disorder may have a tense, high-strung personality, psychological intervention with parental support is sometimes indicated. In the paramyotonic disorders, the treatment is essentially supportive and medical.

MYOPATHIES

Congenital Myopathies

A satisfactory nosological classification of the congenital myopathies is not available. However, through refinement of histochemical and electron-microscopic techniques, many previously ill-defined entities can now be recognized (4). Their inheritance pattern is not always clear and prognosis is variable although, for the most part, relatively benign (12, 32, 80, 89, 90). A

Table 14.5.—*Continued*

Serum Enzymes	EMG	Biopsy	Distribution of Weakness	Other Signs
Normal or elevated	Myopathic, denervation potentials	Large fibers with central fibrillary material in central core	Generalized Legs more than arms	Congenital hip or patellar dislocation Scoliosis
Normal Slightly to moderately elevated	Myopathic	Abnormal rod structure in type I fibers	Generalized or proximal and cervical muscles	Myopathic facies Respiratory problems Pseudohypertrophy
Normal	Myopathic	Concentric lamellar patterns resembling fingerprints	Generalized	Mental retardation Mild tremor of extremities
Normal	Few myopathic potentials	Decreased mitochondria, abnormal sarcomere pattern	Generalized	Ptosis, contractures, scoliosis
Increased CPK	Myopathic Some myotonic discharges	Myotubules, central nuclei	Generalized or proximal	Myopathic facies Exrraocular muscle weakness Ptosis, palate weakness
Normal	Myopathic	Enlarged mitochondria	Proximal	Dysphagia Waddling gait, increased lordosis, Gower's sign
Normal	Myopathic	Increased number of mitochondria	Proximal	Attacks of weakness Waddling gait

potential complication of importance specifically in patients with central core disease and elevated serum enzymes is their susceptibility to malignant hyperthermia in response to potent inhalation anesthetic agents (21, 38). Table 14.5 shows the characteristic clinical and laboratory findings in congenital myopathies. Figures 14.6 and 14.7 show children with nemaline and myotubular myopathy, respectively.

Metabolic Myopathies

Most inherited metabolic myopathies of known etiology are related to enzyme deficiencies involved in glycogen metabolism. Thus, the organ system affected may include muscle tissue, central nervous system, heart, and liver in a variety of combinations as a result of glycogenosis. Myopathy is the leading sign in type II or Pompe disease (42) with 1-4 glycosidase or acid maltase deficiency and in type V or McArdle disease (19, 23) with phosphorylase deficiency. Both are autosomal recessive disorders.

In Pompe disease (42), there is enlargement of the heart, liver, spleen, and the muscles are firm and rubbery. Brain and spinal cord neurons can be affected. The infant is weak, hypotonic, delayed in development, and often appears with cardiorespiratory distress (Fig. 14.8). Deep tendon reflexes are absent and the serum muscle enzymes are markedly elevated. It is a rapidly

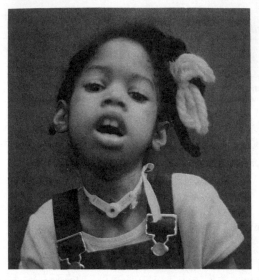

Figure 14.6. Facial weakness in nemaline myopathy.

progressive disorder with death usually before the 2 yr. The electromyogram is bizarre with low-amplitude, short-duration potentials, profuse fibrillations, and many repetitive discharges. Biopsy shows disruption of muscle fibers distended with vacuoles that, on proper staining, prove to be glycogen deposits.

McArdle disease (19, 23) usually becomes manifest in the older child or young adult. Painful muscle cramps precipitated by exertion and accompanied by transient myoglobinuria are the main clinical symptoms. Muscle atrophy and contracture may eventually develop. On ischemic exercise test, there is no rise in blood lactate or pyruvate level and muscle biopsy shows excess glycogen.

Muscle disorders caused by abnormal lipid metabolism have been identified (14, 77). Carnitine palmityl transferase deficiency has been described in some patients who, particularly after periods of fasting, develop muscle weakness, cramps, and myoglobinuria. Recurrent episodes of hepatic and cerebral dysfunction resembling Reye syndrome (53) have been reported in some children with carnitine deficiency demonstrated in the muscle, serum, and liver.

Mitochondrial myopathies or encephalomyopathies involve disorders of electron transport chain resulting in severe neurological deficit and muscle weakness (58). The so-called MELAS syndrome occurs in childhood with periodic vomiting, seizures, and stroke-like episodes. Other disorders involving mitochondrial abnormality can occur in later childhood or adolescence. The reader is referred to the many excellent reviews on this subject (24, 87, 88).

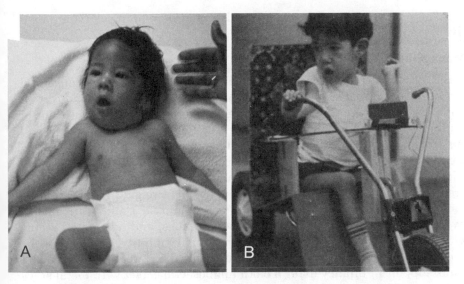

Figure 14.7. Myotubular myopathy. Floppy infant, myopathic facies.

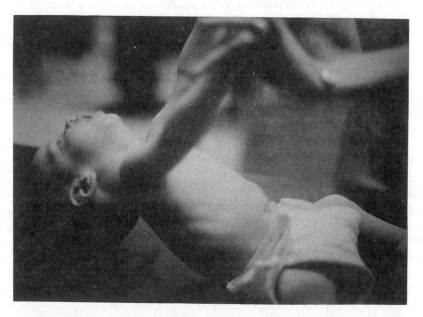

Figure 14.8. Marked hypotonia and weakness in Pompe's disease.

Inflammatory myopathies, polymyositis, and dermatomyositis are relatively common in children. These are discussed in Chapter 12.

Management

Because of the more favorable outcome for the child born with congenital or metabolic myopathies, with the exception of Pompe disease and certain mitochondrial myopathies, treatment can be more aggressive. Prevention of contractures by range of motion exercises, static splints, serial casting, and surgical release may be in order (26). Subluxation and frank hip dislocation are common particularly in the child with central core disease. Preventive adductor release or open hip reduction are sometimes necessary. Initially a prone-board or parapodium, and later long-leg lightweight braces will facilitate upright stance. The use of crawling devices and carts allow early mobility in prone and sitting. Walkers, proper crutches, and adequate bracing with instruction in ambulation can help upright mobility. Scoliosis of the spine should be anticipated in a child with generalized weakness. Adequate trunk support in infancy using a cloth lumbosacral corset with metal stays and a firm spinal orthosis during childhood may prevent rapid progression of scoliosis. The child with nemaline myopathy is particularly prone to respiratory complications. However, for all children with generalized weakness, a program of breathing exercises, postural drainage, and chest physical therapy must be instituted. The use of intermittent positive pressure apparatus in the form of night-time ventilators can allow some children to attend school all day without assistive ventilation. Because of delay in ambulation, some toddlers will need a stroller or other similar devices to provide postural support and easy transport. Wheelchair prescription must be individualized for the occasional child who does not attain ambulation.

DISORDERS OF NEUROMUSCULAR JUNCTION

Myasthenia gravis is a disorder characterized by intermittent weakness usually following sustained muscle activity, with improvement after rest. It is a major autoimmune disease that produces a defect in neuromuscular transmission secondary to many different pathophysiological etiologies (41, 46, 76, 98). There are several types in children: (a) transient neonatal myasthenia in an infant born to a myasthenic mother; (b) congenital or infantile myasthenia of a nonmyasthenic mother; and (c) juvenile myasthenia, which is akin to the adult form of myasthenia gravis. The infants of mothers with myasthenia sometimes will present as weak, lethargic babies who have a poor cry, poor sucking abilities, and respiratory difficulties. Prompt response to edrophonium (Tensilon) will confirm the diagnosis.

Congenital myasthenia gravis has been seen in children at 12 to 14 months of age. Ophthalmoplegia, facial and bulbar weakness may precede limb muscle weakness by many months (Fig. 14.9). Myasthenic crisis may be confused with acute respiratory distress associated with bronchopneumonia. The diagnosis is suspected clinically and confirmed pharmacologi-

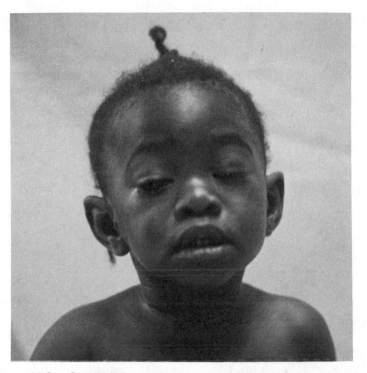

Figure 14.9. Congenital myasthenia gravis. Note facial weakness, ptosis.

cally with edrophonium (Tensilon) and repetitive nerve stimulation. Post-exercise facilitation and exhaustion are difficult to obtain in this age group. Stimulation of the facial nerve in a sedated infant, observing for decrement in the orbicularis oculi, may be more rewarding than stimulation of a limb nerve in the early stages of the disorder.

Muscle biopsy may show denervation atrophy, type II fiber atrophy, mild necrosis, lymphorrhages, and phagocytosis, but often it may be entirely normal. Treatment of this disorder is unpredictable and mostly unsatisfactory in the very young child. In older children, thymectomy, corticosteroids, and plasmapheresis are treatment options (45).

Other etiological agents that may cause problems at the neuromuscular junction include botulism, tick paralysis due to toxins liberated by several Dermacentor species, particularly the female pregnant tick, certain insecticides and crop sprays may induce loss of reflexes and paralysis (18). They represent problems for acute medical management and rarely lead to residual rehabilitation problems.

NEUROPATHIES

In considering childhood neuropathies, the clinician has to separate the acute affections that include traumatic, infectious, immunological, and toxic causes from the chronic disorders of hereditary motor sensory neuropathies (Tables 14.6 and 14.7). Among the acute traumatic lesions, facial and brachial plexus palsies are relatively more common and deserve special emphasis (40).

Facial palsy in a neonate usually follows a complicated delivery sometimes because of extended impingement of the baby's head against the maternal sacrum, or prolonged forceps applications, or secondary to intracranial bleeding. It must be differentiated from absence of the seventh nerve nucleus as in Möbius syndrome, visceral arch maldevelopment, or the more benign condition of hypoplasia of the depressor anguli oris muscle. The infant with true facial palsy is unable to wrinkle his or her forehead, close the eye on the affected side, or suck the nipple without dribbling. Electrodiagnostic studies can elucidate the severity and extent of damage. Most traumatic facial palsies clear spontaneously. In rare cases, reinnervation will occur over a 3- to 4-month period. Supportive management includes the use of methylcellulose drops, taping the affected eye, and massage of the face to prevent contractures and maintain tone.

The brachial plexus can be damaged during delivery when the infant's head is delivered and the shoulders are impinged in the birth canal. Traction of the cervical roots and nerves occurs when the neck is hyperextended. Severity of denervation in the affected extremity can be determined by electromyography. Treatment includes early and meticulous movement of the joints in the paralyzed limb. Use of supportive splints prevents flexion de-

Table 14.6.
Acute Neuropathies

1. *Traumatic*	Kanamycin
Facial Palsy	Gentamycin
Brachial plexus birth injury	Dilantin
Postinjection neuropathy	Penicillin
Sciatic	Apresoline
Radial	Isoniazid
Injury (radial, etc., fractures, etc.)	Furadantin
2. *Infections*	Vincristine
Lyme disease	Streptomycin
Diphtheria	b. *Heavy metals*
Herpes	Lead
Brachial neuritis	Arsenic
Guillain-Barré (?)	Mercury
3. *Allergic (?)*	c. *Insecticides*
Vaccination	DDT
Pertussis	Endrin
Tetanus	Aldrin
Rubella	Pentachlorophenol
Rabies	5. *Metabolic*
4. *Toxic*	Diabetes mellitus
a. *Drugs*	Hypothyroidism
Chloramphenicol	Chronic renal insufficiency

Table 14.7.
Hereditary Motor and Sensory Neuropathies

Type	Genetic	Clinical Findings	Edx	Pathology
MSN type I (Dominantly inherited hypertrophic neuropathy) Charcot-Marie-Tooth type	Autosomal dominant	Symptomatic 2–4 decades Weakness of small muscles of feet and peronei, later hands; enlarged peripheral nerves	Decreased motor and sensory nerve conduction velocities	Axonal atrophy, segmental demyelination and remyelination Onion bulb formation
MSN type II (Neuron type of peroneal muscular atrophy)	Autosomal dominant	Abnormal gait, pes cavus weakness of dorsiflexion and plantar flexion of ankles	Conduction velocities low normal EMG shows large motor unit potentials and fasciculations	Neuronal atrophy and degeneration milder peripheral changes
MSN type III (Hypertrophic neuropathy of infancy, Déjérine-Sottas)	Recessive	Onset in infancy; club feet kyphoscoliosis, generalized muscle weakness, worse distally; areflexia, sensory loss? ataxia; nystagmus	Decreased motor and sensory nerve conduction velocities	Demyelination ?Metabolic abnormality
MSN type IV (Refsum)	Recessive	Onset in childhood; thick nerves; severe sensory abnormality, skin icthyosis, deafness, retinitis	Slow motor and sensory NCV	
MSN type V (Spastic paraplegia)	Dominant	Onset in childhood Spastic paraparesis	Normal motor NCV Abnormal sensory NCV EMG shows large motor unit potentials fasciculations	
MSN type VI (with optic atrophy)	Rare—probably dominant	Peripheral limb weakness and optic atrophy and blindness		

formity of the wrist and dynamic extension splints help avert elbow flexion contracture. As reinnervation proceeds, active exercises are prescribed using equilibrium reactions and bilateral hand activities to assist the child in recognition of the affected extremity. Residual problems include scapular winging, loss of elbow supination, and loss of limb length even in the mild to moderate injuries (Fig. 14.10).

Among the neuropathies of infectious etiology, Guillain-Barré syndrome has been diagnosed as early as 6 months of age. A respiratory or gastrointestinal illness may precede or coincide with onset of polyneuritis. Distal paresthesias, pain, heaviness, and aching of arms and legs may precede overt weakness. Facial palsy can be the initial and only finding. In children, ascending paralysis involving distal limb muscles with gradual development of proximal weakness is not the usual picture. Children often have both proximal and distal involvement from the onset. Bulbar and respiratory paralysis and compromised central cardiac regulation may lead to a rapid demise. Etiology remains obscure, but viruses that have been associated with Guillain-Barré include varicella, herpes zoster, herpes simplex, coxsackie, Echo-6, and mumps. Recovery usually occurs quickly in young children but remyelination as determined by nerve conduction studies may continue for 4 to 5 yr. Nerve conduction studies may show initial proximal delay in terms of prolonged H or F latency determinations. Distal latency prolongation, temporal dispersion, may be visible by the second to third week of the disorder.

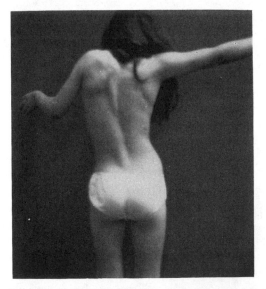

Figure 14.10. Left brachial plexus birth palsy. Underdevelopment of the extremity, scapular winging, and shoulder girdle weakness.

Significant weakness may exist and require long-term rehabilitation in Landry-Guillain-Barré syndrome. It involves proper bed position and range of motion exercises to prevent contractures and respiratory care if upper airway compromise is a problem. Some children have a great deal of pain and suspending them in a tepid whirlpool with gentle active assistive range of motion may be all that they will tolerate. As the disease becomes quiescent, graduated strengthening exercises are in order. Strenuous activities have been reported to cause transient decrease of strength and should be avoided in the early stage of recovery. The use of supportive splints and braces may be necessary as a temporary measure or for permanent residual weakness. Plasmapheresis has provided an aggressive and effective treatment regimen in certain patients who meet specific criteria for this intervention (28).

Metabolic causes of neuropathy, including those associated with thyroid dysfunction, are rare in children. However, the clinician should remember the possibility of diabetic neuropathy in the pediatric age group (96). Studies show that one third of the children affected with diabetes for 5 yr or longer have a peripheral neuropathy (39). Both segmental demyelination and axonal changes have been described.

Among heavy metals, lead poisoning is the most common but only occurs in long-standing poisoning. Children usually manifest central nervous system signs, gastrointestinal symptoms, and anemia before developing a peripheral neuropathy.

The most serious neuropathies in infancy are associated with white matter demyelinization affecting not only peripheral nerves but also the brain, as in Krabbe's disease, metachromatic leukodystrophy, or neuroaxonal dystrophy. In very young infants, pyridoxin deficiency may lead to peripheral neuropathy. Other vitamin B deficiencies can result in neuropathies but are rare in this country except for those associated with problems of gastrointestinal malabsorption.

The chronic hereditary familial neuropathies are seen in very young children, affecting both motor and sensory nerves. Dyck and associates (30, 57) devised a relatively sensible classification of these disorders (Table 14.7).

Hereditary motor sensory neuropathy-Type I, HMSN-type I, (Charcot-Marie-Tooth hereditary distal polyneuropathy) is relatively common in children and affects the distal limb nerves with weakness of the feet and hands and gradual progression over many years. It is usually transmitted as an autosomal dominant disorder. Children first manifest with flat feet and later develop pes cavus with high arch and claw toes. They are most susceptible to ankle sprains because of weak ankle musculature. The hands may be involved causing difficulties with fine motor function. Later, they develop a typical stork-leg appearance with very thin hypotrophic musculature in the lower extremities. Deep tendon reflexes are frequently diminished. There may be some loss of distal sensation.

Of particular importance is the concept that Charcot-Marie-Tooth disease is a spectrum of disorders and the neuropathy may be the peripheral component of more serious disorders involving the cerebellum and spinal cord, as in spinocerebellar degeneration. In a single kindred, one can see a child with only a peripheral neuropathy; the sibling may have peripheral neuropathy and spinal cord involvement, including loss of proprioception and vibration sense; yet another child in the family has the whole disorder in a full-blown picture with ataxia, loss of proprioception, as well as peripheral weakness (31).

Nerve conduction studies are diagnostic and show marked prolongation of distal latencies with diminution of the amplitude and temporal dispersion of the evoked potentials. There is increase in H and F latencies. Sural nerve biopsy shows reduction in the number of nerves on cross-section and onion bulb formation secondary to demyelination and remyelination. Muscle biopsy demonstrates type grouping with mild changes of denervation and reinnervation.

HMSN-type III or neuropathy of Déjèrine and Sottas is a sensory motor neuropathy that is present shortly after birth. The affected infants are late in development and delayed in walking with truncal ataxia and choreiform movements of the hands. They have markedly slow nerve conduction.

HMSN-type IV is a disorder affecting the peripheral nerves with cerebellar abnormalities. Symptoms include ataxia, nystagmus, retinal degeneration, sensorineural hearing loss, ichthyosis, and cardiac pathology. Dietary reduction in phytol seems to result in improvement.

There are many other hereditary neuropathies including those that affect primarily or exclusively the sensory nerves. These disorders are rare and their onset may vary from birth to late childhood (29). Neuropathies associated with mucopolysaccharidoses have also been described (47).

Management

An exercise program should be initiated to prevent contractures resulting from progressive weakness and muscle imbalance; to maintain a good postural alignment and ambulation. Simple lightweight plastic or leather shoe inserts support an early pes cavus, delay rapid development of intrinsic muscle contractures, and provide comfort on weight-bearing. A molded foot orthosis ensures mediolateral stability when varus or valgus attitude develops. Steppage gait can be controlled by polypropylene AFOs. A walkerette or crutches may be needed to assist in ambulation when the child is young or in case of more severe weakness. Scoliosis remains a serious problem in some hereditary neuropathies and surgical treatment is often indicated. The parents and child must be taught to use appropriate precautionary measures to avoid abrasions, excoriations, inadvertent burns, or other injuries when there is a sensory deficit. They should be instructed in meticulous foot care, including nail clipping. When weakness of the hands, particularly of the intrinsic muscles, makes fine motor tasks difficult, adaptive devices may prove helpful in buttoning, writing, cutting, and other similar daily activities. With the exception of cases with progressive ataxia or considerable diffuse weakness, most children retain independent mobility and self-care skills.

Conclusion

Neuromuscular diseases present a variety of symptoms and functional disabilities. Preventive, adaptive, and supportive methods of rehabilitation can assist children with these disorders in making the best possible adjustment to their handicap.

REFERENCES

1. Bach J, Alba A, Pilkington LA, Lee M: Long-term rehabilitation in advanced stage of childhood onset, rapidly progressive muscular dystrophy. *Arch Phys Med Rehabil* 63:328–331, 1981.
2. Bach JR, O'Brien J, Krotenberg R, Alba AS: Management of end stage respiratory failure in Duchenne muscular dystrophy. *Muscle Nerve* 10:177–82, 1987.
3. Banker BQ: Congenital deformities: Arthrogryposis multiplex congenita. Chapter 73. In Engel AG, Banker BQ (eds). *Myology*. New York, McGraw Hill Co. 1986, pp. 2109–2118.
4. Banker BQ: The congenital myopathies. Chapter 51. In Engel AG, Banker BQ (eds). *Myology*. New York, McGraw Hill Co. 1986, pp 1527–1581.
5. Barohn RJ, Levine EJ, Olson JO, Mendell JR: Gastric hypomotility in Duchenne's muscular dystrophy. *N Engl J Med* 7, 319:15–8, 1988.
6. Binder H: New Ideas in the Rehabilitation of Children with Spinal Muscular Atrophy. In Merlini L, Granata C, Dubowitz V (eds). *Current Concepts in Childhood Spinal Muscular Atrophy*. New York, Springer-Verlag Wien, 1989, pp. 117–125.
7. Botwin-Madorsky JG, Radford LM, Neumann, EM: Psychosocial aspects of death and dying in Duchenne muscular dystrophy. *Arch Phys Med Rehabil* 65:79–82, 1984.
8. Bouwsman G, Van Wijngaarden GK: Spinal muscular atrophy and hypertrophy of the calves. *J Neurol Sci* 44:275–279, 1980.
9. Bradley WG, Jones MZ, Mussine JM, Fawcett PRW: Becker type muscular dystrophy. *Muscle Nerve* 1:111–132, 1978.
10. Brooke MH: *A Clinician's View of Neuromuscular Diseases,* 2nd Ed. Baltimore, Williams & Wilkins, 1986.
11. Brooke MH, Fenichel GM, Griggs RC, Mendell JR, Moxley RT 3rd, Miller JP, Kaiser KK, Florence JM, Pandya S, Signore L, et al: Clinical investigation of Duchenne muscular dystrophy. Interesting results in a trial of prednisone. *Arch Neurol* 44:812–817, 1987.
12. Byrnes E, Blumberg PC, Hallpike JF: Central core disease. Study of a family with five affected generations. *J Neurol Sci* 53:77–83, 1982.
13. Cambridge W, Drennan JC: Scoliosis associated with Duchenne muscular dystrophy. *J Pediatr Orthop* 7:436–440, 1987.
14. Carroll JE: Myopathies caused by disorders of lipid metabolism. Review Article: 74 references. *Neurol Clin* 6:563–574, 1988.
15. Charash LI: Psychosocial, educational, and vocational considerations in neuromuscular disease—genetic overview. In Fowler WF Jr (ed). *Physical Medicine and Rehabilitation: State of the Art Reviews:* 2: No. 4, 626–630.
16. Colbert AP, Craig C: Scoliosis management in Duchenne muscular dystrophy: Prospective study of modified Jewett hyperextension brace. *Arch Phys Med Rehabil* 68(5 Ptl):302–304, 1987.

17. Cole CG, Coyne A, Hart KA, et al: Prenatal testing for Duchenne and Becker muscular dystrophy. *Lancet* 1:262–6, 1988.
18. Cornblath DR: Disorders of neuromuscular transmission in infants and children. *Muscle Nerve* 9:606–611, 1986.
19. Cornelio F, Bresolin N, DeMauro S, Mora M, Balestrini MR: Congenital myopathy due to phosphorylase deficiency. *Neurology* 33:1383, 1983.
20. Curran FJ: Night ventilation by body respirators for patients in chronic respiratory failure due to late stage Duchenne muscular dystrophy. *Arch Phys Med Rehabil* 62:270–274, 1981.
21. Denborough MA, Dennett X, Anderson R McD: Central-core disease and malignant hyperpyrexia. *Br Med J* 1:272, 1973.
22. DeSilva S, Drachman DB, Mellits D, Kuncl RW: Prednisone treatment in Duchenne muscular dystrophy. Long-term benefit. *Arch Neurol* 44:818–822, 1987.
23. DiMauro S, Bresolin N: Phosphorylase deficiency. Chapter 52. In Engel AG, Banker BQ (eds). *Myology*. New York, McGraw-Hill Co., 1986, pp 1585–1601.
24. DiMauro S, Zeviani M, Moraes CT, Nakase H, Rizzuto R, Lombes A, Shanske S, Schon EA: Mitochondrial encephalomyopathies. *Prog Clin Biol Res* 306:117–128, 1989.
25. D'Orsogna L, O'Shea JP, Miller G: Cardiomyopathy of Duchenne muscular dystrophy. *Pediatr Cardiol* 9:205–213, 1988.
26. Drennan JC: Orthopedic management of neuromuscular disorders. Philadelphia, JB Lippincott, 1983.
27. Dubowitz V: *Color Atlas of Muscle Disorders in Childhood*. Chicago, Year Book Publishers, Inc., 1989.
28. Dyck PJ: Acute inflammatory demyelinating polyradiculopathy. Diseases of peripheral nerves. Chapter 72. In Engel AG, Banker BQ (eds). *Myology*. New York, McGraw-Hill Co., 1986, pp. 2092–2094.
29. Dyck PJ: Diseases of peripheral nerves. Chapter 72. In Engel AG, Banker BQ (eds). *Myology*. New York, McGraw-Hill, 1986, pp. 2069–2108.
30. Dyck PJ: Inherited neuronal degeneration and atrophy affecting peripheral motor, sensory and autonomic neurons. In Dyck PT, Thomas PK, Lambert EH, Bunge RP (eds). *Peripheral Neuropathy*. Philadelphia, WB Saunders, 1984, p. 1600.
31. Dyck PJ, Ott J, Moore SB, Swanson CJ, Lambert EH: Linkage evidence for genetic heterogeneity among kinships with Hereditary Motor and Sensory Neuropathy Type I. *Mayo Clin Proc* 58:430–435, 1983.
32. Edstrom L, Wroblenski R, Mair WGP: Genuine myotubular myopathy. *Muscle Nerve* 5:604, 1982.
33. Eng GD: Psychosocial issues in the treatment of children with muscular dystrophy. In Heller BW, Flohr LM, Zegans LS (eds). *Psychosocial Interventions with Physically Disabled Persons*. New Brunswick, NJ, Rutgers University Press, 1989, pp. 108–116.
34. Eng GD: Rehabilitation of the child with a severe form of Spinal Muscular Atrophy. In Merlini L, Granata C, Dubowitz V (eds). *Current Concepts in Childhood Spinal Muscular Atrophy*. New York, Springer-Verlag Wien, 1989.
35. Eng GD: Spinal muscular atrophy. Anticipatory rehabilitation based on the natural course of the disease. In Merlini L, Granata C, Dubowitz V (eds). *Current Concepts in Childhood Spinal Muscular Atrophy*. New York, Springer-Verlag Wien, 1989.
36. Eng GD, Binder H: Rehabilitation of infants and children with neuromuscular disorders. *Pediatr Ann* 12:745–754, 1988.
37. Eng G, Binder H, Koch B: Spinal muscular atrophy: Experience in diagnosis and rehabilitation management of 60 patients. *Arch Phys Med Rehabil* 65:549–553, 1984.
38. Eng GD, Epstein BS, Engel WK, McKay DW, McKay R: Malignant hyperthermia and central core disease in a child with congenital dislocating hips. *Arch Neurol* 35:189–197, 1978.
39. Eng, GD, Hung W, August GP, Smokvina MD: Nerve conduction velocity determinations

in juvenile diabetes: Continuing study of 190 patients. *Arch Phys Med Rehabil* 57:1–5, 1976.

40. Eng GD, Koch B, Smokvina M: Brachial plexus palsy in neonates and children. *Arch Phys Med Rehabil* 59:458–464, 1978.
41. Engel AG: Congenital myasthenia syndrome. *J Child Neurol* 3:233–246, 1988.
42. Engel AG: Infantile acid maltase deficiency. Chapter 55. In Engel AG, Banker BQ (eds). *Myology*. New York, McGraw-Hill, 1986, p. 132.
43. Engel AG: Paramyotonia congenita. Chapter 64. In Engel AG, Banker BQ (eds). *Myology*. New York, McGraw-Hill, 1986, pp. 1848–1849.
44. Engel AG: The muscle biopsy. Part 2. In Engel AG, Banker BQ (eds). *Myology*. New York, McGraw-Hill, 1986, pp. 30, 833.
45. Engel AG: Therapy in acquired autoimmune myasthenia gravis. Chapter 67. In Engel AG, Banker BQ (eds). *Myology*. New York, McGraw-Hill, 1986, pp. 1944–1947.
46. Engel AG, Lambert EH, Mulder DM, et al: A newly recognized congenital myasthenia syndrome attributed to a prolonged open time of the acetylcholine-induced ion channel. *Am Neurol* 11:553, 1982.
47. Fowler GW: Neuropathy in mucopolysaccharidosis type 3. Electromyography. *Clin Neurophysiol* 14:29–34, 1974.
48. Fowler WM Jr: Medical rehabilitation of persons with muscular dystrophy and other neuromuscular disorders. *Rehabilitation Research Review Series*. The Catholic University of America, DATA Institute, 1985.
49. Fowler WM Jr: Rehabilitation management of muscular dystrophy and related disorders: II. Comprehensive care. *Arch Phys Med Rehabil* 63:322–328, 1982.
50. Fowler WM Jr, Goodgold J: Rehabilitation management of neuromuscular diseases. In Goodgold J (ed). *Rehabilitation Medicine*. St. Louis, CV Mosby Co, 1988, pp. 278–316.
51. Fowler WM Jr, Taylor M: Rehabilitation management of muscular dystrophy and related disorders: 1. The role of exercise. *Arch Phys Med Rehabil* 63:319–321, 1982.
52. Fukuyama Y, Osaw M, Suzuki H: Congential muscular dystrophy of the Fukuyama type—clinical, genetic and pathological considerations. *Brain Dev* 3:1–29, 1981.
53. Glascow AM, Eng G, Engel AG: Systemic carnitine deficiency simulating recurrent Reye syndrome. *J Pediatr* 96:889–891, 1980.
54. Gomez MR: Motor Neuron Diseases in Children. Chapter 69. In Engel AG, Banker BQ (eds). *Myology*. New York, McGraw-Hill, 1986, pp. 1993–2012.
55. Granata C, Cornelio F, Bonfiglioli S, Mattutini P, Merlini L: Promotion of ambulation of patients with spinal muscular atrophy by early fitting of knee-ankle-foot orthoses. *Dev Med Child Neurol* 29:221–224, 1987.
56. Hackmatt JZ, Dubowitz V: Ultrasound imaging and directed needle biopsy in the diagnosis of selective involvement in muscle disease. *J Child Neurol* 3:205–213, 1987.
57. Harding A: Inherited neuronal atrophy and degeneration of lower motor neurons. In Dyck PJ, Thomas PK, Lambert EH, Bunge RP (eds). *Peripheral Neuropathy*. Philadelphia, WB Saunders, 1984, pp. 1537–1556.
58. Harding AE, Holt IJ: Mitochondrial myopathies. Review Article: 21 references. *Prog Clin Biol Res* 306:117–128, 1989.
59. Harding AE, Thomas PK: Hereditary distal spinal muscular atrophy—A report of 34 cases and a review of the literature. *J Neurol Sci* 45:337–348, 1980.
60. Harper PS: Myotonic dystrophy. In Emery AEH, Rimoin DL (eds). *Principles and Practice of Medical Genetics*. Edinburgh, Churchill-Livingstone, 1983.
61. Hausmanowa-Petrusewicz I, Fidzianska A, Niebroj-Dobosz I, Strugalska H: Is Kugelberg-Welander SMA a fetal defect? *Muscle Nerve* 3:389–402, 1980.
62. Hausmanowa-Petrusewicz I, Karwanska A: Electromyographic findings in different forms of infantile and juvenile proximal spinal muscular atrophy. *Muscle Nerve* 9:37, 1986.
63. Hoffman EP, Fischbeck KH, Brown RH, Johnson M, Medori R, Loike JD, Harris JB,

Waterston R, Brooke M, Specht L, et al: Characterization of dystrophin in muscle-biopsy specimens from patients with Duchenne's or Becker's muscular dystrophy. *N Engl J Med* 318:1363–1368, 1988.

64. Hoffman EP, Kunkel LM, Angelini C, et al: Improved diagnosis of Becker muscular dystrophy by dystrophin testing. *Neurology* 39:1011–1017, 1989.

65. Karagan NJ, Richman LC, Sorenson JP: Analysis of verbal disability in Duchenne muscular dystrophy. *J Nerve Ment Dis* 168:419–423, 1980.

66. Karpati G: Principles and practices of myoblast transfer. *J Neurol Sci* 98: Suppl 33, 1990.

67. Kingston HM, Harper PS, Pearson PL, Davies KE, Williamson R, Page D: Localization of the gene for Becker muscular dystrophy. *Lancet* 2:1200, 1983.

68. Kugelberg E, Welander F: Heredofamilial juvenile muscular atrophy simulating muscular dystrophy. *Arch Neurol Psychiatry* 75:500–509, 1956.

69. Law PK, Fang Q, et al: First clinical trial of myoblast transfer therapy. *J Neurol Sci* 98:Suppl 32, 1990.

70. Leibowitz D, Dubowitz V: Intellect and behavior in Duchenne muscular dystrophy. *Dev Med Child Neurol* 23:577–590, 1981.

71. Leon SH: Schuffler MD, Kettler, Rohrmann CA: Chronic intestinal pseudoobstruction as a complication of Duchenne's muscular dystrophy. *Gastroenterology* 90:455–459, 1986.

72. McMenamin JB, Becker LE, Murphy EG: Congenital muscular dystrophy: A clinical pathologic report of 24 cases. *J Pediatr* 100:692, 1982.

73. Merlini L, Granata C, Bonfiglioli S, Marini ML, Carvellati, Savini R: Scoliosis in spinal muscular atrophy: Natural history and management. *Dev Med Child Neurol* 31:501, 1989.

74. Miller JR, Colbert AP, Schock NC: Ventilator use in progressive neuromuscular disease: Impact on patients and their families. *Dev Med Child Neurol* 30:200–207, 1989.

75. Monaco AP, Berelson CJ, Middlesworth W, Colletti C, Aldridge J, Fischbeck KH, Bartlett R, Pericok-Vance M, Roses AD, Kunkel LM: Detection of deletions spanning the Duchenne muscular dystrophy locus using a tightly linked DNA segment. *Nature* 316:842–845, 1985.

76. Mora M, Lambert EH, Engel AG: Synaptic vesicle abnormality in familial infantile myasthenia (FIM). *Neurology* 35(Suppl 1):100, 1985.

77. Munsat TL: Review of neuromuscular diseases. In *Physical Medicine & Rehabilitation: State of the Art Reviews* 2,4. Philadelphia, Hanly & Belfus, Inc., 1988, pp. 467–479.

78. Noble-Jamieson CM, Heckmatt JC, Dubowitz V, Silverman M: Effects of posture and spinal bracing on respiratory function in neuromuscular disease. *Arch Dis Child* 61:178–181, 1986.

79. Nonaka I, Sugita H, Takada K, Kumagai K: Muscle histochemistry in congenital muscular dystrophy with central nervous system involvement. *Muscle Nerve* 5:102–106, 1982.

80. Norton P, Ellison P, Sulaiman AR, Hart J: Nemaline myopathy in the neonate. *Neurology* 33:351, 1983.

81. Pearn J: Classification of spinal muscular atrophies. *Lancet* 1:919–922, 1980.

82. Pearn JH, Gardner-Medwin D, Wilson J: A clinical study of chronic childhood spinal muscular atrophy. *J Neurol Sci* 38:23–37, 1978.

83. Perloff JK: Cardiac rhythm and conduction in Duchenne's muscular dystrophy: A prospective study of 20 patients. *J Am Coll Cardiol* 3:1263–1268, 1984.

84. Rideau Y, Glorion B, Delaubier A, Torle O, Bach J: The treatment of scoliosis in Duchenne muscular dystrophy. *Muscle Nerve* 7:281–286, 1984.

85. Russman BS, Melchreitt R, Drennan JC: Spinal muscular atrophy: The natural course of the disease. *Muscle Nerve* 6:179–181, 1983.

86. Sarnst HB, O'Connor T, Byrne PA: Clinical effects of myotonic dystrophy on pregnancy and the neonate. *Arch Neurol* 33:459–488, 1976.

87. Schapira AH: Mitochondrial myopathies. Comment. *BMJ* 298:1644–1645, 1989.

88. Schapira AH: Mitochondrial myopathies. Review article. *BMJ* 298:1127–1128, 1989.

89. Shy AM, Engel WK, Somer JE, Wanko T: Nemaline myopathy. A new congenital myopathy. *Brain* 86:793, 1963.
90. Shy AM, Magee KR: A new congenital non-progressive myopathy. *Brain* 79:610, 1956.
91. Siegel IM: Spinal stabilization in Duchenne muscular dystrophy: Rationale and method. *Muscle Nerve* p. 417,1982.
92. Smith AD, Koreska J, Mosely CF: Progression of scoliosis in Duchenne muscular dystrophy. *J Bone Joint Surg* [Am] 71:1066–1074, 1989.
93. Splaingard ML, Frates RC, Jefferson LS, et al: Home negative pressure ventilation: Report on 20 years of experience in patients with neuromuscular disease. *Arch Phys Med Rehabil* 66:239–242, 1985.
94. Steadman H, Sarkar S: Molecular genetics in muscular dystrophy research: Revolutionary progress. *Muscle Nerve* 11:683–693, 1988.
95. Swank SM, Brown JC, Perry RE: Spinal fusion in Duchenne's muscular dystrophy. *Spine* 7:484, 1982.
96. Thomas PK, Eliasson SG: Diabetic neuropathy. In Dyck PJ, Thomas PK, Lambert EH, Bunge RP (eds). *Peripheral Neuropathy*. Philadelphia, WB Saunders, 1984, pp. 173–1810.
97. Vignos PJ Jr: Respiratory function and pulmonary infection in Duchenne muscular dystrophy. *Isr J Med Sci* 13:207–214, 1977.
98. Vincent A, Cull-Candy SG, Newsome-Davis J, et al: Congenital myasthenia: End-plate acetylcholine receptors and electrophysiology in five cases. *Muscle Nerve* 4:306, 1981.
99. Voit T, Lamprecht A, Lenard HG, Goebel HH: Hearing loss in facioscapulohumeral dystrophy. *Eur J Pediatr* 145:280–285, 1986.
100. Walton JN, Gardner-Medwin D: Progressive muscular dystrophy and the myotonic disorders. In Walton JN (ed). *Disorders of Voluntary Muscle*, ed 5. Edinburgh, Churchill Livingstone, 1988.
101. Whelan TB: Neuropsychological performance of children with Duchenne muscular dystrophy and spinal muscular atrophy. *Dev Med Child Neurol* 29:212–220, 1987.
102. Yotsukura M, Miyagawa M, Tsuya T, Ishihara T, Ishikawa K: Pulmonary hypertension in progressive muscular dystrophy of the Duchenne type. *Jpn Circ J* 52:321–326, 1988.

15

Limb Deficiencies in Children

YASOMA CHALLENOR

A youngster with limb deficiency must first be accepted and treated as a child and then, secondarily, as a child with a problem. Parents and clinicians on the therapeutic team must understand that the need for support, nurture, and discipline is the same for these youngsters as for all growing children. Limb deficiency in children represents a marked difference from the usual experience in the adult amputee clinic. Incidence, etiology, prescription, and therapy pose a range of concerns for management that are at variance with problems of adult amputees.

Incidence and Etiology

It has been estimated that 11% to 13% of new amputees are under 21 yr of age, while approximately 5% are under age 11 yr (13, 31). The usual pediatric amputee clinic deals with children under age 15 yr, of whom 50% to 57% have congenital limb deficiency and an additional 10% have anomalies either treated as or resulting in amputation (1, 30, 35). The population with congenital limb loss represents upper extremity loss in 62% of cases: 42%, unilateral upper limb; 27%, unilateral lower limb; and 24%, multiple limb deficiencies (35).

Congenital limb deficiencies are often related to intrauterine maldevelopment during the first 2 months of pregnancy (6, 23). Although limb malformations have been described in a number of genetic syndromes (12, 23, 33), familial occurrence is rare. In addition to the well-documented effect of thalidomide (48, 60), contraceptives (20, 27, 30, 42) and maternal diabetes (67) have also been implicated, as have other drugs suspected to be teratogenic agents (33). Partial limb absence has also been associated with certain autosomal genetic disorders, such as Holt-Oram and Fanconi syndromes, and trisomies 13 and 18 (23, 48). Disseminated intravascular coagulopathy secondary to meningococcemia may also cause limb loss (Fig. 15.1), often in

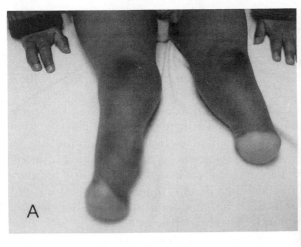
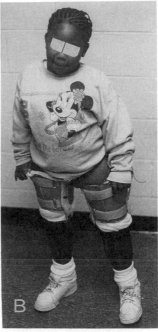

Figure 15.1A, This 6-yr-old has lost both legs below the knees, as well as some digits of the right hand due to disseminated intravascular coagulopathy associated with meningococcemia.
B, Epiphyseal distortion, common in disseminated intravascular coagulopathy, has made tibial osteotomies necessary to achieve adequate limb alignment for prosthetic fitting.

association with superficial skin necrosis, which makes prosthetic management particularly difficult (9, 41).

Trauma is a surprisingly frequent cause of amputation in children; approximately 70% of acquired childhood amputations are related to vehicular accidents and farm equipment mishaps, farm power tool injuries, explosions from firecrackers or homemade bombs, chemical experimentation, and gunshot wounds related to hunting accidents and other missilery mishaps.

Railroad, household, and thermal or electrical injuries account for the remainder of traumatic amputations. There is also a small percentage resulting from recreational activities, playground equipment, and falling from heights. Of all acquired pediatric amputations, 30% are caused by disease or neoplasm (21, 28).

Classification

The International Society of Prosthetics and Orthotics has recently entertained a new classification, which has much merit and will be outlined subsequently. However, there are several classification systems worthy of review, not only because they are still in clinical use, but also because they are frequently found in prosthetic literature. One frequently used system of delineation of amputations follows standard terminology for traumatic injuries: above or below the specific joint in question. Thus, above or below elbow and above or below knee localizations are used. Additionally, several classifications exist for congenitally acquired limb deficiencies. Complete absence of one or more limbs, amelia, is distinguished in one classification from those involving partial absence: meromelia. In the more comprehensive Frantz and O'Rahilly systems (8, 20), deficiencies are subdivided into *terminal* representing complete loss of the distal end of an extremity, or *intercalary,* denoting absence of intermediate parts with preserved proximal and distal components of the limb. Both terminal and intercalary deficiencies can be divided into horizontal or longitudinal deficits.

One often finds mixtures of the older terminology with the newer one, striving for both brevity and accuracy of description. For instance, radial aplasia, radial meromelia, or intercalary longitudinal radial deficit are different descriptions of the same deficiency (34). In an alternate classification (57, 58), common clinical entities of limb deficiency are described by groupings according to limb segments primarily affected by embryological failures of development. The missing parts are named; any osseous part not named is understood to be intact.

In 1988, a most comprehensive classification was proposed to the International Society for Prosthetics and Orthotics (15, 16). Descriptions are based on anatomical level and characterized as transverse or longitudinal and total or partial. According to this system, an above-knee amputation would be a transverse thigh deficiency (upper, middle, or lower third). A radial aplasia would be a longitudinal total radial deficiency. A fibular dysgenesis would be a longitudinal partial fibular deficiency. If, in addition, toes were missing, one would add: tarsus partial rays IV and V. A phocomelia would be a transverse total deficiency of the humerus, radius, and ulna. With this specificity or terminology, with its logical anatomical basis, discrepancies in terminology of complex deficits would be minimized. This could conceivably lead to more accurate statistics as to the incidence of specific combinations of deficits.

Principles of Management

The concept of preservation of residual limb length applies both to congenital and acquired problems, but with different long-range goals. In general, one aims to preserve epiphyses in order to allow maximal limb growth. However, in congenital limb deficiency, it is an added factor that the preservation of phocomelic digits or appendages allows switch control of externally powered prostheses or digital tactile exploration and sensory feedback.

As the child grows, there may be many factors modifying this general principle, as will be illustrated subsequently.

PARENTAL SUPPORT

The parent of a child with congenital limb deficiency is faced with an abrupt and unfortunate contrast between the perfect infant they had visualized and expected and the child who actually exists with a limb deficiency. The parents must be supported and helped in dealing with the infant *as an infant* and seeing the limb deficiency as a handicap, but one for which future compensations do exist. They must see the infant as a child with all the needs and growth requirements of the normal infant to whom they must relate as parents. They must realize that the child can be an intact personality who incidentally happens to have a limb deficiency and that independence commensurate with age and compatible with the level of limb deficiency must be fostered.

The parents need support for dealing with feelings of self-recrimination, indignation, remorse, or anger during the period of adjustment to having a child who is born with a defective limb or has lost an extremity. It may require considerable time until they are able to develop a realistic and practical attitude about the child's functional outlook.

Initially this support will most likely come from the physician, psychologist, or social worker on the prosthetic team. Early questions may relate to the child's future function, so that possible prosthetic options should be presented to the parents when they are amenable to hearing and absorbing this information. The parents should have an opportunity to see other children use their prostheses and function psychologically and socially. As their ability to deal with questions increases, more details of future prosthetic options and/or surgical requirements can be amplified. Sharing of feelings and discussions of the child's future need not occur solely with the professional members of the prosthetic team. A parent support group may be better accepted by some families or it may be a valuable supplement to professional counseling (2, 43, 53, 55)

There is no way of predicting in advance whether parents will accept or reject the idea of a prosthesis for their infant because their reactions are influenced by their own prior experience and/or prejudices about children with handicaps. However, the warm supportive and understanding attention of the rehabilitation team should help to provide and to preserve all possible prosthetic and functional options for the child in the future. The current trend of early prosthetic fitting is consistent with this aim, but also allows youngsters with minimal or unilateral deficits to make their own decisions at a later age as to whether or not they wish to continue using a prosthesis on the basis of functional and psychological considerations. Until that time, the parents must understand what prosthetic and/or surgical possibilities exist so that they can participate in making reasonable decisions about the child's management together with the team (14, 17). It is part of the course of preprosthetic training to demonstrate to parents the types of prosthetic designs and terminal devices that are available for children of different ages. Probably the most variability in parental choice exists in terms of the initial passive prosthetic terminal device for upper extremity amputees. Whether they elect one that looks definitely artificial or prefer a perhaps less functional but more cosmetic design is not always predictable. However, the parents should be made familiar gradually and gently with the range of devices, as well as the advantages and disadvantages of each, so that they are constructive participants in the selection process. On occasion, interchangeable options may be the preferred compromise between function and cosmesis. This is certainly true as the child grows older.

MANAGEMENT OF UPPER LIMB DEFICIENCY

The occupational therapist naturally tends to be primarily involved in the management of children with upper extremity limb deficiency. Preprosthetic training begins with introducing the limb remnant to different textures and shapes for tactile awareness and input as well as to encourage exploration of the environment with the residual limb (Figs. 15.2 and 15.3).

As the child becomes older, games that require those proximal limb motions that will later be used in prosthetic operation are incorporated into cause and effect games (25) (Fig. 15.4). Many of these activities also contribute to increasing trunk control and equilibrium reactions, since balance and stabilization of the torso are necessary to free the residual upper extremity for operation of the prosthesis at a later time (Fig. 15.5). The arms are used for many gross motor developmental tasks that come into play between the 3rd and 6th month, such as propping in prone position to elevate the trunk and holding objects between two hands, even if one or both hands are a passive prosthetic extension of the deficient upper extremity. After 6 months, the arms are needed for aid in achieving sitting. Because of the need for using the arms to attain successive developmental milestones, children with upper extremity limb deficiency should receive a passive prosthesis between 3 to 4 months of age (65).

Through consistent early use, the prosthetic limb extension becomes incorporated into the developing body image and is viewed by the infants as part of their own extremity. Early prosthetic fitting tends to correlate well with continued prosthetic use throughout childhood (37, 46). Increasing use of the prosthesis for developmental tasks encourages parental acceptance of the prosthesis (44). Early fitting enhances natural development of the necessary eye-prosthetic-hand coordination and control. In unilateral upper limb deficiency, bimanual function decreases trunk and shoulder girdle asymmetry and alleviates muscle and bone hypotrophy of disuse. Inefficient means of handling objects between the axilla and humerus or between

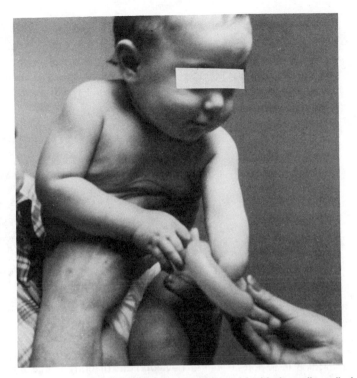

Figure 15.2. This 5-month-old infant is using his residual below-elbow limb to assist the intact right arm for exploration of toys and manipulation of toys between both limbs. At this stage, a prosthesis should begin to extend his grasp and to be of demonstrable use to him in manipulating large objects or two-handed toys.

shoulder and chin are discouraged, as is dental damage from using the mouth as a second hand. Postural and balance training is extremely important in bilateral upper limb deficiency. In the absence of protective arm extension, equilibrium must be maintained by substituting trunk movements and by tone readjustment around the hips and other lower extremity joints for weight shifting (59) (Figs. 15.6 and 15.7).

While the initial prosthesis may have a padded passive mitt, it is helpful to have a passive thumb in which objects can be placed by the parents to encourage visual exploration. As the child becomes older, one may then think of adding an active control to the terminal device that can be manipulated by the youngster. The selection of terminal devices is described in the timetable of fitting (Table 15.1). In general, a prosthesis with a self-activated terminal device is provided between 14 and 18 months of age. Shortly thereafter, actual training in active use of the terminal devices is introduced. It has been suggested that developmental signs of readiness for learning the operation of a cable-controlled terminal device are: (*a*) an attention span of

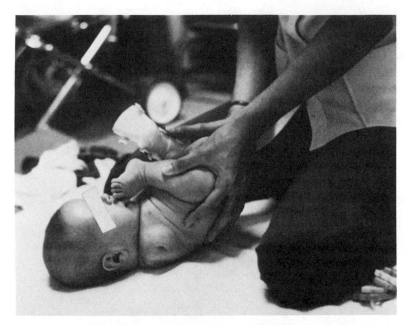

Figure 15.3.   Patients with amelia may miss the stage of tactile exploration of reaching from hands to feet and then secondarily getting hands and feet to the mouth. Yet, tactile and oral exploration is important in the development of body image and must be assisted.

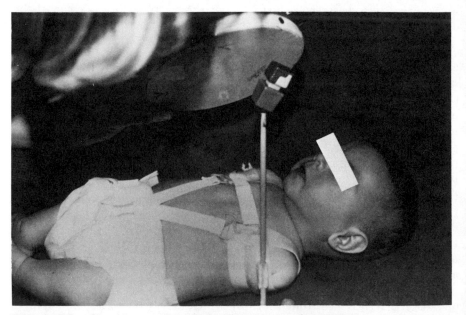

Figure 15.4.   Shoulder muscles which will later be used to operate a prosthesis can be encouraged to develop mobility and controlled quite early at the same time that the infant is learning cause and effect concepts. Photograph courtesy of Challenor Y: In Downey JA, Low NL (eds). *The Child with Disabling Illness.* New York, Raven Press, 1982.

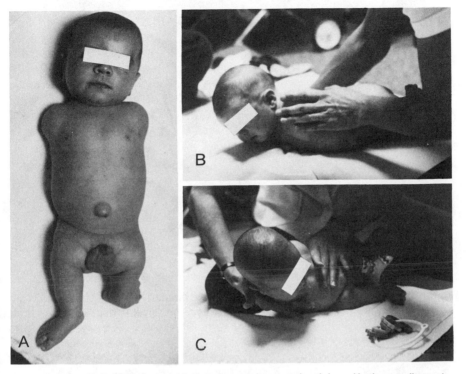

Figure 15.5. Head righting and forward propping may be delayed in the amelic or phocomelic child and must be encouraged with suitable positioning and encouragement of active motion.

at least 10 minutes; (*b*) ability to follow a two-step direction; (*c*) interest in two-handed activities; and (*d*) ability to perform the control motion. Implicit in these prerequisites is the willingness of the child to permit handling by the therapist and awareness of the function of the terminal device once it has been demonstrated (11, 48, 61, 63).

The rapport between the therapist and child during the preprosthetic training period is put to constructive use in the actual prosthetic fitting and training. Parents are encouraged to participate in training sessions since their carryover of similar activities at home is an integral part of the prosthetic management program. It is important that training in the use of the terminal device begin early, before the child develops an overwhelming motivation for gross motor activities, especially before learning to run well, so that interest in the manual dexterity phase of development is maintained.

A standard upper limb prosthesis for a below-elbow amputee comprises a socket fitted to the residual limb and a terminal device substituting for a hand. The socket is held in place by a canvas-webbing harness that loops around the contralateral axilla. A small cable connected to the terminal

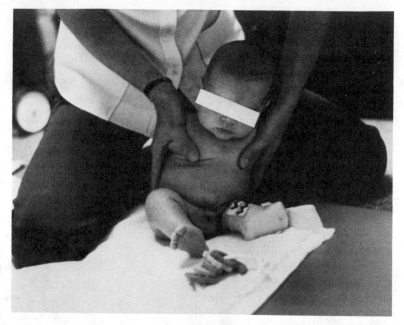

Figure 15.6. Use of truncal muscles is guided and gradually encouraged as the infant grows to the point where he maintains the sitting position independently.

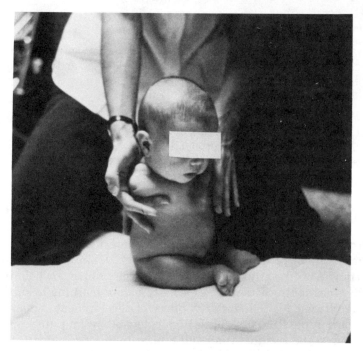

Figure 15.7. Independent sitting expands the infant's range of visual exploration. Using momentum to come independently to a sitting position usually develops at about 2-yr of age when the patient can understand and follow one- and two-stage commands.

Table 15.1.
Timetable of Fitting

Age	Terminal Device Choices (Partial List)	Wrist Units	Elbows
4–6 months	Dorrance 12P hook Passive Mit		CAPP[a] infant modular components with passively positioned elbow
6–12 months	10 AW Wafer Hosmer passive infant hand Dorrance 12P hook CAPP terminal device Centri passive hand		
12–30 months	CAPP terminal device Dorrance 10P hook Variety Village VV 0-3B Electromechanical hand Adept terminal device F III	CAPP adjustable rotation friction wrist	CAPP modular elbow with 4 position lock
3–6 yr	CAPP terminal device Systemteknik electric hand Variety Village VV2-6B Dorrance 10P hook Steeper Electric hand Electromechanical hand Adept terminal device C II	Wrist flexion unit Quick disconnect wrist unit for interchangeable terminal devices	CAPP modular elbow (manually adjustable) OCCC[b] electric elbow

Table 15.1.—*Continued*

Age	Terminal Device Choices (Partial List)	Wrist Units	Elbows
6–8 yr	CAPP terminal device Dorrance 99X hook Dorrance 100 & 101 hand Otto Bock hand Systemteknik hand Steeper electric hand VV5-9B Electromechanical hand		CAPP modular elbow NYU[c] motor lock elbow Variety Village Electric Elbow
8–11 yr	Dorrance 88X Hand Hosmer/Dorrance DH-200 or 201 hand Variety Village 105 hand Greifer terminal device Adept terminal device B 1		CAPP modular elbow Boston electric elbow
11 to adolescent	Dorrance 88X hook Dorrance 99X hook Dorrance 200 or 201 hand Variety Village 107, 109 hands CAPP terminal device size 2 Greifer terminal device		NYU motor lock elbow

[a]CAPP, Child Amputee Prosthetics Project, UCLA, CA.
[b]OCCC, Ontario Crippled Children's Center.
[c]NYU, New York University.

device runs along the socket and attaches to the proximal part of the suspension. Humeral flexion causes tension on the cable and opens the terminal device. On relaxation, strong elastic bands around the terminal device produce closure.

Above-elbow prostheses may have a prosthetic elbow joint that is activated by a second cable. Humeral flexion for this prosthesis initiates elbow flexion, after which shoulder depression locks the elbow in the flexed position desired. Once the elbow is locked, humeral flexion can activate the terminal device. The elbow is unlocked by humeral extension. Both the prosthetic wrist and elbow joints can incorporate rotation. It is accomplished passively by the uninvolved hand and facilitates approaching objects of varied shapes from different positions.

A usual sequence of events in teaching the operation of a prosthetic hook is: (a) maintain hook opening; (b) initiate hook opening for grasp; (c) relax and close hook; and (d) open hook for release (49). Refinement in the use of prosthetic terminal device generally occurs between 2 and 3 yr of age. The child learns to adapt the extent of opening to different sized objects, to place objects appropriately in the terminal device, to preposition it, and to control its opening and release while holding the prosthetic arm in different positions relative to the trunk. Active control of the prosthesis and terminal device is practiced in age-appropriate play activities and by manipulation of toys in order to maintain the child's interest and motivation.

As mentioned previously, the parents play an integral part in the training program. Their acceptance of the prosthesis and encouragement of its wear and use throughout the day and even in a preschool program is essential. Initially, the child is shown the functional use of the prosthesis through play, with the expectation that more spontaneous use will follow. For the unilateral amputee, this predominantly involves bimanual activities. For the bilateral proximal upper extremity amputee, the choice is between using prostheses or the lower extremities. There may be times in the child's life when the prostheses are not available because of needed repairs or when the need for tactile feedback makes the child elect to use the lower extremities for manipulative activities. Thus, part of the preprosthetic and prosthetic training for the child with bilateral upper extremity deficiency is the maintenance of hypermobility at all joints of the lower limbs and the ability to use the toes for manipulation (4, 24).

Between 3 and 4 yr of age, prosthetic elbow control is added and the child begins to learn the motions to activate elbow flexion and to lock the elbow in a desired position (50). Prior to the introduction of active control, an elbow with prelocked, passively set positions is used. The recent development of electrically powered prosthetic components is most often applicable to children who have a proximal amputation, such as shoulder disarticulation. In this type of problem, shoulder elevation or use of a phocomelic digit may activate the electrically driven terminal device. In general, this is much less energy consuming and is learned quite easily by children. At the present time, the weight of electrically powered elbow units makes it less desirable for the very young child, but remains as an option for elbow control when the child is older.

Recently, there has been a trend in some countries to use myoelectrically controlled prostheses, even for distal amputations, for example, below the elbow (52, 53). Children have been fitted with this type of prosthesis as early as 3 yr of age. They generally learn activation of the myoelectric control by having electrodes positioned over the appropriate muscle for opening and closing a remote prosthetic hand in order to grasp or release an object. Once they can reliably control the remote unit, they are then fitted with their own motor-driven hand. Learning is usually natural and rapid, since muscles utilized for prosthetic hand opening and closing are the same as those used for an intact hand. Advantages of the myoelectric hand include cosmesis and the lack of suspension harness and cables necessary for the standard prosthesis. Disadvantages of any fairly complex electrical device relate to the frequency of repairs necessary.

The development of myoelectrically controlled prostheses for children may bring into question many of the traditional features of standard prosthetic use that we have considered acceptable in the past. For example, in viewing the motion picture of a child who initially was fitted with a standard below-elbow cable-control prosthesis and, subsequently, with a myoelectric prosthesis, a marked contrast is noted. With the standard prosthesis, the youngster has excellent use of humeral flexion and, particularly, scapular abduction for control of the prosthesis. Occasionally, in some positions, trunk motion is used to supplement scapular abduction. Within the first day or two after the myoelectric prosthesis is provided, the youngster quickly learns to operate it, but body motions that were used for controlling the cable device are still apparent. Now that these movements serve no functional purpose, their somewhat odd and unphysiological nature is suddenly revealed. With a standard prosthesis, these body motions would be considered excellent prosthetic use and, therefore, worthy of praise. Without the context of the standard prosthesis, the quite unusual nature of these body movements becomes evident. Although the youngsters are able to discard these previously learned motions within a few days, one is left with the perception that what we view with a professional eye as normal function of a cable-activated prosthesis user may be somewhat bizarre to nonprofessional eyes or to peers. Thus, one of the perhaps hidden advantages of early myoelectric prosthetic fitting is the natural appearance of the child during prosthetic use. Acceptance of the myoelectric prosthesis is roughly equivalent to that of the cable-driven prosthesis and may be somewhat more acceptable to the bilaterally upper limb-deficient child (22, 36, 54, 66).

MANAGEMENT OF LOWER EXTREMITY DEFICIENCY

Gross motor activities, the province of the physical therapist, are applied in preprosthetic as well as prosthetic training (29). Postural training is crucial, particularly for children who have unilateral or unequal limb deficiency, discrepancies in leg length, asymmetry or muscle development, and habitual or compensatory postures that encourage uneven body alignment. It is important to preserve motion in the residual limb and to encourage development of muscle strength in both residual and intact limbs for functional compensations. As the child begins to sit, an equal length of the lower extremities gains increasing importance for attaining balance. Symmetry of pelvic control and muscle development is also a reason for early fitting of lower extremity prostheses (32). Children should have a lower extremity device in place at least by the time they are achieving independent sitting balance and very definitely by the time they are ready to pull up to a standing position. In the erect position, weight shifting and balancing are practiced progressing to ambulation and gait training (26) for safety on indoor level surfaces and, later, outdoors, including irregular terrains and inclines. As motor control increases, more complex ambulatory skills are practiced, such as stair climbing, maneuvering in small spaces and around obstacles, changing direction, and varying the speed of walking to the extent permitted by the level of the amputation. Devices that are used by nonhandicapped children should be adapted to the youngster with limb deficiency for use with or without the prosthesis. Thus, a tricycle may have handlebar adaptations to compensate for short limbs or terminal devices or may have pedal adaptations to accommodate a prosthesis. Swimming is generally encouraged as an excellent form of mobility training and exercise (38). This may require adaptations for entering and exiting the pool and special safety devices (64) while, in other cases, a swimming prosthesis may be considered. Refinements in ambulation training should be introduced as early as the child's motor developmental level permits, rather than allowing establishment of ingrained poor gait habits, which may be much less amenable to therapy later.

FITTING TIMETABLE

Upper Extremity

The process of prosthetic fitting and selection of available designs represents a constant balance between proper size and weight of devices on the one hand, and motor skills, developmental abilities and expanding functional needs of the child on the other (Table 15.1). The range of initially applicable upper extremity terminal devices varies in respect to shape, capability to hold a passively inserted object, and overall appearance (45), (Fig. 15.8). The initial terminal device is most frequently a soft mitten-shaped hand into which objects can be passively placed between the thumb and

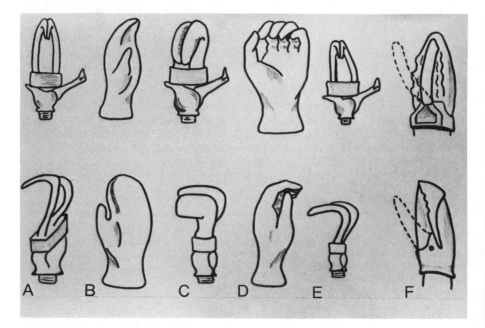

Figure 15.8. Terminal devices. *A*, pediatric 10× size (99× is somewhat larger, and adult size would be twice as large); *B*, molded mitten (passive); *C*, passive "wafer" device; *D*, Variety Village passive molded hand (101); *E*, plastisol-coated hook (12-P); *F*, CAPP device. Fitting schedules are detailed in Table 14.1.

"digits." The rounded, plastisol-coated contour of this mitt is probably safer for a child with imperfect upper extremity control than a hook would be. However, as the child begins more active visual and manual exploration of his or her environment, one may substitute a small plastisol-coated hook. The choice of devices for passive handling of object would then be among the hook, the passive molded hand, such as the Variety Village 101 hand, and the prehensile CAPP terminal device (10). Because the last device has a rel-atively large, rubber-lined, irregular prehensile surface, it offers the most adaptability for grasping and retaining objects of varying sizes and shapes (51, 56).

Growth accommodation is adjustable to a great degree with thin-walled, flexible thermoplastic sockets (for both upper and lower extremity prosthe-ses). These thermoplastic sockets (as contrasted with laminated plastic) are easily heat molded to adjust for comfort and have the added advantage of allowing some heat dissipation through the socket's thin wall (3, 18).

Lower Extremity

Lower limb deficiency, especially if above the knee, may somewhat delay independent achievement of sitting and/or encourage asymmetric sitting posture. The more proximal the limb deficiency, the more likely the delay or asymmetry. It is useful to have a lightweight extension of the limb in place by 6 months of age, with weight-bearing capacity by 9 to 10 months of age when the infant begins to pull to standing position. For above-knee deficiencies, the initial prosthesis may be "monolithic," i.e., without a knee joint. By 2½ to 3 yr of age, a lockable knee joint may allow training and therapy for prosthetic knee control, although the carryover to functional use outside the therapy setting may not occur for quite some time (48). Considering first the most distal amputations, solid ankle cushion heel (SACH) feet are available in a wide range of pediatric sizes and, for the adolescent, can give interchangeability to accommodate shoes with different heel heights. This is a cosmetic benefit for the adolescent. Generally, it is the policy of pediatric amputee clinics to provide below-knee amputees with a modified patellar tendon weight-bearing socket so that this pattern of weight-bearing becomes habitual for future use. However, auxiliary means of suspension are usually needed because of the stresses that juvenile activities place on the prosthesis (Fig. 15.9). This is particularly true for climbing activities, where the suspension must be optimal. A frequently used policy is to add to a patellar tendon-bearing socket lateral knee joint with a thigh corset for suspension and knee stabilization. Later, when cosmesis becomes more important to the child, a simple patellar tendon-bearing prosthesis without auxiliary suspension aids may be used. Of note is that approximately ⅓ of below-knee

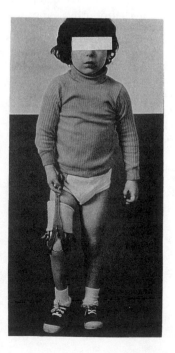

Figure 15.9. A conventional below-knee prosthesis usually stands the wear and tear of active pediatric use, as well as providing an additional suspension for the climbing activities in which most young children engage. Photograph courtesy of L. Rangaswamy.

limb-deficient children develop dislocatable patellae, a factor that must be taken into consideration when evaluating knee pain in limb-deficient youngsters (39, 40).

Training for using a prosthetic knee joint may begin between ages 2 ½ to 4 yr, depending on the aptitude of the toddler and the nature of the limb deficiency. This follows the use of the monolithic prosthesis, which is the initial extension of the limb when sitting balance is achieved. The first knee joint for a unilateral above-knee amputee may be lockable either by friction during weight-bearing or by a manual lock for security. As erect activities, including standing, stair climbing, and pivoting become secure, more time may be spent with the knee unlocked. Because of the energy requirements of walking with unlocked knee joints, the bilateral above-knee amputee may choose to ambulate with knees locked either reciprocally or with crutches using a swing-through gait. The option to preserve ambulation is necessary because of architectural barriers that might preclude entrance of a wheelchair into many locations to which the child desires access. However, for bilateral above-knee or more proximal bilateral amputations, the high energy for ambulation may lead to spending a fair amount of time in a wheelchair as the child becomes older and heavier.

The use of flexible socket for the above-knee amputee should be considered as a desirable option to accommodate growth or a residual limb that is undergoing changes in contour (19). The adolescent unilateral above-knee amputee may benefit from the hydraulic knee units that are available for adolescent age and size. This type of knee unit provides a smoother gait and, to some extent, allows a greater adaptation for varying the speed of walking. "Energy storing" designs, such as the Flex-foot, Sten-foot, or Carbon-copy foot, also facilitate a smooth gait and enhance some prosthetic sports uses.

For any amputee, walking on uneven or inclined surfaces can be a problem in adjustment of balance. There is also a change in the stresses applied to the residual limb when walking over irregular ground. The standard SACH foot allows minimal compensation for uneven surfaces. The single axis ankle, available for adolescents, can adapt to inclined surfaces although not to lateral irregularities onto which the amputee may step. A new development in foot-ankle units to accommodate irregular grounds is being explored at the California Amputee Prosthetic Project and may expand the functional options of amputees with better adaptation to various terrains in the future (26).

Congenital amputees often present odd combinations of absence of portions of the extremities with deformity of the remaining segments. One current trend for management of such lower limb congenital deficiencies is to allow maximal growth of the limb prior to any surgical revision or reconstruction. However, prosthetic adaptations to accommodate the deformities of the residual limb may be difficult or uncosmetic (Fig. 15.10). Surgery for cosmesis of limb fitting may be performed just before school age or earlier if

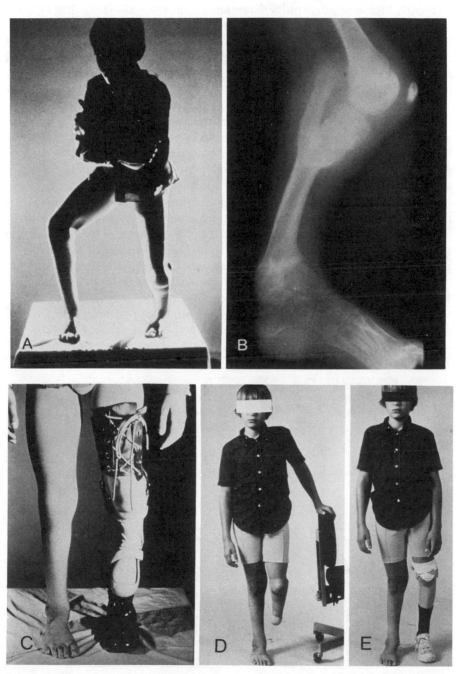

Figure 15.10. *A* and *B*, congenital absence of the tibia produces more shortening and deformities than absence of the fibula. Obtaining adequate alignment and cosmetic fit with the standard prosthesis can be difficult. *C, D,* and *E*, after surgical revision, a more cosmetic and lighter weight prosthesis can be supplied. Photographs courtesy of Y. Challenor and L. Rangaswamy.

a steadily increasing deformity threatens to limit function (Fig. 15.11). Generalizations in managing congenital limb deficiencies can, however, be misleading. The great multiplicity of deformities and deficiencies, compounded by the variability of the child's developmental and emotional status as well as family attitudes, make surgical and prosthetic individualization of planning of prime importance.

Deformities that occur in a single limb or prominently in a hemisomatic distribution represent a challenge for maintaining symmetrical function as well as for preventing or alleviating scoliosis and other postural deviations (Fig. 15.12A). Part of the continuous monitoring and maintenance therapy program is aimed at preservation of good postural alignment, particularly in the preschool child and during growth spurts (26) (Fig. 15.12B).

Probably one of the greatest challenges to prosthetic fitting is represented by bilateral hip disarticulations, bilateral amelia of the lower limbs, or by ablation of deformed lower limbs in a child with agenesis of the lumbosacral spine, where there may not be well-developed ischial tuberosities for weight-bearing. In such an instance, the socket would be a modified sitting bucket that distributes weight over the abdomen and lower thoracic area (Fig. 15.13).

The frequency with which protheses are adjusted or changed because of growth may vary with the nature of the congenital deformity. Some congen-

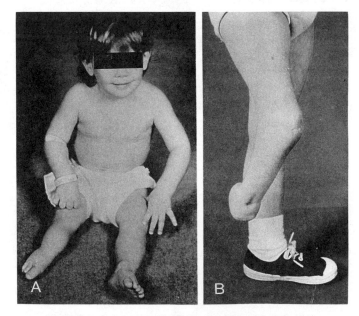

Figure 15.11. Congenital absence of the fibula after ablation of the remnants of the foot constitutes an easy below-knee fitting problem. Same child with prosthesis shown in Figure 15.12. Photographs courtesy of L. Rangaswamy.

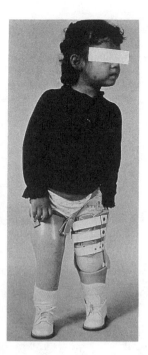

Figure 15.12. Deformities in a hemisomatic distribution may cause problems with truncal alignment and possible scoliosis. Symmetry of function during sitting activities and walking must be observed continuously and attended to in therapy as far as is possible.

ital deformities treated as limb deficiencies (e.g., proximal femoral focal deficiencies) may result in marked impairment of growth so that the prosthesis need not be changed as frequently as for the acquired amputation with normal epiphyses in the residual limb. It can be anticipated that because of growth a child will probably need a new prosthesis annually until age 5 yr; every 2 yr between ages 5 and 12 yr; and then every 3 to 4 yr until adulthood

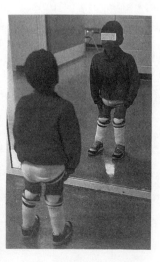

Figure 15.13. This 5-yr-old boy is independently ambulatory with prosthesis following foot ablation surgery because of the malalignments imposed by fibular dysgenesis. Because he is now normal height-for-age and age-appropriately mobile, his self-esteem and confidence have soared.

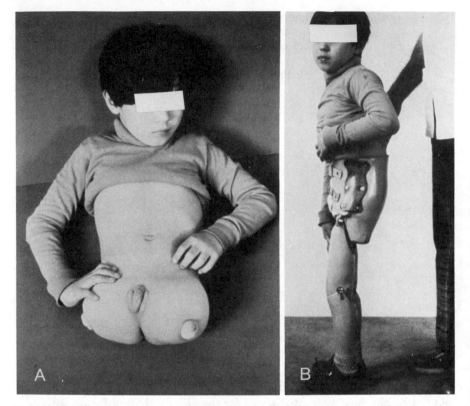

Figure 15.14. A sitting bucket type of socket with modified Canadian prosthesis alignment (as in a hip disarticulation) is used for stability. The child then ambulates with a swing-through gait just as a paraplegic would.

(31). This is a rule-of-thumb to use as a guideline, but, again, it must be emphasized that the planning for each child must be individualized according to his or her growth pattern and other needs.

Computer-aided designed and manufactured sockets, or CAD/CAM sockets (not to be confused with CAT/CAM sockets (contoured adducted trochanteric/controlled alignment method), hold promise for more comfortable and appropriate socket fitting, especially in the presence of atypical anatomical features. CAD/CAM systems have recently become commercially available, but remain to be fully evaluated, especially for the pediatric population (62).

The Role of the Physiatrist

The management of the limb-deficient child requires a carefully planned and sensitively coordinated intervention by many professionals, each with a carefully trained area of expertise. Thus, the pediatrician may be the initial person to see the congenitally limb-deficient infant after birth, but may not have the prosthetic expertise to give the parents a knowledgeable introduction to the child's functional outlook and prosthetic future. While this knowledge may be part of the training of one or more of the therapists who are integral to the ongoing management of the child in the future, it requires a singularly placed person in terms of knowledge and expertise to have the total overview of the management possibilities for the infant, functionally, surgically, prosthetically, and emotionally. It is the role of the physiatrist to integrate all of the many separate areas of medical and other professional expertise and to orchestrate constantly the contributions of these experts over a period of years in a manner that is acceptable to the parents, with a minimum amount of confusion and certainly without conflict between the members of this orchestrated therapeutic team. The conductor of an orchestra learns the dynamics and contributions of each of the instruments even though he may be an artist in only one or two. Correspondingly, the physiatrist knows the unique contribution to be gained at varying points in time from each of the members of the therapeutic team, as well as how to assemble these experts into a dynamic and constructive, but never intrusive unit. The activities of the prosthetic team should be supportive in leading parents to realize that they are not alone in handling the child's problem. At the same time, they must be made to feel an integral part in planning and accomplishing the child's habilitation.

New Developments

Throughout this chapter, newer developments in pediatric prosthetics have been mentioned in the context of the material covered. Other developments are being explored but are not yet commercially available. NASA has recently developed an artificial leg with a fairly natural gait caused by energy transfer of hydraulically displaced fluid from the normal leg to the amputated side. The pressurized fluid moves with the normal leg to artificially rotate a linkage arm that lifts the artificial leg in a motion similar to that of a natural leg (7). Another area of exploration is the use of multiple control sites for myoelectric control in patients with proximal dysmelia. Computerized recognition of patterns of muscular control around the shoulder transmits energy to motorized control of the elbow and terminal device so that shoulder motions are translated into function at the elbow and hand (68). The recent expansion of a microprocessor technology should enable miniaturization of the computers needed for controlling such devices. Similar technology should make it possible for myoelectric signals to have lighter weight electrical control (47). Historically, progress in prosthetic development has been slow, to say the least. Within the past decade, however, the developing specialty of rehabilitation engineering has led to an expansion of technology and promising devices available to handicapped persons, including the amputee. Integration of the rehabilitation engineer into the prosthetic team is viewed as a desirable augmentation of expertise and should lead to more rapid prosthetic development as a promising area for the future.

REFERENCES

1. Aitken GT: Surgical amputations in children. *J Bone Joint Surg* 45:1735, 1963.
2. Alexander J: The child amputee: summary of a forum. *Arch Phys Med Rehabil* 56:169, 1975.
3. Banziger E: Surlyn socket designs for the young child. *J Assoc Child Prosth-Orth Clin* 24:12–13, 1989.
4. Bender LF: *Prostheses and Rehabilitation After Arm Amputation.* Springfield, IL, Charles C Thomas, 1974.
5. Bergholz SG: Patient census at child amputee clinics—1971. *Interclin Information Bull* XII 6:4, 1973.
6. Blechschmidt E: The early stages of human limb development. In Swinyard C (ed): *Limb Development and Deformity: Problems of Evaluation and Rehabilitation.* Springfield, IL, Charles C Thomas, 1969.
7. Burch L: Artificial leg with natural gait. *NASA Tech Briefs* 3:246, 1978.
8. Burtch RL: Nomenclature for congenital skeletal limb deficiencies. A revision of the Frantz and O'Rahilly classification. *Artif Limbs* 10:24–35, 1966.
9. Challenor Y: Amputation secondary to disseminated intravascular coagulopathy. Presented at the Annual Meeting of the Assoc of Children's Prosth-Orth Clin June 8, 1990, NY.
10. Challenor Y, Rangaswamy L, Katz J: Limb deficiency in infancy and childhood. In Downey JA, Low NL (eds): *The Child with Disabling Illness,* ed. 2, New York, Raven Press, 1982.
11. Clarke SD, Patton JG: Occupational therapy for the limb-deficient child. *Clin Orthop* 148:47–54, 1980.
12. Cohlan SQ: A review of teratogenic agents and human congenital malformations. In Swinyard C (ed): *Limb Development and Deformity: Problems of Evaluation and Rehabilitation.* Springfield, IL, Charles C Thomas, 1969.
13. Committee on Prosthetics Research and Development: Report on the Sixth Workshop Panel on upper extremity prosthetic components of the subcommittee on design and development. *Orthot Prosthet* 23:81–115, 1969.
14. Cowie V, Swinyard C: Counseling parents of children with congenital limb deformities. In Swinyard C (ed): *Limb Development and Deformity: Problems of Evaluation and Rehabilitation.* Springfield, IL, Charles C Thomas, 1969.
15. Day HJB: Nomenclature and classification in congenital limb deficiency. In Murdoch G (ed). *Amputation Surgery and Lower Limb Prosthetics.* Edinburgh, Blackwell, 1988, pp. 271–278.
16. Day HJB: Nomenclature and classification in congenital limb deficiency. Presented at the First International Symposium on Limb Deficiency of the Internat'l Soc for Prosth & Orth. Aug 1988, Heidelberg.
17. Fishman S: Behavioral and psychological reactions of juvenile amputees. In Swinyard C (ed): *Limb Development and Deformity: Problems of Evaluation and Rehabilitation.* Springfield, IL, Charles C Thomas, 1969.
18. Fishman S, Berger N, Edelstein J: ISNY flexible sockets for upper-limb amputees. *J Assoc Child Prosth-Orth Clin* 24:8–11, 1989.
19. Fishman S, Edelstein JE, Krebs DE: Icelandic-Swedish-New York above-knee prosthetic sockets: Pediatric experience. *J Pediatr Orthop* 7:557–562, 1987.
20. Frantz C, O'Rahilly R: Congenital skeletal limb deficiencies. *J Bone Joint Surg* 43A:1202–1224, 1961.
21. Glaty HW: A preliminary report on the amputee census. *Artif Limbs* 7:5–10, 1963.

22. Glynn MK, Galway HR, Hunter G, Sauter WF: Management of the upper-limb deficient child with a powered prosthetic device. *Clin Orthop* 209:202–205, 1986.

23. Goldberg MJ, Bartoshesky LE, O'Toole D: The pediatric amputee: An epidemiologic survey. *Orthop Rev* 10:49–54, 1981.

24. Guerrero V, Epps CH: Early prosthetic rehabilitation of the child with unilateral below elbow congenital deficiency. *Interclin Information Bull* XI 12:9, 1972.

25. Hart MD: Classroom aids for a child with severe upper limb deficiencies *Am J Occup Ther* 41:467–469, 1987.

26. Hoy MG, Whiting WC, Zernicke RF: Stride kinematics and knee joint kinetics of child amputee gait. *Arch Phys Med Rehabil* 63:74–82, 1982.

27. Janerich DT, Piper JM, Glebatis DM: Oral contraceptives and congenital limb reduction defects. *N Engl J Med* 291:697, 1974.

28. Kay HW, Fishman S: 1018 children with skeletal limb deficiencies. *Monogr NY Post Grad Med Sch Prosthet Orthot* 1967, p 71.

29. Kitabayashi B: The physical therapist's responsibility to the lower extremity child amputee. *Phys Ther Rev* 41:722–727, 1961.

30. Lambert CN: Limb loss through malignancy. In Aitken GT (ed): *The Child with an Acquired Amputation.* Washington DC, National Academy of Sciences, 1972.

31. Lambert CN, Hamilton RC, Pellicore RJ: The juvenile amputee program: Its social and economic value—A follow-up study after the age of twenty-one. *J Bone Joint Surg* 51:A:1135–1138, 1969.

32. Lambert CN, Sciora J: The incidence of scoliosis in the juvenile amputee population. *Interclin Information Bull* XL 2:1, 1971.

33. Lamy M, Marateauz P: The genetic study of limb malformation. In Swinyard C (ed): *Limb Development and Deformity: Problems of Evaluation and Rehabilitation.* Springfield, IL, Charles C Thomas, 1969.

34. Marquardt E: The management of infants with malformation of the extremities. In Swinyard C (ed): *Limb Development and Deformity: Problems of Evaluation and Rehabilitation.* Springfield, IL, Charles C Thomas, 1969.

35. McDonnell PM, Scott RN, McKay LA: Incidence of congenital upper-limb deficiencies. *J Assoc Prosth-Orth Clin* 23:8–14, 1988.

36. Mendez MA: Evaluation of a myoelectric hand prosthesis for children with a below-elbow absence. *Prosthet Orthot Int* 9:137–140, 1985.

37. Menkveld SR, Novotny MP, Schwartz M: Age-appropriateness of myoelectric prosthetic fitting. *J Assoc Child Prosth-Orth Clin* 22:60–65, 1987.

38. Michael JW, Gailey RS, Bowker JH: New developments in recreational prostheses and adaptive devices for the amputee. *Clin Orthop Relat Res* 256:64–75, 1990.

39. Molvor JB, Gillespie R: Patellar instability in juvenile amputees. *J Pediatr Orthop* 7:553–556, 1987.

40. Mowery CA, Herring JA, Jackson D: Dislocated patella associated with below-knee amputation in adolescent patients. *J Pediatr Orthop* 6:299–301, 1986.

41. Nogi J, Cohen L, Mayhew J, Sharps C: Multiple amputees: complications of meningococcemia/purpura fulminans—Medical, surgical, and prosthetic Treatment. *J Assoc Prosth-Orth Clin* 23:28, 1988.

42. Nora JJ, Nora AH: Birth defects and oral contraceptives. *Lancet* 2:941, 1973.

43. O'Donnel P: Structured parent interaction. *Interclin Information Bull* 16:10–12, 1977.

44. Patton J: Developmental approach to pediatric prosthetic evaluation and training. In Atkins DJ, Meier RH (eds). *Comprehensive Management of the Upper-Limb Amputee.* New York, Springer-Verlag, 1989, pp. 138–142.

45. Patton J: Prosthetic components for children and teenagers In Atkins DJ, Meier RH (eds). *Comprehensive Management of the Upper-Limb Amputee.* New York, Springer-Verlag, 1989, pp. 99–118.

46. Reid D, Fay L: Survey of Juvenile Hand Amputees. *J Assoc Child Prosth-Orth Clin* 22:51–56, 1987.

47. Schmidl H: The I.N.A.IL. Experience fitting upper-limb dysmelic patients with myoelectric control. *Bull Prosthet Res* 27:17–42, 1977.

48. Setoguchi Y, Rosenfelder R: *The Limb Deficient Child.* Springfield, IL, Charles C Thomas, 1982.

49. Shaperman J: Early learning of hook operation. *Interclin Information Bull* 14–18, 1975.

50. Shaperman J: Learning patterns of young children with above-elbow prostheses. *Am J Occup Ther* 33:299–305, 1979.

51. Shaperman J, Sumidal CT: Recent advances in research in prosthetics for children. *Clin Orthop* 148:26–33, 1980.

52. Sorbye R: Myoelectric controlled hand prostheses in children. *Int J Rehabil Res* 1:15–25, 1977.

53. Sorbye R: Myoelectric prosthetic fitting in young children. *Clin Orthop* 148:34–40, 1980.

54. Sorbye R: Upper extremity amputees: Swedish experience concerning children. In Atkins DJ, Meier RH: *Comprehensive Management of the Upper Limb Amputee.* New York, Springer-Verlag, 1989, p. 229.

55. Sullivan RA, Celikyol F: An ongoing seminar for parents of amputee children. *Interclin Information Bull* 15:9–14, 1976.

56. Sumida W, Shaperman J: Clinical application of the infant modular below-elbow prosthesis. *Interclin Information Bull* 13:1–14, 1974.

57. Swanson AB: A classification for congenital limb malformations. *J Hand Surg* 1:8–22, 1976.

58. Swanson AB, Barsky AJ, Entin MA: Classification of limb malformation on the basis of embryological failures. *Surg Clin North Am* 48:1169, 1968.

59. Sypniewski BL: Questionnaire survey concerning age of initial fitting. *Interclin Information Bull* 6:1, 1972.

60. Taussig GB: A study of the German outbreak of phocomelia. *JAMA* 180:1106, 1962.

61. Tervo RC, Leszczynski J: Juvenile upper-limb amputees: early prosthetic fit and functional use. *Interclin Information Bull* 18:11–15, 1983.

62. Topper AK, Fernie GR: Computer-aided design and computer-aided manufacturing (CAD/CAM) in prosthetics. *Clin Orthop Relat Res* 256:39–43, 1990.

63. Trefler E: An evaluation of the 1970 summer training program for children with upper extremity amputations. *Interclin Information Bull* XI 4:10, 1972.

64. Vollradt G: Physiotherapeutic treatment of dysmelic children. *Interclin Information Bull* 5:1–13, 1970.

65. Watts HG, Corideo CP, Dow M: An upper limb prosthesis for infants. *J Assoc Child Prosth-Orth Clin* 20:55–56, 1985.

66. Weaver SA, Lange LR, Vogts VM: Comparison of myoelectric and conventional prostheses for adoloescent amputees. *Am J Occup Ther* 42:87–91, 1988.

67. Williamson DAJ: A syndrome of congenital malformations possibly due to maternal diabetes. *Dev Med Child Neurol* 12:145–152, 1970.

68. Wirta R, Taylor DR, Finley FR: Pattern-recognition arm prosthesis—A final report. *Bull Prosthet Res* 10:8–35, 1978.

16

Rehabilitation of the Burned Child

HELGA BINDER

Burns are the third leading cause of accidental death and injury in children in the United States. Approximately 1300 are killed each year (53, 72) and the number of injuries is estimated to be in the ten thousands. The highest incidence is between 0 and 4 years of age and in half the cases is due to scalding. Until preadolescence, the accident usually occurs at home and could have been prevented in the majority of cases. In contrast to the adult population where the cause of injury is frequently negligence at work or during leisure time, in the case of young children, it is their most endearing qualities, boundless curiosity and healthy playful exploration, that usually cause them to be terribly hurt and often physically and psychologically scarred for life. The introduction of flame-retardant night clothes and smoke detectors in the 1970s have not significantly changed the number of pediatric burn victims, most likely because of the prevalence of scald burns in children, but also because preventive measures are least observed by the at highest risk population groups, which tend to be the underprivileged (13). One study found that burned children tended to be the younger or youngest child in a larger-than-expected and economically disadvantaged family with only one parent (53). Most of the accidents are due to momentary or constant negligence by the caretakers of infants and toddlers. A large number of burns in this age group is unfortunately also due to child abuse (2, 59, 76, 87, 98). In older children, the risk of accidents is often compounded by emotional instability attracting them to danger (18) or, occasionally, to suicidal attempts.

Public education about burn prevention has been ongoing over the past decade and has taken many forms (65). Population awareness to burn prevention is the theme of the 1990 "Safe Kids" campaign with the emphasis on legislation stipulating the lowering of hot water temperature in the home to 120°.

As shown in Table 16.1, certain types of thermal injuries are characteristic

Table 16.1.
Typical Burns of Childhood

Age	Cause	Body Areas
6–36 months	Scalds—hot liquid splash —hot bath water negligence or abuse	Shoulder, arm, head, face, upper trunk One or both lower extremities, buttocks, perineum lower abdomen.
12–36 months	Contact burns from touching stove, radiator, iron, hotplate	Palms and fingers
	Contact burn—child abuse, placement on hot object	Hands, feet, buttocks
9–24 months	Electrical burns from chewing on electrical cord	Mouth, lips, commissures, tongue, alveolar ridge
6–14 years	Flame burns due to play with matches, gasoline, fire crackers, etc.	Face, anterior neck and trunk, hands, arms, thighs
Adolescent boys	Electrical burns from play around high tension power source	Entrance most frequently upper extremities, exit anywhere

to children of certain ages. Of interest is also that the boy to girl ratio increases from 3:2 in infants and toddlers to almost 4:1 in adolescents. This is no doubt due not only to the higher physical activity level of boys but, particularly in high tension electric injuries, it is also due to recklessness and the wish to prove manly fearlessness.

Due to constant advances in critical burn care and the establishment of specialized burn centers and burn units in some pediatric hospitals, the survival rate of pediatric burn patients has continued to improve dramatically over the past 20 years (33, 72, 79). Comprehensive rehabilitation services for these patients have been established simultaneously, since it became clear that a careful rehabilitation program can prevent many plastic reconstructive surgical procedures (7, 36, 101).

The task of rehabilitation medicine in treating burned children consists of:

1. Contracture preventing positioning and splinting alternating with a gentle range of motion exercise program to the involved joints in the acute and healing or pregrafting stage;
2. Prevention of hypertrophic scar formation by early and prolonged consistent pressure application to the healed wound, together with massage and vigorous stretching exercises to the involved body parts;
3. Prevention of generalized debility by means of a strengthening and general conditioning program, beginning in the early stage with the uninvolved body parts and progressing in vigorousness as the child's condition improves;

4. Long-term follow-up of the growing child to prevent recurrent contractures and deformities, but also to address possible emotional problems.

The degree of involvement of rehabilitation medicine depends on the severity and the location of the burns.

Classification of Burns

According to the classification of the American Burn Association, thermal injuries are designated as minor, moderate, or major burns based on size, depth, and the age of the patient. Criteria for classification are shown in Table 16.2.

It must be remembered that calculation of burn size relative to total body surface area varies with age. Because of the changing body proportions, the relative surface area of the head decreases, while those of the trunk and lower extremities increase with growth as illustrated in Figure 16.1.

Preschool children, particularly those under 2 yr of age, have a higher risk of developing circulatory compromise, fluid, and electrolyte imbalance than older children or adults. Therefore, partial- or full-thickness burns of relatively smaller size must be treated as major burns in this age group (Table 16.2).

Burn depth is interchangeably described as first, second, and third degree or superficial, partial- and full-thickness. In addition, the second degree or partial-thickness burns are divided into superficial and deep burns (Fig. 16.2).

SUPERFICIAL BURNS

Erythema, mild edema, and intense pain characterize first degree burns and only the epidermis is involved. They are usually caused by brief scalding or overexposure to sunlight or ultraviolet rays. They heal within 5 to 7 days

Table 16.2.
Burn Classification by Degree of Severity in Children[a]

Minor	=	Up to 10% TBSA superficial and superficial partial-thickness burn
	=	Up to 2% full-thickness burn not involving eyes, ears, face or genitalia
Moderate	=	10–20% TBSA partial-thickness burns
	=	2–10% full-thickness burns not involving eyes, ears, face, or genitalia
Major	=	More than 20% TBSA partial-thickness burns; more than 10% TBSA full thickness
		In children less than 2 yr old, any partial or full-thickness burn involving more than 5% TBSA
		Any burn involving eyes, ears, face, hands, feet or genitalia
		All inhalation injuries
		All electrical burns
		All burns complicated by other medical problems

[a]TBSA, total body surface area.

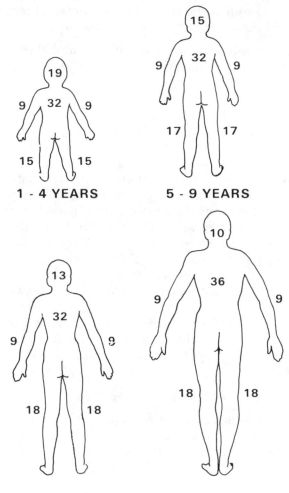

Figure 16.1. Calculation of the extent of burned area relative to total body surface at different ages.

with peeling of the injured epidermal cells, but without scarring or skin discoloration.

SUPERFICIAL PARTIAL-THICKNESS BURNS

These are characterized by severe pain and blisters; they involve the epidermis and the superficial part of the dermis. The causes are scalding, hot grease, chemicals, or touching of hot metal or flames. In uncomplicated cases, they heal in 7 to 14 days without scarring but with transient or permanent discoloration of the skin.

DEEP PARTIAL-THICKNESS BURNS

These involve the epidermis and most of the dermis and are characterized by tough red skin with blisters. Pain decreases with depth. The causes are the same as in superficial burns. Healing without complications occurs in 3 to 4 weeks with hypertrophic scarring. Grafting is frequently required and these burns often convert to full-thickness or third degree injuries.

FULL-THICKNESS BURNS

Full-thickness burns involve all skin layers and may include the subcutaneous tissue as well as muscle and bone. They are characterized by leathery white, brown, black, or mahogony-colored painless skin with easily extractable hairs. The causes are identical to those responsible for partial-thickness burns and, in addition, include electrical injuries. Healing takes weeks to months and is always associated with scarring. Grafting is required in all except very small full-thickness burns.

Treatment

MINOR BURNS

Most minor burns can be treated on an outpatient basis unless there is evidence of child abuse or incompetence of the child's caretakers. All minor burns, except for superficial burns, are treated with topical antibacterial agents and bulky dressings with the goal of preventing infection and encouraging rapid healing. No functional limitations are expected unless the burn crosses a joint or is in the vicinity of it. In these cases, the caretakers are instructed to perform gentle active-assistive range of motion exercises, which are carefully monitored during each clinic visit. Immediate splinting

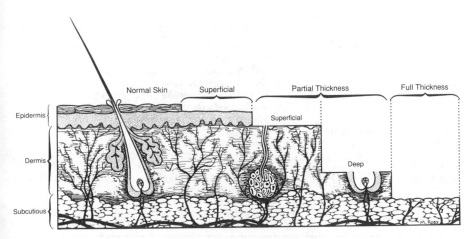

Figure 16.2. Burn depth.

is rarely necessary unless the hand is involved. Healing with scar formation calls for pressure application, splinting, and stretching as in the treatment of major burns. Close follow-up is necessary until maturation of the scar for a minimum of 9 months and then at yearly intervals if critical body areas, such as the hands or major joints, are involved, since burn scars may not keep up with bone growth.

MODERATE AND MAJOR BURNS

Most moderate and all major burns have to be treated in a hospital. Resuscitation measures and prevention of medical complications are of primary concern in the acute phase. However, positioning and splinting may be needed already in the first 24 to 48 hours to counteract the tendency of resting the injured part in a position of comfort, which tends to lead to contractures. These measures may be used regardless whether the choice of wound care and cleansing procedures is topical antibacterial agents with exposure or dressing of the wound, or surgical treatment consisting of early excision of the damaged tissues and grafting. Circumferential burns of the extremities or trunk frequently lead to compression syndromes or respiratory problems requiring escharotomies in the first 48 hours. Except for burns of the face and perineum, dressing of the wounds is the preferred approach in children because it permits comforting contact with parents and caretakers.

POSITIONING

Positioning of the child is outlined in Table 16.3 and illustrated in Figure 16.3. It is the extreme opposite of the position burn victims will naturally assume, namely, the fetal position with flexion of the trunk and all major

Table 16.3.
Positioning of the Burned Patient[a]

Area Involved	Contracture Preventing Position
Anterior neck	Slight extension
Shoulders	90° abduction, 15–20° adduction, neutral rotation
Arms	Elbows extended, forearms supinated
Hand, dorsal burn	Wrist 15–20° extension, MCP joints 60–90° flexion
	IP joints full extension
	Thumb in 45° abduction and opposition
Exposed extensor tendons	As above, but MCP joints in 30–40° flexion
Palmar burn	Wrist in 15–20° extension
	Fingers in full extension, including MCP joints
	Thumb in wide palmar abduction
Anterior chest	Shoulders in 90° abduction and slight external rotation; beware of anterior dislocation
Perineum	Symmetrical hip abduction of 10–15°
	Full extension, neutral rotation
Leg	Knee in full extension, ankle at 90° dorsiflexion

[a]MCP, metacarpophalangeal; IP, interphalangeal.

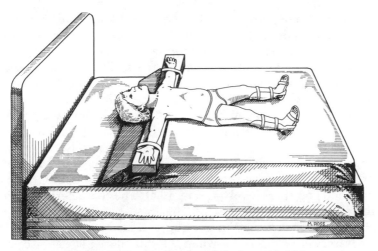

Figure 16.3. Positioning of the burned child.

joints. In addition to preventing contractures, positioning also aids drainage of the rapidly forming edema from the involved body parts during the first 48 hours following the burn and, thus, prevents subsequent interstitial fibrosis and scarring. Positioning can be achieved with the help of pillows, foam rubber blocks, towel rolls, sandbags, boards, or thermoplastic splints.

In anterior neck burns, the proper position is slight neck extension by hanging the head over a short mattress or towel roll. For anterior chest burns, towel rolls along the spine result in slight retraction and external rotation of the shoulders. This position has to be carefully monitored to avoid anterior shoulder dislocation. Hip abduction can be achieved with the help of a foam rubber wedge or a cross-bar attached to boots. The latter serve the double purpose of maintaining the ankles at 90° dorsiflexion. Alternative means of ankle positioning are posterior ankle foot splints, a bedboard, or, in prone position, hanging the feet over a short mattress. For prevention of edema, it is particularly important to elevate the hands and feet and, in boys with perineal burns, the scrotum. The positioning must be coupled with passive- or active-assistive range of motion exercises to prevent extension contractures. In case of very ill or circumferentially burned children, a 2-hourly turning schedule may be used. More frequently, these children are placed in airflow or Clinitron beds, which, however, markedly limit any active movement and should, therefore, be discontinued as soon as the child's condition permits. Detailed illustrated positioning and splinting instructions should be left at bedside to guarantee continuous optimal care.

SPLINTING

Children frequently need to be positioned with the help of splints since they cannot be expected to stay in a desired position for any length of time.

In acute burns, three-point or gutter elbow and knee extension splints as well as hand and ankle-foot splints are the most frequently used. In anterior neck burns, a neck conformer can be applied over a thin dressing as soon as the edema has subsided. A difficult problem is splinting to maintain abduction in burns around the shoulder, particularly in the axilla. Pillows or sling suspension in the acute phase and an airplane splint in the healing stage or after grafting are the usual approaches, but the results are not uniformly satisfactory. Since burns of the hand require special considerations, their management, including splinting, will be discussed separately.

The availability of various thermoplastic materials allows a great versatility of custom-molded splints in sizes and shapes appropriate for the child's age and body part involved (Fig. 16.4). The characteristics of some of these materials are shown in Table 16.4.

Splints are applied over a thin dressing and held in place with gauze bandage. They are worn at all times when the child does not exercise or use the burned limb in functional or play activities, particularly if contractures appear unavoidable or the child is uncooperative in range of motion exercises. Frequent evaluation to ensure proper fit and application is needed especially in small children to avoid decubiti or nerve compression. Damage to the ulnar nerve in its groove at the elbow and to the peroneal nerve at the fibular head are well-known examples of pressure neuropathy. Early on, frequent remolding may be necessary because of subsiding edema.

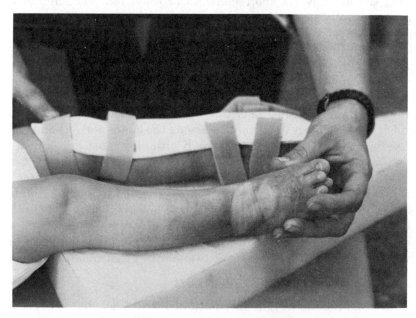

Figure 16.4. Anterior leg conformer for dorsal foot burns.

Table 16.4.
Materials for Thermoplastic Splints[a]

Brand Name	Water Temperature	Pliable In	Setting Time
Kay Splint	160°F	90–120 seconds	8–10 minutes
Orthoplast			
Aquaplast	140°F	120 seconds	2–5 minutes (2% shrinkage)
Polyform	150–160°F	60 seconds	2–5 minutes
Polyflex		120 seconds	

[a]All materials can be washed with soap and water, alcohol, or gas sterilized.

Serial splinting is also used for treatment of joint contractures in the subacute and chronic phases. In contractures of the ankles and feet and, particularly, of the hands, fiberglass casting has proven very effective.

RESPIRATORY THERAPY

In severely ill children and especially in those with inhalation injuries and chest burns, breathing exercises, chest physical therapy, and postural drainage are immediately instituted and continued until the danger of pulmonary complications have subsided.

HYDROTHERAPY

Hydrotherapy is an important part of burn treatment in the majority of burn units (92) and is used for wound debridement as well as range of motion exercises. Because of the danger of electrolyte imbalance and sepsis by infants under 6 months of age, children 6 to 18 months old with more than 15% total body surface area (TBSA) burns, children 18 to 36 months old with more than 20% TBSA burns, and older children with more than 30% TBSA burns are not receiving hydrotherapy. In all children, immersion in tap water is the usual mode and salt with iodine is added in larger burns to achieve an isotonic solution (Table 16.5).

Disposable tub liners are universally used to prevent contamination, but sterile conditions cannot be achieved. Some centers prefer rinsing, which is less likely to cause contamination and is also less stressful than a tub bath. Bathing is done once or twice daily and usually for 10- to 20-minute periods. The water temperature must be 98° and can be slightly higher if only an extremity is immersed. The room is warmed with heat lamps. Tub time is also used for gentle active-assistive range of motion exercises to the involved joints and spontaneous play activity is encouraged.

PAIN MANAGEMENT

Children are generally medicated prior to tubbing as well as before other dressing changes and physical therapy. Patients with extensive burns who commonly receive medication for background pain are boosted with intravenous short-acting opiates (usually Fentanyl) in addition to Valium for

Table 16.5.
Hydrotherapy Guidelines[a]

Age (months)	TBSA Burned	
0–6		No tubbing
6–18	0–10%	Tub
	10–15%	Tub with isotonic salt water solution
	Stable condition	
	NA+ >130	
	>15%	No tub
18–36	0–10%	Tub
	10–20%	Tub with isotonic salt water solution
	Stable condition	
	NA+ >130	
	>20%	No tub
>36	0–10%	Tub
	0–30%	Tub with isotonic salt water solution
	Stable condition	
	Na+ >130	
	>30%	No tub
		No iodized salt!

[a]TBSA, total body surface area; NA+, serum sodium level

procedures. If there is no venous access, Dilaudid is most commonly used. Intramuscular drugs are avoided at all costs because of the added stress. Children with smaller burns receive Tylenol with codeine. Weaning from pain medication is generally no problem and permanent addiction in burned children has not been described (71).

In addition to medication, behavior modification is routinely used. Most accepted is that of patient participation in all dressing changes or other painful procedures, including stretching of tight joints. Complete information is given and unpleasant surprises are avoided (8, 23, 49, 71). Music, toys, and other enjoyable distractions are used additionally if they appear helpful.

The usefulness of hypnosis for burned children remains unproven (81). In older children, transcutaneous electrical nerve stimulation (TENS) is worth trying if the location of the burn is appropriate (71).

EXERCISE PROGRAM IN ACUTE AND SUBACUTE PHASES

The principal aims of maintaining strength and joint mobility dictate the choice of active and active-assistive range of motion exercises. Exceptions are those cases when the child is too small or too sick to cooperate and, therefore, passive exercises are required to avert progressive loss of motion. In some cases of uncooperative patients, it is helpful to assess the range of motion in a joint under anesthesia prior to a surgical procedure in order to set realistic goals. Treatment should be administered at least twice daily and should combine the traditional forms of exercise with functional activities.

All children who are medically stable should be encouraged to use the burned body parts as much as possible provided there are no surgical contraindications. Participation in self-care and play activities incorporating those movements that may be compromised by the injury provide a natural and most acceptable way for inducing upper extremity use in children. Playing with a busy-box type wall or ball games are some of the most suitable ways to mobilize joints of the arms. Use of the hands is encouraged by playing with putty, action toys that require squeezing (Ping Pong), or by devising special levers that can be used in video games (1). Unless the burns are severe, ambulation can be started usually on the 3rd or 4th day after the injury. Minor or moderate burns of the lower extremities do not contraindicate walking. However, the legs must be wrapped with supportive bandages over the dressing in a figure-eight fashion to prevent edema. For the same reason, the legs are kept elevated during prolonged sitting. Tricycling, playing with push carts or similar toys are enjoyed by children and offer suitable active exercise for lower extremity burns. Walking is preferable to sitting when the shoulder, neck, and trunk are burned. Some centers limit or avoid sitting altogether because of the difficulties encountered in trying to control the habitually assumed posture of neck flexion, shoulder protraction, and consequent kyphosis. Other centers use equipment like a tall cerebral palsy walker, which forces the child to extend the arms overhead to walk. Activities that emphasize elongation of the trunk, chest expansion, and shoulder retraction are indicated to prevent spinal deformities, including scoliosis, especially in asymmetrical burns of the torso, shoulder, or pelvic girdle (Fig. 16.5).

MANAGEMENT OF GRAFTED BURNS

Immediate or early wound excision and grafting of deep partial- and full-thickness burns has become a common practice (33, 34, 102, 103). However, in young children, demarcation of nonviable from viable tissue is often unclear and viable tissue may be inadvertently removed. Particularly in large burns, temporary grafting using homografts, xenografts, or commercially available skin substitutes may be used to cover the area until final skin grafting can be performed (33). Full-thickness skin grafts are used for the face, neck, and hands if at all possible. Split-thickness sheet or meshed grafts are used in other areas, with the latter providing the poorest cosmetic effect. Autologous cultured epithelium has also become available for use in extensive burns with inadequate donor sites, but it provides only epidermal coverage and not much experience with this technique has been gained. Postoperative treatment of a final skin graft generally consists of a bulky occlusive dressing and immobilization with a thermoplastic splint applied

Figure 16.5. Mobilization of upper extremity joints by play. Pressure garment on the arms, figure-eight elastic wrapping of the trunk.

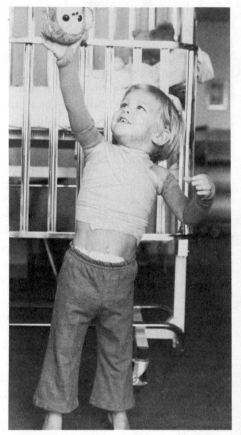

in the operating room. In circumferential extremity or hand burns, immobilization can be achieved by skeletal suspension with or without traction to hold the grafted body part in the desired position while the uninvolved joints can be freely exercised and actively moved (34, 102).

Minimal immobilization time is 5 days, but may vary according to the surgeon's preference. Mobility after grafting is achieved by gentle active-assistive range of motion exercises and functional use. All movements must be performed carefully to avoid bleeding, injury, and detachment of the still fragile tissues. There may be a need for reinstituting hydrotherapy if open areas remain.

As in other phases of burn care, functional use in self-care and play activities is preferable to formal exercises and compliance is much better. Detailed instuctions should be left at the bedside so that everyday activities can be used continuously and in a purposeful manner to keep all joints as limber as possible.

PREVENTION OF HYPERTROPHIC SCAR FORMATION AND CONTRACTURES

Children, particularly Black and Oriental youngsters, tend to heal with an abundance of scar tissue which exceeds that observed in adults. Slow healing wounds with a great deal of inflammatory response, like those occurring in burns, tend to form raised, engorged, angry-looking, painful, and itching scars with a relentless tendency to contract for at least 6 to 12 months (69).

Nodules containing increased numbers of myofibroblasts and/or fibroblasts that produce an abundance of collagen arranged in whorls are the basis for the appearance of the fresh hypertrophic scar. Due to capillary sprouting, the nodules are initially very vascular, but eventually become internally avascular as they increase in size. This is thought to lead to hypoxia and eventual degeneration of the fibroblasts, which marks the beginning of the maturation phase of the scar and the forming of contractures (45). Pressure application leading to capillary occlusion appears to affect fibroblast activity negatively and seems to permit more physiological linear alignment of the collagen (69). The beneficial pressure effect had been noted first by Fujimori and associates (29) who used industrial sponge under wraps to produce more pliable scar tissue. It was confirmed by Cronin in 1961 (21) who first advocated splinting of grafted neck burns to prevent otherwise inevitable contractures in this difficult body area and found that a well-conforming splint produced also a smoother scar. Splinting of burned body parts combined with continuous pressure application after spontaneous healing or firm take of an autograft was pioneered in the USA at the Shriners Burn Institute in Galveston, Texas in the late 1960s and early 1970s (40, 48, 73, 100). In the meantime, this measure has become common practice and has led to a marked decline in the number of surgical scar release procedures (7, 36). It has also reduced the itching and burning sensation so commonly associated with healing and freshly healed burn wounds.

For effective control of hypertrophic scar formation, an even pressure of 25 to 30 mm Hg, which leads to blanching of the raised red areas, must be used for 24 hours a day with time out only for hygiene and therapy. This is achieved by pressure garments, thermoplastic splints, pressure inserts, or any combination of these methods. Materials used for pressure garments vary in elasticity and firmness as shown in Table 16.6. Therefore, the amount of pressure can be controlled to a degree by the choice of garment. It can be further increased by the addition of splints and pressure inserts, particularly over areas where even firm pressure is otherwise difficult to achieve.

The use of pressure application can be started when wound healing is almost complete or 2 to 3 weeks following a successful graft take. Initially, elastic bandages are used in a figure-eight pattern in order to keep the shearing forces low (Fig. 16.5). Each body part is wrapped separately to permit

Table 16.6.
Pressure Wraps and Garments

1. Used in early healing period to provide minimal pressure and shear forces Ace Wrap-trunk, extremities in figure-eight style Elastic Net —————— Tubigrip ————————————————	Trunk in small children; extremities of all sizes, face, and head
2. Used in the intermediate period for healed burns to provide increased pressure and shear forces Lycra Spandex Garments-fashioned by occupational therapist and fastened with Velcro closures, Jobst Interim	
3. Used in the chronic period for well-healed burns to provide optimal pressure and highest tolerable shear forces Jobst —————————— Bioconcept ———————— Barton & Carey————	Custom-made skintight garments with zippers

active function. On the face, several layers of gauze and tubular netting may be used. As the skin becomes less fragile, temporary pressure clothing can be tailored or custom ordered (Jobst Interim) and the final step is skintight fitting with a custom-made garment (46). Outside seams and zippers considerably decrease the stress of donning and minimize skin irritation (Fig. 16.6). The child wearing a pressure garment has to be checked at monthly intervals to ensure skintight fit. Several garments may have to be ordered in succession as long as the scars change rapidly, particularly in the first 6 months. For hygienic reasons, two sets should be provided to guarantee continuous wearing. The garment will have to be worn for a minimum of 9 months but, more often, for 12 to 18 months. Its use should be maintained until the scar remains soft and pale and no contractures occur between follow-up visits at 2- to 3-week intervals after wearing has been discontinued. Simultaneously, the skin is massaged with softening and moisturing agents such as Eucerin cream, cocoa butter, or mineral oil. Good results have been reported from warm paraffin application prior to passive stretching, but this method is not generally used in children (36). Prolonged immersion in water or sun exposure should be avoided in order to prevent maceration of the skin or development of dry, cracked skin or fissures.

Patients with burns over the anterior aspect of the neck, lower face, and upper chest are in great danger of losing the normal anatomic contours. The chin may become drawn onto the chest by scarring and, subsequently, severe distortion of the facial features can develop in severe cases with inability to close the mouth. In this area, pressure garments are ineffective. In addition to proper positioning in the acute phase, various ways of immobilization immediately after grafting have been developed. Some institutions use conventional halo fixation with hyperextension of the neck (84); others use thermoplastic head splints to prevent neck flexion and rotation (5, 14). These devices are especially helpful in children who cannot cooperate with immobilization efforts. Following graft take, low or high temperature thermoplastic neck conformers are used for the double purpose of maintaining normal neck and shoulder contours and applying pressure. A one-piece splint can be used for burns limited to the neck without extension to the lower face and will prevent flexion of the neck primarily (26). In children, this purpose is also satisfactorily achieved by use of variations of the Watusi (82) collar. Semirigid tubes, such as radiator hose, are stacked to the necessary height to provide a good chin shelf and are covered with Elastinette and tied snugly around the neck (Fig. 16.7). Two- and three-piece thermoplastic splints have been developed in an effort to provide upward pressure to the chin and upper neck and downward pressure to lower neck and shoulders, but to permit eating and speaking and acceptable appearance in burns that extend over the lower face and entire neck (51). In young children, a detrimental effect on mandibular growth and alignment of the teeth is of concern with use of the two- and three-component neck splints and they are, therefore, not used until adolescence. In the first few weeks, weekly adjustments of the splint may be needed to guarantee total contact as the scar changes. The splint has to be reformed after 3 to 6 months. Since the splint is worn directly on the

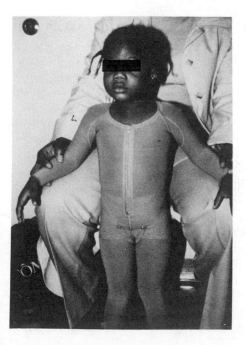

Figure 16.6. Whole body pressure garment.

Figure 16.7. Watusi collar fabricated from radiator hose. Courtesy of Brian Burne, OTR, Children's Hospital, Denver.

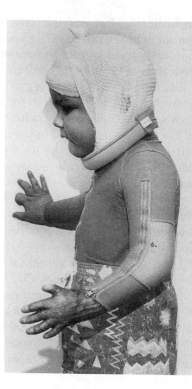

skin, it has to be taken off at regular intervals to prevent maceration of the skin; continuous use for a minimum of 6 months is the rule.

In burns of the axilla, immobilization in a small child after grafting can be achieved with the help of a foam "papoose" (55). After graft take, the most successful device for maintaining range of motion is the airplane splint, which rests on the iliac crest and is closely contoured to the axillary space. It is usually fabricated with a separate forearm trough to prevent pressure on the elbow and a handgrip for good positioning of the wrist and hand in case of burns over these areas. The airplane splint must be anchored with a harness or strap across the chest and around the opposite shoulder and can be worn over a pressure garment (Fig. 16.8). This splint is commonly worn at night alternating with axillary foam or Spenco pressure pads secured by figure-eight elastic wrapping during the day. A recent approach is using foam and silicone gell pads, which exude some silicone oil and make the skin pliable at the same time (78). They are again held in place with figure eight elastic wrapping. The silicone deteriorates quickly and needs to be replaced frequently.

It is notoriously difficult to achieve the necessary even distribution of firm pressure over the face, neck, clavicle, axilla, anterior chest wall, groin, dorsum of the foot, and finger web spaces. These areas require the application of additional pressure inserts under tight fitting garments or in the shoe. Products used range from foam over Spenco to silicone rubber. They have to be frequently remolded, especially in the first 6 months because of the rapidly changing contours effected (3).

The importance of preventing hypertrophic scarring and contractures in the first 6 months after healing cannot be emphasized enough. Continuous use of splints and pressure application must be followed strictly since contractures have been found to increase within hours after removal of positioning devices, particularly in the neck and the axilla.

Burns Requiring Special Consideration

HAND BURNS

Burns may affect the dorsal or volar aspect of the hand or they may be circumferential. Full-thickness burns, though relatively rare in the pediatric age group, may be due to scalding or flame burns. They are frequently associated with major burns affecting other parts of the body and usually involve the dorsal aspect. On the other hand, partial-thickness burns more frequently occur over the palm. Palmar burns are often isolated injuries from accidental touching of hot objects or as a result of child abuse (10, 103). In all hand burns, the tendency to assume the position of comfort and rapid development of considerable edema very quickly leads to claw hand deformity with hyperextension of the metacarpophalangeal and flexion of the interphalangeal joints. The thumb will be adducted, thus rendering the hand functionally useless (41, 67, 103). Treatment in the acute period depends on

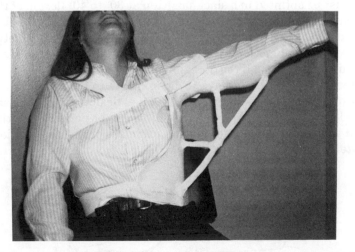

Figure 16.8. Airplane splint for axillary burns. Courtesy of C. Leman, OTR, Washington Hospital Center, Washington DC.

the location and severity of the burn and the general condition of the child. Superficial partial-thickness burns or small palmar burns will be treated with topical antibacterial agents and dressings. Each finger is wrapped separately to maintain the web spaces and to allow functional use throughout the day. A static resting splint, shown in Figure 16.9, is applied with gauze bandage during all rest periods and at night. Metacarpophalangeal flexion, extension of the interphalangeal joints, wide abduction, and opposition of the thumb must be maintained and frequently checked (36). Elevation can be achieved by pillows or a sling in older and cooperative youngsters and with the help of skin traction in small children. The hand should be raised to about the level of the heart in the first few days to prevent edema and to decrease consequent fibrosis and scar formation. If the general condition of the child permits, deep, partial-, or full-thickness dorsal hand burns are frequently treated with immediate early excision and autografting (103). After grafting, the hand is secured in a paddle or racket-type thermoplastic splint with external fixation at the fingernails (68) or internal fixation through the distal phalanges (Fig. 16.10). Some centers use internal fixation and place the hand in special surgical apparatus, such as the banjo or hay rake (34, 102) with exposure of the graft. Other centers report good success with casting of the hand immediately after grafting. Children under 5 yr of age are casted with all joints extended; older children in metacarpophalangeal joint flexion and interphalangeal joint extension, just as in the splint. This permits excellent immobilization without having to restrict the child's general mobility. Range of motion exercises are begun at the individual surgeon's discretion as early as 5 days after grafting. Great care has to be taken to keep the finger extensor tendons moist and well protected in case of exposure. The fingers must be splinted in a slack position at 30° to 40° flexion of the metacarpophalangeal joints to prevent tendon rupture until successful wound coverage can be accomplished. At the individual surgeon's discretion, gentle, passive range of motion exercises of individual joints can be safely performed during this time. If the dorsal hood mechanism is exposed, the proximal interphalangeal joints have to be splinted in extension until wound coverage or for as long as 4 to 6 weeks. Isolated flexion exercises of the metacarpophalangeal and distal phalangeal joints can be performed in the meantime and gentle, active range of motion exercises of the involved joints can begin after wound coverage has been achieved. Boutonniere deformity rep-

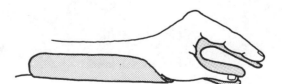

Figure 16.9. Resting splint for hand burn.

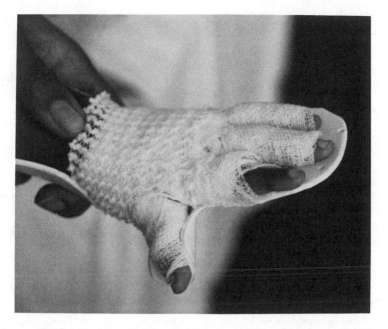

Figure 16.10. Paddle splint for skeletal suspension of hand after grafting.

resents the most common late complication of dorsal hand burns and is difficult to repair. It is caused by destruction of the extensor hood and slipping of the lateral bands, which then act as flexors of the proximal and extensors of the distal interphalangeal joints. In severe dorsal burns that affect the joint, fusion in a functional position may have to be considered in late childhood.

Volar burns generally involve partial skin thickness. As long as they are limited to the palm, severe contractures rarely develop. On the other hand, burns of the fingers and interdigital spaces can lead to severe webbing and syndactyly unless prevented by the use of spacers during scar formation (32, 77). In the acute stage, the hand and fingers are splinted in full extension with palmar abduction of the thumb (Fig. 16.11). Although some occupational therapists have become very skillful in making hand splints even for infants, casting, use of the sandwich splint (95), or, in rare cases, a silicone rubber mitten seem to be the most common approaches for hand burns in small or uncooperative children. After graft healing, a dynamic splint may be needed to facilitate finger flexion. Pressure application to prevent hypertrophic scarring and webbing is especially difficult in the hand. Coban, a self-adherent elastic tape, can be used for decrease of edema and pressure application. It is carefully wrapped distally to proximally and in fragile areas over thin gauze to decrease friction. Various inserts, such as foam or silicone rubber, are used therafter in conjunction with elastic pressure gloves partic-

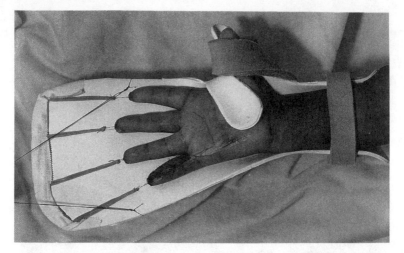

Figure 16.11. Fingers and thumb are splinted in full extension and abduction in palmar burn.

ularly to maintain the web spaces. Although gloves and spacers must be worn continuously until the scars mature, the child is encouraged to use the hand as much as possible. Leaving the fingertips free improves dexterity and will gradually alleviate hypersensitivity of the skin. The use of static splints is commonly continued at night. A frequent late complication is a flexion contracture of the fifth digit, which can be treated by splinting. In small children, serial casting is more effective. In very severe burns with charring of the fingers, early amputation is indicated to avert infection.

It is well recognized that the treatment of hand burns with casting, splinting, and exercises has decreased the incidence and recurrence of hand deformities in children. However, the need for successive surgical procedures cannot be prevented in all cases, especially in those with very extensive burns (27, 61). Hand function may sometimes be good, even though appearance is poor (62).

FACIAL BURNS

In the pediatric age group, facial burns are treated mostly with elastic pressure masks and inserts. However, full facial silicone elastomere molds (57) and high temperature plastic transparent face masks (86) are gaining more acceptance. Children as young as 7 weeks have been fitted with the latter. The need for anesthesia during initial fabrication and, later, frequent adjustments in young children and concern about stunting mandibular growth are the negative aspects. Adjustments are, therefore, commonly made if anesthesia is required for other reasons and strapping over the top of the head and occiput rather than around the head has largely eliminated dental problems. Cosmetic results reportedly are excellent. Just as with the neck conformers, these splints will have to be worn 23 hours for many months.

ELECTRIC BURNS

Two kinds of electric burns are typical for the pediatric age group: (*a*) electric burns of the mouth, which remain virtually limited to infants and toddlers; and (*b*) high tension injuries of preadolescent or adolescent boys.

Electric burns of the mouth are caused by arcing between two wires carrying 110 to 220 V of household current and occur in infants or toddlers who chew on an electric cord. Despite the low tension current, the arc creates very high temperatures and severe tissue coagulation, most often of the lips and lateral commissures, ensues. Systemic reactions other than elevated temperature appear to be rare. The initial signs may, therefore, be deceptive. However, massive edema will develop quickly and there is usually extensive necrosis with clear tissue demarcation about 10 to 14 days after the injury. At this stage, life-threatening bleeding from the corroded labial artery may occur. For this reason, the usual practice is to admit the child unless the parents appear eminently qualified to provide care at home and are instructed in pressure application to stop the hemorrhage until the child can be transported to the hospital. The approach in most burn centers is conservative, at least until demarcation takes place. The child's activity is restricted to prevent further injury. Diet is adjusted to tolerance and, in severe cases, nasogastric tube feeding is instituted. Oral hygiene is extremely important. Elbow extension splints may be used to keep the child from touching the wound. Depending on the prevailing school of thought, further treatment consists of early excision and immediate reconstruction, spontaneous wound healing and late reconstruction, or early, continuous oral splinting (50, 70). There seems to be no difference in the eventual outcome to the surgical approaches. However, the conservative approach by splinting seems to have gained wider acceptance in recent years. A plastic orthodontic retainer was first described by Colcleugh and Ryan in 1976 (17) and many others have been developed since. Some are removable (22) and some are cemented to the teeth (88). These retainers have to be fabricated by an orthodontist, need to be remodeled every 3 to 4 months, and must be worn a minimum of 6 months or often for a year. They will maintain the natural contours of the mouth in addition to stretching the lips. They seem to be very effective for extensive burns to the mouth.

For small burns to the lips and microstomia associated with facial burns, commercially available mouth conformers consisting of two high temperature plastic pieces connected by metal expanders are commonly used (50). They are light and quite well tolerated by older cooperative children.

HIGH TENSION INJURIES

This type of burn occurs on coming in contact with electric power of more than 500 V. It is most common in preadolescent or adolescent boys while trying to retrieve a ball or kite from a high tension wire or while they are knowingly engaged in dangerous activities (11, 42). The injuries are caused by the current traversing the body and by ignition of clothing with resultant flame burns. In addition, trauma to the bones and muscles can occur due to powerful tetanic contractions from low frequency alternating currents. Bone, cartilage, and skin are most resistant and least conductive, while nerves and blood vessels are the least resistant and most conductive of electric current. Due to these differences in tissue properties, the current tends to travel along nerves and blood vessels which are also very sensitive to heat. Therefore, massive tissue destruction marks the path of the current despite relatively small entry and exit wounds. If the child does not succumb to cardiac fibrillation and respiratory arrest due to the current traversing the heart or brain stem, the injuries and rehabilitation problems are generally serious with rapid development of marked edema that leads to severe ischemic changes and often necessitates extensive fasciotomies and exploration for relief of compartmental compression syndromes. Amputations are frequently inevitable. The child can sustain long bone or vertebral fractures as a result of tetanic contractions or falling from considerable height. Unconsciousness, convulsions, spinal cord injury, and head injury are neurological complications that can become evident immediately after the injury.

EXERCISE PROGRAM IN THE CHRONIC PHASE

Massage and stretching of the scarred areas should be continued throughout the chronic stage, preferably twice daily. These sessions also serve to monitor and adjust the pressure garments, inserts, and splints. A burn injury with its metabolic sequelae, suffering from pain, subsequent immobilization, and restrictions in the usual activity level inevitably leads to a decrease in the child's state of physical well-being and fitness. General conditioning and strengthening exercises, including noninvolved parts, are a part of the rehabilitation program to restore endurance and tolerance of physical activities appropriate for the child's age. An important aspect of management is to work with the child and family so that, at the time of discharge, they are familiar with the recommended home exercise program, proper donning and wearing of splints and pressure garments, skin care and precautions necessitated by these devices. They must be aware that a conscientious home maintenance program is part of the long-range rehabilitation process. In contrast to adults, a growing child is prone to develop recurrent contractures until full growth has been achieved, particularly when the burns and scars involve the hand, foot, or extend over a joint. After discharge, follow-up visits are needed at regular and gradually increasing intervals.

Systemic Complications

SKELETAL SYSTEM

Osteoporosis appears to be a rather uniform finding in all major burns. It may be diffuse or localized underlying the burn area. The latter type is usually more severe. In most cases, inflammatory changes and immobilization of a limb are the initiating factors. However, reflex sympathetic dystrophy has also been observed at the site of some full-thickness burns.

Early complications, which occur primarily in children, are joint destruction and ankylosis apparently caused by bacteremia and sepsis (24).

Heterotopic ossification with ankylosis appears to occur equally rarely in children as in adults and seems to affect primarily patients with extensive full-thickness burns. Retrospectively, the incidence is reported as 1% to 2% in severe burns (74), but since there is a high rate of spontaneous resolution, the true incidence may actually be higher (66, 91). The most common sites of ectopic ossifications are the elbow and hip joint. Increasing pain and decreasing range of motion are the first signs that tend to occur several months after injury. Calcium, phosphorus, and alkaline phosphatase studies do not seem to be helpful, but bone scans tend to show the lesion as much as 3 weeks earlier than x-rays (91). As in other patients with heterotopic ossification, passive range of motion exercises are avoided but active range of motion exercises within or below pain limits do not appear to be harmful (19, 74). In addition, splinting must continue. The usefulness of Didronel in these patients is uncertain. Similar to adults, gradual absorption of the ectopic bone seems to be the usual course in children.

In the pediatric age group, growth retardation of the affected extremity may accompany severe burns. It can be related to premature closure of the epiphysis (28) or to restrictive scar formation that interferes with epiphyseal growth (80). Surgical release of the scar tissue may lead to resumption of growth. In extensive burns of the hand, premature fusion of the metacarpal and phalangeal epiphyses was observed leading to significant permanent growth reduction (64).

Spinal deformities are initiated by the protective positions that a child with burns of the torso will assume. Later, asymmetrical scarring over the thorax or lumbosacral area gives rise to scoliosis, while scar formation of the anterior aspect of the chest can lead to kyphosis.

Anterior dislocation of the shoulder, posterior dislocation of the hips, and metacarpophalangeal and phalangeal joint dislocations of the hands and feet do occur if strict positioning coupled with range of motion exercises and splinting are not carried out.

NERVOUS SYSTEM

Neurological symptoms ranging from confusion to convulsions and coma are known to occur during the acute stage of burns in children even when the injury is relatively minor (96). Electrolyte imbalance (60, 63), hyperglycemia, hypoxia, or hypovolemia (4) have been implicated. In some cases, children appear to have had true febrile seizures (79). Some authors attribute these complications to concurrent cerebral edema (75) or encephalopathy (63). However, in some cases, the cause remains obscure (96).

Iatrogenically caused neurological symptoms were recognized with many topically applied agents, especially hexachlorophene, which causes an encephalopathy. Respiratory arrest and seizures have been noted with the use of topical anesthetic agents like lidocaine and tetracaine (97). However, the incidence of neurological complications seems to be decreasing with increasingly sophisticated burn management. Recovery without neurological sequelae has been the usual course in most cases.

Complications affecting the central nervous system are most frequently encountered with electric burns (89). They may become evident immediately after the injury but the onset of signs may be delayed for months or years. Spinal cord dysfunction, brought on by current traversing from arm to arm or leg, is manifested as flaccid or spastic paraparesis or quadriparesis and can be transient or permanent. Progressive muscle atrophy and signs of amyotropic lateral sclerosis may follow in some cases (25, 35). Cerebral damage with hemiplegia and symptoms of striatal and brain stem dysfunction have also been described (20). In fatal cases, thrombosis of major arteries, hemorrhage, perivascular cavitation, focal demyelination, and neuronal chromatolysis were demonstrated in the spinal cord and brain.

Peripheral neuropathies associated with distal weakness, lack of endurance, and easy fatigability have been described in adults with flame burns over greater than 20% and children with burns over more than 30% TBSA as well as in patients with smaller electrical burns (38). The exact etiology remains unclear, although it may be related to metabolic disturbances or neurotoxic drugs administered for burn care (35). Patients with peripheral neuropathy tend to improve significantly over time, but adult patients may complain about easy fatigability for many years (37). In children, this complaint would most likely be impossible to elicit. On the other hand, neuropathy of the eighth cranial nerve seems to affect young children more commonly after systemic or topical application of neurotoxic antibiotics (6, 31). The resulting high frequency hearing loss is progressive and irreversible leading to severe hearing impairment as an additional handicap.

Focal neuropathies are encountered directly due to the burn injury, compression from edema and scarring (35, 42), repeated intramuscular injections, poor positioning, and too heavy dressings (37). They affect most commonly the brachial plexus, the median, radial, and ulnar nerves in the upper extremities, and the peroneal nerves in the lower extremities. These complications are preventable.

Psychosocial Problems

It is a well-known fact that the majority of children with burns come from a stressed home environment and have emotional problems preceding the injury. Some reports suggest that the frequency of these problems approaches 80%. Older boys who sustained their injuries while knowingly engaging in dangerous forbidden activities often perceive the pain and extensive wounds as just punishment. They see the nurses, physicians, and other caretakers as persecutors who try to "skin them alive" (54). These problems persist despite good psychological management of burn patients. Often, the parents harbor severe guilt feelings as well (15). Victims of neglect and abuse were found to have a high incidence of depression, which appears plausible (13). Social workers, psychiatrists, and psychologists are most valuable members of the burn team as they can explore premorbid problems and assist the staff in selecting the best approach to handle the patient and family as well as permitting nurses to vent their pain and frustration in dealing with a severely burned child (43). Counseling parents and child about necessary procedures that may appear unwarranted and cruel helps gain more cooperation (8).

The inevitable pain associated with dressing changes, hydrotherapy, and exercises remains a difficult problem despite improved pain management. Relaxation techniques, biofeedback, and stress management approaches were found to be useful for some older children (47, 85). Withdrawal and depression in the younger child often respond best to art and play therapy (52, 56).

Many children develop regressive unacceptable behavior during the long hospitalization required for grafting and healing. Behavior modification with consistent participation of all staff and team members may be needed. Refusal to eat is a frequent serious problem (99). Letting the children select their own menu, making meals a feeding game, and sharing meals in the company of other children are helpful approaches to this problem.

Discharging the child from the sheltered environment of the burn unit has to be planned with care (58). This is particularly important for children with visible burn scars and for those who have to wear pressure garments, masks, and splints. Nurses, child life, and social workers should visit the school before the child returns. Explaining the problems to teachers and classmates with visual props, such as puppets, helps minimize teasing and creates a warm and accepting environment (44, 93). Day or weekend home visits before final discharge are therapeutic for the child and family and often discover unforeseen difficulties.

The emotional support must continue after discharge and takes many forms. In an effort to address the cosmetic problems associated with burns, Jobst is offering pressure garments in many different shades for children. In one clinic, a make-up artist offers children the same services that are available to adults with facial disfigurements. Children with hair loss can receive hair pieces or whole wigs if they wish. Burn camps are springing up all over the USA with former burn victims frequently working as counselors (94).

Psychological sequelae in patients with major burns have to be expected. Studies have demonstrated that an educated and accepting mother or family and a stable, cohesive home are better predictors of long-term emotional adjustment than site or extent of the burn (9, 12). Young children appear to adjust better than adolescents (83). Fear, anxiety, phobias, and psychosomatic complaints were found in one third of children who had survived major burns, but all showed a great deal of energy in trying to adjust to their disabilities (12, 39). Another study found considerably more overanxious disorders, phobias, and regressive behavior in burned children and adolescents compared to normal controls, but there was no increase in depressive disorders (90).

Burn clinics now generally offer long-term comprehensive follow-up including counseling and emotional support for patients and families. A permanent decline of school performance was reported in 25% of children and adolescents who had sustained burn injuries (16). Visible scars were found to have a profound negative influence on educational adjustment and career planning at adolescence (30).

The management of children with burns requires, therefore, close cooperation between team members with the goal not only of restoration of physical function, but also of emotional recovery and adjustment.

I am indebted to the members of the Burn Team at Children's National Medical Center, Washington, D.C. and to the Occupational Therapists, Cheryl J. Leman, Elizabeth A. Rivers, Mary Beth Daugherty, and Brian Burne, for their valuable suggestions and criticism.

REFERENCES

1. Adriaenssens P, Eggermont E, Pyck K, Boechx W, Gilles B: The video invasion of rehabilitation. *Burns* 14:417, 1988.
2. Alexander RC, Surrell JA, Cohle SD: Microwave oven burns to children: An unusual manifestation of child abuse. *Pediatrics* 79:255, 1987.
3. Alston DW, Kozerefski P, Quan PE, Luterman A: Materials for pressure inserts in the control of hypertrophic scar tissue. *J Burn Care Rehab* 2:40, 1981.
4. Antoon AY, Volpe JJ, Crawford JD: Burn encephalopathy in children. *Pediatrics* 50:609, 1972.
5. Apfel LM, Wachtel TL: Halo neck splint. *J Burn Care Rehab* 8:140, 1987.
6. Bamford MFM, Jones LF: Deafness and biochemical imbalance after burn treatment with topical antibiotics in young children. *Arch Dis Child* 53:326, 1978.
7. Bartlett RH, Wingerson E, Simonton S, Allyn PA, Martinez S, Feinberg SD: Rehabilitation following burn injury. *Surg Clin North Am* 58:1249, 1978.

8. Beales JG: Factors influencing the expectation of pain among patients in a children's burns unit. *Burns* 9:187, 1983.
9. Blakeney P, Herndon DN, Desai MH, Beard S, Wales-Seale P: Longterm psychosocial adjustment following burn injury. *J Burn Care Rehab* 9:661, 1988.
10. Brandt KA: Isolated burn of the palm: A typical injury in the young child. *Handchirurgie* 10:207, 1978.
11. Burke JF, Quinby WC, Bondoc C, McLaughlin E, Trelstad RL: Patterns of high tension electrical injury in children and adolescents and their management. *Am J Surg* 133:492, 1977.
12. Byrne C, Love B, Browne G, Brown B, Roberts J, Streiner D: The social competence of children following burn injury: A study of resilience. *J Burn Care Rehab* 7:247, 1986.
13. Campbell JL, La Clave LJ: Clinical depression in pediatric burn patients. *Burns* 13:213, 1987.
14. Carlow DL, Gelfant B: Head splint for immobilization of the neck post grafting. *J Burn Care Rehab* 7:257, 1986.
15. Cella DF, Perry SW, Poag ME, Amand R, Goodwin D: Depression and stress responses in parents of burned children. *J Pediatr Psychol* 13:87, 1988.
16. Chang FC, Herzog B: Burn morbidity: A follow-up study of physical and psychological disability. *Ann Surg* 183:34, 1976.
17. Colcleugh RG, Ryan JE: Splinting of electrical burns of the mouth in children. *Plast Reconstr Surg* 58:239, 1976.
18. Cole M, Herndon DN, Desai H, Abston S: Gasoline explosions, gasoline sniffing: An epidemic in young adolescents. *J Burn Care Rehab* 7:532, 1986.
19. Crawford CM, Varghese G, Mani MM, Neff JR: Heterotopic ossification: Are range of motion exercises contraindicated? *J Burn Care Rehab* 7:323, 1986.
20. Critchley M: Electrical injuries. *Trans Med Soc Lond* 59:19, 1936.
21. Cronin TD: The use of a molded splint to prevent contracture after split skin grafting of the neck. *Plast Reconstr Surg* 27:7, 1961.
22. Dado DV, Polley W, Kernahan DA: Splinting of oral commissure electrical burns in children. *J Pediatr* 107:92, 1985.
23. Elliott CH, Olson RA: The management of children's distress in response to painful medical treatment for burn injuries. *Behav Res Ther* 21:675, 1983.
24. Evans EB, Smith R: Bone and joint changes following burns. *J Bone Joint Surg* 41A:785, 1959.
25. Farrell DF, Starr A: Delayed neurological sequelae of electrical injuries. *Neurology* 18:601, 1968.
26. Feldman AE, MacMillan BG: Burn injury in children: Declining need for reconstructive surgery as related to the use of neck orthoses. *Arch Phys Med Rehabil* 61:441, 1980.
27. Foerster W: Sequelae of hand burns in early childhood. *Unfallheilkunde* 82:379, 1979.
28. Frantz CH, Delgado S: Limb-length discrepancy after third degree burns about the foot and ankle. *J Bone Joint Surg* 48A:443, 1966.
29. Fujimori R, Hiramoto M, Ofugi S: Sponge fixation method for treatment of early scars. *Plast Reconstr Surg* 42:322, 1968.
30. Goldberg RT: Rehabilitation of the burn patient. *Rehabil Lit* 35:73, 1974.
31. Graham WC: Survival of a severely burned child with bilateral sensorineural deafness from topical antibiotics. *Panminerva Med* 11:44, 1969.
32. Gunn AL: Late complications of burns of the hand in children and their treatment. *Guys Hosp Rep* 119:71080, 1970.
33. Harmel RP Jr, Vane DW, King DR: Burn care in children: Special considerations. *Clin Plast Surg* 13:95, 1986.
34. Harnar T, Engrav L, Heimbach D, Marvin JA: Experience with skeletal immobilization after excision and grafting of severely burned hands. *J Trauma* 25:299, 1985.

35. Helm PA: Neurological involvement in burn injuries. *Arch Phys Med Rehabil* 61:488, 1980.
36. Helm PA, Kevorkian CG, Lushbaugh M, Pullium G, Head MD, Cromes GF: Burn injury: Rehabilitation management in 1982. *Arch Phys Med Rehabil* 63:6, 1982.
37. Helm PA, Pandian G, Heck E: Neuromuscular problems in the burn patient: Cause and prevention. *Arch Phys Med Rehabil* 66:451, 1985.
38. Henderson B, Koepke GH, Feller I: Peripheral polyneuropathy among patients with burns. *Arch Phys Med Rehabil* 52:149, 1971.
39. Herndon DN, LeMaster J, Beard S, Bernstein N, Lewis SR, Rutan TC, Winkler JB, Cole M, Bjarnason D, Gore D, Burke Evans E, Desai M, Linares H, Abston S, Van Osten T: The quality of life after major thermal injury in children: An analysis of 12 survivors with >80% total body, 70% third degree burns. *J Trauma* 26:609, 1986.
40. Huang T, Blackwell SJ, Lewis SR: Ten years experience in managing patients with burn contractures of axilla, elbow, wrist, and knee joint. *Plast Reconstr Surg* 61:70, 1978.
41. Huang T, Larson DL, Lewis SR: Burned Hands. *Plast Reconstr Surg* 56:21, 1975.
42. Hunt JL, Sato RM, Baxter CR: Acute electric burns. *Arch Surg* 115:434, 1980.
43. Kavanagh C: Psychological intervention with the severely burned child: Report of an experimental comparison of two approaches and their effects on psychological sequelae. *J Am Acad Child Psychiatry* 22:145, 1983.
44. Kibbee E: Life after severe burns in children. *J Burn Care Rehab* 2:44, 1981.
45. Kischer CW, Shetlar MR, Chvapil M: Hypertrophic scars and keloids: A review and new concept concerning their origin. *Scanning Electron Microscopy* 4:1699, 1982.
46. Kloeti J, Pochon JP: Conservative treatment using compression suits for second and third degree burns in children. *Burns* 8:180, 1982.
47. Knudson-Cooper MS: Relaxation and biofeedback training in the treatment of severely burned children. *J Burn Care Rehab* 2:102, 1981.
48. Larson DL, Abston S, Evans EB, Dubrkovsky M, Linares H: Techniques for decreasing scar formation and contractures in the burned patient. *J Trauma* 11:807, 1971.
49. Lasoff EM, McEttrick MA: Participation versus diversion during dressing change: Can nurses attitudes change? *Iss Comp Ped Nurs* 9:391, 1986.
50. Leake JE, Curtin JW: Electrical burns of the mouth in children. *Clin Plast Surg* 11:669, 1984.
51. Leman CJ: The triple component neck splint. *J Burn Care Rehab* 7:357, 1986.
52. Levinson P, Ousterhout DK: Art and play therapy with pediatric burn patients. *J Burn Care Rehab* 1:42, 1980.
53. Libber SM, Stayton DJ: Childhood burns reconsidered: The child, the family, and the burn injury. *J Trauma* 24:245, 1984.
54. Long RT, Cope C: Emotional problems of burned children. *N Engl J Med* 264:1121, 1961.
55. Macdonald LB, Covey MH, Marvin JA: The papoose: Device for positioning the burn child's axilla. *J Burn Care Rehab* 6:62, 1985.
56. Mahaney NB: Restoration of play in a severely burned three-year-old child. *J Burn Care Rehab* 11:57, 1990.
57. Malick MH: Flexible Elastomer molds in burn scar control. *Am J Occup Ther* 34:603, 1980.
58. Manger G, Speed E: A coordinated approach to the discharge of burned children. *J Burn Care Rehab* 7:127, 1986.
59. McLoughlin E, Crawford JD: Types of burn injuries. *Pediatr Clin North Am* 32:61, 1985.
60. McManus WF, Hunt JI, Pruitt BA: Postburn convulsive disorders in children. *J Trauma* 14:396, 1974.
61. Meissl G: Primary treatment of electrical burns in children. *Z Kinder Chir* (Suppl) 30:133, 1980.
62. Melhorn JM, Horner RL: Burns of the upper extremity in children: Longterm evaluation of function following treatment. *J Pediatr Orthop* 7:563, 1987.

63. Mohnot D, Snead DC III, Benton JW: Burn encephalopathy in children. *Ann Neurol* 12:42, 1981.
64. Mooney WR, Reed MH: Growth disturbances in the hands following thermal injuries in children. *J Can Assoc Radio* 39:91, 1988.
65. Morrison MIS, Herath K, Chase C: Puppets for prevention: "Playing safe is playing smart". *J Burn Care Rehab* 9:650, 1988.
66. Munster AM, Bruck HM, Johns LA, von Prince K, Kirkman EM, Remig RL: Heterotopic calcification following burns: A prospective study. *J Trauma* 12:1071, 1973.
67. Newmeyer WL, Kilgore ES: Management of the burned hand. *Phys Ther* 57:16, 1977.
68. Newton N, Bubenickova M: Rehabilitation of the autografted hand in children with burns. *Phys Ther* 57:1383, 1977.
69. Noordhoff MS: Control and prevention of hypertrophic scarring and contracture. *Clin Plast Surg* 1:49, 1974.
70. Ortiz-Monasterio F, Factor R: Early definite treatment of electric burns of the mouth. *Plast Reconstr Surg* 65:169, 1980.
71. Osgood PF, Szyfelbein SK: Management of burn pain in children. *Pediatr Clin North Am* 36:1001, 1989.
72. Parish RA, Novack AH, Heimbach DM, Engrav LH: Pediatric patients in a regional burn center. *Pediatr Emerg Care* 2:165, 1986.
73. Parks DH, Evans EB, Larson DL: Prevention and correction of deformity after severe burns. *Surg Clin North Am* 58:1279, 1978.
74. Peterson SL, Mani MM, Crawford CM, Neff JR, Hiebert JM: Postburn heterotopic ossification: Insights for management decision making. *J Trauma* 29:365, 1989.
75. Prekop R, Bardosova G, Simko S, Varady L: Brain oedema in burned children. *Acta Chirurg Plast* 26:184, 1984.
76. Purdue GF, Hunt JL, Prescott PR: Child abuse by burning—an index of suspicion. *J Trauma* 28:221, 1988.
77. Quan PE, Rau SE, Alston DW, Curreri W: Control over scar tissue in the finger web spaces by use of graded pressure inserts. *J Burn Care Rehab* 1:27, 1980.
78. Quinn KJ: Silicone gel in scar treatment. *Burns* 13:533, 1987.
79. Raine PAM, Azmy A: A review of thermal injury in young children. *J Pediatr Surg* 18:21, 1983.
80. Ritsilae V, Sundell B, Alhopuro S: Severe growth retardation of the upper extremity resulting from burn contracture and its full recovery after release of the contracture. *Br J Plast Surg* 29:53, 1976.
81. Rivlin E: The psychological trauma and management of severe burns in children and adolescents. *Br J Hosp Med* 3:210, 1988.
82. Sandel E, Rath Khaleeli C: Use of the thermoplastic total contact and the foam Watusi ring neck splints. Rockville MD, *Am Occ Ther Assoc Newsletter* 2:2, 1981.
83. Sawyer MG, Minde K, Zuker R: The burned child—scarred for life? *Burns* 9:205, 1983.
84. Schubert W, Kuehn C, Moudry B, Miyamoto S, Ahrenholz DH, Solem LD: Halo immobilization in the treatment of burns to the head, face, and neck. *J Burn Care Rehab* 9:187, 1988.
85. Schubert-Walker LJ, Healy M: Psychological treatment of a burned child. *J Pediatr Psychol* 5:395, 1980.
86. Shons AR, Rivers EA, Solem LD: A rigid transparent face mask for control of scar hypertrophy. *Ann Plast Surg* 6:245, 1981.
87. Showers J, Garrison KM: Burn abuse: a four-year study. *J Trauma* 28:1581, 1988.
88. Silverglade D: Splinting electrical burns utilizing a fixed splint technique: A report of 48 cases. *J Dentistry Child* 50:455, 1983.
89. Silversides J: The neurological sequelae of electrical injury. *Can Med Assoc J* 91:195, 1964.

90. Stoddard FJ, Norman DK, Murphy JM, Beardslee WR: Psychiatric outcome of burned children and adolescents. *J Am Acad Child Adolesc Psychiatry* 28:589, 1989.
91. Tepperman PS, Hilbert L, Peters WJ, Pritzker KPH: Heterotopic ossification in burns. *J Burn Care Rehab* 5:283, 1984.
92. Thomson PD, Bowden ML, McDonald K, Smith DJ, Prasad JK: A survey of burn hydrotherapy in the United States. *J Burn Care Rehab* 11:151, 1990.
93. Walls Rosenstein DL: A school reentry program for burned children part I: Development and implementation of a school reentry program. *J Burn Care Rehab* 8:319, 1987.
94. Walls Rosenstein DL: Camp celebrate: A therapeutic weekend camping program for pediatric burn patients. *J Burn Care Rehab* 7:434, 1986.
95. Ward RC, Schnebly WA, Kravitz M, Warden GD, Saffle JR: Have you tried the sandwich splint? A method of preventing hand deformities in children. *J Burn Care Rehab* 10:83, 1989.
96. Warlow CP, Hinton P: Early neurological disturbances following relatively minor burns in children. *Lancet* 2:978, 1969.
97. Wehner D, Hamilton GC: Seizures following topical application of local anesthetics to burn patients. *Ann Emerg Med* 13:456, 1984.
98. Weimer CL, Goldfarb W, Slater H: Multidisciplinary approach to working with burn victims of child abuse. *J Burn Care Rehab* 9:79, 1988.
99. White S, Kamples G: Dietary noncompliance in pediatric patients in the burn unit. *J Burn Care Rehab* 11:167, 1990.
100. Willis BA: Positioning and splinting in the burned patient. *Heart Lung* 2:696, 1973.
101. Wright PC: Fundamentals of acute burn care and physical therapy management. *Phys Ther* 64:1217, 1984.
102. Youel L, Burke Evans E, Heare TC, Herndon DN, Larson DL, Abston S: Skeletal suspension in the management of severe burns in children. *J Bone Joint Surg* 68A:1375, 1986.
103. Zamboni WA, Cassidy M, Eriksson E: Hand burns in children under 5 years of age. *Burns* 13:476, 1987.

17

Skeletal Disorders, Musculoskeletal Pain, and Trauma in Children

JANE C. S. PERRIN AND PHOEBE SATUREN

Physicians responsible for evaluation and management of infants and children at risk for developmental delay must know how to recognize dysmorphic features and how to appraise skeletal abnormalities and trauma as to their prognosis and management or their significance as markers of other pathology.

Deformities in the Neonate

Although skeletal anomalies may be discussed in the literature as isolated problems, it must be recognized that they may represent just part of a multiple malformation syndrome. Deformities arise from a variety of factors. Some stem from heredofamilial influences, including recognizable chromosome defects, or from defined syndromes whose dominant or recessive inheritance is described. Others are due to intrauterine causes. An adverse influence occurring at one point in time may affect several structures at a vulnerable developmental stage causing a collection of associated defects called an anomalad. Evaluation must be complete before definitive information is supplied to the family for similar phenotypes may result from either genetic or prenatal environmental etiologies (20, 32).

The infant must be carefully examined for minor dysmorphic markers, such as low-set ears, transverse palmar creases, or digital defect. The pattern of pathology can warrant additional studies for visceral or metabolic disorders. For example, maldevelopment of the radial side of the forearm varying from mild hypoplasia of a proximally located thumb to total aplasia of the radius can be associated with cardiac defects (Holt-Oram syndrome), thrombocytopenia, renal defects, and many other anomalies. In contrast, deficiencies of the ulna are usually sporadic.

An example of a skeletal defect attributed to a single gene disorder with Mendelian inheritance is cleidocranial dysostosis (aplasia of the clavicles with other osseous and dental abnormalities), an autosomal dominant defect with incomplete penetrance. A male infant with hydrocephalus manifested at birth, who has thumbs flexed at the metacarpophalangeal joint, can have the sex-linked syndrome; there is a poor developmental prognosis for the infant and predictable recurrence rate far greater than the usual types of congenital hydrocephalus.

In contrast, isolated anomalies, if genetic, such as clubfoot, often have multifactorial inheritance patterns. Statistical probability of recurrence is based on the number of known affected relatives. Recurrence risk in an isolated case is slightly greater than the general population, depending on the gene frequency of the defect.

The teratogenetic effects of maternal exposure to viral infection, such as rubella or toxoplasmosis, are well described. Maternal alcohol ingestion results in the more subtle features of the fetal alcohol syndrome—an infant with developmental delay and characteristic facies including short palpebral fissures and broad nasal bridge. Limb defects can be minor, such as mild digit contractures and hypoplastic toenails, or, occasionally, more severe, including radioulnar dystosis or hip dislocation (51).

A variety of abnormalities, usually asymmetric and atypical, have been attributed to early fetal compression from amniotic fluid loss or entanglement by fibrotic amniotic bands. Deep grooves encircling an extremity (Streeter's bands) occasionally produce postnatal compression. Limb deficiencies and facial clefts have been described.

Some abnormalities that are more benign but may look startling at birth are caused by intrauterine molding, especially where there has been oligohydramnios. Examples include a hollow in the neck and apparent mandibular defect when a shoulder has compressed the side of the chin or hyperextension of the knees after frank breech presentation. The baby can usually be "folded," i.e., positioned to reproduce the uterine posture that caused the compression. These deformities are usually transient and will respond to simple passive range of motion or serial splinting.

Neonates born prematurely or with multiple malformations may need intensive care for respiratory or other life-threatening problems and it may be necessary to defer therapy for a skeletal defect. However, the joint laxity of the neonate offers an opportunity for effective correction of an abnormality by simple conservative means, such as splinting or range of motion, during the first few weeks that is never regained.

Even when the outlook for independence is guarded, early intervention for treatment of abnormalities such as talipes equinovarus can spare the child from repeated surgeries later in life, causing disruption of schooling programs or deferral of standing or ambulation. Now that rehabilitation intervention is becoming routine in neonatal units, physiatrists have an opportunity to institute early treatment or to encourage their orthopaedic colleagues to initiate early serial casting. Padded splints can be used, even for tiny premature infants and can be effective even though they are applied intermittently on a 2-hour on-off schedule to protect their tender skin.

Later, orthopaedic management of skeletal disorders must be incorporated into a total plan or care. Hospitalization must be timed in relation to therapeutic intervention for other problems and to school attendance. Postoperative therapy must be planned, splinting as well as range of motion and activation begun as early as possible, orthoses and mobility aids planned for and funded, and, above all, hospital stays kept short by providing home or outpatient rehabilitation services as soon as feasible.

Gait Deviations

Infants just beginning to toddle have a stiff, broad-based, and slightly flexed-knee gait that may evolve into patterns that are the cause of much parental concern but that are actually normal variants or somewhat delayed evolution of mature skeletal alignment. Sometimes malalignment can be multiple in femur, tibia, and foot. Children with hypotonia and ambulation delay are even more likely to exhibit deviant gait patterns, possibly due to prolonged and atypical postures in supine and prone positions and to late weight-bearing as a stimulus to osseous molding. For adequate evaluation, the child must be fully undressed and the gait observed, looking for the width of supporting base, line of progression, symmetry, and attention paid, in succession, to the hip, knee, and foot (62).

FEMORAL ANTEVERSION

In normal infant development, the angle made by the neck of the femur with the shaft increases from relative coxa valga to coxa vara, delayed when standing and walking are not achieved. The transcervical angle of the femur in the frontal plane related to the transcondylar axis is normally 40° at birth decreasing to 15° by adolescence (Fig. 17.1). When this angle caused by the torsion of the femoral shaft remains increased, the child walks with hips in internal rotation and patellae facing medially. Passive internal rotation of the hips, best tested in the prone position, is increased. X-ray measurement is difficult, although a CAT scan can assess the degree.

Prolonged sleeping postures with the feet tucked under the buttocks or "kneel" sitting or "W" sitting have been incriminated. Exercises and orthoses, such as cable twisters, cannot correct the deformity and are believed to cause external tibial torsion. The alignment improves with growth (66) and the deviation is rarely handicapping (30, 61). Surgical correction (63), which requires femoral osteotomy, is very rarely justified although it may be indicated when cerebral palsy and risk of hip dislocation are present as well.

HEAD-NECK ANGLE:

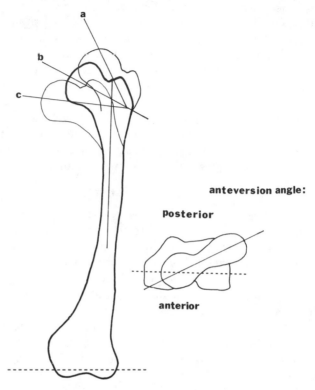

Figure 17.1. Angle of neck-shaft and anteversion of the femur. *A,* increased, coxa valga; *B,* normal; *C,* decreased, coxa vara. The *smaller diagram* shows a top view relating a line drawn from left to right through the greater trochanter and femoral head *(solid line)* to the transcondylar femoral axis distally *(dotted line).*

FEMORAL RETROVERSION

Familial patterns of out-toeing gait caused by hip external rotation stemming from femoral retroversion are common. Obesity and conditions associated with hypotonia, such as Down's syndrome, can also be causative factors; genu valgum can be an additional problem. Discouraging contributory sitting or sleeping patterns can be tried but the deviation usually should be accepted without wasteful attempts at therapy.

INTERNAL TIBIAL TORSION

The normal infantile inward rotation of the tibia—a twisting of the shaft—may persist in the toddler years producing a unilateral or bilateral toe-in gait pattern. It can be tested with the child prone, with knees flexed, observing the relationship of the femoral shaft to the midline of the plantar surface of the foot. The child can also be sitting with knees at 90° over the table edge. With the patella in midline, the lateral malleolus will be *anterior* to the frontal plane of the distal tibia; the medial malleolus is more posterior. Normal maturation will eventually result in the adult configuration with the lateral malleolus about 15° posterior to the medial malleolus.

This common problem is frequently treated by or in fact, overtreated by shoe modifications, such as wedges, special inserts, straight lasts, torque heel, or by twisters or night braces.

Efficacy of any of these interventions is unproven (61).

LATERAL TIBIAL BOWING

Although usually physiological in the infant and likely to resolve in time, tibia vara associated with a localized abnormality of the proximal medial tibial epiphysis and metaphysis (Blount's disease) is not likely to self-correct. Intrinsic bone pathology, such as rickets or epiphyseal trauma, should be ruled out.

If the diagnosis is made and confirmed by x-ray, bracing, with night-time trial initially followed by use during the day may resolve the problem and surgery will be avoided. Knee-ankle orthoses with lateral proximal tibial pullers and free ankle joints can be prescribed when the child is under 3 yr but are not likely to be effective later. Tibial osteotomies should be considered only after follow-up reveals insufficient spontaneous improvement (19).

Abnormalities of the Foot

PES PLANUS

The infant's foot may look flat because of the fat pad along the medial arch. Later, mobile flattening of the plantar arch is very common and not handicapping. It is not altered by orthopaedic shoes, scaphoid pads, or heel cups (75).

Children with hypotonia, however, can have such laxity that pronation of the foot eventually becomes severe enough to cause weight-bearing on the medial malleolus. Progression to hallux valgus and bunions in adult life cause problems with shoe fitting and foot pain. Prescription of sturdy shoes with firm counters and molded inserts to support the talus can be useful for toddlers. During early standing, therapists can fashion small ankle-foot orthoses (AFOs) of aquaplat. More supportive AFOs or supramalleolar orthoses can be prescribed for fabrication by an orthotist after the child is age 3 yr. Children are likely to find orthotics that can be used with sneakers more acceptable than orthopaedic shoes.

CONGENITAL PES VALGUS

Congenital rigid flatfoot with vertical talus is associated with other malformations in 50% of cases. In infancy, the sole of the foot is convex, the heel is in equinus and is not correctable manually. Later, during stance, angulation of the medial border of the foot with weight-bearing on the midfoot causes "rockerbottom" deformity. Although a normal heel-toe pattern is not possible, the foot is relatively stable. Correction requires surgery. Shoe inserts should be prescribed only to relieve pressure areas. The abnormality can be accepted and should be when ambulation is limited, when the foot is painless, or when intervention is delayed (59).

CONGENITAL CLUBFOOT

Talipes equinovarus presents, as the name implies, with inversion and adduction of the forefoot, inversion of the heel, and equinus. The talus is malformed, the navicular is displaced medially, leg and foot muscles are atrophic, and shortening is common. Malformation syndromes should be looked for and hips checked for subluxation. Later, untreated equinovarus deformity caused by muscle imbalance secondary to neuromuscular disorders, such as cerebral palsy, muscular dystrophy, or myelodysplasia can be confused with primary talipes. Correction can be difficult if arthrogryposis is a factor.

Serial casting, begun as early as possible after birth, is the most common orthopaedic treatment, with multiple soft-tissue releases performed after 3 to 6 months if tight structures prevent successful manipulation (75). Maintenance of correction by the use of Dennis-Brown bars or dynamic AFOs is essential and must be continued throughout early childhood. Although recurrent deformity may be caused by inadequacy of surgery or postoperative care, it is important to be sure that an occult neurological disorder, such as diastomatomyelia with tethering of the spinal cord, has not been overlooked.

Persistent equinovarus results in an unstable foot, liable to pain due to pressure on the outer sole border and recurrent ankle sprains. Even nonambulatory children are further handicapped because of problems with shoe fitting, difficulty with weight-bearing transfers, or pressure areas on the lateral malleoli from wheelchair pedals. Early splinting and surgical correction can spare the child from much discomfort later, even in the presence of progressive impairments.

PES CAVUS

The presence of a high rigid arch due to fixed equinus of the forefoot on the hindfoot accompanied by flexed "clawed" toes is occasionally seen as a congenital malformation but is more common in neurological disorders resulting in weakness of intrinsic foot musculature. Spinocerebellar syndromes and occult diastomatomyelia are examples. Shoe prescriptions providing support just behind the metatarsal heads by pads or bars on the outside of the soles and high toe box to create adequate toe room can prevent development of painful calluses. An AFO may be necessary for stability. Surgery can be considered, even in slowly progressive conditions.

Affections of the Hip Joint

SUBLUXATION AND DISLOCATION

Of congenital hip subluxations, 90% are the *typical* type, affecting girls seven times more often than boys. The left hip is more often involved and there is a frequent history of breech delivery. The acetabulum is normal at birth and the subluxation is possibly related to the custom of keeping the infant swaddled with hips extended.

However, the *teratological* type is associated with a malformed, shallow acetabulum filled with fibrofatty tissue; it presents a more difficult treatment problem and is associated with other anomalies, especially with arthrogryposis.

Neonatal screening, either clinically or by ultrasound, has markedly reduced the need for complex salvage surgery and the incidence of late complications of acetabular dysplasia such as surgically related avascular necrosis of the femoral head, shortening and osteoarthritis in adult life.

Initially, the instability of the hip may only be evident clinically by the palpable sensation of a "click" as the hip is gently flexed and abducted (Ortolani's sign) or slowly maneuvered into adduction bringing the head over the acetabular rim (Barlow's sign) (28).

With progression toward complete dislocation, hip abduction becomes limited, and asymmetry of thigh creases and apparent femoral shortening are noted. A toddler will walk with a *Trendelenburg* gait, shifting the trunk laterally over the affected hip during the stance phase. If bilateral, the gait deviation has been described as a "duck waddle."

X-rays may show poor development of the femoral head. Signs of displacement of the head from its normal position in the acetabulum include an increased acetabular index, discontinuity of the Shenton's line, or location outside of the lower medial quadrant of the joint space (Fig. 17.2). In neonates, ultrasonography can show dysplasia in the presence of a normal clinical examination. Later, arthrogram or CAT scan can verify displacement and show the presence of a redundant capsule that can interfere with conservative means of reduction.

Treatment in the neonate begins as soon as the clinical diagnosis is suspected since initial x-rays may not be helpful (44). A device should be utilized that places the hips in 90° flexion and 45° abduction. Wider abduction has been incriminated as a cause of avascular necrosis of the femoral head. The Pavlik harness, made of adjustable webbing straps, is commonly used and is effective provided the mother is carefully instructed in its application (24).

Persistent subluxation after 3 to 4 months usually requires reduction

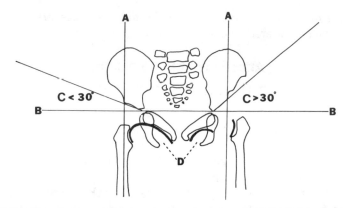

Figure 17.2. Roentgenographic evaluation in congenital hip dislocation. *A,* Perkins vertical line, perpendicular dropped from the lateral acetabular margin. *B,* Hilgenreiner's line, through the "Y" cartilages. The femoral head should lie in the lower medial quadrant formed by the intersection of the two lines. *C,* acetabular index, the angle formed by a line through the acetabular roof and Hilgenreiner's line; normal below 30°. *D,* Shenton's line, the arc will appear broken in the presence of dislocation. The abnormal hip appears on the right.

under anesthesia and tenotomy of tight musculature followed by application of a spica cast. Management of a child in a spica requires careful monitoring for evidence of pressure areas. An adapted infant seat or floor scooter that allows the child some mobility to explore, continued participation in developmental programs, or use of home services can minimize the deprivation and emotional consequences of prolonged immobilization.

Dysplasia or displacement persisting after age 2 yr calls for further orthopaedic intervention. Realignment of the acetabular roof using a wedge of iliac bone (Salter innominate osteotomy) and proximal femoral varus derotation osteotomy to correct coxa valga are commonly used procedures.

Late-onset subluxation and eventual dislocation accompany muscle imbalance caused by spasticity or weakness in many neuromuscular conditions, especially when strong hip flexor and adductor muscles overpower weak extensors and abductors and when delayed weight-bearing prevents the maturation of the neck-shaft alignment toward coxa vara. The importance of clinical examination of the hip joint whenever an infant or child with a developmental disorder is seen cannot be overemphasized. Early therapeutic intervention for congenital or paralytic hip dislocation can prevent either a painful, awkward gait deviation in the ambulatory child or avoid pressure problems caused by asymmetrical sitting posture in the wheelchair-bound individual (8, 29).

LEGG-CALVÉ-PERTHES DISEASE (JUVENILE COXA PLANA)

Avascular necrosis of the femoral capital epiphysis usually begins between 4 and 8 years of age and is five times more frequent in boys than girls. Affected youngsters may have histories of lower birth weights, short stature, or delayed bone age. Although vascular causes have been postulated, etiology is unknown. Effusion in the hips, such as occurs in idiopathic transient synovitis, may cause tamponade of the retinacular vessels of the joint capsule, compromising blood supply.

Stages in the natural course are summarized in Table 17.1. Prognosis for reconstitution of the femoral head depends on the age of onset. It is better if the child is younger than 5 yr and when the head is only partially involved and does not undergo severe collapse. Although healing invariably occurs, persistent deformation of the femoral head leads to late degenerative hip disease.

Differential diagnosis during the early synovitis stage includes sepsis of the hip. Other diagnostic possibilities include sickle cell anemia, slipped capital femoral epiphysis, congenital hip dislocation, rheumatoid arthritis and other collagen diseases, steroid therapy, and, if bilateral, multiple epiphyseal dysplasia. Some authors recommend Technetium-99 bone scintigraphy for diagnostic purposes (13).

Onset can be insidious with a limp, pain in the hip referred to the medial thigh or knee, and limitation of abduction, internal rotation, and extension.

During the early *synovitis* stage, while diagnostic studies are underway, bedrest in traction should be accompanied by daily active and active-assistive exercises until pain and spasm subside, usually requiring up to 3 weeks.

Once there is *full range of passive motion*, containment therapy is planned. Older systems of treatment by prolonged bedrest or nonweight-bearing crutch-walking have been discarded. Children between 4 and 8 yr old are candidates for using orthotics to achieve acetabular coverage of the femoral head while permitting ambulation. The efficacy of any device must be checked by serial standing anteroposterior x-rays to verify that the head is well seated.

Petrie casts, long-leg plasters with an abducting broomstick, are inexpensive and cannot be removed but can stress medial knee ligaments after prolonged use. With a qualified orthotist and cooperative family available, the Tachdjian orthosis with its molded thigh socket and Patten bottom can maintain the hip in desired abduction-internal rotation. The Atlanta Scot-

Table 17.1.
Clinical Course of Legg-Perthes Disease

	Duration	X-Ray Findings
Synovitis	1–3 weeks	Effusion only
Necrosis	1 month–1 yr	Increased density of head
Regeneration or fragmentation	3 months–2 yr	Areas of variable density, collapse of all or part of head, subluxation
Residual or healed		Restoration of sphericity or coxa magna and late degenerative arthritis

tish Rite orthosis, consisting of pelvic band, hip joints set in abduction, and thigh cuffs is well accepted (16). Other braces, such as the Toronto or Newington orthoses, are bulkier and require the use of a gait aid.

When necrosis is severe or the child is past age 8 years, containment is achieved surgically, utilizing either Salter innominate osteotomy or femoral osteotomy. Surgery can compress a 2- or 3-yr treatment program into 8 to 12 weeks, but complications including permanent shortening and limp can result (74). Postoperatively, physical therapy is important to restore full motion and strength to the hip joint. Follow-up is essential because, if the hip fails to remodel postoperatively, further orthotic management may be warranted (57, 69).

SLIPPED CAPITAL FEMORAL EPIPHYSIS

Posteroinferior displacement of the femoral capital epiphysis can occur acutely after trauma or a fall or, gradually, with progressing limp, pain radiating down the medial thigh to the knee, and limitation of internal rotation and adduction. Boys are more usually affected during rapid, early adolescent growth with peak incidence at 13 yr. Involvement is bilateral in about 25% of the cases. Obesity or, conversely, a tall-thin habitus may be associated, implicating endocrine factors. The epiphysis may become more vulnerable at a time when its orientation changes from a horizontal to a more oblique plane. Slippage can complicate hypothyroidism, renal osteodystrophy, and Prader-Willi syndrome.

X-rays done in the preslip stage show widening and rarefaction of the epiphyseal plate. Early evidence of slip shows loss of projection of the curve of the head above the neck and alteration of Shenton's line. Frog lateral films are essential to see early changes. CT scan can quantify displacement of the head and the degree of closure of the epiphysis. With chronic displacement, a hump may appear in the anterosuperior margin of the femoral neck producing a mechanical impediment to range of motion.

The best results in treatment occur when the head and neck can be fixed in situ and slip is minimal. Outcome is poorer in severe slips (more than ⅔ displacement of the head) or when manipulation of the epiphysis to relocate is needed.

Postoperatively, vigorous active-assistive exercise to restore flexion, abduction, and internal rotation should be prescribed. Curtailment of full weight-bearing for up to three months and contact sports participation until the epiphysis has closed, is recommended. A weight reduction regimen and follow-up of the status of the opposite hip are important.

Chondrolysis or acute cartilage necrosis can be the cause of persistent postoperative pain and increasing loss of motion. X-ray shows narrowing of the joint space. Prolonged vigorous range of motion therapy can result in gradual improvement of mobility. Another complication seen after surgical manipulation of the epiphysis is avascular necrosis (15).

Leg Length Discrepancy

Leg-length discrepancies can result from congenital malformations, such as absence of the fibula, infections, or trauma affecting the epiphyses, or neurologic disorders with asymmetric involvement, such as poliomyelitis.

Minor shortening has not been proven as a cause of back disorders, structural scoliosis, or degenerative arthritis. In fact, mild shortening, as occurs in early onset spastic hemiplegia can be an advantage, facilitating swing-through of a weaker leg during the gait cycle. If more severe, there is some increase in energy cost of walking and cosmesis of ambulation can be impaired (25).

Discrepancy of less than 2 cm can be accepted and shortening from 2 to 5 cm can be managed by shoe lift. When epiphyseal disruption is known, serial measurements of discrepancy correlated with bone age are essential for planning of future management. Clinical measurement of length whether "actual"—from anterosuperior iliac spines to medial malleoli—or "apparent"—from umbilicus to medial malleoli—are prone to error (6). Correlation of x-ray scanogram or CT scan measurements with estimates of predicted growth using the Greulich-Pyle or Tanner-Whitehouse Atlases based on hand films are done.

Moderate discrepancies of 5 to 10 cm can be treated by epiphysiodesis of distal femoral or proximal tibia on the normal side. Although potential for complications is great and morbidity is prolonged, lengthening the involved limb using techniques, such as developed by Wagner and Ilizarov, permit ambulation following osteotomy and external fixation with gradual distraction of severed bone ends (53).

Decision-making cannot be based dogmatically on numbers of centimeters involved but are related to overall height, associated deformities, weakness, and social factors. When shortening will ultimately be severe (over 15 cm), ablation of the foot by Symes or below-knee amputation and prosthetic fitting is an option, preferably in infancy. Bulky, awkward shoe build-ups and prolonged or multiple surgeries are avoided; a functional and cosmetic gait will result (48).

SCOLIOSIS

Progressive spinal curvature is idiopathic in over 85% of cases, but can be secondary to neuromuscular, generalized skeletal, or connective tissue pathology. Table 17.2, abridged from the Scoliosis Research Society classification, shows the wide variety of disorders that can affect the growing spine.

Infantile Idiopathic Scoliosis

Spinal curvature present before three years of age is designated as infantile scoliosis. Spontaneous improvement is the usual course unless there are

Table 17.2.
Classification of Scoliosis

Nonstructural	
Postural	
Compensatory due to leg-length discrepancy, hip flexion contracture, nerve root irritation, extravertebral irritation, hysterical	
Structural	
Idiopathic (genetic)	Infantile, juvenile, adolescent
Congenital	Vertebral defects—spina bifida, fused, wedged, hemivertebrae
Neuromuscular	Upper motor neuron—cerebral palsy, spinocerebellar disorder
	Lower motor neuron—spinal muscular atrophy
	Myopathic—muscular dystrophy
Neurofibromatosis	
Mesenchymal	Marfan's syndrome, Ehler's-Danlos syndrome
Traumatic	Postfracture, early laminectomy, thoracic burns
Osteochondrodystrophies	
Miscellaneous	Metabolic disorders, tumors

congenital spinal malformations, such as fused or hemivertebrae, that can produce a severe progressive curve. These cases require aggressive treatment (36).

Adolescent Idiopathic Scoliosis

Adolescent idiopathic scoliosis (43) has a female to male ratio of 8 to 1 and is thought to be of genetic origin. The most common inheritance pattern is autosomal dominant with incomplete penetrance. Now that intervention is done for most scoliosis, the outcome of untreated curves in adult life is not entirely clear, but it appears that although the incidence of back pain is not increased, progression of a thoracic curve beyond 60° is associated with impaired cardiopulmonary function in adult life. Curves beyond 50° at skeletal maturity continue to progress over the years. School screening programs for scoliosis have certainly led to earlier intervention than ever before but may have resulted in a significant number of over-referrals of youngsters with curves of little or no significance (42).

Inspection for scoliosis should be part of all routine physical examinations. Observation of the back with the child standing should include notation of shoulder asymmetry, pelvic obliquity, elevation of the iliac crest or an exaggerated crease in the flank. Anteriorly, a breast may appear enlarged because of rotational deformity of the thorax. On forward bending, a rib hump appears on the convexity of the thoracic curve and paraspinal muscles are prominent on the lumbar convexity.

Complete neurological evaluation and inspection for skin lesions, such as café-au-lait spots indicative of neurofibromatosis, or a midline hairy patch overlying a spinal anomaly, leg-length discrepancy, or hip or knee contracture are essential (34).

An x-ray consisting of a standing anteroposterior view with breast shielding usually suffices. The Cobb technique is commonly used to measure a curve (Fig. 17.3). All curves include some rotation, with right thoracic and right thoracic-left lumbar patterns being most common.

The most rapid progression occurs during the peak pubertal growth spurt—about 1 yr before onset of menses in girls and when testicular enlargement begins in boys so that Tanner staging and estimation of skeletal maturity are essential for treatment planning. Spine growth is complete when the iliac apophyses have united to the crests and vertebral ring epiphyses have fused—after age 16 to 17 yr.

Treatment cannot be based on rigid criteria as to the number of degrees in a curve since variation in growth rates, years of growth remaining at the time of diagnosis, potential for progression of different curve patterns, the diagnosis of an underlying etiology, such as neuromuscular disease, and the likelihood of compliance with therapy all affect decision-making. For example, a thoracic curve with associated neurofibromatosis requires early fusion, while fusion of a long curve before maturity carries an increased risk of pseudoarthrosis. As a rule of thumb, curves less than 20° can be observed, with studies at 6-month intervals while curves more than 50° cannot be managed by brace treatment. The orthopedist must be primarily responsible for following the patient from the time of initial diagnosis since he/she is responsible for the timing as well as the performance of surgery (37).

Molded thoraco-lumbosacral orthoses (TLSO) are now commonly prescribed for curves with apices below T7 while the Milwaukee brace is indicated for higher curves and for adolescent kyphosis. Acceptance of brace treatment requires close supportive counseling of these teenagers and com-

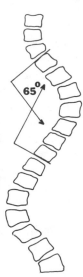

Figure 17.3. The Cobb method of measuring the curvature in scoliosis. The angle measured is formed by perpendicular lines dropped from the lines drawn through the superior border of the upper vertebra and the inferior border of the lowest vertebra of the given curve.

pliance has improved in clinics where braces are prescribed for 16-h use, permitting school attendance during the day without the appliance. Implanted or transcutaneous electrical stimulation of paraspinal muscles has not proven to be of benefit (77).

Exercise alone *cannot* correct a scoliotic curve, but it is an integral part of brace treatment, maintaining flexibility and strength of the trunk musculature. Abdominal muscle strengthening, pelvic tilts, flattening of the lumbar lordosis, and segmental exercise to teach the patient how to pull away from the corrective pads should be taught. The youngster in a brace can participate in many sports other than contact sports; swimming is especially recommended.

Some curves will progress despite consistent brace use, so the patient should never be promised that surgery can be avoided. Surgery for idiopathic scoliosis most commonly consists of fusion with posterior instrumentation. Correction of neuromuscular scoliosis has now become feasible, even in the face of marked weakness and severe curvature by the use of the Luque segmental spine stabilization and combinations of anterior and posterior stabilization utilizing instrumentation developed by Dwyer, Zielke, and Cotrel-Dubousset. Patients with progressive conditions, such as muscular dystrophy or juvenile spinal muscular atrophy, should be considered for intervention when curves increase beyond 30° if they are sufficiently mature, since bracing alone cannot stabilize a neurogenic curve. Maintenance of stable sitting and pulmonary function can be achieved even as weakness progresses.

Constitutional or Intrinsic Bone Disease

Some 100 osseous disorders of probable heritable etiology have been described. They are classified as to the variability in body proportions, i.e., whether limbs alone or the skull and trunk are also affected or as to the nature of the metabolic abnormality in skeletal development (76). Achondroplasia is an example of abnormal head and limb growth manifested at birth, while osteogenesis imperfecta exemplifies an abnormality of density, diaphyseal and metaphyseal modeling due to impairment of osteoid formation. Disorders of calcium-phosporus metabolism, whether caused by vitamin D deficiency, either dietary or from a genetic defect in its metabolism, parathyroid disease, or renal osteodystrophy, produce generalized abnormalities in bone formation, short stature, or susceptibility to progressive deformity with growth.

Secondary complications are common in many types of dwarfing syndromes and should be thought of in the evaluation of any youngster with skeletal dysplasia (60).

Susceptibility to fracture is most dramatic in osteogenesis imperfecta but occurs in fibrous dysplasia and whenever there is osteopenia secondary to neurological, rheumatological or hematological disorders, such as thalassemia or sickle cell anemia. In the severe form of osteogenesis imperfecta, fractures can occur in the course of ordinary handling and, although they heal, sometimes with exuberant callus, multiple angular deformities and dwarfing occur as the breaks continue. Hypotonia, hypermetabolism with increased seating, capillary fragility, and hearing loss due to otosclerosis are associated problems.

The infant can be nursed on a padded bed with longitudinal splinting of the extremities and padded head support. As the child grows, protective orthoses that encase the limb with either plastic shells or extended leather cuffs can provide protection. When bones are very fragile, weight-bearing may not be feasible until adolescence, when frequency of fractures diminishes. Mat exercises to develop muscle strength and wheelchair training should be prescribed. Intramedullary rodding of the long bones helps preserve alignment but may need to be repeated. Extensible rods are now available.

The cervical spine is often affected in skeletal disorders. There may be maldevelopment of the odontoid, excessive laxity of the transverse odontoid ligament or accumulation of an abnormal substance within, or hypertrophy of the longitudinal ligaments.

Atlantoaxial instability is seen in the short-trunked syndromes, such as Morquio's disease. Asymptomatic instability has been reported in up to 20% of children with Down's syndrome although clinical symptoms are rare. Onset of symptomatic C1-C2 subluxation may be insidious with fatigability as the only early sign. Later evidence of spasticity appears, first in the lower extremities, and the child may refuse to walk. Lateral views of the cervical spine in extension and flexion must be taken, with CAT scan for verification. The ambulation difficulty should not be attributed to lower extremity deformities since timely posterior fusion of C1-C2 can prevent disastrous progression to quadriplegia.

Thoracolumbar kyphoscoliosis can appear early and bracing can be difficult due to the short trunk and rigid curves. Insertion of distraction rods without spine fusion may gain time before skeletal maturity. Lumbar spine deformity can be associated with symptoms of spinal stenosis.

Hip deformities, such as limited extension, and x-ray findings resembling avascular necrosis may occur, but the abnormal architecture seen on films may not be associated with much functional limitation. Bracing for angular and rotational limb deformities is poorly tolerated and not often successful. Surgical intervention, such as osteotomy, must be carefully planned, since any resulting limitation of range of motion can compound disability, interfering with stair climbing and dressing activities.

Most individuals with short stature are of normal intelligence but, too often, are perceived by others as either younger than their chronological age or as retarded. It is important that there be recognition of the child's maturity and capacities and of the emotional problems that can ensue when a child must deal with a very visible impairment.

Skeletal Neoplasms

Advances in diagnosis, staging of disease, and chemotherapy have markedly altered the prognosis for survival in childhood malignancy. Primary osseous malignant tumors had a cure rate below 20% before 1970, while, at present, disease-free 5-yr survival rates as high as 85% are being reported from centers where vigorous treatment regimens are offered (18).

Osteosarcoma occurs most often during the adolescent growth spurt, with a male to female ratio of 1.5 to 1. The initial presenting complaint is usually pain, followed in frequency by the presence of a mass. Sites of predilection are the distal femur, proximal tibia, and proximal humerus, with metastases to the lung the most likely cause of death. Classical x-ray findings consist of a mixed lytic and sclerotic lesion near the metaphysis, cortical invasion, periosteal elevation, and soft tissue extension with spicules radiating out from the bone, producing a "sunburst" appearance. Ewing's tumor, also more common in boys but rare in black children, is seen in the long bone diaphyses and the pelvis. Tumor growth can be so rapid that the center becomes necrotic and osteomyelitis is diagnosed.

Differential diagnosis, staging, and evaluation of histopathology require special expertise available in centers where there is a well-developed oncology program. In addition to x-ray, angiography, CT scan, and Technetium-99 scintigraphy, MRI (26) is useful to delineate the intramedullary and soft tissue involvement. Biopsy study may include electron microscopy. Before surgery is performed, an initial course of chemotherapy can document the tumor's sensitivity to the chosen combination. The use of high-dose methotrexate with citrovorum rescue combined with multiple agents has revolutionized osteogenic sarcoma treatment, while Ewing tumor still includes radiation among the therapeutic options. The prolonged, intermittent cycles of treatment extending over a year are associated with many side effects, alopecia, bone marrow depression, nausea, peripheral neuropathy requiring close supervision. Children, however, tolerate the therapies remarkably well, and often spend intervals at home and can even return to school.

Because of the improved resectability of lesions following preoperative treatment, limb-sparing procedures are now available as alternatives to amputation. The physiatrist can assist in family counseling when treatment options are available. Damage to epiphyses from irradiation or resection makes amputation more appropriate for children under 8 yr. An amputation can be a more realistic decision for some youngsters, permitting rapid mobilization, cosmesis, and decreased morbidity.

Interim rehabilitation services can be given in the home community when a cancer center is at a distance. Liaison among treatment agencies is essential and a child's activities must be monitored so that symptoms of complications can be noted, but overprotection and isolation can be avoided (35).

Musculoskeletal Pain and Trauma

Spine or extremity pain from injury or disease in childhood usually presents with tenderness, decreased range of motion, swelling, weakness, or altered function, such as refusal to walk.

Causes of childhood musculoskeletal pain, which may be difficult to diagnose, are sickle cell infarcts, reflex sympathetic dystrophy (RSD) after minor injury (4), bilateral nocturnal leg pain gone by morning (growing pain), fibromyalgia with sleep disturbance and morning stiffness, recurrent extremity pain in children with ligamentous laxity (juvenile episodic arthritis-arthralgia) (21), and conversion symptoms producing pain in a nonanatomic distribution.

Pain response varies with age and family. Young children react with crying, refusal to move the painful part, clinging to a parent from whom separation causes fear and anxiety. The 3-yr-old to 4-yr-old can describe and localize the pain if encouraged. By age 6 yr, the child can score pain on a 10-cm line from zero to ten, no pain to worst possible pain (71).

Pain treatment requires careful explanation to the child and parent. As with adults, treatment of chronic pain ranges from medications, physical modalities, transcutaneous nerve stimulation (TENS), to behavior techniques including muscle relaxation, meditation/mental imagery, and biofeedback. Nonsteroidal anti-inflammatory drugs, analgesics, antidepressants, and narcotics including patient control analgesia (PCA) for older children and adolescents with unremitting pain should be given in adequate doses and frequency based on body weight or surface area and age (71).

INJURIES

Children suffer intentional and unintentional injuries. Intentional trauma is inflicted or self-inflicted from risk-taking (hood surfing on cars), inappropriate sports, such as boxing, suicide attempts, or child abuse.

Of the 22 million children injured each year in the United States, more than one million are abused (9, 14). The leading causes of death from child abuse are head and abdominal hollow viscus injuries, but injuries range from scalds and burns to retinal detachment of the shaken baby syndrome, sexual abuse, soft tissue trauma, avulsions, and fractures in various stages of healing.

Reporting suspicion of child abuse to authorities is obligatory. The preschooler with young, previously abused parents is at greatest risk. Handicapped infants and children are especially vulnerable. Careful follow-up of abused children who are returned home is imperative.

Even unintentional serious injuries occur disproportionately in some families, with school-aged boys 6 to 14 yr at greatest risk (58). Most common causes of trauma are falls from stairs (31), windows (47), roofs, walls, trees, or horses (5); accidents with farm machinery (67); vehicular injuries, including pedestrian, motor vehicle, motorcycle, bicycle (10), and all terrain vehicles (2); and sports.

In high school sports, football and gymnastics have the highest injury rates (46): 10 thousand head and neck injuries per year in football (72); spine and upper extremity injuries predominate in gymnastics (79). Head and spinal cord injuries are discussed elsewhere in this text. Major spine trauma is the purview of the orthopaedist (49, 68).

Acute Injuries: Fractures, Sprains, Strains, Contusions

FRACTURES

Growth plate (physis) tenderness after trauma is likely to be growth plate injury, not a sprain. The cartilaginous physis and epiphysis will separate before a ligament tears (12). The Salter-Harris classification of epiphyseal plate fractures is a guide for treatment and prognosis for growth impairment. Type I epiphyseal separation without displacement and Type II epiphyseal separation with a fragment of metaphysis are usually stable or easily reducible and growth is usually unimpaired. Type III and Type IV are intra-articular fractures with partial plate injuries usually requiring open reduction to prevent disturbance of growth and promote joint mobility. Type V from axial compression may also disturb growth (Fig. 17.4).

Management of the child with suspected fracture includes neurovascular examination, splinting for radiographs, and referral to the orthopaedist.

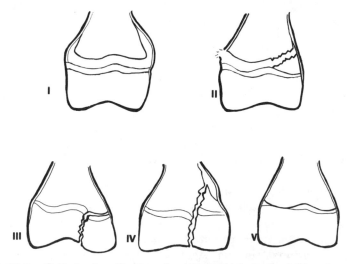

Figure 17.4. Salter's classification of epiphyseal injuries in children types I to V.

Traction or compression neuropathies are most common with compartment syndromes and with distal humeral supracondylar fractures.

Fracture healing is rapid and joint stiffness of an intact joint after casting is unusual in the child. Remolding of well-aligned metaphyseal fractures in adolescents with at least 2 yr of growth remaining can be anticipated.

Physiatric management postfracture, while the child is casted, puts priority on return to school rather than using the option of limited home teaching. Emphasis is on crutch walking or wheelchair transfers and mobility and safe transport to and from school. During the period of limb immobility, electric stimulation techniques may limit strength loss (38). After removal of cast or cast brace, a program of stretching and strengthening is ordered, if needed, using land therapy techniques or pool (22).

CONTUSIONS, STRAINS, AND SPRAINS

Although contusions, sprains, and strains occur less frequently overall in children than in adults, incidence in pediatric athletes is as high as 50% (46). Contusions are muscle injuries by blunt trauma, most commonly in the quadriceps. If severe bleeding occurs, myositis ossificans sometimes develops and may resemble osteogenic sarcoma radiographically such that biopsy is necessary (73). In fact, any injury with prolonged swelling or pain requires assessment for tumor.

Strains are disruption at the musculotendinous junction, although, in childhood, the alternate injury often is apophyseal avulsion. Strains are most common in the hamstrings and a preventive program includes warm-up stretches and strengthening and correction of faulty running technique.

Sprains are ligamentous tears diagnosed by ruling out undisplaced growth plate fracture. These most often involve the ankle, but in twisting knee injuries, medial collateral and anterior cruciate ligament tears can be coincident with fracture of the femoral physis or avulsion of the tibial tubercle (65).

Both sprains and strains are classified as first, second, or third degree disruption with third degree being complete tearing and instability. For the latter, casting, air casting, or cast bracing may need to precede the rehabilitation program.

Treatment is RICE (rest, ice, compression, elevation), range of motion, weight-bearing, stretching and strengthening, and graduated return to the sport. For the ankle, RICE therapy is followed by active range of motion achieved by tracing the letters of the alphabet on the floor with foot and ankle motion, progressive weight-bearing, jogging, and broken field running.

Overuse Syndromes: Sports Injuries

Overuse injuries result from repetitive microtrauma causing inflammation of joints, stress fractures, avulsions and apophysitis, tendonitis, and bursitis. Vulnerable sites are the epiphyseal plate and articular cartilage of joints, and nonarticular apophyses that provide major muscle group attachments: proximal radius, iliac crest and spine, tibial tubercle, and calcaneous.

During growth spurts, soft tissue elongation lags behind bone growth resulting in decreased joint flexibility. Other predisposing factors in overuse injury are thought to be rotational and angular deformities; bone density; type of sport, training intensity and errors; equipment; coaching and supervision (52, 79).

SPINE

After the knee, the most common area of overuse injury in girls is the back (33). Causes of pain range from lumbar hyperlordosis, spondylolysis, and spondylolithesis, and herniated disc to thoracolumbar apophysitis (atypical Scheuermanns) (52). Sports most likely to cause back pain are gymnastics, dance, riding, running, football, and ice hockey.

Vertebral osteomyelitis and tumors, diskitis, spondylitis, and sacroiliitis can be confused with sport injury. Localized tenderness, kyphosis, step-off sign, radicular signs combined with the sport history, and radiographs or bone scintigraphy usually clarify diagnosis. Experience in interpreting pediatric spine films is needed to distinguish vertebral ossification centers from fractures (41).

Patients with atypical Scheuermann's disease or spondylolisthesis sometimes need a Boston brace body jacket for 3 months for pain control. Rehabilitation methods for overuse back pain include rest from the sport; nonsteroidal anti-inflammatory drugs, icing, or heat; a flexibility program, and water jogging.

Pediatric athletes with skeletal dysplasias and ligamentous laxity are at risk for atlantoaxial subluxation (Down, Ehlers Danlos, Marfan, Morquio syndromes); or predisposed to spinal stenosis and disc herniation (achondroplasia, spondyloepiphyseal, and spondylometaphyseal dysplasia) (41). These children should be diverted from collision and diving sports and from power weight lifting.

LOWER EXTREMITY

While pelvic apophyses are subject to overuse injury (hip pointers), gymnasts and dancers may develop iliopsoas tendonitis or slipped capital femoral epiphysis. Both can refer pain to the knee. The iliotibial band becomes painful at its insertion, over the greater trochanter (snapping hip), and at the lateral femoral condyle especially with long distance hill running. Management is to decrease the running program, stretch the iliotibial band, and use shoe orthotics to control foot pronation.

KNEE

The knee is the most common site of athletic trauma to joint and ligaments and of overuse injury. Examination maneuvers and signs have been summarized (54).

If a knee buckles, medial or lateral collateral ligament instability is tested with a patient supine, the ankle stabilized, and the knee in 15° flexion applying valgus or varus stress on the knee to open the medial or lateral knee joint.

Examination for anterior cruciate ligament tear is the Lachman anterior drawer sign with the knee at 15° flexion and the leg externally rotated: the thigh is stabilized with anterior force applied on the tibia. Posterior tibial force for the posterior drawer test or sag sign delineates a posterior cruciate ligament tear. MRI and arthroscopy aid in the diagnosis. Suspected joint derangement (football, skiing) requires orthopaedic management (78).

Patellofemoral stress joint pain (chondromalacia patellae) and tender apophysitis of the inferior patella (Sinding-Larsen syndrome) or tibial tubercle (Osgood-Schlatter disease) (39) are common examples of traction overuse microtrauma on the extensor mechanism. This set of symptoms, known as Jumper's knee, increases with frequency of training sessions for the long jump, basketball, football, or volleyball, progressing from pain after practice to pain during the activity (11). There is compression tenderness of the patella or a tender tibial tubercle. Symptoms also occur with quadriceps overuse in the crouched gait of cerebal palsy. Sonogram demonstrates an enlarged tendon and bone scan increased uptake at injury sites of apophysitis.

Rest from the sport or a short period of immobilization in a posterior splint may be necessary for relief and should be followed by quadriceps strengthening exercises. Efficacy of prophylactic knee bracing is in doubt and not recommended by the American Academy of Pediatrics Committee on Sports Medicine (3).

Recurrent patellar dislocation is associated with ligamentous laxity and causes the knee to give out when stepping down. The 'Q' angle (patellar femoral tibial angle) is greater than 15° and the apprehension test is positive as the child pushes away the examiner's hand when medial to lateral patellar pressure is applied to displace the knee cap.

The locking knee is evaluated for torn meniscus by the McMurray test, which is begun with the knee fully flexed, then slowly extending the leg while applying maximal internal rotation, repeating with external rotation, to observe for pain and clunk. A loose joint body from a detached bone fragment of osteochondritis dissecans may cause locking as well.

LEG, ANKLE, AND FOOT

Shin splints or medial tibial stress syndrome follow increased training intensity and repeated traction at the origin of the posterior tibial or medial soleus. There is diffuse distal posteromedial tibial pain and tenderness and a linear pattern on bone scintigraphy. Skeletal immaturity, obesity, pronated feet, and leg length discrepancy predispose.

Stress fractures are most common in the proximal tibia, second and third metatarsals, and the lateral malleolus. Chronic compartment syndrome is uncommon in children. Presentation is diffuse anterior leg pain and dorsal foot paresthesias.

Tendonitis of the heel cord, calcaneal apophysitis (Sever's disease), and stress fractures cause heel pain and tenderness, while plantar fasciitis and metatarsal stress fractures present as plantar pain in dancers and runners.

Bone scans are positive the 1st day after onset in 95% of stress fractures and 100% by the 3rd day. Radiation exposure from one bone scan is the equivalent of five chest x-rays or 3/4 of a gastrointestinal series (50). Bone single-photon emission computed tomography (SPECT) is a nuclear medicine technique that allows discrete localization of injury even including rhabdomyolysis (50).

The child with stress fractures must be nonweight-bearing and walk with crutches until the pain stops. Substituting water for land training with running motions in the deep end of the pool maintains conditioning. For the described foot problems, heel cord stretching, heel elevation of the shoe, soft shoe orthotics, and foot taping (70) are useful.

UPPER EXTREMITY

Overuse injuries of the shoulder, elbow, and wrist happen from throwing and racquet sports, swimming, and the arm weight-bearing sports, such as gymnastics and cheerleading.

Overuse injury to the shoulder (little league and swimmer's shoulder) causes anterior pain from proximal humeral growth plate injury, often including coracoacromial impingement of the supraspinatous tendon and anterior humeral subluxation.

Nursemaid's elbow or radial head subluxation from yanking the child's extended pronated arm is the most common elbow injury to preschoolers. The child refuses to use the arm until reduction is achieved by the maneuver of forearm supination and elbow flexion.

Little league elbow is due to repetitive traction and compression causing proximal radial physis injury, osteochondritis dissecans of the capitellum, apophysitis, and avulsion of the medial epicondyle. Valgus or flexion deformity and nerve entrapment at the elbow or forearm may be secondary (7).

Selective muscle testing to dislocate/relocate the humerus, sonogram, and MRI (23) of shoulder joint or elbow aid in diagnosis.

Treatment of shoulder pain demands limiting swim distance or the innings pitched. Little league rules allow no more than six innings with 3 days rest between pitching games. Therapy is aimed at increasing the range of internal rotation, stretching the rotator cuff and scapular rotators, strengthening the shoulder girdle followed by throwing lobs at reduced speed before full return to the sport. Throwing technique is modified to reduce valgus stress on the elbow (64).

Although overuse injuries of the wrist and hand in children are less common than those of the shoulder and elbow, persistent wrist pain after a fall or handstand requires serial radiographs or a bone scan for possible scaphoid or hamate hook fracture, carpal subluxation, or aseptic necrosis of the lunate (Kienbock's disease). Ball players are subject to epiphyseal fractures of phalanges or ligament and tendon disruption, which usually requires casting or splinting (45).

SPORTS-RELATED NERVE INJURIES

A fall on the outstretched arm with the neck flexed toward the opposite side in football or a collison against the boards in hockey may cause "stinger" or "burner" pain from cervical root or brachial plexus compression or traction. The child should not return to play that day or until pain and weakness is resolved. Entrapment neuropathies of the arm and wrists are experienced by both athletes and musicians (40).

Screening Examination and Training for Sports

Medical preassessment of the pediatric athlete emphasizes counseling on injury prevention. Physical examination includes maturity assessment (because of chronological age 12 yr, physical maturity varies from 9 to 15 yr), maneuvers to bring out asymmetries of joint motion and strength, and testing of balance and concentration.

Abnormalities that disqualify children and adolescents from sports participation have been classified by body system and type of sport (collision, contact, endurance). Acute infections, cyanotic congenital heart disease, and unhealed earlier injuries disqualify a child from all competitive sport participation, while deafness and seizures eliminate participation from collision sports only (27). Such exclusion could *not apply* to sports modified appropriately. In addition, children with poor concentration or who are easily distracted are said to do better with individual sports, such as karate, wrestling, and fencing, than with team sports (1).

The Academy of Pediatrics has recommended bans on all-terrain vehicles, trampolines, boxing, power weight lifting, and long distance running for children because of the risk of injury (2).

Physical training should be geared to children and adolescents. For warmups, static stretching is the method of choice for flexibility development. These exercises are detailed elsewhere (31). Weight training with light weights is a method of conditioning by repetitive exercises as opposed to power weight lifting techniques which demand one maximal effort. Weight training is considered safe for the prepubescent. Whether free weights or machines are used, supervision is essential (56). The prescription for aerobic exercises for endurance training of children is the same as for adults: 20 to 30 minutes of aerobic exercise three times weekly.

Wheelchair Sports Injuries

Therapeutic and competitive sports for the handicapped child and adolescent have proliferated and, with these programs, the role for the physician in teaching conditioning and injury prevention, classification for meets, and injury treatment (55). Wheelchair track and basketball athletes are especially prone to soft tissue and nerve entrapment overuse injuries of the upper extremity, decubiti, fractures from wheelchair falls, and hypothermia and hyperthermia during marathon racing (17).

REFERENCES

1. Alexander JL: Hyperactive children: Which sports have the right stuff? *Phys Sports Med* 18:5–108, 1990.
2. American Academy of Pediatrics Committee on Accident and Poison Prevention: All-terrain vehicles: Two,-three,-and four-wheeled unlicensed motorized vehicles. *Pediatrics* 79:306–308, 1987.
3. American Academy of Pediatrics Committee on sports medicine: Knee brace use by athletes. *Pediatrics* 82:228, 1990.
4. Ashwal S, Tomasi L, Neumann M, Schneider S: Reflex sympathetic dystrophy in children. *Pediatr Neurol* 4:38–42, 1988.
5. Barone GW, Rodgers BM: Pediatric equestrian injuries: A 14-year review. *J Trauma* 29:245–247, 1989.
6. Beattie P, Isaacson K, Riddle D, et al: Validity of derived measurements of leg-length differences obtained by use of a tape measure. *Phys Ther* 70:150, 1990.
7. Bennett JB: Athletic injuries of the elbow. *Surg Round Orthop* 4:35–40, 1990.
8. Bennett JT, MacEwen GD: Congenital dislocation of the hip. *Clin Orthop* 247:15, 1989.
9. Boyce W, Sobelewski S: Recurrent injuries in school children. *Am J Dis Child* 143:338–342, 1989.
10. Cass DT, Gray AJ: Pediatric bicycle injuries. *Aust NZ J Surg* 59:719–724, 1989.
11. Colosimo AJ, Basset III, FH: Jumper's knee diagnosis and treatment. *Orthop Rev* 19:139–149, 1990.
12. Conrad EU, Rang MC: Fractures and Sprains. *Pediatr Clin North Am* 33:1523–1540, 1986.
13. Conway JJ: Radionucleide bone scintigraphy in pediatric orthopedics. *Pediatr Clin North Am* 33:1313, 1986.
14. Council on Scientific Affairs: American Medical Association diagnostic and treatment guidelines concerning child abuse and neglect. *JAMA* 254:796–800, 1985.
15. Crawford, AH: Current concepts review: Slipped capital femoral epiphysis. *J Bone Joint Surg* 70-A:1422, 1988.
16. Crawford, AH: Symposium: Legg-Calvé-Perthes disease. *Contemp Orthop* 11:65, 1985.
17. Curtis KA, Dillon DA: Survey of wheelchair and athletic injuries: Common patterns and prevention. *Paraplegia* 23:170–175, 1985.
18. Enneking WF, Conrad EU: Common bone tumors. *Clin Sympos* 41:3, 1989.
19. Ferriter P, Shapiro F: Infantile tibia vara. *J Pediatr Orthop* 7:1, 1987.
20. Friedman JM: A practical approach to dysmorphology. *Pediatr Ann* 19:95, 1990.
21. Gedalia A, Person DA, Brewer EJ Jr, Giannini EH: Hypermobility of the joints in juvenile episodic arthritis/arthralgia. *J Pediatr* 107:873–876, 1985.
22. Genuario SE, Vegso JJ: The use of a swimming pool in the rehabilitation and reconditioning of athletic injuries. *Contemp Orthop* 20:381–387, 1990.
23. Greenberg DA, Jones JD, Zink WP, Price CT: Anatomy and pathology of the pediatric elbow using magnetic resonance imaging. *Contemp Orthop* 19:345–351, 1989.
24. Grill F, Bensahel H, Candell J, et al: The Pavlik harness in the treatment of the congenitally dislocating hip: report on a multicenter study of the European Pediatric Orthopedic Society. *J Pediatr Orthop* 8:1, 1988.
25. Gross R: Leg length discrepancy: How much is too much? *Orthopaedics* 1:307, 1978.
26. Hall TR, Kangarloo H: Magnetic resonance imaging of the musculoskeletal system in children. *Clin Orthop* 244:119, 1989.

27. Harvey J: The participation examination of the child athlete. *Clin Sports Med* 1:353–369, 1982.
28. Hensinger R: Congenital dislocation of the hip. *Orthop Clin North Am* 18:597, 1987.
29. Herring JA: Congenital dislocation of the hip. In Morrissy RT (ed): *Lovell and Winter's Pediatric Orthopedics,* ed 3. Philadelphia, JB Lippincott Co, 1990.
30. Hubbard DD, Staheli LT, Chen D, et al: Medial femoral torsion and osteoarthritis. *J Pediatr Orthop* 8:540, 1988.
31. Jaffe M, Ludwig S: Stairway injuries in children. *Pediatrics* 82:457–461, 1988.
32. Jones KL: *Smith's Recognizable Patterns of Human Malformation,* ed 4. Philadelphia, WB Saunders Co, 1988.
33. Kannus P, Niittymaki S, Jarvinen M: Athletic overuse injuries in children. *Clin Pediatr* 27:333–337, 1988.
34. Keim H, Hensinger R: Spinal deformities. *Clin Symposia* 41:4, 1989.
35. Klein MJ, Kenan S, Lewis MM: Osteosarcoma: Clinical and pathological considerations. *Orthop Clin North Am* 20:327, 1989.
36. Koop SE: Infantile and juvenile idiopathic scoliosis. *Orthop Clin North Am* 19:331, 1988.
37. Kostiuk JP: Current concepts review: Operative treatment of idiopathic scoliosis. *J Bone Joint Surg* 72A:1108, 1990.
38. Kramer JF: Muscle strengthening via electric stimulation. *Crit Rev Phys Med Rehabil* 1:97–133, 1989.
39. Krause BL, Williams JPR, Catterall A: Natural history of Osgood-Schlatter disease. *J Pediatr Orthop* 10:65–68, 1990.
40. Lederman RJ: Peripheral nerve disorders in instrumental musicians. *Ann Neurol* 22:125, 1987.
41. Letts M, MacDonald P: Sports injuries to the pediatric spine. *Spine: State Art Rev* 4:49–83, 1990.
42. Lonstein J: Natural history and school screening for scoliosis. *Orthop Clin North Am* 19:227, 1988.
43. Lonstein J, Winter RB: Adolescent idiopathic scoliosis, *Orthop Clin North Am* 19:239, 1988.
44. MacEwen GD, Mason B: Evaluation and treatment of congenital dislocation of the hip in infants. *Orthop Clin North Am* 19:815, 1988.
45. McCue FC, Mayer V: Rehabilitation of common athletic injuries of the hand and wrist. *Clin Sports Med* 8:731–776, 1989.
46. McLain LG, Reynolds S: Sports injuries in high school. *Pediatrics* 84:446–450, 1989.
47. Meller JL, Shermeta DW: Falls in urban children. *Am J Dis Child* 141:1271–1275, 1987.
48. Moseley CF: Leg length discrepancy. *Orthop Clin North Am* 18:529, 1989.
49. Morissy RT (ed): *Lovell and Winter's Pediatric Orthopaedics,* 3rd ed. Philadelphia, JB Lippincott, 1990.
50. Nagel C: William Beaumont Hospital Royal Oak MI. Personal communication, 1990.
51. Nyhan WL: Structural abnormalities: A systematic approach to diagnosis. *Clin Sympos* 42:2, 1990.
52. O'Neill DB, Micheli LJ: Overuse injuries in the young athlete. *Clin Sports Med* 7:591–610, 1988.
53. Paley D. Current techniques of limb lengthening. *J Pediatr Orthop* 8:73, 1988.
54. Perrin JCS, Badell A, Binder H, et al: Pediatric rehabilitation. Musculoskeletal and soft tissue disorders. *Arch Phys Med Rehabil* 70:S183–S189, 1989.
55. Perrin JCS, Johnstone K: Handicapped sports and sports injuries. *State Art Rev: Phys Med Rehabil.* June, 1991.
56. Rooks DS, Micheli LJ: Musculoskeletal assessment and training: The young athlete. *Clin Sports Med* 7:641–677, 1988.
57. Schoenecker PL: Legg-Calvé-Parthes disease. *Orthop Rev* 15:561, 1986.
58. Schor EL: Unintentional injuries. *Am J Dis Child* 141:1280–1284, 1987.

59. Seiman LP: Surgical correction of congenital vertical talus under the age of two years. *J Pediatr Orthop* 7:405, 1987.
60. Shapiro F: Medical progress: Epiphyseal disorders. *N Engl J Med* 317:1702, 1987.
61. Staheli LT: Lower positional deformity in infants and children. *J Pediatr Orthop* 10:559, 1990.
62. Staheli LT: Rotational problems of the lower extremities. *Orthop Clin North Am* 18:503, 1987.
63. Staheli LT, Clawson DK, Hubbard D: Medial femoral torsion: experience with operative treatment. *Clin Orthop* 146:222, 1988.
64. Stanitski CL: Management of sports injuries in children and adolescents. *Orthop Clin North Am* 19:689–698, 1988.
65. Steiner ME, Grana WA: The young athlete's knee: Recent advances. *Clin Sports Med* 7:527–546, 1988.
66. Svennigan S, Apulset K, Terjesen T: Regression of femoral anteversion: a prospective study of intoeing children. *Acta Scand Orthop* 60:170, 1989.
67. Swanson JA, Sachs MI, Dahlgren KA, Tinguely SJ: Accidental farm injuries in children. *Am J Dis Child* 141:1276–1279, 1987.
68. Tachdjian MO: *Pediatric Orthopedics,* 2nd ed. Philadelphia, WB Saunders, 1990.
69. Thompson GH, Salter RB: Legg-Calve-Perthes Disease: current concepts and controversies. *Orthop Clin North Am* 18:617, 1987.
70. Torg JS, Pavlov H, Torg E: Overuse injuries in sport: The foot. *Clin Sports Med* 6:291–320, 1987.
71. Tyler DC, Smith M, Womack W, Pomietto M: Pain management in infants, children, and adolescents. In Loeser JD, Egan KJ (eds): *Managing the Chronic Pain Patient.* New York, Raven Press, 1989, pp. 161–177.
72. United States Consumer Product Safety Commission Sports Estimates Reports. National Electronic Injury Surveillance System, 1986.
73. Webber A: Acute soft-tissue injuries in the young athlete. *Clin Sports Med* 7:611–624, 1988.
74. Wenger DR: Selective surgical containment for Legg-Perthes disease: Recognition and management of complications. *J Pediatr Orthop* 1:153, 1981.
75. Wenger DR, Leach J: Foot deformities in infants and children. *Pediatr Clin North Am* 33:1141, 1986.
76. Wilson GN: Pediatric approach to the skeletal dysplasias. *Pediatr Ann* 19:141, 1990.
77. Winter RB: In Morrissy RT (ed). *Lovell and Winter's Pediatric Orthopedics,* ed 3. Philadelphia, JB Lippincott Co, 1990.
78. Zarins B, Adams M: Knee injuries in sports. *N Engl J Med* 318:950–961, 1988.
79. Zito M: Musculoskeletal injuries of young athletes: The new trends. In Gould JA (ed). *Orthopaedic and Sports Physical Therapy.* St. Louis, CV Mosby, 1990, pp. 627–650.

18

Cerebral Palsy

GABRIELLA E. MOLNAR

Cerebral palsy is a collective term that encompasses a spectrum of clinical syndromes. Etiological factors and the resultant central nervous system lesions are diverse. The common diagnostic criteria that are shared by the variety of clinical syndromes classified as cerebral palsy are: *disorder of movement and posture* caused by *nonprogressive lesion* or injury that affects the *immature brain* (11, 100).

The definition of cerebral palsy implies that the underlying neurological lesion or lesions must be static and that the process that led to brain dysfunction is no longer active. A further implication is that the central nervous system damage occurred in early life before brain maturation was completed (11, 100, 210). Although the essential diagnostic sign of cerebral palsy is a motor deficit, the possibility that there may be other associated symptom complexes of cerebral dysfunction is implicit in the stipulation of central nervous system pathology.

Despite advances in the understanding, treatment, and prevention of events that predispose to brain damage, cerebral palsy continues to be the most frequent childhood disability. Epidemiological studies in the United States during the 1940s and 1950s showed a prevalence of 1.6 to 5.8/1000 live births or 500 cases/100,000 population (166). A door-to-door survey of case finding method and inclusion of previously undetected cases probably accounted for the higher rates in some of these studies. The most recent and largest number of American data originated from the Collaborative Perinatal Project, which included observations of 54,000 pregnancies and the outcome of their offspring (156). In this study, Nelson and Ellenberg found a prevalence rate of 5.2/1000 live births at 12 months of age. However, the same authors reported that as much as 50% of the children showed resolution of neuromuscular dysfunction on follow-up at 7 yr of age (157). Early assessment apparently included suspected and/or mild cases without persistent motor disability and overestimated the prevalence of cerebral palsy. Kitchen et al. (114) from Australia, also indicated that a number of children classified as cerebral palsy at 2 yr of age showed no signs consistent with this diagnosis by 5 yr.

Advances in obstetric and neonatal care raised the hopes of reducing neurological morbidity among the survivors. Hagberg et al. (85) reported that the incidence of cerebral palsy in Sweden declined between 1958 and 1970. However, by 1976, the incidence has again increased (210). From Western Australia, Stanley and her group described a similar temporary reduction of incidence rate in 1979, with subsequent increase by 1982 (210, 211). These changes are attributed to a higher survival rate of sick neonates, especially in the group of low birth weight premature infants who would have previously succumbed to perinatal complications (86, 210). Despite such transient fluctuations, the frequency of cerebral palsy remained remarkably constant at a rate of 2 to 3 cases/1000 live births during the last four decades (113). In a review of secular epidemiological trends, Paneth and Kiely concluded that the overall prevalence of cerebral palsy has not changed since the 1950s and that, at school age, a rate of 2/1000 live births is a reasonable estimate for industrialized countries (166).

Etiology

Damage to the central nervous system may occur: (a) prenatally; (b) perinatally during labor or the neonatal period; and (c) postnatally in early life. The antecedents of cerebral palsy have been the subject of intensive studies in recent years. Correlative analyses of large samples of pregnancy in populations with cerebral palsy led to the recognition that prenatal causes have a more important contribution than previously assumed (153, 155, 156). Furthermore, it became evident that even when multiple risk factors are considered, a large proportion of cases is unexplained (158). Conversely, combinations of similar or identical adverse antecedents do not result in uniform morbidity (156).

Prenatal factors that pose a risk for cerebral palsy are summarized in Table 18.1 (153, 156, 210). Maternal risk factors unrelated to pregnancy include mental retardation, hyperthyroidism, estrogen, or thyroid use. Alcohol ingestion produces an identifiable syndrome and smoking leads to intrauterine growth retardation. Other known adverse effects of maternal intake of drugs or toxic substances are illustrated by anticonvulsant therapy (210) and by the fetal Minamata disease due to methylmercury (33). Infections during gestation, especially of the TORCH group, are among prenatal causes. Severe cardiorespiratory compromise and abdominal trauma in the pregnant woman (172) can injure the fetus or jeopardize fetal circulation and oxygen supply resulting in prenatal anoxic damage. Complications of pregnancy and placental abnormalities affect fetal development and this risk is increased with previous histories of reproductive inefficiency (155, 156, 179, 210). Genetic factors have been implicated in nonprogressive ataxic, diplegic, and dystonic syndromes of unexplained origin with familial disposition (100, 143, 144, 210).

Prenatal factors may lead to premature birth and/or intrauterine growth

Table 18.1.
Prenatal Risk Factors and Markers

Maternal mental retardation, seizures, hyperthyroidism, estrogen, or thyroid use
Reproductive inefficiency, history of previous abnormal pregnancies and fetal wastage, death, or
    stillbirth
    Placental complications (chorionitis, low placental weight, placental infarcts)
    Third trimester bleeding
    Breech presentation
    Severe proteinuria with preeclampsia or eclampsia
Maternal/intrauterine fetal infections
    Toxoplasmosis, rubella, cytomegalovirus, herpes simplex
Maternal illness with severe cardiorespiratory compromise
Abdominal trauma during pregnancy
Toxic/teratogenic agents from maternal ingestion or environment, anticonvulsant treatment dur-
    ing pregnancy
Genetic disposition
    Familial history, motor deficit in older sibling (?)
Gestational age 32 weeks or less, low birth weight
Small-for-gestational age (SGA), intrauterine growth retardation, fetal deprivation or malnutrition,
    chronic intrauterine anoxia
Multiple birth, twin pregnancy
Congenital malformations
    CNS anomalies—primary microcephaly or porencephaly, other CNS anomalies
    Malformations and dysmorphism other than CNS
Socioeconomic factors—late/inadequate prenatal care

---

retardation of both term and preterm infants (51, 210). Prematurity remains the most common antecedent of cerebral palsy and its prevalence is inversely related to birth weight and gestational age (6, 50, 51, 210). Ellenberg and Nelson estimated that there is an approximately 20-fold increased risk when birth weight is under 1500 g (52). Studies of premature infants born between the late 1970s and mid-1980s show that prevalence rates per 1000 live births ranged from 8% to 10% in the 1500 to 2499-g low birth weight group (LBW) to 18% to 20% in the under 1500 gm very low birth weight (VLBW) cohort (82, 175, 210). On an optimistic note, Saigal et al. (193) reported a decreased disability rate in the 500 to 1000-g birth weight cohort in infants who were born between 1977 and 1980 and assessed at 3 yr of age. Small-for-gestational age (SGA) birth weight is an indication of intrauterine growth retardation (51). SGA infants have a high incidence of major and minor congenital defects (17); however, brain maturation is consistent with their gestational age (51). In the Vancouver study, the frequency of cerebral palsy and other neurological deficits was identical in preterm infants regardless whether they were SGA or appropriate for gestational age (AGA) (51). Term SGA infants with severe fetal deprivation may suffer brain impairment from chronic prenatal hypoxia, but the neuorological lesions differ from those seen in the immature brain of preterm neonates (51). Developmental disabilities in fetal deprivation are usually learning and attention deficits rather than cerebral palsy.

Dental enamel dysplasias of the deciduous and permanent teeth are markers for identifying the time of prenatal damage. Because of their common ectodermal origin, both neural tissues and dental enamel are affected by the same intrauterine insult (14). In autopsy studies, neuropathological changes indicate the time of insult since the evolution of specific reactive neural tissue responses requires a defined interval (54).

Perinatal intrapartum asphyxia has been considered the major etiological factor in cerebral palsy since the article of Little in 1862 on this subject (134). Freud (71) refuted this contention and recent studies support his viewpoint (69, 99, 221). Using the Apgar score as a measure of asphyxia, a score of 3 at 10 to 15 minutes presents a 10% to 15% risk for cerebral palsy; the majority of children with this score have no cerebral palsy; more than 75% of cases with cerebral palsy have normal Apgar scores (154, 155). Nelson and Ellenberg (53, 155) found that Apgar scores of 3 or lower at 1 minute were associated with 80% survival rate and 1.7% morbidity at 1 yr of age. With the same scores at 20 minutes, death rate reached 87% in the 1st year; morbidity among the survivors was 36%. The American Academy of Pediatric stated that, in addition to Apgar scores, other signs should be present to support the diagnosis of encephalopathy from asphyxia, including hypotonia lasting at least several hours and neonatal seizures (5, 25). Metabolic acidosis in the umbilical cord blood is a confirmation of perinatal asphyxia (5, 68). The uncertainty of attributing cerebral palsy to intrapartum asphyxia is compounded by the vulnerability of prenatally compromised infants to the stress of delivery (177, 210). The nature and pathomechanism of obstetric complications as perinatal antecedents of cerebral palsy has been widely scrutinized (157, 210, 214). Nelson and Ellenberg found that the rate of cerebral palsy did not exceed 2% following placenta previa, abruptio placentae, breech delivery, cord prolapse, nuchal cord, mid or high forceps delivery, and Pitocin augmentation (157).

The time of onset of perinatal cerebral palsy may be during the postpartum period. In sick neonates, systemic complications, especially those affecting pulmonary and circulatory function, can lead to brain hypoxia (206). Intraventricular-periventricular bleeding and/or hypoxic infarcts are typical of prematures (210). In isoimmune or hemolytic disease of the newborn, brain damage results from bilirubin encephalopathy (230). Neonatal infections with septicemia and meningitis may also cause central nervous system damage in newborns (210).

Neuromuscular deficit caused by a disease or insult to the brain may be designated as postnatal cerebral palsy after the acute stage has passed and the pathological process brought under control. The generally accepted time frame is a central nervous system impairment sustained after the neonatal period and before postnatal brain maturation is complete, or from 4 weeks up to 5 yr of age (210). Cerebrovascular accidents, encephalopathies, poisoning or any illness complicated by anoxia, ischemia, hemorrhage, or other

Table 18.2.
Timing of Pathogenetic Periods in Cerebral Palsy[a]

	Term births N = 457 (%)	Premature births N = 224 (%)
Obvious prenatal cause or risk factor	24	6
Combined prenatal and perinatal factors	20	23
Purely perinatal factors	19	51
No identifiable risk factors	30	17
Obvious postnatal cause	8	2

[a]Adapted from Hagberg B and Hagberg G (210, pp. 116–134).

types of nonprogressive neuronal damage are contributory factors in postnatally acquired cases. Despite similarities in neurological consequences, traumatic head injury, including child abuse under 5 yr of age, are now usually classified under that category rather than as postnatal cerebral palsy.

Prenatal and perinatal events are responsible for two thirds or more of cases in both term and preterm infants. However, as seen in Table 18.2, premature infants are more susceptible to suffer perinatal complications because of the physiological immaturity of their organ systems and brain. Cerebral palsy of postnatal origin constitutes only a small number of cases in either group. Consistent with general experience in 20% to 30% of cases where symptoms of early onset are present, no apparent etiology can be ascertained. A search for progressive neurological conditions, familial diseases, malformations of the brain, and possible genetic anomalies must be conducted in these instances before the diagnosis of cerebral palsy as a nonprogressive, nonfamilial condition is accepted.

Clinicopathological Correlations

Neuropathological lesions in cerebral palsy show a great deal of diversity, depending on the nature and severity of insult and on the stage of central nervous system development when it occurred. This brief description concentrates only on the most frequent characteristic clinicopathological correlations; for detailed discussion, readers are referred to monographs and reviews addressing this subject (34, 167, 210, 219, 230). Ischemic hypoxic encephalopathy may develop prenatally, intrapartum, or in the neonate from a variety of events that interfere with cerebral blood flow and oxygen supply. Periventricular leukomalacia is an ischemic lesion that occurs with predilection in premature newborns before or shortly after birth (185). Infarcts in the periventricular region affect the white matter with cystic lesions as a late residual consequence. In the mature brain of term infants, the cortex, white matter, basal ganglia, and cerebellum are more vulnerable to ischemia (210, 230). Table 18.3 lists the different types of lesions in hypoxic ischemic encephalopathy and their clinical correlates.

Various types of intracranial bleedings associated with cerebral palsy are shown in Table 18.4. Massive intracranial hemorrhage as a result of trau-

Table 18.3.
Neonatal Hypoxic-Ischemic Encephalopathy[a]

Neuropathology	Site of Lesion	Clinical Correlates	Predisposing factors
Selective neuronal necrosis	Cerebral cortex	Spastic quadriparesis	Border zone between major cerebral arteries
	Deep layers	Mental retardation	
Most common		Seizure disorder	
Primarily full-term neonates	Diencephalon	Visual, auditory discrimination deficits(?)	
	Thalamus	Unknown	
	Hypothalamus	Rigidity(?)	Asphyxia in experimental animals
	Basal ganglia		
	Midbrain		
	Oculomotor, trochlear nuclei		
	Red nucleus		
	Substantia nigra		
	Reticular formation	Attention deficit	
		Hyperactivity	Prematurity-anoxia, acidosis
	Pons		
	Reticular formation		
	Trigeminal, facial, pontine nuclei	Bulbar, pseudobulbar palsy	
	Medulla		
	Cuneate, gracilis, dorsal vagal nuclei		
	Cerebellum	Ataxia	
	Purkinje cells		
	Dentate and roof nuclei		
Parasagittal cerebral injury	Cerebral cortex	Probable	"Watershed" infarct
Principal ischemic lesion of full-term asphyxiated infants	Subcortical white matter	Spastic quadriparesis	Border zones of major arteries
		Less frequent spastic hemiparesis	Decreased blood flow at extreme circulatory branches
	Superomedial parasagittal aspects of covexity		Posterior region watershed of all three major vessels
	Posterior or anterior		Asphyxia
	Parieto-occipital area	Associated visual motor deficits	Impaired vascular autoregulation, systemic hypotension, hypoxemia, acidosis
	Bilateral, often asymmetrical	Dyslexic syndrome (?)	
		Perceptual disturbances	

Periventricular leukomalacia Principal ischemic lesion of premature infants with impaired cerebral perfusion	White matter adjacent to external angle of lateral ventricles At level of occipital radiation Around foramen of Monro Hemorrhage into anoxic lesion, serious complication	Spastic diplegia Small lesion—legs affected More extensive lesion to centrum semiovale and corona radiata—legs and arms affected Subtle visual, auditory, somesthetic deficits	Border zones between penetrating branches of three major arteries Endotoxin? Bacteremia Septicemia Relative sparing of cortex and subcortical white matter due to persistent meningeal artery anastomoses in preterm
Focal and multifocal ischemic brain necrosis Incidence increases with gestational age	Localized areas of necrosis in the distribution of major vessels Half in area of middle cerebral artery Unilateral Porencephalic cyst or cysts Progressive enlargement possible	50% of congenital hemiparesis	Focal cerebrovascular compromise Vascular maldevelopment Thrombus Embolization General circulatory insufficiency, hypoxia/ischemia Inflammation/infection Toxoplasma, cytomegalovirus, herpes, bacterial meningitis Trauma Ventricular rupture Intracranial hemorrhage
Status marmoratus Least frequent Premature or full-term	Caudate nucleus, globus pallidus, putamen, thalamus Neuronal loss, gliosis, hypermyelination	Choreoathetosis Mental retardation Dystonia, resting tremor—less frequent Spastic quadriparesis with rigidity	Unclear Asphyxia

[a]Adapted from various sources (167, 210, 219, 230).

Table 18.4.
Intracranial Hemorrhage[a]

Periventricular—Intraventricular Hemorrhage
  Most significant in premature infants less than 32 weeks of gestational age
  Bleeding into subependymal germinal matrix
  Immature development of arterial and capillary bed in subependymal plate
  Increased venous pressure, systemic blood pressure fluctuations, impaired vascular
    autoregulation
  Hypoxia, hypercapnia
  May be associated with periventricular leukomalacia, selective neuronal necrosis, venous
    infarction or focal brain injury
Primary subarachnoid hemorrhage
  Pathogenesis unclear, hypoxia or trauma probable
  Premature: hypoxia, trauma
  Full term: trauma, hypoxia
  Slowly developing hydrocephalus may follow
Intracerebellar hemorrhage
  Small premature infants
  Traumatic laceration of cerebellum and/or rupture of major veins or occipital sinus
  Hemorrhagic venous infarctions
  Primary intracerebellar hemorrhage
  Extension of bleeding from intraventricular or subarachnoid hemorrhage
  Germinal matrix present with poorly supported vascular bed
Subdural hemorrhage
  Least common
  Trauma with laceration of tentorium, falx
  Infratentorial or supratentorial bleeding from large veins and venous sinuses
  Large full-term or premature
  Primaparous or older multiparous mother
  Small birth canal; precipitous or prolonged labor; breech, foot, or brow presentation; high for-
    ceps extraction

---

[a]Adapted from various sources (167, 219, 230).

matic birth with vascular tears and subdural hematoma is very rare with current obstetric practices. The most frequent type among hemorrhagic lesions is intraventricular-periventricular bleeding. This neuropathology is the most significant contributor to mortality and morbidity in premature infants. Propensity for this lesion in the group of less than 32 weeks of gestational age is related to the poorly developed vascular bed in the germinal matrix of the subependymal plate of the immature brain. Grading system for the severity of pathology consists of isolated subependymal hemorrhage (grade I), bleeding into the ventricle without dilatation (grade II), with ventricular dilatation (grade III), and intraventricular hemorrhage with extension to the surrounding white matter parenchyma (grade IV) (230). Grade I and II bleedings do not result in cerebral palsy. The range of late sequelae includes subependymal pseudocyst following small isolated bleedings, ventricular enlargement or hydrocephalus, and paraventricular porencephalic cyst when the bleeding extends to the parenchyma (210).

Bilirubin is a neurotoxic agent that interferes with the cellular metabolism of neurocytes. Its passage through the blood-brain barrier occurs only when it is not bound to serum albumin (230). As seen in Table 18.5, bilirubin encephalopathy may develop for several reasons that directly or indirectly raise the free serum bilirubin fraction and increase the permeability of the blood-brain barrier or, perhaps, neuronal susceptibility. In neonatal isoimmune hemolytic disease, the free serum bilirubin fraction rises because the rate of production exceeds the available serum albumin-binding capacity. A similar situation may occur in the rather rare cases of congenital biliary atre-

Table 18.5.
Bilirubin Encephalopathy[a]

Mechanism of neurotoxicity
    Interference with intracellular enzymatic oxydation and phosphorylation
    Impairment of mitrochondrial functions
    Binding to cell membrane phospholipids
Parthegenesis
    Elevated free serum bilirubin fraction
    Increased production—isoimmune or other hemolytic disease of the newborn
    Decreased excretion—biliary atresia
    Reduced albumin binding capacity
    Small birth weight, premature
    Decreased serum albumin
    Decreased binding capacity or affinity—acidosis, asphyxia
    Increased competition for binding—endogenous or exogenous anions
    Increased permeability of blood-brain barrier
    Small birth weight
    Asphyxia, infections, vasculitis
    Possible increased neuronal susceptibility
    Asphyxia, acidosis
    Intracranial hemorrhage
Pathology
    Bilirubin deposits and staining of specific nuclei
    Basal ganglia—globus pallidus, subthalamic nuclei
    Hippocampus
    Geniculate bodies
    Brainstem nuclei—inferior colliculi, inferior olivary nuclei, oculomotor, vestibular, cochlear
        nuclei
    Cerebellum—vermis, dentate nucleus
    Neuronal necrosis—Purkinje cells
    Diffuse brain damage in associated hypoxic-ischemic injury
Clinical Correlates
    Extrapyramidal movement disorder
    Basal ganglia—athetosis, dystonia, chorea, ballismus, tremor, or incoordination of volitional
        movements
    Facial dyskinesia
    Pseudobulbar palsy—swallowing, phonation, articulation impairment
    Gaze abnormalities
    Brainstem nuclei—paralysis of conjugate vertical eye movements
    Auditory impairment
    Cochlear nuclei—hearing deficit, high freqency sensorineural hearing loss, auditory
        imperception
    Intellectual function preserved in pure kernicterus, may be impaired with associated hypoxic-
        ischemic injury

---

[a]Adapted from Volpe (230).

sia. In these instances, the risk of kernicterus is proportionate to the elevated total serum bilirubin level over 16 to 18 mg/ml. In contrast, among small birth weight premature infants, asphyxia, acidosis and other factors lead to decreased albumin binding capacity (184, 227). Thus, there is a disproportionate rise of unbound bilirubin fraction or in blood-brain transport and bilirubin encephalopathy may develop at total serum concentrations below 16 mg/ml. Bilirubin has a selective affinity to specific structures in the brain, especially the basal ganglia and other subcortical nuclei; hence the term kernicterus. Consistent with the discrete basal ganglion lesions, dyskinesias are the typical motor deficit in cerebral palsy of this etiology. When bilirubin toxicity is the sole etiological agent, intellectual functioning is usually unaffected; however, in premature infants, associated hypoxic ischemic injury with more diffuse brain damage increases the risk of cognitive impairment. Prenatal testing of pregnant mothers and exchange transfusion for the newborn have eliminated bilirubin encephalopathy caused by isoimmunization. Phototherapy is a preventive measure in small birth weight premature infants (184).

Classification

In an historical review, Ingram (100) described different classifications of cerebral palsy proposed since the 19th century. Although no uniform internationally accepted classification exists, functional categorizations based on the nature and distribution of neuromuscular abnormalities are the most widely used in clinical practice (11, 55) (Table 18.6).

Spastic paresis represents the most commonly encountered neuromuscular dysfunction. As a rule, in hemiparesis, the upper extremity is more affected. Occasionally, neurological signs are so mild in the leg that it justifies a functional designation of monoparesis. Diplegia is the preferred term for spastic paresis affecting both lower extremities. This clinical type occurs most often in prematurity as a result of hemorrhage or ischemic leukomalacia in the periventricular region (178). Mild incoordination of the upper extremities is not unusual; frank signs of spasticity are present with more extended lesions that affect both the medially and laterally located pyramidal tracts subserving the lower and upper extremities, respectively (230). Less frequently, diplegic distribution of spasticity follows hypoxic ischemic encephalopathy in term infants, although the underlying pathological lesion is usually different from that associated with prematurity (230). Spastic quadriparesis involves all extremities with greater impairment of the lower limbs. In general, it indicates a more extensive diffuse damage. Spastic quadriparesis can occur in both preterm and term infants. By convention, the term of double hemiplegia is used when spasticity is more severe in the arms (100). Reflecting the changes in obstetric and neonatal care, there is some shift in the relative frequency of different spastic types of cerebral palsy. Hemiparesis caused by traumatic delivery was more prevalent in the

Table 18.6.
Clinical Classification of Cerebral Palsy

Type	Frequency %
Spastic	75–85
Hemiparesis (monoparesis)	10–15
Diplegia	35–45
Quadriparesis (double hemiplegia)	25–30
Dyskinetic	5–10
Athetosis	5–8
Dystonia	2–3
Chorea	Rare
Ballismus	Rare
Tremor	Rare
Mixed and other types	10–15
Spastic-dyskinetic	5–10
Spastic-ataxic	3–5
Rigid-spastic	Rare
Ataxic	3–5
Atonic (hypotonic)	Rare

past; on the other hand, spastic diplegia seems to be on the increase with greater survival rate of prematures.

Dyskinetic cerebral palsy includes a number of movement disorders (42). Athetosis, dystonia, or their combination are predominant. Tremor, choreiform, and ballistic movement disorders are relatively rare. Table 18.7 describes the characteristic clinical signs that distinguish these movement disorders. With successful preventive treatment of neonatal isoimmune disease, the overall frequency of dyskinetic cerebral palsy has been reduced. The classic kernicteric athetosis of Rh incompatibility is seen in older teenagers and adults but not in young children. Hypoxic ischemic encephalopathy affecting the basal ganglia is a more likely cause of dyskinetic cerebral palsy in the young age group (124–126).

Table 18.7.
Clinical Characteristics of Dyskinetic Movement Disorders

Athetosis	Slow writhing movements Face and extremities Distal musculature more affected
Dystonia	Rhythmic twisting distortions and tone changes Trunk and proximal parts of the limbs Slow uncontrolled movements with fixed postures
Chorea	Rapid irregular jerky movements Face and extremities
Ballismus	Coarse wide amplitude flailing or flinging movements Mostly extremities

Other types of cerebral palsy comprise a small number of cases. In the ataxic type, signs of cerebellar dysfunction include incoordinated gait, head titubation, intention tremor, nystagmus, and scanning speech. Ingram (100) distinguishes ataxic diplegia with associated spasticity from the pure ataxic type. Etiological factors in the former are similar to diplegia of term infants, including congenital malformations and hydrocephalus, whereas in the latter, genetic factors seem to play a role and mental retardation is frequent (143, 144, 210). Some classifications include rigidity as a separate clinical type. Distinction of rigidity from severe spasticity or the coexistence of these signs is often a matter of the examiner's judgment. Hypotonia is a frequent early sign and may precede spasticity of dyskinesia as transient symptom (42, 101). A small number of children show persistent considerable tone decrease and may be classified as hypotonic or atonic cerebral palsy. There may be a combination of neurological signs, usually spasticity, and some form of dyskinesia (42, 101).

Diagnosis

HISTORY

Complications of pregnancy, labor, and neonatal course are risk factors that alert the clinician to the possibility of cerebral palsy. Postnatal causes that may result in nonprogressive residual motor disability and justify the label of cerebral palsy in children under 5 yr of age have been discussed previously. Historical information should include a complete inventory of the earliest and advanced motor milestones to ascertain that development was not arrested at a certain stage since, in the absence of an intercurrent illness, that would suggest an evolving neurological disease rather than cerebral palsy of pre- or perinatal origin.

LABORATORY EXAMINATIONS

Cranial ultrasonography is the method of choice in neonates and infants to visualize hemorrhagic and hypoxic ischemic insults (130). CAT scan is another well-established neuroradiological method for detecting and localizing central nervous system lesions when brain damage is suspected (2, 58, 119). Magnetic resonance imaging (MRI) can demonstrate small lesions missed by other methods and also abnormalities of myelination associated with developmental delay (15, 88, 103, 115). Positron emission tomography (PET) (35, 36) and single photon emission computed tomography (SPECT) visualize brain metabolism and perfusion (46). PET scan studies showed that there is a sequential order of maturational changes in the infant's brain that correlates with developmental achievements known from clinical behavioral observations (35). SPECT studies of children with hemiplegic cerebral palsy demonstrated hypoperfusion in the hemisphere contralateral to the motor deficit. In mild diplegia, no abnormalities were present. Children with moderate diplegia or quadriparesis had bilateral hypoperfusion in the superior motor cortex, whereas in severe cases, these changes involved the superior and inferior motor cortex and cortical areas of the parietal and frontal lobes as well. Age range of the children studied was 13 months to 12 years (46). At present, PET and SPECT are available only for selected studies.

Cerebral evoked potential responses assess the functional integrity of the central nervous system (13, 118, 230, 237). Brainstem-auditory evoked potentials detect injury to the nuclei of the eighth cranial nerves and the inferior colliculi, which are sensitive to hypoxic ischemic encephalopathy, and to bilirubin neurotoxicity. Lesions of the cortical, somesthetic, and visual structures occur in hypoxic ischemic encephalopathy, especially with selective neuronal necrosis (230). Periventricular leukomalacia extending into the white matter parenchyma may damage the visual and auditory radiation. Increased latency and abnormal response patterns in the newborn correlate with the degree of perinatal asphyxia and persistent abnormalities are accompanied by other signs of brain damage. Visual evoked-potential latencies are prolonged in premature infants with hydrocephalus following periventricular-intraventricular hemorrhage due to encroachment on the optic radiation, but reversal to normal after shunt placement has been reported (230). Event-related potentials (ERP) measured by computer-averaged EEG showed delayed maturation and abnormal responses in some high risk and neurologically impaired infants on tasks that entail visual and auditory attention (229).

CLINICAL EXAMINATION

Close follow-up of infants at risk for having cerebral palsy has provided better insight into the prognostic significance of neonatal neurological abnormalities (70, 231). Early signs with predictive value include tone abnormalities of limbs, neck, and trunk, weak cry and suck (29), the need for tube feeding, and diminished activity level lasting for more than 1 day. However, data from the Collaborative Perinatal Project showed that the incidence of cerebral palsy was only 16% among the infants who exhibited a combination of these signs as neonates (156). Touwen (223) suggests that there are differences in the quality of movements in preterm infants who are neurologically damaged compared to those who are unimpaired on follow-up at age equivalent to full-term gestation. Because, in many cases, neurological abnormalities of the newborn period resolve, at least as far as neuromuscular dysfunction is concerned, there is a need for caution to avoid early unjustified labeling of infants as having cerebral palsy. As noted earlier, a similar course of improvement may ensue during early childhood, particularly when abnormal signs are subtle (114, 157).

Since movement control is acquired gradually during infancy, impairments of volitional motion, such as spastic paresis or dyskinesia, may be difficult to recognize until after 4 months of age, unless the neurological abnormalities are striking. Perinatally acquired hemiparesis may be an exception if asymmetry of limb movements and posture is significant (42). The suspicion of cerebral palsy can be usually confirmed by the second half of the 1st year as unequivocal signs of neuromuscular deficit evolve and motor development continues to lag behind. However, in mild cases, subtle symptoms may be overlooked until the age when more advanced milestones should be attained and delayed or abnormal standing and walking become evident. Using the Bayley Scales of Infant Development and the Motor Assessment of Infants, Harris (89) found that, in premature infants at 4 months corrected age, quadriplegia was more consistently predictable compared to hemiparesis or diplegia. The Bayley Motor Scale at 1 year corrected age was a highly sensitive indicator of all three diagnostic categories. The mean age of clinical diagnosis for spastic diplegia was 12 ½ months; for hemiparesis, 21 months; and for quadriparesis, 5 months of corrected age in this study.

Early signs and symptoms that should arouse suspicion can be categorized in five general groups; established diagnosis of cerebral palsy rests on the presence of unequivocal abnormalities in several areas.

TONE ABNORMALITIES

While alterations of muscle tone are the earliest signs, mild aberrations may be difficult to detect. Interpretation of tone abnormalities should be weighed in context of the infant's general state as discussed in Chapter 1. Abnormal tone can be manifested as decreased, increased, or fluctuating resistance to passive movements.

Most infants with cerebral palsy undergo an early stage of hypotonia preceding the appearance of definitive neurological signs (20, 42, 101, 130). The duration and degree of hypotonicity tends to be related to the type of neuromuscular dysfunction and its severity. Generally, the hypotonic stage is more prolonged as a precursor of dyskinesia than of spasticity. Long-lasting and significantly reduced tone tends to augur a rather severe motor deficit in either type of neuromuscular dysfunction. Persistent tone decrease is the leading sign of hypotonic cerebral palsy. In the ataxic type, there is hypotonia of cerebellar origin. The differential diagnosis of hypotonic infants is discussed in Chapters 1 and 14.

Hypertonicity is characteristic of the spastic and rigid clinical types (20, 42, 101). Aside from increased resistance to passive motion, a number of clinical observations are indicative of hypertonicity. A tendency of opisthotonic posturing signals heightened extensor tone (222) and may be interpreted by the parents as precocious head raising and rolling over from prone to supine (Fig. 18.1). Increased resistance and stiffness when the infant is pulled to sit suggests hip extensor hypertonicity and is one of the earliest signs of spasticity (Fig. 18.2). Some parents may report difficulties with separating the legs on diaper changes, an indication of spastic hip adductors.

Fluctuating tone, which changes from hypotonia to hypertonicity, depending on the phase of involuntary movements, is typical of dyskinesias

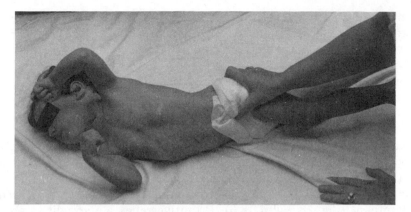

Figure 18.1. A 16-month-old infant, with spastic athetosis, opisthotonus, fisting of the hands.

(20). It can be perceived on passive movements or during rest when the examiner's hand is placed on a limb. Tone fluctuations are often evident before visible signs of dyskinesia appear.

REFLEX ABNORMALITIES

In spastic cerebral palsy, hyperreflexia with expanded reflexogenic zone, clonus, overflow, enhanced stretch reflex activity and other well-known

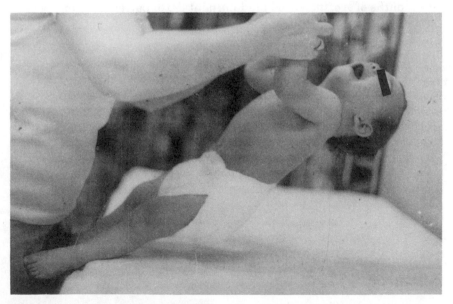

Figure 18.2. A 14-month-old infant, with severe quadriparesis, hip extensor spasticity.

signs of upper motor neuron lesion are present. One of the most readily evoked stretch reflexes and a frequent, though not specific, sign of cerebral palsy is adductor catch, which can be elicited by sudden passive abduction of the hips.

Persistent and predominant primitive infantile reflexes offer some of the earliest clues of suspicion or diagnosis (20, 42, 64, 101, 219). For a description of these reflexes, the reader is referred to Chapter 2. Obligatory tonic neck reflexes at any age or persistent nonobligatory activity after 6 months indicates a central nervous system impairment affecting the motor structures (Fig. 18.3). The Moro (Fig. 18.4), palmar, and plantar grasp reflexes often remain evident and hyperactive beyond the expected age. Likewise, tonic labyrinthine reflexes and positive supporting reaction may become predominant (Fig. 18.5 and 18.6). Primitive reflex abnormalities are not restricted to any one type of cerebral palsy, but tonic labyrinthine, positive supporting, and grasp reflexes generally persist in spasticity, while in dyskinesia, the Moro and tonic neck reflexes are more frequent. The clinical manifestations of abnormal reflexes extend over a spectrum from overt obligatory movement patterns that impede volitional motor control, to vestigial forms with subtle influence on muscle tone.

POSTURAL ABNORMALITIES

Influenced by primitive reflex activity and tone aberrations, infants with spastic cerebral palsy assume abnormal positions at rest and respond with predictable postural changes when moved about in space (20, 64, 101). After 3 to 4 months of age, increased predominant flexor pattern in prone position

Figure 18.3. A 1½-yr-old child, with athetosis. Persistent obligatory asymmetric tonic neck reflex. Pseudobulbar palsy, tongue thrust, and lateral deviation toward the side of head rotation. Athetoid posturing of the fingers in the left hand.

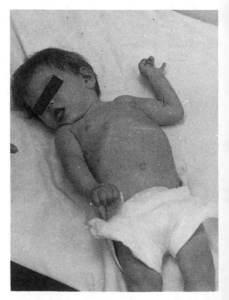

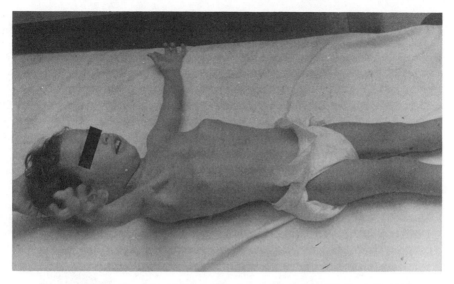

Figure 18.4. Persistent Moro reflex in an 18-month-old athetoid child.

with arms and legs drawn under the body is a sign of increased muscle tone and is attributed to tonic labyrinthine reflex. In supine, extensor posture, scissoring at the hips, and plantar flexion at the ankles indicate spasticity (Fig. 18.5). This pattern becomes more pronounced in vertical suspension and on weight-bearing (Fig. 18.6). The diagnosis of lower extremity spasticity is definitely confirmed when this postural response can be consistently elicited on lifting the child into vertical position. In milder cases, only a partial response may be evoked consisting of leg extension with plantar flexion or only equinus attitude of the ankles.

The typical upper extremity posture in spastic quadriparesis is an exaggeration and persistence of the infantile sleeping and resting arm position.

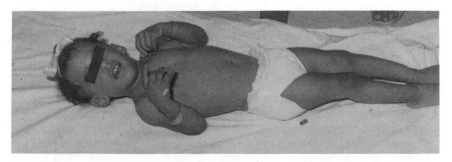

Figure 18.5. Young child with spastic quadriparesis. Abnormal posture of arm flexion, hip adduction, leg extension, and ankle plantarflexion attributed to tonic labyrinthine reflex.

Figure 18.6. Same child as in Figure 18.5 in vertical position, hyperactive positive supporting reaction, scissoring.

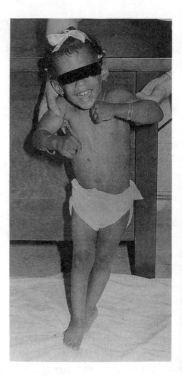

The shoulders are abducted, elbows flexed, hands fisted, a posture that is descriptively called the strap hanger sign. Habitual posturing of this type in a fully awake infant after 4 to 5 months, or a consistently fisted hand after 6 months, particularly with the thumb drawn into the palm, are signs of upper extremity spasticity. Abnormal fisting of the hand may be the only indication of increased tone in mild cases.

In perinatally acquired hemiparesis, asymmetrical arm position may be quite striking from early age (42). In contrast to the infantile posture of the sound extremity, the affected arm is adducted, the forearm is pronated, and the fingers are closed in a fist.

Hypotonic infants lie in the pithed frog position with abduction, external rotation, and partial flexion of the hips; the arms lie limply alongside the body. Unusual and changeable joint and extremity postures are characteristic of dyskinesia. Spooning of the hands with hyperextended fingers is especially suggestive of athetosis (Fig. 18.7).

DELAYED MOTOR DEVELOPMENT

Late attainment of motor milestones is a universal symptom (21, 42, 48, 101). As a rule, delay in sitting is the first sign to attract attention and concern. The discrepancy in motor development tends to increase with successive milestones. Its extent is related to the degree of neuromuscular dysfunction. Isolated or predominant delay in motor milestones compared to other areas of development differentiates a neuromuscular deficit from other types of disabilities in high-risk infants.

ATYPICAL MOTOR PERFORMANCE

The manner in which the infant or child performs various motor skills provides important diagnostic information (21, 63, 64, 101). Asymmetrical upper extremity use or apparent hand preference in the 1st year is an early sign of hemiparesis. Misinterpreting its significance, parents often attribute this symptom to natural dominance. However, preferential hand function does not emerge under normal circumstances until the 2nd year.

A history of abnormal crawling, stance, or gait is frequent. Infants with hemiparesis propel themselves only with the unaffected arm and leg. Forward progression by reciprocal arm movements while the pelvis and legs are dragged on the floor or hiked along without alternating motion is the usual crawling pattern of children with diplegia. It is described as combat crawl or bunny hop (21). Instead of crawling, some children with diplegia scoot on their abdomen, while those with hemiparesis move around sitting on their buttocks and propel themselves with the unaffected extremities. More severely impaired children with quadriparesis or athetosis may substitute rolling for prone progression. Standing and walking on the toes are well-known symptoms of lower extremity spasticity.

Facial grimacing and writhing movements of the tongue, fingers, and toes are early manifestations of athetosis (Fig. 18.3 and 18.7) (21, 42, 101). Incoordinated reaching, withdrawal, and fanning of the fingers on approaching an object suggest dyskinetic movements. Intention tremor, head titubation, and truncal instability are discernible in the ataxic type.

Sucking and feeding difficulties, lack of jaw and lip closure, tongue thrust (Fig. 18.3), drooling, and poor mobility of the oral musculature indicate pseudobulbar palsy and are frequently the earliest signs of dyskinetic neuromuscular deficit or bilateral spasticity (21, 152, 173, 207).

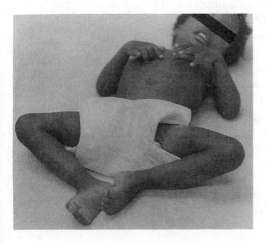

Figure 18.7. A 16-month-old child with hypotonia, incipient athetosis of both hands.

Differential Diagnosis

In the hypotonic stage, other causes of floppy infant syndrome must be considered as differential diagnostic possibilities. Infants with spinal muscular atrophy, congenital myopathy, or hereditary sensorimotor neuropathy of early onset present with hypotonicity and weakness. Family history points toward a genetic nature of the problem in some cases. On the other hand, the history can be misleading since neonates with severe weakness due to a disease of the motor unit may suffer from perinatal distress, suggesting the possibility of a static encephalopathy. Unlike in cerebral hypotonia where deep tendon reflexes are usually hyperactive, a floppy infant with lower motor neuron paralysis or muscle weakness has diminished or absent response to tendon tap. In case of considerable weakness, physiological infantile reflexes, such as Moro, tonic neck, and grasp reflexes, are likely to be absent, whereas in cerebral palsy, they can be easily evoked even in the hypotonic stage. Benign congenital hypotonia and a variety of genetic syndromes, metabolic diseases, and infantile botulism may be associated with reduced tone. Electrodiagnostic studies, muscle biopsy, and other laboratory examinations identify hypotonia of neurogenic or myopathic origin as discussed in Chapters 6 and 14.

Birth trauma of the spinal cord is initially manifested by decreased tone, often affecting all extremities because of its frequent location at the lower cervical, high thoracic segments. A history of breech delivery, brisk stereotypic flexor withdrawal, and other spinal responses to noxious stimuli without indication of discomfort, lack of spontaneous extremity movements, absent infantile reflexes mediated by supraspinal areas, and distended bladder will differentiate this injury from cerebral hypotonia.

The differential diagnosis of brachial plexus birth palsy and hemiparesis rarely presents a problem despite some resemblance in arm posture. Localized flail paralysis and absent motor and grasp reflexes help distinguish brachial plexus injury from evolving signs of prenatal or perinatal hemiparesis.

Degenerative diseases of the central nervous system may simulate cerebral palsy. Slowly progressive familial spastic paraparesis can be mistaken for diplegia. Lack of pre- and perinatal risk factors and the history of similar symptoms in other family members may provide diagnostic clues. The relatively fast pace of early development can mask a progressive neurological course in degenerative gray or white matter diseases. The strictest caution should be exercised in accepting the diagnosis of nonprogressive neuromuscular deficit as cerebral palsy when the presenting sign is ataxia and particularly when there is associated spasticity. A considerable number of these cases prove to be insidiously progressive spinocerebellar diseases. On occasion, a slowly growing tumor of the central nervous system with early onset has been erroneously diagnosed as cerebral palsy (34).

Clinical Course of the Motor Disability

As it can be expected in a group of syndromes as diverse in their manifestations as cerebral palsy, the differences in clinical course are considerable (42, 47, 48, 101, 195, 219). Dysfunction of the neuromuscular system and the presence of associated nonphysical deficits share equal roles in determining the natural history, anticipated complications, and outcome (70).

A fundamental diagnostic criterion of cerebral palsy is that the neurological lesion is not progressive. Yet, the clinical course is characterized by changing function and dysfunction over the long years of growth and development. The natural history can be envisioned as a summation of competing favorable and adverse developmental lines represented by the preserved innate potential, on one hand, and by the organic deficits and their secondary consequences, on the other.

The first few years are marked by changing neurological signs as continuing, although defective maturation of the central nervous system proceeds (42, 48, 101, 219). While development is delayed and limited by the brain damage, maturation works in favor of new functional accomplishments. Spasticity or dyskinesia tend to evolve gradually with an apparent intensification of clinical signs as part of the natural course. When the brain injury is less extensive, functional compensation continues for many years despite an evident spastic paresis or other type of movement disorder. In case of severe neuromuscular deficit, motor function remains arrested on a low level.

At a later age, changing clinical manifestations are related to the secondary musculoskeletal sequelae of a long-standing neurological deficit (18, 94, 161, 194, 215). Children with moderate to severe disability have a greater propensity for developing such complications, but contractures and deformities can occur in any child rather rapidly during the accelerated phases of growth, especially in adolescence. When the neurological deficit is compounded by progressive musculoskeletal deformities, mechanical limitations of mobility and deteriorating function will follow.

Regardless of the extent of motor handicap, a psychosocial disability may also lead to failure of achieving maximal expectations or to a regression of function (42, 231). Both physical and/or behavioral complications can diminish the effect of natural development thrust.

Spastic Types of Cerebral Palsy

After the initial hypotonic state, spasticity usually appears around 6 months (42, 101, 133, 219). Significant tone increase prior to this age or persistence of hypotonicity beyond 1 yr generally suggests a rather severe neuromuscular dysfunction.

The clinical features of pathological motor behavior in spastic cerebral palsy may be viewed as increased and abnormally distributed tone with postural deviations largely under the influence of disinhibited reflexes; absent, poorly developed, or delayed control of postural mechanism; and spastic paresis with inability to perform coordinated volitional movements (21, 42, 101). Unbalanced muscle action leads to soft tissue contractures and, in the pediatric age group, leaves an indelible mark on the growing skeleton. The risk of bone and joint deformities is directly related to the severity of spastic muscle imbalance (18, 194, 219). Hip dislocation and scoliosis constitute the most serious complications (39, 60).

SPASTIC HEMIPARESIS

The initial hypotonic stage is usually short-lived and often unnoticed (42, 101). Most cases are recognized around 6 months of age and all but the very mildly affected ones by 1 yr or later (226).

Early gross motor milestones are generally delayed by 4 to 6 months. The outlook for ambulation is universally favorable and virtually all children walk by 3 yr of age (42, 147, 149). Unequal stride length and stance phase, triceps surae spasticity with diminished or absent heel strike, and ineffective toe clearance are the prominent features of hemiparetic gait. Heel-cord tightness or contracture and foot deformities, particularly equinus or equinovarus, are the most frequent complications.

Abnormal arm posture tends to be quite evident and it increases on physical activities as a result of disinhibited spastic overflow (Fig. 18.8). Assistive function of the affected hand depends on the degree of paresis and sensory feedback. Cortical sensory deficit is a unique feature of this clinical type and should be suspected when the child tends to ignore the hemiparetic arm (42). Impaired sensation, including astereognosis, defective position sense, two-point discrimination, graphesthesia and topagnosia, is attributed to parietal lobe damage and occurs in approximately 50% of cases. Despite the limited function of the hemiparetic hand, these children are expected to become independent in daily activities unless perceptual or cognitive deficits interfere with learning self-care and adaptive skills. Contractures of the spastic forearm pronators and of the elbow and wrist flexors may occur. Thumb in palm, finger flexion, or hyperextension of the interphalangeal joints are characteristic of the spastic hand.

A frequent symptom is underdevelopment of the hemiparetic extremities (96) (Fig. 18.9). It is unusually commensurate with the extent of spastic paresis but tends to be greater in association with a sensory deficit. Delayed appearance of carpal ossification centers suggests that a neurogenic trophic effect may play a role (95). Growth discrepancy tends to be greater in the arm and rarely exceeds 1 inch in the leg. A mild nonstructural and nonprogressive scoliosis may develop due to unequal leg lengths, asymmetrical function, and body alignment.

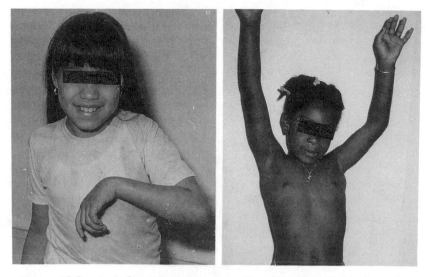

Figure 18.8.   *Left,* Characteristic arm posture of a child with hemiparesis.
Figure 18.9.   *Right,* Left hemiparesis, underdevelopment of the arm.

SPASTIC DIPLEGIA

Hypotonia is followed by spasticity usually in the second half of the 1st year (42, 101). Early predominant extensor hypertonicity may revert to excessive flexor tone at a later age.

The course of motor development and ultimate functional outcome varies (19, 128). In a prospective study of children with diplegia, maintenance of sitting by 2 yr was a good predictive sign of eventual ambulation. Children who did not sit by 4 yr did not achieve ambulation. Similarly, persistent obligatory infantile reflex activity beyond 18 months implied poor prognosis for ambulation. In this series, approximately 20% of children required assistive devices for walking. An additional 15% relied on using a wheelchair because of severe neuromuscular dysfunction, intellectual deficit, or both (149). Watt and his co-workers (234) confirmed that sitting at 2 yr has a high prognostic value but found that adding other variables did not increase predictive strength on a multivariate analysis. Badell-Ribera (7) reported that motor control on sitting and crawling at 1 ½ and 2 ½ yr predicts the ambulatory potential of diplegic children.

Postural and gait deviations range from mild to severe, affecting mostly the ankles or all lower extremity joints (18, 159, 174, 215). Figure 18.10 illustrates the characteristic early spastic posture seen in infants and young children. Postural abnormalities may change over the years, particularly in ambulatory children, as shown in Figures 18.11 and 18.12 (21, 101, 194).

Severe spastic muscle imbalance or contractures of the hip flexors and

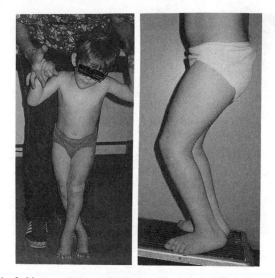

Figure 18.10. *Left,* Young diplegic child. Predominant extensor posture, scissoring.
Figure 18.11. *Right,* School-age ambulatory child with diplegia. Crouch posture.

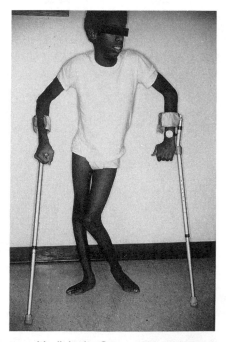

Figure 18.12. Teenager with diplegia. Community ambulator. Vase stance, internally rotated left leg, genu valgum, bilateral pes planovalgus, pelvic obliquity. Note neurogenic atrophy of the legs compared to well-developed torso, shoulder girdle, and arms.

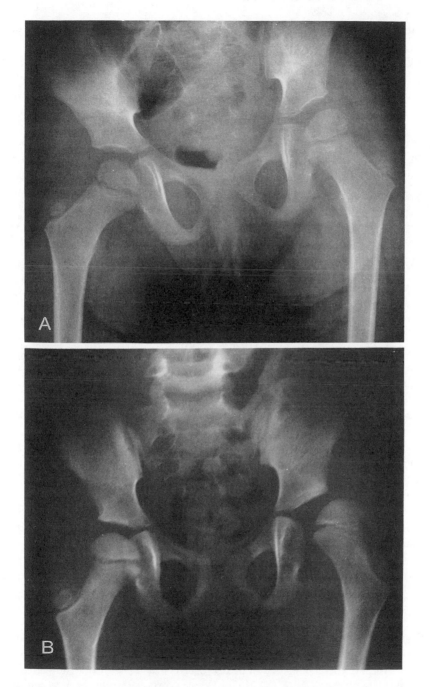

Figure 18.13. *A,* Coxa valga, partial subluxation of the left hip, pelvic obliquity. *B,* Progression to dislocation.

adductors result in persistence of infantile coxa valga and femoral anteversion (Fig. 18.13). Subluxation, acquired acetabular dysplasia, and eventual hip dislocation follow, particularly in the severely affected, nonambulatory child (18, 39, 215, 219). Pelvic obliquity and scoliosis are inevitable consequences of unilateral hip dislocation. Spasticity is enhanced by a painful dislocated hip. Progressive scoliosis can compromise the ability to sit, upper extremity use, cardiopulmonary status, and independent wheelchair function.

Children with diplegia have adequate control of the arms and hands. However, in some cases, there may be a mild and, at times, asymmetrical neurological dysfunction with hyperreflexia, slight tone increase, incoordination or fine tremor in the upper limbs. From the viewpoint of physical disability, independence in daily living is a reasonable expectation. However, functional achievements are also contingent on the child's intellectual ability (147).

SPASTIC QUADRIPARESIS

While spasticity tends to be greater in the legs, neuromuscular dysfunction affects the upper limbs as well. An asymmetrical deficit with more pronounced paresis on one side of the body is not unusual. Because of the extensive cortical and hemispheric lesions, this clinical type has the highest incidence of severe physical and associated handicaps. However, the extent of damage varies and there is a spectrum of mild to severe cases with considerable differences in functional outcome (19, 42, 48, 101).

Early signs and symptoms, their course of evolution, and abnormalities of stance and gait are similar to those described in diplegia. Musculoskeletal complications are more frequent and severe due to the extensive motor disability (18, 194, 219). Children with spastic quadriparesis must be closely monitored for hip dislocation and scoliosis (39, 60, 183). As a result of bilateral central nervous system lesions, a supranuclear impairment of the lower cranial nerves occurs (42). Sucking, swallowing and chewing difficulties, drooling, and dysarthric speech are clinical signs of the resultant pseudobulbar palsy (135, 152).

As in diplegia, maintenance of sitting by 2 yr and suppression of obligatory infantile reflexes by 18 months are good prognostic indicators of eventual walking (19, 149). Approximately one fourth of the children with spastic quadriparesis never become ambulatory and are dependent for care because of upper extremity impairment, intellectual deficit or both. About one third of the children can walk only with assistive devices; some of them become limited community ambulators. An additional one third of the group is mildly affected and has minimal or no restrictions in walking, self-care, and other aspects of daily life. As a rule, children who walk independently or with assistive devices have adequate motor control of the upper extremities for self-sufficiency in other areas of physical function, but the overall outcome is also contingent on mental abilities (147).

Dyskinetic Types

A neonate with acute bilirubin encephalopathy is hypotonic in the first few days. Hypertonicity and opisthotonus appear thereafter (42, 101). In a period of days or weeks, tone will again diminish. Hypotonicity, persistent, and, at times, obligatory tonic neck and neonatal neck righting reflexes represent the initial signs of motor dysfunction. The characteristic extrapyramidal movement disorder does not become evident until 12 months or occasionally as late as 3 yr (42, 101). Dyskinetic pseudobulbar palsy affects swallowing, mastication, phonation and articulation, and results in drooling and dysarthric speech (42, 101, 152). Dyskinesia or paralysis of conjugate upward gaze is an additional sign in kernicterus (42, 101). Unlike most other types of cerebral palsy, in dyskinesia, the upper extremities may be more involved than the lower limbs. Athetosis is the most common symptom and can be first noticed in the fingers, toes, and facial musculature (Fig. 18.3). There may be a combination of various types of dyskinesias or the nature of movement disorder may change over time; for example, athetosis may evolve into dystonia or into a combination of both by adolescence (Figs. 18.14 and 18.15).

During childhood, contractures rarely develop with athetosis since involuntary movements contribute to preservation of joint mobility. In dystonia, where fixed postures are maintained most of the time, the likelihood of deformities is increased. Equinovarus foot deformities and scoliosis are the most likely musculoskeletal complications (Figs. 18.15 and 18.16). Carpal tunnel syndrome and cervical spondylosis with progressive radiculomyelopathy have been described in adults with dyskinetic cerebral palsy and are attributed to continuous torsion movements and joint instability (112).

The outlook for ambulation is favorable in the majority of cases. Although walking may be awkward, three fourths of the children become ambulatory, one half of them before 3 yr of age. The age of sitting and development of infantile reflexes are useful for predicting whether a child will be able to walk (149). Because the neuromuscular dysfunction can be more severe in the arms than in the legs, some children who are ambulatory may need partial or considerable assistance in self-care and other daily activities.

Clinical Types with Mixed Neurological Signs

The distribution of neurological deficit is generally quadriplegic in the spastic athetoid type (42, 101). Neuromuscular dysfunction is often severe and its functional consequences reflect spastic paresis and dyskinetic incoordination. Approximately one half of the children attain walking, most of them after 3 yr of age (149). In the ambulatory children, upper extremity function is generally adequate for performing daily activities, while most of the wheelchair-confined youngsters need considerable or complete care (147). Musculoskeletal complications may develop as a result of spastic muscle imbalance but at a somewhat slower pace on account of dyskinetic

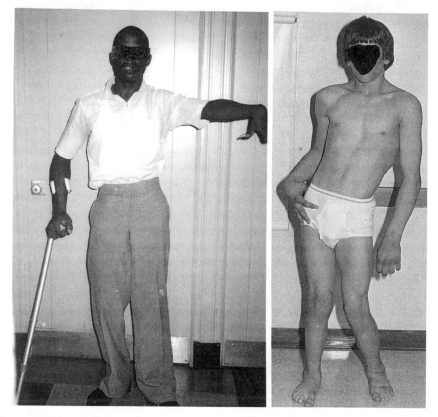

Figure 18.14. *Left,* Dystonic posturing of the left arm.
Figure 18.15. *Right,* Teenager with dystoria of trunk and extremities, asymmetrical posture, and scoliosis from dystonic movements.

movements. Nonambulatory children are at risk for developing acquired hip dysplasia and scoliosis.

Other Clinical Types

Early motor development usually proceeds at a very slow pace in the ataxic type of cerebral palsy. Nevertheless, the long-term prognosis for ambulation is good. Cerebellar signs tend to decrease; gait and hand function improve over the years (101).

The rigid and atonic types have poor prognosis (42, 101). The severe neuromuscular dysfunction and associated intellectual deficit preclude ambulation and independence in self-care. Lack of active movement control contributes to the development of musculoskeletal complications in both types. In rigidity, deformities are related to increased tone and neurogenic muscle imbalance. Severe generalized extensor tone causes progressive restriction of hip and knee flexion and limits sitting in a wheelchair. In the atonic type,

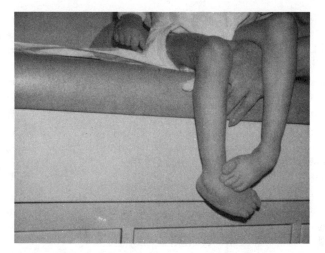

Figure 18.16. Dystonic athetosis, equinovarus attitude of the ankles.

postural alignment and deformities are influenced by gravity. Hip abduction, external rotation, and flexion contractures can be quite severe in children who lie in the pithed frog position, typical of hypotonicity. In some cases, anterior hip dislocation may develop over the years, and hip abduction contractures can make it impossible to place a child in a wheelchair.

Associated Disabilities

Reports about the incidence of associated disabilities vary (42, 48, 101, 194, 219). With some exceptions, the likelihood of multiple handicaps tends to be proportionate to the severity of neuromuscular dysfunction.

From a composite of many studies on intelligence in cerebral palsy, several trends emerge (42, 48, 70, 101). Compared to the general population, the proportion of high normal and superior intellectual endowment is lower. The overall incidence of mental retardation is approximately 50%. Severe to profound mental deficiency comprises about one half of the retarded group in cerebral palsy compared to 10% in the overall retarded population (116, 117). Approximately one third of cases with mental retardation have mild cognitive deficits. Microcephaly, seizure disorder, and, with some exceptions, severe neuromuscular dysfunction are associated with an increased risk of intellectual deficit. There is some correlation between the frequency and degree of mental deficiency and the clinical type of neuromuscular dysfunction. Retardation occurs most frequently and has the highest rate of severe deficits in spastic quadriparesis, and in the rigid and atonic types. A lower incidence of mental retardation, presenting as mild intellectual deficit in the majority of cases, is seen in spastic hemiparesis and diplegia. In the classic isoimmunization athetosis, where discrete lesions are confined to the basal ganglia, intellectual prognosis is generally favorable regardless of the severity of neuromuscular dysfunction. However, this trend does not apply to combined bilirubin and anoxic encephalopathy, a more common cause of athetosis in recent years. The correlation between specific perinatal complications and the incidence of retardation is a subject of epidemiological and clinical studies (51, 70, 210).

Difficulties encountered on the psychological assessment of children with cerebral palsy and the consistency of results on repeated examinations are addressed in the literature (117) and in Chapter 3. For clinical purposes, language development, especially speaking in two- to three-word sentences by 3 yr of age, is a good indication of intellectual potential (47). However, lack of speech resulting from severe hearing deficit or from impaired motor control of speech production should not be interpreted as mental deficiency. Conversely, overestimation of cognitive abilities in mildly retarded children with good verbal and social skills is a pitfall to be kept in mind. Clinical impressions of intelligence can be misleading and psychological evaluation is warranted before the child reaches school age.

Children with cerebral palsy are at a high risk for seizure disorders (42, 48, 101). The overall incidence is approximately 50% with a variable frequency in different clinical types (3, 4, 212, 219). Seizures were reported in 70% of cases in postnatally acquired hemiparesis compared to 50% in the congenital type. More than one half of the cases with spastic quadriparesis have epilepsy with an increasing rate among the severely handicapped. Seizures are less frequent in diplegia and dyskinetic cerebral palsy and occur in one fourth to one third of these cases. The clinical manifestations of epilepsy include various kinds of generalized and focal, minor motor, or partial seizures. Grand mal with tonic-colonic convulsions is a frequent type. Focal motor seizures may occur in hemiparesis. Infantile spasm with myoclonic jerks and minor motor epilepsy that produce continuous or frequent seizure activity have serious prognostic implications for both intellectual and motor function. Clinical seizures may resolve eventually or they may be absent despite an abnormal EEG.

Deficits of extraocular movements and vision are more common in cerebral palsy than among nonhandicapped children (74, 77, 219). Strabismus is the most frequent abnormality (77) reported in 20% to 60% of all cases, with the highest rates in spastic diplegia and quadriparesis. Esotropia seems to be more prevalent than exotropia. Suppression of vision and progressive amblyopia of one eye develops when nonalternating strabismus is uncorrected or treated late. Strabismus may interfere with depth perception and stereopsis. Defective visual fixation and tracking without overt strabismus were observed on electro-oculographic examinations (107). Paralysis of conjugate upward gaze is one of the clinical manifestations of kernicterus. Nystagmus is present in the ataxic type. Refractive errors severe enough to warrant correction occur in approximately 50% of cases. Hyperopia appears to be more characteristic of children with cerebral palsy, but there is also an increased incidence of myopia and astigmatism. A homonymous hemianopsia accompanies hemiparetic cerebral palsy in 25% of cases and is especially common with cortical sensory deficit resulting from a parietal lobe syndrome. Retinopathy of prematurity occurs in preterm infants. Hydrocephalus can lead to optic atrophy with progressive loss of vision and eventual blindness; a neurological consultation is mandatory when the cause of optic atrophy is unexplained. Cortical blindness may follow a severe anoxic encephalopathy and can be confirmed by visual evoked potential studies.

Communication disorders may be related to hearing impairment, defective motor control of speech production, central language dysfunction, or cognitive deficit (42, 48, 219). The characteristic hearing loss in cerebral palsy is a sensorineural impairment (219). It was estimated at 12% among children under 15 yr old, with a four times higher prevalence in athetosis than in spasticity. Kernicterus has been the most common cause of sensorineural hearing loss in athetosis. Intrauterine infections, especially rubella, cytomegalovirus, toxoplasmosis, and syphilis, as well as perinatal hypoxia, meningitis, encephalitis, and ototoxic drugs are some other potential etiological factors.

Defective or slow language acquisition often reflects an intellectual disability (42, 48, 101). However, developmental language disorders unrelated to mental retardation also occur. Disorders of verbal and written communication may be encountered, including various syndromes of dysphasia and dyslexia. After 1 ½ to 2 yr of age, insults to the dominant hemisphere lead to aphasia. Although most children show significant recovery from aphasia acquired before 8 to 10 yr, they rarely regain premorbid level of function. Differences between the language competence of children with congenital right versus left hemiparesis have been demonstrated. For further discussion of the characteristics of speech and language disorders, the reader is referred to Chapter 4.

Early feeding difficulties, excessive drooling, and defective speech are manifestations of pseudobulbar palsy resulting from supranuclear spastic paralysis or dyskinetic incoordination of the muscles controlled by the lower cranial nerves (42, 101, 150, 207). Speech defects due to impaired coordination of articulation, phonation, and respiration may range from slightly distorted sound production to complete anarthria (135). Nearly all children with athetosis and approximately one half of those with bilateral spasticity have some degree of dysarthria (42, 101). Severe speech impediment was reported in 40% of cases with athetosis. On occasion, mild athetosis of the skeletal musculature may be associated with severe pseudobulbar palsy, making speech impairment the most significant disability in a child who is independent in other areas of physical function.

Drooling is another manifestation of pseudobulbar palsy and represents a serious social disability. Feeding difficulties due to oral motor incoordination may lead to inadequate caloric intake and poor weight gain (75, 108, 228). Maldevelopment of the oropharyngeal structures and dental malocclusion tend to accompany pseudobulbar palsy and can further impede the effectiveness of sucking, chewing, and swallowing. Recurrent aspirations are not unusual and compound other pulmonary complications. Gastroesophageal reflux occurs mostly in severe motor disabilities and is another source of aspiration.

Defective control of the respiratory muscles may compromise the efficiency of pulmonary ventilation. Decreased vital capacity and aerobic working capacity was demonstrated both in spastic and athetoid neuromuscular dysfunction (12, 16, 136, 137). Lack of adequate cough and minor aspirations may lead to obstructive pulmonary disease. Restrictive pulmonary disease accompanies scoliosis. These problems are responsible for the frequent recurrent acute and chronic respiratory infections in children with severe handicaps. Bronchopulmonary dysplasia in former premature infants compounds the effects of these complications. Chronic pulmonary disease is a major cause of shortened life expectancy in the severely disabled group.

Perceptual dysfunction is widely documented in cerebral palsy (48, 70, 97, 219). A variety of complex agnosic problems were described that demonstrate an impairment of interpreting visual, auditory, and other sensory information and suggests defective intersensory integration. Agnosic and apraxic difficulties can interfere with learning to read, write, and even with simple daily activities, such as dressing, since these skills entail perceptual discrimination and a properly executed motor plan. The diagnosis and consequence of perceptual dysfunction is elaborated in more detail in Chapter 3.

Disorders of behavior have significant implications for learning, functional achievements, and life adjustment. Organic behavior syndrome may present with a spectrum of symptoms, including attention deficit, distractibility, disturbances of impulse control, and overt hyperkinesis (42, 48). The origin and remediation of psychosocial dysfunction and reactive emotional maladjustments are discussed in Chapter 5.

Management

The rehabilitation of children with cerebral palsy calls for a developmentally oriented plan that includes but is not limited to the treatment of neuromuscular disability (47, 48, 133, 146, 216). Fostering the acquisition of new skills and anticipatory treatment of potential complications are the two fundamental aspects of intervention. The implementation of a rehabilitation plan is a joint endeavor by the family, physician, and all other professionals working with the child (138, 224). Success of this undertaking rests on mutual understanding and agreement on realistic expectations.

EARLY INTERVENTION

Early intervention programs originated in the 1970s. PL 99–457 enacted in 1986 mandates that all states must establish services for infants and toddlers at risk or with known developmental disabilities (49). Eligibility for early intervention is based on delays in physical, language, or cognitive function, as a result of medical or environmental factors. A multidisciplinary approach and a focus on working through the family are organizational features shared by these programs.

The rationale of early intervention stems from research data on the intricate and mutually reinforcing effect of infant-caregiver interaction and its influence on early development (27, 80, 140). Infants who show limited interactive responses may receive less cuddling, handling, and playing from their caregivers (232). A physical disability that curtails active exploration of the surrounding world may create a degree of experiential deprivation and compound the existing organic deficits. Infants and young children with cerebral palsy require modified ways of physical handling to allow full use of their limited motor ability (62, 173). Some families have a natural resourcefulness to adapt the customary ways of parenting to the special needs of their handicapped child, but others face considerable difficulties in making such adjustment on their own (26, 133). Observations of mothers and children with cerebral palsy in their home showed that inappropriate toys, environmental and other obstacles often enhance the child's physical limitations (202, 203). Family-focused early intervention helps establish effective parenting so that the family can create an environment more suitable for the handicapped child. Professional advice reassures the family that they are not abandoned without hope (216). Confidence gained from understanding and helping the child's problems provides support during the process of grieving and promotes constructive coping.

Despite many favorable reports, the efficacy of early intervention has not been supported by strong experimental evidence (27, 84, 164). In a meta-analysis of 31 studies, Shonkoff and Hauser-Cram (204) concluded that the performance of children who were enrolled in such programs was only slightly superior to those who were not. The fundamental and unanswered question is whether nurturing environmental conditions can produce changes in brain organization, especially in the presence of central nervous system damage (41, 56, 61, 110). Animal experiments that demonstrated environmentally induced changes in neuronal differentiation support early intervention for infants with developmental disabilities by inference (120, 139).

Treatment of the Motor Disorder

Overall objectives for the rehabilitation of motor deficit must be formulated in the context of realistic long-range expectations. The extent of neuromuscular disability serves as a guide for defining the maximal potential in physical accomplishments. However, fulfillment of these expectations may be hindered by other coexistent deficits, such as blindness, significant agnosic and apraxic difficulties, and, especially, mental retardation or social maladjustment (67).

In general terms, the purpose of treating the physical disability is to promote the development of postural and movement control, to improve fine and gross motor skills, and to prevent musculoskeletal complications (9, 18,

21, 132, 133, 173). Short-term goals are based on evaluation and periodic reassessment of the child's functional status and musculoskeletal system.

Treatment of the motor dysfunction should be eclectic, using *appropriately selected* and *well-timed combinations* of therapeutic exercises, orthoses, surgical procedures, and other modes of intervention. A dogmatic adherence to any single therapeutic system or method with the exclusion of others is not justified by controlled studies or clinical experience in the perspective of many years (163, 220).

THERAPEUTIC EXERCISES

Chapter 7 describes various types of therapeutic exercises and pertinent controversial issues (141, 220). Details of techniques used in cerebral palsy are addressed in a number of papers and monographs on the subject (9, 21, 173, 195, 197, 219). This discussion is a general overview of the role of and indications for physical and occupational therapy.

Improvement in gross motor function is one of the principal aims of therapy. The child's current function determines which skills he needs to refine, is able to learn, and can be prepared for as a potential future accomplishment (192). The prevailing practice is to combine various forms of facilitation techniques with training in functional motor activities along the developmental sequence from head control to walking. This approach reflects the continuing search for means to alleviate the clinical abnormalities of an underlying movement disorder without losing sight of function as the primary goal of therapy (10, 21, 131, 132, 173, 195, 197). In infancy or for children with severe delay in gross motor development, head control may be the initial goal of therapy. Stimulation of head righting in response to postural changes is reinforced by toys or other items of interest to induce active lifting and holding of the head in prone, supine, and sitting position. Rolling and moving about in prone position should be encouraged as the first stage of mobility. Protective extension and equilibrium reactions are stimulated to help attain sitting, crawling, standing, and walking. Training in each gross motor milestone is advanced gradually from assisted control of posture and movements to independent practice as the child acquires the necessary coordination. Treatment to enhance upper extremity function and manual dexterity should start in infancy (34, 47, 131, 132, 173, 195). As it has been so aptly said, infants reach with their eyes before reaching with their hands. Eye-hand coordination is a prerequisite of manual skills. Stability of the torso and control of the shoulder girdle are additional requirements to consider. Initially, therapy may consist of encouraging arm movements; subsequent steps follow the maturational stages of palmar prehension, differentiation of pincer grasp, graduated release, and precise fine manipulatory skills. Expectations for bimanual or unilateral hand function depend on the motor deficit. Children will naturally select the unimpaired or less affected limb as the dominant extremity. Impaired sensation as seen in the parietal lobe syndrome of hemiparesis predicts poor hand use. Encouraging the use of hemiparetic arm through bilateral play activities, such as catching a large ball, is a reasonable approach to decrease the often striking neglect in these cases. However, continuous insistence by verbal reminders or by restriction of the unaffected arm only provokes resistance and resentment on the part of the child. Increased spontaneous use of the affected hand was reported in hemiparetic children after repeated presentation of "multisensory stories" when a verbal narrative was accompanied by actual objects placed close to the hemiparetic extremity (106). Therapy is conducted in the form of play and games. Toys and other objects are selected with a variety of shapes, textures, consistency, and functional use (38, 173, 195). Aside from the practice of motor skills, learning about object permanence, cause and effect, sensory and perceptual discrimination are additional therapeutic aims.

Integrity of the musculoskeletal system must be maintained to prevent deterioration of function and increasing disability (18, 94, 194, 215). Spastic muscle imbalance creates a tendency for soft tissue contractures in a rather predictable distribution. Progressive tightening of elbow, wrist, and finger flexors can further compromise the use of a spastic upper limb. In the legs, flexion deformities of the hips and knees, contracture of the hip adductors, and ankle plantar flexors are the most common. Gravity and positioning are additional predisposing factors for the development of progressive deformities. Well-known examples are the virtually inevitable hip and knee flexion contractures in children who sit all day. Stretching, passive, or active assistive range of motion exercises performed regularly may prevent or delay progressive loss of soft tissue and joint mobility. However, when active muscle function is severely limited, passive exercises alone are often unsuccessful to maintain range of motion. Accelerated growth rate, particularly in adolescence, enhances the progression of deformities (161).

Biofeedback (5, 155) and functional electrical stimulation (FES) have been recommended to train control of specific muscle groups. In a follow-up study of children with hemiplegia, initial gait improvement was not maintained 6 to 12 months after discontinuation of biofeedback (198, 199). Study on long-term effectiveness of FES is not available in cerebral palsy.

Although physical therapy is the most often used treatment in cerebral palsy, efficacy studies are scarce and, for the most part, lack controls (8, 24, 44, 109, 163, 165, 176, 193, 208, 238). In 1989, Tirosh and Rabino found only nine studies during the preceding 15 years pertaining to the efficacy of physical therapy (220). They noted that experimental design was often inadequate and only two investigations used statistical analysis. The authors concluded that the effect of this therapeutic modality has yet to be demonstrated. Palmer et al. (164) compared the results of an early stimulation program and physical therapy in young diplegic children. They found no differences in motor accomplishments between the two groups, but children who received early stimulation did better in language and social development. Unresolved issues are how long should therapy continue, what level of intensity would yield optimal results, and what form of preventive maintenance is justified for the severely affected child with no functional goals. Most children achieve a maximal level of gross motor function, including ambulatory potential, by 6 to 7 years. After this age, physical therapy, regardless of its intensity, is unlikely to produce further functional gains. However, the child will continue to improve in strength, endurance, and coordination if a proper life-style of activities is maintained. Adaptive physical education and sports can achieve this goal while providing more enjoyable experience and contact with peers (104, 146). Preventive maintenance therapy for severely affected children is difficult to obtain and frequently unsuccessful.

FUNCTIONAL TRAINING

Gross motor abilities and hand dexterity are physical determinants for planning a program in activities of daily life. The choice of tasks is guided by developmental expectations appropriate for age and for the individual child's cognitive function. Although training in visual-motor and perceptual skills may be used as a complimentary treatment, only a direct task-oriented approach with practice and repetition will lead to proficiency in specific functional activities (9). When complete independence is not realistic, the child should be encouraged to learn any part of the task he or she can master. Compensatory functional techniques and adaptive devices are aids to independence. No functional training will be successful unless the child is expected to perform consistently at home, in school, and in all other situations of life.

HOME PROGRAM

Advice and education of the family is an important phase of treatment and represents an extension of therapeutic goals to the home. Modifications in physical transactions of daily care are based on observations which show that abnormal tone, posture, and movements may be enhanced or decreased by the way the child is handled, positioned, or moved (62). Education in home management includes techniques for carrying, dressing, seating, locomotion, and other physical activities. Feeding problems caused by pseudobulbar palsy are a frequent cause of concern and source of frustration for the family (62, 152). Desensitization of hyperactive gag, bite reflex, and tongue thrust; facilitation of sucking, swallowing, and chewing; proper positioning; and seating are some aspects of the feeding technique to improve oral motor coordination. Practice of self-care skills, crutch walking, wheelchair locomotion, or a set of simple exercises may be part of the home program at a later age. All recommendations should be carefully weighed and considered with a view of family dynamics to avoid increased parental anxiety or already existing tension between the child and family.

ORTHOSES AND ADAPTIVE DEVICES

The application of resting or night splints is an adjunctive measure to maintain range of motion. Most frequently used are splints to prevent ankle plantar flexion and contractures of the wrists and fingers. A hip abduction orthosis is recommended to delay adduction contractures and progressive subluxation of the hips or to prevent their postoperative recurrence in the severely affected child (148). Temporary ankle-foot splints can be made from thermoplastic materials using the same constructional features as permanent orthoses. A knee extension splint has been recommended for genu recurvatum in conjunction with gait training (43).

Orthoses are prescribed to improve function and/or for the prevention of soft tissue deformities (148, 151). Children with hemiparesis often require an ankle-foot orthosis (AFO) for spastic equinus attitude, which may be associated with supination, or less frequently, pronation of the foot (189). In most cases, an AFO also controls excessive knee extension in stance phase by restricting undue plantar flexion. Ambulatory children with bilateral spasticity generally do not require or benefit from extensive bracing. However, AFOs are often needed for abnormal alignment of the feet when the child pulls to stand and begins to cruise. Selection of solid ankle or hinged AFO is contingent on kinesiological considerations and proximal joint stability (142). Pes planovalgus is a frequent and often severe foot abnormality in this group (Fig. 18.17). Well-fitting plastic AFOs, which incorporate the features of inhibitory casting, are used in these cases. Supramalleolar orthoses (SMO) may be sufficient when plantar flexor spasticity is mild and mediolateral malalignment is the main concern. There is no universally successful orthosis for crouch gait. Knee-ankle-foot orthoses (KAFO) do not

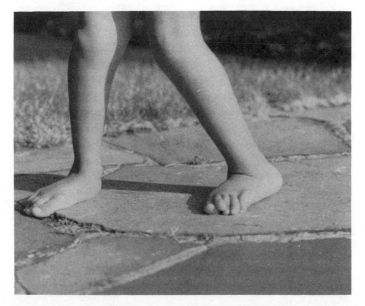

Figure 18.17. Pes planovalgus and hallux valgus in a diplegic child.

eliminate knee flexion in stance phase unless the joints are locked. Ambulation becomes more cumbersome with stiff knees, despite a more pleasing appearance of posture. In some cases, postural improvement can be achieved if knee extension moment is increased by limiting dorsiflexion of the ankles. The floor reaction orthosis with adjustable pretibial shell is another option to correct excessive knee flexion (239). For internal rotation gait, twister orthoses were recommended. However, enthusiasm for their use is dampened by concerns about the development of rotational knee instability and external tibial torsion. The hip action brace restricts adduction but allows free abduction. It is an option to consider when mediolateral hip stabilization is desired for vase stance or lesser degrees of adducted gait. Orthoses have limited application in dyskinetic cerebral palsy. A notable exception is dystonic equinovarus posturing of the ankle, which can interfere with safe ambulation and may be controlled by an AFO (Fig. 18.16).

In recent years, inhibitory and progressive casting has gained popularity and is used as an alternative to an AFO for alleviating abnormal ankle-foot alignment (43, 87, 92, 217). The rationale is that inhibition of persistent hyperactive tonic foot reflexes would restore balanced muscle action, thus permitting the development of physiological equilibrium reactions in the feet (233). The essential component is a molded footplate that stabilizes the hindfoot and controls excessive toe flexion caused by hyperactive plantar grasp reflex. The footplate is incorporated into a bivalved short leg cast or boot. Clinical observation suggest that, in many cases, there is improved postural control around proximal joints with snugly fitting casts that provide a stable, secure supporting base.

The principles and indications of scoliosis bracing apply to cerebral palsy. However, because the majority of children who develop spinal deformities are severely and often multiply handicapped, the value and efficacy of orthotic treatment has been questioned. Refuting these reservations, several reports show satisfactory results in controlling the spinal curvature and no significant problems with tolerating the orthosis (102, 219).

Because of the intent to simulate the developmental sequence of motor milestones, orthoses may be prescribed for ambulation as an exercise or only for passive standing. Prevention of contractures is an additional aim of this approach. The parents must be counseled about realistic expectations and the purpose of orthoses in these instances. A prone stander or standing table to control abnormal postures and to provide greater stability is usually preferred over extensive orthoses for the limited purpose of passive standing.

For a discussion of wheelchairs, seating, nonverbal communication devices, and other types of adaptive equipment in cerebral palsy, the reader is referred to the appropriate chapter (83, 111).

ORTHOPAEDIC SURGERY

In the overall plan of rehabilitation, there is an important role for judiciously used and well-timed surgical treatment (18, 194, 215, 219). Surgery

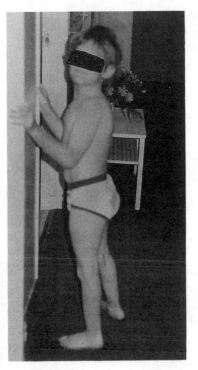

Figure 18.18. Young diplegic boy shown in Figure 18.10 following bilateral surgical lengthening of hip adductors and tendo Achilles.

may be indicated to improve function and appearance, to prevent or correct deformities, or for a combination of these reasons.

Spastic muscle imbalance can be decreased by tendon lengthening or transfer (Fig. 18.18). Improved posture and gait after correction of a spastic equinus foot is an example of functional gains from surgery (72, 105, 186). Alleviation of deforming muscle forces for preventive purposes is an equally important aim and, in severely impaired children, the main indication for surgery. Skeletal complications of spastic muscle imbalance can be anticipated long before their appearance and may be avoided by early soft tissue surgery. Acquired hip dislocation may be prevented in some severely affected children by release of spastic hip flexors and adductors (39). However, soft tissue procedures are not always successful in preventing bone deformities. Osteotomy and arthrodesis may be needed to correct progressive subluxation or dislocation of the hip, torsional deformity of the femur, or severe foot abnormalities.

Surgical procedures are less frequently recommended for the upper extremities (78, 121). Due to the central motor and sensory impairment (22), improved cosmetic appearance is a more consistent gain after surgery than enhanced volitional movement control and functional use.

Opinions often differ regarding the procedure of choice for achieving optimal surgical correction. Postoperative deterioration of ambulatory function is a concern but can be avoided by careful analysis of the presenting postural and gait abnormalities. Electromyographic assessment of spastic gait can be used to identify abnormal muscle activity and to select the most appropriate surgical intervention (1, 174, 201, 213). Postoperative immobilization leads to a temporary setback of function. It is important to realize that many months may be required until disuse weakness and lack of practice are corrected and the maximal benefit of surgery becomes evident. Range of motion exercises in warm water are most effective to overcome joint stiffness and pain immediately after a cast is removed. Physical therapy to regain strength and movement control will shorten the time needed to achieve the functional improvement expected after surgery. A most difficult and often unsuccessful task is to prevent recurrence of surgically corrected deformities in children who are nonfunctional ambulators or who do not walk at all. Surgery is rarely advisable or necessary before 3 yr of age since neurological signs may be still in a flux and maturation of motor function is in a stage of evolution.

To avoid unrealistic expectations and disappointments, the purpose of surgery must be carefully explained to the family and, when possible, to the child. They must also understand postoperative care, the time and effort needed to reach the projected functional benefits, and possible problems with long-range maintenance of gains.

NEUROSURGICAL PROCEDURES

Stereotaxic ablation of selected thalamic nuclei (79), chronic electrical stimulation of the cerebellum (40, 45) or posterior column of the cervical cord (98) are neurological procedures that have been tried and abandoned for treating spastic cerebral palsy.

Selective posterior rhizotomy is the only surgical treatment currently in use (171). Foerster (65) proposed the technique of severing L2-S2 posterior roots entirely except for sparing L4 or L5 to preserve quadriceps function for the treatment of spasticity in cerebral palsy and other neurological diseases. He reported the results of 159 cases of which 88 were cerebral palsy. In the 1970s, Fasano and associates (59) revived and modified the technique of surgery by performing partial rhizotomy of only those rootlets that, on electrical stimulation, produced a spread and prolonged activation of several muscle groups. Peacock and associates (168, 170) further modified this method by selective posterior rhizotomy using L2-L5 laminectomy and localizing the posterior roots in the cauda equina. During the procedure, muscle responses to electrical stimulation of the rootlets are monitored electromyographically. Those rootlets, which generate increased, clonic, or sustained muscle contractions are selectively divided. The proposed neurophysiological mechanism is to alleviate spasticity by eliminating the influence of excitatory rootlets, which presumably contribute to disinhibition of reciprocal innervation through their spinal interneuronal connections. Patients for the procedure are selected on the basis of having pure spasticity, without signs of any other type of neuromuscular dysfunction. Children with spastic diplegia who can walk, have good intelligence, adequate strength, motor control, and balance are said to derive maximal benefit from the procedure. Intensive, preferably five times a week, physical therapy is recommended postoperatively for 6 to 12 months to regain strength. In cases of contractures, orthopaedic surgery is advised after but not prior to the rhizotomy. Follow-up studies up to 7 yr indicate persistent weakness in some children. Postoperative gait analysis showed increased stride length and speed of ambulation and some improvement of electromyographic gait abnormalities (30). H-reflex studies indicated a decrease of spasticity (31). Landau and Hunt (127) questioned the justification and efficacy of selective posterior rhizotomy on several grounds. They postulated that the neurophysiological mechanism is not proven; and lack of volitional control is a more significant contributor to the range of motor disabilities in upper motor neuron syndromes than spasticity per se. Since children with cerebral palsy do improve throughout childhood, particularly the preferentially selected mild diplegic population, controlled studies are needed to prove the effectiveness and superiority of selective posterior rhizotomy over other methods of treatment; the risks of diminished sensation and possible other long-term adverse effects have not been addressed. As with other neurosurgical procedures that have been enthusiastically endorsed in the past, it remains to be seen whether selective posterior rhizotomy will withstand the test of time.

PHARMACOLOGICAL TREATMENT

A number of drugs have been recommended to decrease spasticity (76). The general tranquilizing effect of diazepam usually counteracts its value as an antispasticity agent and limits the use of the drug in children who function independently. Dantrolene sodium, acting on the muscle tissue, has a more specific effect on spastic hypertonicity. Most children and their parents report decreased stiffness and greater ease of movement, although objective functional improvement is difficult to measure. Untoward reactions are generally transient and not significant. Temporary elevation of liver enzymes may occur, but hepatotoxicity has not been reported in children. Baclofen, which is currently recommended for spinal cord spasticity, may produce relaxation of predominant extensor hypertonicity in some cases (76). The use of levodopa in dyskinetic cerebral palsy has been abandoned.

Injection of phenol or alcohol solution into the peripheral nerve or motor points of a spastic muscle results in tone decrease by creating a chemical neurolysis (76). The effect is transient, lasting several months. Good results and no significant side effects were reported with repeated injections. The procedure is useful primarily as a temporizing measure.

Medical Management

Seizure disorders must be treated with anticonvulsants (3, 219), although an abnormal EEG without history of clinical episodes does not necessarily require drug treatment. However, the parents should be informed about this finding and the possibility that seizures may develop. Laboratory tests to monitor adverse reactions and therapeutic blood level are performed regularly during anticonvulsant therapy. In addition to the clinical type of seizures, behavioral side effects should be kept in mind when selecting the appropriate medication. Some children eventually become seizure-free. Gradual discontinuation of drug therapy is considered in the absence of recurrent episodes after 2 to 4 yr, particularly when EEG is no longer abnormal (219).

All children with cerebral palsy should undergo periodic assessment of visual and auditory function in view of the high incidence of these deficits. Early correction of impaired vision and hearing is essential to alleviate developmental consequences of such additional disabilities (48, 74, 77, 219). Speech and language disorders and their treatment, including nonverbal communication devices (219), are discussed in Chapter 4.

Head circumference is measured on every examination. A continuing downward shift reflects decreased brain growth and raises concerns about intellectual outlook. A relative increase of head circumference suggests the possibility of hydrocephalus for which premature infants with intraventricular-periventricular hemorrhage are especially at risk. Children with shunted hydrocephalus should be observed for signs of malfunction.

Height and weight measurements are taken serially to determine physical growth. A tendency for relatively smaller body size was shown in cerebral palsy as a group, but significant growth retardation is most frequent in severely disabled children (209). Additional discrepancy between stature and weight suggests inadequate nutrition. When oral motor dysfunction compromises adequate food intake, high caloric supplemental feeding and/or gastrostomy are required (75, 169, 181, 200). Allowance for the increased cost of physical activity should be taken into consideration in active children.

Dental anomalies, malocclusion, oral motor dysfunction, and gingival hypertrophy caused by some anticonvulsant drugs make proper dental care essential (14, 152). For the treatment of drooling, behavioral, pharmacological, and surgical methods offer several options (28, 90, 180).

The treatment of bronchopulmonary dysplasia in premature infants with cerebral palsy is in the expertise of pediatric pulmonary specialists. With the higher survival rate of small prematures, the number of ventilator and tracheostomy-dependent children with cerebral palsy seems to be increasing. A preventive intervention for obstructive lung disease from aspiration in mild oral motor dysfunction is proper feeding and positioning techniques. Swallowing studies are advisable in more severe cases to rule out aspiration of food and secretions from the pharynx or gastroesophageal reflux, and to determine whether gastrostomy and fundoplication are indicated (66, 81, 236). Assisted coughing, chest percussion, and postural drainage should be performed regularly when difficulties with clearing upper airway and bronchial secretions are present. The treatment of respiratory infections is antibiotics, bronchodilators, and other appropriate medications. Restrictive pulmonary disease develops from weakness and incoordination of respiratory muscles. Thoracic deformities, especially scoliosis and poor sitting posture, enhance the mechanical efficiency of breathing. Nwaobi and Smith reported improved vital capacity with adapted wheelchair seating as a result of good postural support (160). Spinal orthosis or, for curvatures above 40°, surgical stabilization are temporary and definitive treatment methods of scoliosis (60, 183). Pulmonary function studies should be performed prior to surgery to assess the risk of postoperative mechanical ventilatory dependency (123).

It is well-documented that motor deficits increase the energy expenditure of physical activities (32, 187, 188). On the other hand, work physiological studies demonstrated that, in cerebral palsy, pulmonary function and working capacity are below normal (12, 16, 136, 137). Rothman found that exercises increased vital capacity (190). Despite these considerations, the issue of promoting optimal cardiopulmonary conditioning in mild to moderately affected mobile children has not been systemically addressed. The importance of encouraging a reasonable activity level seems evident. Participation in adapted sports contributes to achieving physical fitness through enjoyment and recreation (104).

Urinary incontinence in cerebral palsy used to be attributed to behavioral causes or intellectual limitation. However, recent data indicate that micturition problems, possibly of neurogenic origin, occur in older children and adults (23). Cystometric studies demonstrated spastic bladder and detrusor sphincter dyssynergy in some cases. The exact mechanism of these abnormalities is unclear. Anoxic spinal cord dysfunction associated with the cerebral insult has been proposed as one potential cause. The long-term effect of bladder abnormalities on upper urinary tract function is currently unknown.

Osteoporosis, although less marked than in lower motor neuron paralysis, develops in severely affected, nonambulatory children. Neuropathic fractures are rare but may occur, especially after immobilization for surgery or other reasons. Weight-bearing in the form of passive standing intends to alleviate bone loss. Heterotopic ossification has not been described in cerebral palsy until a recent report of three cases during postoperative immobilization (129).

Educational and Vocational Considerations

Psychosocial and education issues are discussed in the preceding chapters. Therefore, this subject is addressed briefly, nonetheless emphatically. Physicians must look beyond the problems of physical disability and assist the family in providing a life experience for the child that will prepare him or her for the role of adulthood (73, 93, 145, 182, 235). Planning of education, vocational future, and recreation are equal in importance to caring for the child's physical well-being (37, 42, 91, 147, 162, 219, 225). The primary consideration in educational placement is intellectual ability. Physical assistance and classroom adaptations can compensate for motor dysfunction (205). Support for emotional help and social adjustment is often a more complex and difficult undertaking than rehabilitation of the physical disability (42, 47, 48, 146).

Long-term studies show a 30% to 50% vocational success rate among adults with cerebral palsy, including competitive and sheltered employment (42, 101). Physical ability, cognitive function, and psychosocial skills were three factors influencing ultimate life achievements. Surveys of adults with cerebral palsy demonstrated medical complications related to the neuromuscular dysfunction (191, 218). In profoundly impaired individuals with very severe motor disability and mental retardation, shortened life expectancy is reported (57, 122).

REFERENCES

1. Adler N, Bleck EE, Rinsky LA: Gait electromyograms and surgical decisions for paralytic deformities of the foot. *Dev Med Child Neurol* 31:287–292, 1989.
2. Adsett DB, Fitz DR, et al: Hypoxic ischemic cerebral injury in the term newborn: Correlation of CT findings with neurologic outcome. *Dev Med Child Neurol* 27:155–160, 1985.
3. Aicardi J: Epilepsy in brain-injured children. *Dev Med Child Neurol* 32:191–202, 1990.
4. Aksu F: Nature and prognosis of seizures in patients with cerebral palsy. *Dev Med Child Neurol* 32:661–668, 1990.
5. American Academy of Pediatrics. Committee on Fetus and Newborn. Use and abuse of Apgar score. *Pediatrics* 78:1148–1149, 1986.
6. Astbury J, Orgill AA, et al: Neurodevelopmental outcome, growth and health of extremely low-birthweight survivors: How can we tell? *Dev Med Child Neurol* 32:582–589, 1990.
7. Badell-Ribera A: Cerebral palsy: Postural-locomotor prognosis in spastic diplegia. *Arch Phys Med Rehabil* 66:614–619, 1985.
8. Banham KM: Progress in motor development of retarded cerebral palsied infants. *Rehabil Lit* 37:13–14, 1976.
9. Basmajian JV (ed): *Therapeutic Exercises*, ed 4. Baltimore, Williams & Wilkins, 1984.
10. Bax M: Aims and outcomes of physiotherapy for cerebral palsy. *Dev Med Child Neurol* 29:689–692, 1987.
11. Bax MCO: Terminology and classification of cerebral palsy. *Dev Med Child Neurol* 6:295, 1964.
12. Berg K: Adaptation in cerebral palsy of body composition, nutrition and physical working capacity at school age. *Acta Paediatr Scand (Suppl)*:204, 1970.
13. Beverly DW, Smith IS, et al: Relationship of cranial ultrasonography, visual and auditory

evoked responses with neurodevelopmental outcome. *Dev Med Child Neurol* 32:210-222, 1990.

14. Bhat M, Nelson KB: Developmental enamel defects in primary teeth in children with cerebral palsy, mental retardation or hearing defects: A review. *Adv Dental Res* 3:132-142, 1989.

15. Bigler ED, Yeo RA, Turkheim E: *Neurophysiological Function and Brain Imaging*. New York, Plenum Press, 1989.

16. Bjure J, Berg K: Dynamic and static lung volumes of school children with cerebral palsy. *Acta Paediatr Scand (Suppl)* 204:35, 1970.

17. Blair E, Stanley FJ: Minor morphogenetic anomalies in cerebral palsy. *J Pediatr* 113:955, 1988.

18. Bleck E: *Orthopedic Management in Cerebral Palsy*. Philadelphia, JB Lippincott, 1987.

19. Bleck EE: Locomotor prognosis in cerebral palsy. *Dev Med Child Neurol* 17:18, 1975.

20. Bobath B: *Abnormal Postural Reflex Activity Caused by Brain Lesions*, ed. 3. Frederick MD, Aspen Systems Pub, 1985.

21. Bobath K: *A Neurophysiological Basis for the Treatment of Cerebral Palsy*. Clinics in Developmental Medicine Series, No. 75, ed 2. Philadelphia, JB Lippincott, 1985.

22. Bolanos AA, Bleck EE , et al: Comparison of stereognosis and two-point discrimination testing of the hands of children with cerebral palsy. *Dev Med Child Neurol* 31:371-376, 1989.

23. Borzyskowski M: Cerebral palsy and the bladder. *Dev Med Child Neurol* 31:687-689, 1989.

24. Brandt S, Lonstrup H, et al: Prevention of cerebral palsy in motor-risk infants by treatment ad modum Vojta. *Acta Paediatr Scand* 69:283-296, 1980.

25. Brann AW: Hypoxic ischemic encephalopathy (asphyxia). *Pediatr Clin North Am* 33:451-464, 1986.

26. Brazelton TB, Cramer BG: *The Earliest Relationship. Parents, Infants and the Drama of Early Attachment*. New York, Addison-Wesley Publ Co, 1990.

27. Bricker D (ed): *Intervention with At-Risk and Handicapped Infants: From Research to Application*. Baltimore, University Park Press, 1982.

28. Brundage SR, Moore WD: Submandibular gland resection and bilateral duct ligation as a management of chronic drooling in cerebral palsy. *Plast Reconstruct Surg* 83:443-446, 1989.

29. Bu'Lock F, Woolridge MW, Baum JD: Development of coordination of sucking, swallowing, and breathing: Ultrasound study of term and pre-term infants. *Dev Med Child Neurol* 32:669-678, 1990.

30. Cahan LD, Adam JM, et al: Instrumented gait analysis after selective dorsal rhizotomy. *Dev Med Child Neurol* 32:1037-1043, 1990.

31. Cahan LD, Kundi MS, et al: Electrophysiologic studies in selective dorsal rhizotomy in spastic children with cerebral palsy. *Appl Neurophysiol* 50:459-460, 1987.

32. Campbell J, Ball J: Energetics of walking in cerebral palsy. *Orthop Clin North Am* 9:374, 1978.

33. Choi BH, Lapham LW, et al: Abnormal neuronal migration, deranged cerebral cortical organization, and diffuse white matter astrocytosis of human fetal brain: A major effect of methylmercury poisoning in utero. *J Neuropath Exper Neurol* 37:719-733, 1978.

34. Christensen E, Melchior J: *Cerebral Palsy—A Clinical and Neuropathologic Study*. Clinics in Developmental Medicine Series No. 25. JB Lippincott, 1967.

35. Chugani HT, Phelps ME: Maturational changes in cerebral function of infants determined by FDG Positron emission tomography. *Science* 231:840-846, 1986.

36. Chugani HT, Phelps ME, Mazziotta JC: Positron emission tomography study of human brain functional development. *Ann Neurol* 22:487-497, 1987.

37. Connor FP: Education for the handicapped child. In Downey JA, Low NG (Eds): *The Child with Disabling Illness, Principles of Rehabilitation*. Philadelphia, WB Saunders, 1983.

38. Connor FP, Williamson GG, Siepp JM: *Program Guide for Infants and Toddlers with Neuromuscular and Other Developmental Disabilities.* New York, Teachers College Press, 1978.
39. Cooke PH, Cob WG, Carey RPL: Dislocation of the hip in cerebral palsy: Natural history and predictability. *J Bone Joint Surg* 71B:441–447, 1989.
40. Cooper IS (ed): *Cerebellar Stimulation in Man.* New York, Raven Press, 1978.
41. Cotman CW (ed): *Neuronal Plasticity.* New York, Guilford Press, 1988.
42. Crothers BS, Paine RS: *The Natural History of Cerebral Palsy.* Cambridge, MA. Harvard Press, 1959.
43. Cusick BD: *Progressive Casting and Splinting for Lower Extremity Deformities in Children with Neuromuscular Dysfunction.* Tucson, AZ, Therapy Skill Builders Publ, 1990.
44. D'Avignon MD, Noren L, Arman T: Early physiotherapy ad modum Vojta or Bobath in infants with suspected neuromotor disturbances. *Neuropediatrics* 12:232–241, 1981.
45. Davis R, Schulman J, et al: Cerebellar stimulation for spastic cerebral palsy—double blind quantitative study. *Appl Neurophysiol* 50:451–452, 1987.
46. Denays R, Tondeur M, et al: Cerebral palsy: Initial experience with Tc-99m HMPAO SPECT of the brain. *Radiology* 175:111–116, 1990.
47. Denhoff E: *Cerebral Palsy, the Preschool Years.* Springfield, IL, Charles Thomas, 1967.
48. Denhoff E, Robinault IP: Cerebral Palsy and Related Disorders. New York, McGraw-Hill, 1960.
49. Downey WS: Public Law 99-457. *Clin Pediatr* 29:158–161, 1990.
50. Drillien CM, Thomson AYM, Burgoyne K: Low birthweight children at early school age. A longitudinal study. *Dev Med Child Neurol* 22:26, 1980.
51. Dunn HG: *Sequelae of Low Birthweight: The Vancouver Study.* Clinic Devel Med, No. 95/96, Philadelphia, JB Lippincott, 1986.
52. Ellenberg J, Nelson KB: Birthweight and gestational age in children with cerebral palsy or seizure disorder. *Am J Disease Child* 133:1044–1048, 1979.
53. Ellenberg JH, Nelson KB: Cluster of perinatal events identifying infants at high risk for death or disability. *J Pediatr* 113:546–552, 1988.
54. Ellis W, Goetzman BW, Lindenberg JA: Neuropathologic demonstration of prenatal brain damage. *Am J Dis Child* 142:858–866, 1988.
55. Evans P, Johnson A, et al: Standardized recording of central motor deficit and associated sensory and intellectual deficits. *Dev Med Child Neurol* 31:117–129, 1989.
56. Evrard P, Minkowski A (eds): *Developmental Neurobiology.* New York, Raven Press, 1989.
57. Eyman RK, Grossman HJ, et al: The life expectancy of profoundly handicapped people with mental retardation. *N Eng J Med* 323:584–589, 1990.
58. Faerber EN: *Cranial Computed Tomography in Infants and Children.* Clinics in Developmental Medicine Series No. 93. Philadelphia, JB Lippincott, 1986.
59. Fasano VA, Broggi G, et al: Long-term results of posterior functional rhizotomy. *Acta Neuroclin (Suppl)* 30:435–439, 1980.
60. Ferguson RL, Allen BL: Considerations in the treatment of cerebral palsy patients with spinal deformities. *Orthop Clinic North Am* 19:419–426, 1988.
61. Finger S, Stein DJ: *Brain Damage and Recovery: Research and Clinical Perspectives.* Orlando, Academic Press, 1982.
62. Finnie N: *Handling the Young Cerebral Palsied Child At Home.* New York, Dutton Publ, 1975.
63. Fiorentino M: *A Basis for Sensorimotor Development—Normal and Abnormal.* Springfield, IL, Charles Thomas, 1981.
64. Fiorentino M: *Normal and Abnormal Development—The Influence of Primitive Reflexes on Motor Development.* Springfield, IL, Charles Thomas, 1980.
65. Foerster O: Uber eine neue operative Methode der Behandlung spastischer Lähmungen mittels Resektion hinterer RM Wurzeln. *Z Ortho Chir* 22:202–208, 1922.

66. Foglia RP, Fonkalsrud EW, et al: Gastroesophageal fundoplication for the management of chronic pulmonary disease in children. *Am J Surg* 140:72–79, 1980.
67. Fraser B, Hensinger R: *Physical Management of Multiple Handicaps*. Baltimore, Brooks Publ Co, 1982.
68. Freeman JM, Avery G, et al: National Institutes of Health report on causes of mental retardation and cerebral palsy. Assessment of prenatal and perinatal factors associated with brain disorders. *Pediatrics* 76:457–458, 1985.
69. Freeman JM, Nelson KB: Intrapartum asphyxia and cerebral palsy. *Pediatrics* 82:240–249, 1988.
70. French JN, Harel S, Casear P: *Child Neurology and Developmental Disabilities*. Baltimore, Paul H. Brooks, 1989.
71. Freud S: *Infantile Cerebral Paralysis*. Coral Gables, University of Miami Press, 1968.
72. Fulford GE: Surgical managment of ankle and foot deformities in cerebral palsy. *Clin Orthop* 253:55–61, 1990.
73. Garrison WT, McQuiston S: *Chronic Illness During Childhood and Adolescence: Psychological Aspects*. Dev Clin Psychiat, Vol 19, London, Sage, 1989.
74. Gibson NA, Fielder AR, et al: Opthalmic findings in infants of very low birthweight. *Dev Med Child Neurol* 32:7–13, 1990.
75. Gisel EG, Patrick J: Identification of children with cerebral palsy unable to maintain a normal nutritional state. *Lancet* 1:283–286, 1988.
76. Glenn MB, Whyte J (eds): *The Practical Management of Spasticity in Children and Adults*. Philadelphia, Lea Febiger, 1990.
77. Goble JL: *Visual Disorders in the Handicapped Child*. New York, Marcel Dekker Inc, 1984.
78. Goldner JL: Surgical reconstruction of the upper extremity in cerebral palsy. *Hand Clin* 4:233–266, 1988.
79. Gornall P, Hitchcock E, Kirkland IS: Stereotaxic neuro ourgery in the management of cerebral palsy. *Dev Med Child Neurol* 17:279, 1975.
80. Greenough WT, Juraska JM (eds): *Developmental Neuro-psychobiology*. Orlando, Plenum Press, 1986.
81. Griggs CA, Jones PM, Lee RE: Videofluoroscopic investigations of feeding disorders of children with multiple handicaps. *Dev Med Child Neurol* 31:303–308, 1989.
82. Grögaard JB, Lindstrom DP, et al: Increased survival rate in very low birthweight infants (1500 grams or less): No association with increased incidence of handicaps. *J Pediatr* 117:139–146, 1990.
83. Gulford GE, Cairns TP, Sloan J: Sitting problems of children with cerebral palsy. *Dev Med Child Neurol* 24:48, 1982.
84. Guralnick MJ, Bennett FC: *The Effectiveness of Early Intervention for At-Risk and Handicapped Children*. Orlando, Academic Press, 1987.
85. Hagberg B, Hagberg G, et al: The changing panorama of cerebral palsy in Sweden. V: The birth year period 1979–1982. *Acta Paediatr Scand* 78:283–290, 1989.
86. Hagberg B, Hagberg G, Zetterstrom R: Decreasing perinatal mortality—Increase in cerebral palsy morbidity. *Acta Paediatr Scand* 78:664–670, 1989.
87. Hanson CJ, Jones LJ: Gait abnormalities and inhibitive casts in cerebral palsy: Literature review. *J Pediatr Med Assoc* 79:53–59, 1989.
88. Harbord MG, Finn JP: Myelination pattern on magnetic resonance imaging in children with developmental delay. *Dev Med Child Neurol* 32:295–303, 1990.
89. Harris SP: Early diagnosis of spastic diplegia, spastic hemiplegia, and quadriplegia. *Am J Dis Child* 143:1356–1360, 1984.
90. Harris SP, Purdy AH: Drooling and its managment in cerebral palsy. *Dev Med Child Neurol* 29:807–811, 1987.
91. Haskell B, Barrett EK: *The Education of Children with Motor and Neurological Disabilities*. London, Chapman and Hall, 1989.

92. Hinderer KA, Harris SR, et al: Effects of "tone-reducing" versus standard plaster casts on gait improvement of children with cerebral palsy. *Dev Med Child Neurol* 30:370–377, 1988.
93. Hirst M: Pattern of impairment and disability related to social handicap in young people with cerebral palsy and spina bifida. *J Biosoc Sci* 28:1–12, 1989.
94. Hoffer MM, Knoebel RT, Roberts R: Contractures in cerebral palsy. *Clin Orthop* 219:70–77, 1987.
95. Holt KS: *Disturbances of Carpal Growth.* Clinics in Developmental Medicine Series, No. 4. London, Spastics Society/Heinemann, 1961.
96. Holt KS: Growth Disturbances. *Hemiplegic Cerebral Palsy in Children and Adults.* Clinics in Developmental Medicine Series, No. 4. London, Spastics Society/Heinemann, 1961.
97. Howard EM, Henderson SE: Perceptual problems in cerebral palsied children: A real-world example. *Hum Move Sci* 8:141–160, 1989.
98. Hugenholtz H, Humphreys P, et al: Cervical cord stimulation for spasticity in cerebral palsy. *Neurosurgery* 22:707–714, 1988.
99. Illingworth R: A pediatrician asks—Why is it called birth injury? *Br J Med Obstet Gynecol* 92:122–130, 1985.
100. Ingram TTS: A Historical Review of the Definition and Classification of the Cerebral Palsies. In Stanley F, Alberman E (eds): *The Epidemiology of the Cerebral Palsies.* Clinics in Developmental Medicine Series No. 87, Philadelphia, JB Lippincott, 1984.
101. Ingram TTS: *Paediatric Aspects of Cerebral Palsy.* Edinburgh, ES Livingston, 1964.
102. James WV: Spinal bracing for children with atonic cerebral palsy. *Prosthet Orthot Int* 1:105, 1977.
103. Jernigan TL, Tallal P: Late childhood changes in brain morphology observable on MRI. *Dev Med Child Neurol* 32:379–385, 1990.
104. Johnstone K, Perrin JCS: Sports for the handicapped child and sports injuries of the disabled athlete. In Molnar GE (ed): *Physical Disabilities of Children.* State of the Art Reviews. Rehabilitation. Philadelphia, Hanley & Dreyfus, 1991.
105. Jones ET, Knapp RB: Assessment and management of the lower extremity in cerebral palsy. *Orthop Clin North Am* 18:725–738, 1987.
106. Jones MH, Barrett ML, Olonoff C, Anderson E: Two experiments in training handicapped children. Clinics in Developmental Medicine Series, No. 30. London, Spastics Society/Heinemann, 1969.
107. Jones MH, Dayton GO, Limpaecher R, Murphy TV, Hirsch P: Electro-oculographic studies in cerebral palsied children. In *Aspects of Developmental and Pediatric Ophthalmology.* Clinics in Developmental Medicine Series, No. 32. London, Spastics Society/Heinemann, 1969.
108. Jones PM: Feeding disorders in children with multiple handicaps. *Dev Med Child Neurol* 31:404–406, 1989.
109. Kanda T, Yuge M, et al: Early physiotherapy in the treatment of spastic cerebral palsy. *Dev Med Child Neurol* 26:438–444, 1984.
110. Kaplan MS: Plasticity after brain lesions: Contemporary concepts. *Arch Phys Med Rehabil* 69:984–991, 1988.
111. Katz K, Liebertal M, Erken EHW: Seat insert for cerebral palsied children with total body involvement. *Dev Med Child Neurol* 30:222–226, 1988.
112. Kidron D, Steiner I, Melamed E: Late-onset progressive radiculomyelopathy in patients with cervical athetoid dystonic cerebral palsy. *Europ Neurol* 27:164–166, 1987.
113. Kiely M, Lubin RA, Kiely JZ: Descriptive epidemiology of cerebral palsy. *Public Health Rev* 12:79–101, 1984.
114. Kitchen WH, Ford GW, et al: Children of birthweight < 1000 grams: Changing outcome between ages 2 and 5 years. *J Pediatr* 110:283–288, 1987.
115. Kjos BO, Umansky R, Barkovich AJ: Brain MR imaging in children with developmental retardation of unknown cause: Results in 76 cases. *Am J Neuroradiol* 11:1035–1040, 1990.

116. Klapper ZS, Birch HG: A fourteen year follow-up study of cerebral palsy: Intellectual change and stability. *Am J Orthopysch* 37:540–547, 1967.
117. Klapper ZS, Birch HG: The relation of childhood characteristics to outcome in young adults with cerebral palsy. *Dev Med Child Neurol* 4:643, 1966.
118. Klimach VJ, Cooke RWI: Short latency cortical somatosensory evoked responses of preterm infants with ultrasound abnormality of the brain. *Dev Med Child Neurol* 30:215–221, 1988.
119. Kolawole TM, Patel PJ, Mahdi AH: Computed tomographic (CT) scan in cerebral palsy (CP). *Pediatr Radiol* 20:23–27, 1989.
120. Kolb B, Wishaw IQ: Plasticity of the neocortex: Mechanisms underlying recovery from early brain damage. *Progress Neurobiol* 32:235–276, 1989.
121. Koman AL, Gelberman RH, et al: Cerebral palsy. Management of the upper extremity. *Clin Orthop Relat Res* 253:62–74, 1990.
122. Kudrjacev T, Schoenberg BS, et al: Cerebral palsy. Survival rates, associated handicaps and distribution by clinical subtype (Rochester, MN 1956-1976). *Neurology* 35:900–903, 1985.
123. Kumano K, Tsuyama N: Pulmonary function before and after surgical correction of scoliosis. *J Bone Joint Surg* 64A:242–248, 1982.
124. Kyllerman M: Dyskinetic cerebral palsy. II: Pathogenetic risk factors and intrauterine growth. *Acta Paediatr Scand* 71:551–559, 1982.
125. Kyllerman M: Reduced optimality in pre- and perinatal conditions in dyskinetic cerebral palsy—Distribution and comparison to controls. *Neuropediatrics* 14:29–36, 1983.
126. Kyllerman M, Bager B, et al: Dyskinetic cerebral palsy. I: Clinical categories, associated neurological abnormalities and incidences. *Acta Paediatr Scand* 71:543–550, 1982.
127. Landau WM, Hunt CC: Dorsal rhizotomy, a treatment of unproven efficacy. *J Child Neurol* 5:174–178, 1990.
128. Largo RH, Molinari L, Weber M, et al: Early development of locomotion: Significance of prematurity, cerebral palsy and sex. *Dev Med Child Neurol* 27:183–191, 1985.
129. Lee M, Alexander M, et al: Postoperative heterotopic ossification in cerebral palsy. *Arch Phys Med Rehabil* 72:792–796, 1991.
130. Levene MI, Williams JL, Fawer CL: *Ultrasound of the Infant Brain.* Clinics in Developmental Medicine Series, No. 92, Philadelphia, JB Lippincott, 1985.
131. Levitt S: *Pediatric Developmental Therapy.* St. Louis, Mosby Year Book Publ, 1984.
132. Levitt S: *Treatment of Cerebral Palsy and Motor Delay.* Oxford, Blackwell Scientific Publications, 1982.
133. Lewis M, Taft LT (eds): *Developmental Disabilities, Theory, Assessment and Intervention.* Jamaica, New York, Spectrum Publications, 1982.
134. Little WJ: On the influence of abnormal parturition, difficult labor, premature birth and physical condition of the child, especially in relation to deformities. *Trans Obstet Soc* 3:293, 1862.
135. Love RJ, Hagerman EL, Taimi EG: Speech performance, dysphasia and oral reflexes in cerebral palsy. *J Speech Hear Disord* 85:59, 1980.
136. Lundberg A: Longitudinal study of physical working capacity of young people with spastic cerebral palsy. *Dev Med Child Neurol* 26:328–334, 1984.
137. Lundberg A: Maximal aerobic capacity of young people with spastic cerebral palsy. *Dev Med Child Neurol* 20:205–210, 1978.
138. MacKeith R: The restoration of the parents as the keystone of the therapeutic arch. *Dev Med Child Neurol* 18:825, 1976.
139. Mahajan DS, Desiraju T: Alterations of dendritic branching and spine density of hippocampal CA3 pyramidal neurons induced by operant conditioning in the phase of brain growth spurt. *Exper Neurol* 100:1–15, 1988.
140. Marfo K (ed): *Parent-Child Interaction and Developmental Disabilities.* New York, Praeger, 1988.

141. Matthews DJ: Controversial therapies in the management of cerebral palsy. *Pediatr Ann* 17:762–765, 1988.

142. Middleton EA, Huri GR, McIlwain JS: The role of rigid and hinged polypropylene ankle-foot orthoses in the management of cerebral palsy: A case study. *Prosthet Orthot Internat* 12:129–135, 1988.

143. Miller G: Minor congenital anomalies and ataxic cerebral palsy. *Arch Dis Child* 64:557–562, 1989.

144. Miller G, Cala LA: Ataxic cerebral palsy—Clinico-radiologic correlations. *Neuropediatrics* 20:84–89, 1989.

145. Milunski A (ed): *Coping with Crisis and Handicap.* New York, Plenum Press, 1981.

146. Molnar GE: A developmental perspective for the rehabilitation of children with physical disabilities. *Pediatr Ann* 17:766–777, 1988.

147. Molnar GE: Cerebral palsy: Prognosis and how to judge it. *Pediatr Ann* 8:596, 1979.

148. Molnar GE: Orthotic management of children. In Redford J (ed): *Orthotics, Etc.* Baltimore, Williams & Wilkins, 1986.

149. Molnar GE, Gordon SU: Cerebral palsy: Predictive value of selected clinical signs for early prognostication of motor function. *Arch Phys Med Rehabil* 57:153, 1976.

150. Morris S: *The Normal Acquisition of Oral Feeding Skills.* Santa Barbara, Therapeutic Media Inc., 1982.

151. Mossberg KA, Linton KA, Friske K: Ankle-foot orthoses: Effect on energy expenditure of gait in spastic diplegic children. *Arch Phys Med Rehabil* 71:490–494, 1990.

152. Mueller HA: Facilitating feeding and prespeech. In Pearson P, Williams CE (eds): *Physical Therapy Services in the Developmental Disabilities.* Springfield, IL, Charles C Thomas, 1980.

153. Naeye RL, Peters EC, et al: Origins of cerebral palsy. *Am J Dis Child* 143:1154–1161, 1989.

154. Nelson KB: What proportion of cerebral palsy is related to birth asphyxia? *J Pediatr* 112:572–574, 1988.

155. Nelson KB, Ellenberg JH: Antecedents of cerebral palsy. I: Univariate analysis of risk. *Am J Dis Child* 139:1031–1038, 1985.

156. Nelson KB, Ellenberg JH: Antecedents of cerebral palsy: Multivariate analysis of risk. *N Eng J Med* 315:81–86, 1986.

157. Nelson KB, Ellenberg JH: Children who "outgrew" cerebral palsy. *Pediatrics* 69:529–536, 1982.

158. Nelson KB, Ellenberg JH: The asymptomatic newborn at risk for cerebral palsy. *Am J Dis Child* 141:1333–1335, 1987.

159. Norlin R, Odenrick P: Development of gait in children with spastic cerebral palsy. *J Pediatr Orthop* 6:674–680, 1986.

160. Nwaobi OM, Smith PD: Effect of adaptive seating on pulmonary function in children with cerebral palsy. *Dev Med Child Neurol* 28:351–354, 1986.

161. O'Dwyer NJ, Neilson PD, Nash J: Mechanisms of muscle growth related to muscle contracture in cerebral palsy. *Dev Med Child Neurol* 31:543–547, 1989.

162. O'Grady RS, Nishimura DM, et al: Vocational predictions compared with present vocational status of 60 young adults with cerebral palsy. *Dev Med Child Neurol* 27:775–784, 1985.

163. Paine RS: On the treatment of cerebral palsy: The outcome of 177 patients, 74 totally untreated. *Pediatrics* 29:605, 1962.

164. Palmer FB, Shapiro BK, et al: Infant stimulation curriculum for infants with cerebral palsy: Effect on infant temperament, parent-infant interaction and home environment. *Pediatrics* 85:411–415, 1990.

165. Palmer FB, Shapiro BK, et al: The effects of physical therapy on cerebral palsy: A controlled trial in infants with spastic diplegia. *N Eng J Med* 315:803–808, 1988.

166. Paneth N, Kiely J: The frequency of cerebral palsy: A review of population studies in

industrialized nations since 1956. In Stanley F, Alberman E (eds): *The Epidemiology of Cerebral Palsies.* Clinics in Developmental Medicine Series, No. 87. Philadelphia, JB Lippincott, 1984.

167. Pape KE, Wigglesworth JS: *Hemorrhage, Ischemia and Perinatal Brain.* Clinics in Developmental Medicine Series, No. 69/70. Philadelphia, JB Lippincott, 1979.

168. Park TS, Phillips LH, Peacock W (eds): *Management of Spasticity in Cerebral Palsy and Spinal Cord Injury.* State of the Art Reviews. Neurosurgery. Vol. 4. Philadelphia, Hanley & Belfus Inc., 1989.

169. Patrick J, Boland M, et al: Rapid correction of wasting in children with cerebral palsy. *Dev Med Child Neurol* 28:734–739, 1986.

170. Peacock WJ, et al: Electrophysiologic studies in selective dorsal rhizotomy for spasticity in children with cerebral palsy. *Appl Neurophysiol* 50:459–466, 1987.

171. Peacock WJ, Staudt LA: Spasticity in cerebral palsy and the selective posterior rhizotomy procedure. *J Child Neurol* 5:179–185, 1990.

172. Pearlman MD, et al: Blunt trauma during pregnancy. *N Eng J Med* 323:1609–1613, 1990.

173. Pearson P, Williams C (eds): *Physical Therapy Services in the Developmental Disabilities.* Springfield, IL Charles C Thomas, 1980.

174. Perry J: Cerebral palsy gait. In Samilson RL (ed): *Orthopaedic Aspects of Cerebral Palsy.* Clinics in Developmental Medicine Series, No. 52/53. Philadelphia, JB Lippincott, 1975.

175. Pharoah POD, Cooke T, et al: Effects of birthweight, gestational age, and maternal obstetric history on birth prevalence of cerebral palsy. *Arch Dis Child* 62:1035–1040, 1987.

176. Piper M, Kunos VL, et al: Physical therapy effects on the high risk infants: A randomized controlled trial. *Pediatrics* 76:216–224, 1986.

177. Powell TG, Pharoah POD, et al: Cerebral palsy in low-birthweight infants. I. Spastic hemiplegia: Associations with intrapartum stress. *Dev Med Child Neurol* 30:11–18, 1988.

178. Powell TG, Pharoah POD, et al: Cerebral palsy in low-birthweight infants. II. Spastic diplegic: Association with fetal immaturity. *Dev Med Child Neurol* 30:19–25, 1988.

179. Prechtl HFR: The optimality concept. *Early Human Devel* 4:201–204, 1980.

180. Reddihough, D, Johnson H, et al: Use of benzhexol hydro-chloride to control drooling of children with cerebral palsy. *Dev Med Child Neurol* 32:985–989, 1990.

181. Rempel GR, Colewell SO, Nelson RP: Growth in children with cerebral palsy fed via gastrostomy. *Pediatrics* 82:857–862, 1988.

182. Richardson SA: People with cerebral palsy talk for themselves. *Dev Med Child Neurol* 14:524, 1972.

183. Rinsky LA: Surgery of spinal deformity in cerebral palsy. Twelve years in the evolution of scoliosis management. *Clin Orthop* 253:100–109, 1990.

184. Ritter DA, Kenny JD, Norton HJ, et al: A prospective study of free bilirubin and other risk factors in the development of kernicterus in premature infants. *Pediatrics* 69:260, 1982.

185. Rodriquez J, Claus D, et al: Periventricular leukomalacia and neuropathological correlations. *Dev Med Child Neurol* 32:347–352, 1990.

186. Root L: Varus and valgus foot in cerebral palsy and its management. *Foot Ankle* 4:174–179, 1984.

187. Rose J, Gamble JG, et al: Energy cost of walking in normal children and in those with cerebral palsy: Comparison of heart rate and oxygen uptake. *J Pediatr Orthop* 9:276–279, 1989.

188. Rose J, Gamble JG, et al: Energy expenditure index of walking for normal children and for children with cerebral palsy. *Dev Med Child Neurol* 32:333–340, 1990.

189. Rosenthal RK: The use of orthotics in foot and ankle problems in cerebral palsy. *Foot Ankle* 4:195–200, 1984.

190. Rothman JG: Effects of respiratory exercises on the vital capacity and forced expiratory volume in children with cerebral palsy. *Phys Ther* 4:421–425, 1978.

191. Rubin L, Crocker A: *Developmental Disabilities: Delivery of Medical Care for Children and Adults.* Philadelphia, Lea & Febiger, 1989.

192. Russell DJ, Rosenbaum PL, et al: The gross motor function measure: A means to evaluate the effects of physical therapy. *Dev Med Child Neurol* 31:341–352, 1989.

193. Saigal S, Rosenbaum P, et al: Decreased disability rate among 3-year-old survivors weighing 501-100 grams at birth and born to residents of a geographically-defined region from 1981 to 1984 compared with 1977 to 1980. *J Pediatr* 114:839–846, 1989.

194. Samilson RL (ed): *Orthopaedic Aspects of Cerebral Palsy.* Clinics in Developmental Medicine Series, No. 52/53. Philadelphia, JB Lippincott, 1975.

195. Scherzer A, Tscharnuter I: *Early Diagnosis and Therapy in Cerebral Palsy.* New York, Marcel Dekker Inc., ed 2. 1990.

196. Scherzer AL, Mike V, Ilson J: Physical therapy as a determinant of change in the cerebral palsied infant. *Am J Dis Child* 143:552–555, 1989.

197. Scrutton D (ed): *Management of the Motor Disorders of Children with Cerebral Palsy.* Clinics in Development Medicine Series, No. 90. Philadelphia, JB Lippincott, 1984.

198. Seeger BR, Caudrey DJ: Biofeedback therapy to achieve symmetrical gait in children with cerebral palsy: Long-term efficacy. *Arch Phys Med Rehabil* 64:160–166, 1983.

199. Seeger BR, Caudrey DJ, Scholes, JR: Biofeedback therapy to achieve symmetrical gait in hemiplegic cerebral palsied children. *Arch Phys Med Rehabil* 62:634, 1981.

200. Shapiro B, Green P, et al: Growth of severely impaired children: Neurological versus nutritional factors. *Dev Med Child Neurol* 28:729–733, 1986.

201. Shapiro A, Susak Z, et al: Preoperative and postoperative gait evaluation in cerebral palsy. *Arch Phys Med Rehabil* 71:236–240, 1990.

202. Shere ES: Patterns of child rearing in cerebral palsy, effects upon the child's cognitive development. *Pediatr Digest* 23:28, 1971.

203. Shere ES, Kastenbaum R: Mother-child interaction in cerebral palsy, environmental and psychosocial obstacles to cognitive development. *Gen Psychol Monogr* 73:255, 1966.

204. Shonkoff JP, Hauser-Cram P: Early intervention for disabled infants and their families: A quantitative analysis. *Pediatrics* 80:650–658, 1987.

205. Singer JD: Mainstreaming children with handicaps: Applications for pediatricians. *J Dev Behav Pediatr* 10:151–156, 1989.

206. Skidmore MD, Rivers A, Hack M: Increased risk of cerebral palsy among very low-birth-weight infants with chronic lung disease. *Dev Med Child Neurol* 32:325–332, 1990.

207. Sochaniwsky AE, Koheil RM, et al: Oral motor functioning, frequency of swallowing, and drooling in normal children and in children with cerebral palsy. *Arch Phys Med Rehabil* 67:866–874, 1986.

208. Sommerfeld D, Fraser BA, et al: Evaluation of physical therapy services for severely mentally impaired students with cerebral palsy. *Phys Ther* 61:338–343, 1981.

209. Spender QW, Cronk CE, et al: Assessment of linear growth of children with cerebral palsy: Use of alternative measures to height and length. *Dev Med Child Neurol* 31:206–214, 1989.

210. Stanley F, Alberman E (eds): *The Epidemiology of the Cerebral Palsies.* Clinics in Developmental Medicine Series, No. 87, Philadelphia, JB Lippincott, 1984.

211. Stanley FJ, Watson L: The cerebral palsies in Western Australia: Trends 1968-1981. *Am J Obstet Gynec* 158:89–92, 1988.

212. Süssova' J, Seidl Z, Faber J: Hemiparetic forms of cerebral palsy in relation to epilepsy and mental retardation. *Dev Med Child Neurol* 32:792–795, 1990.

213. Sutherland DH, Olshen RA, Biden EN, Wyatt MP: *The Development of Mature Walking.* Clinics in Developmental Medicine Series, No. 104/105. Philadelphia, JB Lippincott, 1988.

214. Svenningsen NW, Westgreen M, Ingemarsson I: Modern strategy for the term breech delivery—A study with a 14-year follow-up of the infants. *J Perinat Med* 13:117–126, 1985.

215. Tachdjian MO: *Pediatric Orthopedics, ed.2.* Philadelphia, WB Saunders, 1990.

216. Taft LT, Matthews WS, Molnar GE: Pediatric management of the physically handicapped child. In Barness LA (ed): *Advances in Pediatrics*. Chicago, Year Book Medical Publishers, 1983.
217. Tardieu C, Lespargot A, et al: For how long must the soleus muscle be stretched each day to prevent contracture? *Dev Med Child Neurol* 30:3–10, 1988.
218. Thomas AP, Bax MCO, Smyth DPL: *The Health and Social Needs of Young Adults with Physical Disabilities*. Clinics in Developmental Medicine Series, No. 106, Philadelphia, JB Lippincott, 1989.
219. Thompson GH, Rubin IL, Bilenker RM: *Comprehensive Management of Cerebral Palsy*. New York, Grune & Stratton, 1983.
220. Tirosh E, Rabino S: Physiotherapy for children with cerebral palsy. *Am J Dis Child* 143:552–555, 1989.
221. Torfs CP, Van Den Berg B, et al: Prenatal and perinatal risk factors in the etiology of cerebral palsy. *J Pediatr* 116:615–619, 1990.
222. Touwen BC, Hadders-Algra M: Hyperextension of neck and trunk, and shoulder retraction in infancy—A prognostic study. *Neuropediatrics* 14:202–205, 1983.
223. Touwen BCL: Variability and stereotypy of spontaneous motility as a prediction of neurologic development of preterm infants. *Dev Med Child Neurol* 32:501–508, 1990.
224. Turnbull A, Rutherford H: *Families, Professionals and Exceptionality: A Special Partnership*. Riverside NJ, McMillan Publ, 1986.
225. Usdane WM: Vocational planning for the handicapped child. In Downey JA, Low NL (eds): *The Child with Disabling Illness, Principles of Rehabilitation*. Philadelphia, WB Saunders, 1983.
226. Uvebrandt P: Hemiplegic cerebral palsy. *Acta Paediatr Scand (Suppl)* 345:1–100, 1988.
227. Van De Bar M, Van Zeben-Van Der AA TM, et al: Hyperbilirubinemia in preterm infants and neurodevelopmental outcome at 2 years of age. Results of a national collaborative study. *Pediatrics* 83:915–920, 1989.
228. Vaughan CW, Neilson PD, O'Dwyer NJ: Motor control deficits of orofacial muscles in cerebral palsy. *J Neurol Neurosurg Psychiat* 51:534–539, 1988.
229. Vietze PM, Vaughan H: *Early Identification of Infants With Development Disabilities*. Philadelphia, Grune & Stratton, 1988.
230. Volpe JJ: *Neurology of the Newborn*. Philadelphia, WB Saunders, 1981.
231. Wallace HM, Biehl R, Taft LT, Oglesby AC (eds): *Handicapped Children and Youth*. New York, Human Sciences Press, 1987.
232. Walsh RN, Greenough WT (eds): *Environments as Therapy for Brain Dysfunction*. Advances in Behavioral Biology. Vol. 17, New York, Plenum Press, 1976.
233. Watt J, Sims D, et al: A prospective study of inhibitive casting as an adjuct to physiotherapy for cerebral palsied children. *Dev Med Child Neurol* 28:480–488, 1986.
234. Watt JM, Robertson CMT, Grace MGA: Early prognosis for ambulation of neonatal intensive care survivors with cerebral palsy. *Dev Med Child Neurol* 31:766–773, 1989.
235. Wehman P, Conley S, et al: *Vocational Education for Multihandicapped Youth with Cerebral Palsy*. Baltimore, Paul H. Brooks, 1988.
236. Weissbluth M: Gastroesophageal reflux: A review. *Clin Pediatr* 20:7–14, 1981.
237. Willis J, Duncan MC, et al: Somatosensory evoked potentials predict neuromotor outcome after periventricular hemorrhage. *Dev Med Child Neurol* 31:435–439, 1989.
238. Wright T, Nicholson J: Physiotherapy for the spastic child: An evaluation. *Dev Med Child Neurol* 15:146, 1973.
239. Yang GW, Chu DS, et al: Floor reaction orthosis: A clinical experience. *Orthot Prosthet* 40:33–37, 1986.

Index